Practical Perioperative Transoesophageal Echocardiography

OXFORD CLINICAL IMAGING GUIDES

Published and Forthcoming

Acute and Critical Care Echocardiography
Edited by Claire Colebourn and Jim Newton

Focused Intensive Care Ultrasound
Marcus Peck and Peter MacNaughton

Point of Care Ultrasound for Emergency Medicine and Resuscitation
Edited by Paul Atkinson, Justin Bowra, Tim Harris, Bob Jarman, and David Lewis

Practical Perioperative Transoesophageal Echocardiography, Fourth edition
Edited by A. Stephane Lambert, Sara Jane Allen, and Surita Sidhu

Practical Perioperative Transoesophageal Echocardiography

FOURTH EDITION

Edited by

A.Stephane Lambert MD, MBA, FRCPC

Professor, Department of Anesthesiology and Pain Medicine, University of Ottawa
Cardiac Anesthesiologist, University of Ottawa Heart Institute
Ottawa, Ontario, Canada

Sara Jane Allen BHB, MBChB, FANZCA, FCICM, GChPOM, MSt Cambridge

Anaesthetist and Service Clinical Director
Department of Cardiothoracic and ORL Anaesthesia
Intensivist Cardiothoracic and Vascular Intensive Care Unit
Auckland City Hospital, Auckland, New Zealand
Honorary Senior Lecturer, University of Auckland, Auckland, New Zealand

Surita Sidhu MD, FRCPC, FASE

Clinical Professor, Department of Anesthesiology and Pain Medicine
Mazankowski Alberta Heart Institute, University of Alberta
Edmonton, Alberta, Canada

OXFORD
UNIVERSITY PRESS

OXFORD
UNIVERSITY PRESS

Great Clarendon Street, Oxford, OX2 6DP,
United Kingdom

Oxford University Press is a department of the University of Oxford.
It furthers the University's objective of excellence in research, scholarship,
and education by publishing worldwide. Oxford is a registered trade mark of
Oxford University Press in the UK and in certain other countries.

Published in the United States of America by Oxford University Press
198 Madison Avenue, New York, NY 10016, United States of America.

British Library Cataloguing in Publication Data
Data available

Library of Congress Control Number: 2025936993

ISBN 978-0-19-887368-6

DOI: 10.1093/med/9780198873686.001.0001

Printed in Great Britain by
Bell & Bain Ltd., Glasgow

Foreword

In 2003, at the time the first edition of PPTOE was published, perioperative transoesophageal echocardiography had only recently entered mainstream practice. For the first time, anaesthetists were using transoesophageal echocardiography in the cardiac operating room to help guide surgical decision-making and puzzled hospital administrators were receiving capital expenditure requests for echocardiography machines from anaesthesia departments. It was an exciting time to be a young cardiac anaesthetist and the right time to write a practical, how-to guide.

As a young cardiac anaesthetist, I was fortunate to have willing co-authors, cardiologists who supported our endeavours, and a clinical director with a clear-eyed view of the future. Not only did that clinical director (Alan Merry) encourage me to develop the first edition of PPTOE but he took a deep dive and came on board as a co-editor. Malcolm Legget, a wonderful echocardiologist and echo researcher, willingly gave his time and expertise, and in doing so demonstrated that cardiologists and anaesthetists could collaborate for the benefit of patients.

And now, some 20-years later, much has changed. Perioperative transoesophageal echocardiography is performed routinely the world over. Several organisations publish evidence-based guidelines and offer credentialling examinations. No cardiac anaesthetist would expect to be hired without demonstrating competence in perioperative transoesophageal echocardiography. At the time of the second edition in 2011, three-dimensional echocardiography was sufficiently novel that it was afforded a standalone chapter. Now, in 2024, three-dimensional imaging is sufficiently routine that it is integrated across all sections of the book and the standalone chapter is gone. Perhaps the only thing that hasn't changed over the last two decades is the speed of ultrasound in soft tissue, which remains stubbornly fixed at 1540 ms^{-1}.

In life, as in physics, momentum is hard to maintain. So, I am thrilled to introduce a new editorial team for the fourth edition. Stephane, Sara, and Surita bring a wealth of knowledge, experience, and – perhaps most importantly – enthusiasm to the latest edition. The new editors have done a superb job of preserving those aspects of PPTOE that proved popular in earlier editions – notably, a concise and consistent style – while updating the content to reflect the latest evidence and current practices. In particular, key developments in interventional cardiology and in the management of thoracic aortic disease have led to major updates in those chapters. The fourth edition provides a concise, readable, evidence-based summary of the very latest developments in perioperative transoesophageal echocardiography. The library of online clips has also been extensively updated. An aspect of the fourth edition that I think will prove extremely popular is the inclusion of numerous expert tips in every chapter. I wish we had thought of doing that at the outset.

The new editors have assembled a highly-respected team of authors, involving experts from multiple countries and across several continents. The content has been crafted with an eye to the US, UK, and European examinations. While the spelling remains in UK English, the book will appeal equally to readers in Europe, the Americas, Asia, India, and Oceania. An international collaboration for an international audience.

I have had the privilege of observing the fourth edition evolve and develop and borne witness to the huge amount of time and energy required to complete the project. I think you will agree with me that the effort has been worthwhile. I am extremely proud of the new book and congratulate the editors and authors on a splendid job.

David Sidebotham

Editor of first, second, and third editions of

Practical Perioperative Transoesophageal Echocardiography

Preface

Since its introduction in the 1980's, Transoesophageal Echocardiography (TOE) has become a standard of care in operating rooms across the world and it has redefined the role of the cardiac anaesthetist/anesthesiologist, from facilitators of surgery to an integral part of the surgical decision-making team. TOE is also an essential tool in the arsenal of intensivists and cardiologists, in critical care units and echocardiography labs across the world.

Practical Perioperative Transoesophageal Echocardiography, 4th Edition builds upon the popular 3rd edition, which received positive reviews in many countries. This edition brings in a fresh team of experienced editors, who relied on a mix of new and returning authors to share their expertise in perioperative TOE. The book focuses on the perioperative environment and is part of a series by the same publisher, targeting various aspects of echocardiography practice.

Powerful as TOE may be, its diagnostic yield is dependent on the proficiency of the operator, so echocardiographers must develop and maintain high levels of cognitive and technical skills. We hope that *PPTOE 4th Edition* will be a great resource for clinicians of all disciplines who use TOE in their practice. They may be trainees or fellows beginning to learn TOE, or more advanced readers preparing for certification (or *re*-certification) exams. More seasoned practitioners will also find information that may fill some gaps in their knowledge and expert tips that will help them progress to the next level.

With a refreshed look and updated text and references reflecting the latest literature and practice guidelines, this edition addresses the rapid evolution of TOE in the field of 3D imaging. It also covers new applications of TOE, notably in the areas of surgical valve repair and percutaneous techniques, where high-level 2D and 3D TOE imaging is now an essential part of the procedures and a key determinant of clinical outcomes.

Above all, this book is meant to be practical. Like its predecessor, *PPTOE 4th Edition* is richly illustrated, and every chapter is sprinkled with expert tips and "tricks of the trade", which we hope will benefit novice and experienced readers alike. These are tips that we would give our trainees in the operating room, and our hope is that this book will feel to the reader like an informal one-on-one teaching session.

The extensive online content was also refreshed and updated, with each of the 680 videos and 689 figures hand picked to bring our readers the broadest possible exposure to the field of perioperative TOE.

This edition continues in a line of TOE textbooks dating back 20 years. It is the legacy of David Sidebotham, Allan Merry and Malcolm Legget, whose decades-long contributions permeate this edition and without whom none of this would have been possible. We are indebted to them. Our editorial team also acknowledges the past contributions of legacy authors who did not return for this 4th edition. Their work influenced the content of the book and we are thankful for their indirect participation.

Finally, a little wink at our North American readers who may need a few minutes to get used to "TOE" instead of "TEE", and to terms like "anticlockwise" vs." counter-clockwise". With authors spread on four continents and an international audience, there are regional differences in spelling, practices and/or equipment, but the core principles are truly universal.

TOE or TEE, we hope that *PPTOE 4th Edition* will help you develop knowledge and skills that will benefit your patients for years to come, and that you will enjoy reading this book as much as we enjoyed preparing it!

A. Stephane Lambert
Surita Sidhu
Sara Jane Allen

Contents

Abbreviations

2D	two-dimensional
3D	three-dimensional
AR	aortic regurgitation
AS	aortic stenosis
ASD	atrial septal defect
ASE	American Society of Echocardiography
AV	aortic valve
CM	cardiomyopathy
CPB	cardiopulmonary bypass
CT	computed tomography
CW	continuous wave
EACVI	European Association of Cardiovascular Imaging
ECG	electrocardiogram
EOA	effective orifice area
FAC	fractional area change
IVC	inferior vena cava
IVS	inter-ventricular septum
LA	left atrium, left atrial
LV	left ventricle, left ventricular
LVEDA	left ventricular end-diastolic area
LVEDD	left ventricular end-diastolic dimension
LVESA	left ventricular end-systolic area
LVESD	left ventricular end-systolic dimension
LVEF	left ventricular ejection fraction
LVOT	left ventricular outflow tract
MRI	magnetic resonance imaging
MR	mitral regurgitation
MS	mitral stenosis
MV	mitral valve
PA	Pulmonary Artery
PHT	pressure half time
PV	pulmonary valve
PW	pulsed-wave
RA	right atrium, right atrial
RV	right ventricle, right ventricular
RVOT	right ventricular outflow tract
SVC	superior vena cava
SWMAs	segmental wall motion abnormalities
TDI	tissue Doppler imaging
TOE	transoesophageal echocardiogram/ echocardiographic
TR	trisuspid regurgitation
TTE	transthoracic echocardiogram/ echocardiographic
TV	tricuspid valve
VSD	ventricular septal defect
VTI	velocity time integral

Contributors to the fourth edition

A. Stephane Lambert Professor of Anesthesiology, University of Ottawa. Cardiac Anesthesiologist, University of Ottawa Heart Institute, Ottawa, Ontario, Canada *Chapters 1, 2, and 8*

Surita Sidhu Clinical Professor, Department of Anesthesiology and Pain Medicine, Mazankowski Alberta Heart Institute, University of Alberta, Edmonton, Alberta, Canada *Chapters 4 and 19*

Sara Allen Anaesthetist and Service Clinical Director, Department of Cardiothoracic and ORL Anaesthesia, Intensivist Cardiothoracic and Vascular Intensive Care Unit, Auckland City Hospital, Auckland, New Zealand *Chapters 3 and 20*

Ahmad Alli Department of Anesthesiology and Pain Medicine, St. Michael's Hospital, University of Toronto, Toronto, ON, Canada *Chapter 14*

Marie-Eve Chamberland Anesthesiologist, Montreal Heart Institute, Assistant Professor, Université de Montréal, Montreal, Quebec, Canada *Chapter 10*

Mike Charlesworth Consultant in Cardiothoracic Anaesthesia, Critical Care and ECMO, Wythenshawe Hospital, Manchester, UK *Chapter 20*

Michael Cutrone Assistant Professor of Anesthesiology, Duke University Hospital, Durham, NC, USA *Chapter 7*

Jean Deschamps Department of Intensive Care and Resuscitation, Integrated Hospital Institute, Cleveland Clinic Foundation, Cleveland, Ohio, USA *Chapter 6*

Daniel Drake Department of Cardiac Surgery and Extracorporeal Life Support Laboratory, University of Michigan Medical School, Michigan Society of Thoracic and Cardiovascular Surgery Mitral Initiative, Ann Arbor, Michigan, USA *Chapter 9*

Adam Dryden Division of Cardiac Anesthesiology, University of Ottawa Heart Institute, Ottawa, Ontario, Canada *Chapter 17*

Alison Duncan Associate specialist in Cardiology and Transcatheter Valves, The Royal Brompton Hospital, London, UK *Chapter 15*

Joachim Mathias Erb Chair Cardiothoracic and Vascular Anaesthesia, Clinic for Anaesthesiology, Intermediate Care, Prehospital Emergency Medicine and Pain Therapy; University Hospital Basel, Basel, Switzerland *Chapter 11*

Abimbola Faloye Associate Professor, Department of Anesthesiology, Emory University, Atlanta, GA, USA *Chapter 7*

Shelley Rahman Hayley Royal Brompton Hospital, London, UK *Chapter 16*

Mark Hynes Division of Cardiac Anesthesiology, University of Ottawa Heart Institute, Ottawa, Ontario, Canada *Chapter 17*

Wing Lam Anesthesiologist, Associate Clinical Professor, University of Alberta Hospital, Mazankowski Alberta Heart Institute, Edmonton, Alberta, Canada *Chapter 19*

John-Paul Larkin Division of Cardiac Anesthesiology, University of Ottawa Heart Institute, Ottawa, Ontario, Canada *Chapter 8*

Eric Benedet Lineburger Anesthesiology Residency Program Supervisor, Hospital São José, Criciúma-SC, Professor of Anesthesiology, University of the Extreme South of Santa Catarina – Brazil *Chapter 13*

Feroze Mahmood Network Chief Cardiac Anesthesia, Beth Israel Lahey Health, Professor of Anesthesiology, Harvard Medical School, Boston, MA, USA *Chapter 12*

Alan Forbes Merry Professor Emeritus, Department of Anaesthesiology, University of Auckland, Auckland, New Zealand. *Chapters 1, 2, 3, and 4*

Vinodh Bhagyalakshmi Nanjayya Senior Intensive Care Consultant & Head of Cardiothoracic ICU, Department of Intensive Care and Hyperbaric Medicine, Alfred Hospital, Melbourne, Australia *Chapter 21*

Donna Nicholson Division of Cardiac Anesthesiology, University of Ottawa Heart Institute, Ottawa, Ontario, Canada *Chapter 17*

Fabio Papa Department of Anesthesia/ St. Michael's Hospital, Department of Anesthesiology & Pain Medicine - University of Toronto, Toronto, Ontario, Canada *Chapter 13*

Meggie Raymond Anesthesiologist, Montreal Heart Institute, Assistant Professor, Université de Montréal, Montreal, Quebec, Canada *Chapter 10*

Taha Rehman Postdoctoral Research Fellow, Anesthesia, Critical Care & Pain Medicine, Beth Israel Deaconess Medical Center, Harvard Medical School, Boston, MA, USA *Chapter 12*

David Sidebotham Cardiac anaesthetist and intensivist, Department of Anaesthesia and the Cardiothoracic and Vascular Intensive Care Unit, Auckland City Hospital, Auckland, New Zealand. Honorary Associate Professor, Department of Anaesthesiology, Faculty of Health Sciences, University of Auckland, Auckland, New Zealand. *Chapters 1, 2, 3, 4, 8, and 9*

Madhav Swaminathan Thomas Irving Professor and Chair, Department of Anesthesiology, Atrium Health Wake Forest Baptist, Wake Forest University School of Medicine *Chapter 7*

Claude Tousignant Department of anesthesia and critical care, St Michael's Hospital, University of Toronto, Toronto, Ontario, Canada *Chapter 14*

Brett Wakefield Staff Cardiac Anesthesiologist and Intensivist, Cleveland Clinic, Cleveland, OH, USA *Chapter 6*

Benedict Waldron Department of Anaesthesiology and Perioperative Medicine, Alfred Hospital, Melbourne, Australia *Chapter 5*

Jonathan Windram Staff Cardiologist, Associate Professor of Medicine, Mazankowski Alberta Heart Institute, University of Alberta of Hospital, Edmonton, Alberta, Canada *Chapter 18*

Karen G. Zimmerman Department of Anesthesiology, Perioperative Echocardiography Project Manager, Michigan Medicine, University of Michigan, Ann Arbor, Michigan, USA *Chapter 9*

Acknowledgments

The editors thank the following people for their contribution to previous editions:

Cyril Charron France

Rob Doughty New Zealand

Mark Edwards New Zealand

Sarah Fitzsimons New Zealand

Ivor Gerber New Zealand

Andrew Hilton Australia

Mario Kalpokas Australia

Roman Kluger Australia

Cornelis Kruger New Zealand

Malcolm Legget New Zealand

Andrew McKee New Zealand

James Pemberton New Zealand

Susanna Price UK

Colin Royse Australia

David Scott Australia

Andrew Silvers Australia

Damon Sutton Australia

Tim Sutton New Zealand

Guido Tavazzi Italy

Antoine Vieillard-Baron France

Jonathan Wallace New Zealand

Selwyn Wong New Zealand

Gavin Wright UK

Online content accompanying the book

Individual purchasers of this book are entitled to free personal access to additional online content. These online ancillary materials, where available, are noted with iconography throughout the book.

Videos and figures

Multiple choice questions

There are over 680 TOE video clips and a similar number of annotated still frames. These demonstrate the full range of normal and abnormal cardiac structures and functions relevant to the perioperative management of cardiac surgical patients. The material is designed to teach you how to recognize standard views and interpret cardiac pathology. The material is arranged into the following sections:

Appendix 1: Standard views

Appendix 2: Anatomical variants

Appendix 3: Cardiac masses and abnormal structures

Appendix 4: Pericardial and pleural collections

Appendix 5: The left ventricle

Appendix 6: The mitral valve

Appendix 7: The aortic valve and thoracic aorta

Appendix 8: The right heart

Appendix 9: Valve replacement and repair

Appendix 10: Congenital heart disease

Appendix 11: Transplantation and mechanical cardiorespiratory support

Appendix 12 contains over 160 self-assessment questions to help you retain what you have read and revise for exams.

Search for this book's title or ISBN (9780198873686) at https://academic.oup.com/ and go to the online appendix at the end of the book. Use your scratch-off code on the inside cover to access the material.

If you are interested in access to the complete online edition, or are interested in accessing other titles, please consult with your librarian.

1
Physical principles

This chapter reviews the physical principles underpinning the use of ultrasound in clinical echocardiography, including the formation of ultrasound images, the principles of Doppler, and the effect of ultrasound on tissue.

Ultrasound imaging

Ultrasonic transducers work by the piezoelectric effect (from the Greek *piezein*, 'to press tight or squeeze'), whereby certain crystals or ceramics deform slightly when stimulated by electric fields and, reciprocally, generate electric signals when deformed mechanically. The energy of the vibrating crystal is transferred to the molecules of the adjacent medium, creating ultrasound waves. The ultrasound beam travels through tissue and interacts with structures by reflection, refraction, scattering, and absorption. Reflected sound waves return to the transducer and create vibrations that generate electric waveforms, which are processed electronically to derive information about the distance and nature of the reflectors. Multiple ultrasound beams are typically fired sequentially to form a *sector scan*. Successive frames of the sector scan show changes over time, providing moving images of cardiac structures in real time.

Sound waves

Sound can be defined as vibrations transmitted through an elastic medium (e.g. air or water) that can be detected by the ear and interpreted by the brain or detected by a receiver and interpreted by electronic devices. Sound waves that are outside the audible range are called infrasound or ultrasound (Box 1.1).

The piezoelectric crystals vibrate and produce alternating areas of compression and rarefaction (increases and decreases in pressure and density) in the medium adjacent to the ultrasound transducer (Figure 1.1). Energy is transferred to the medium in the form of heat, and the energy of the wave dissipates as it travels away from its source. Unlike electromagnetic waves, sound cannot travel in a vacuum.

Higher-frequency (lower-wavelength) ultrasounds dissipate energy into tissue faster; therefore, they cannot penetrate deeply. By contrast, longer-wavelengths (i.e. lower-frequency) ultrasound can penetrate deeper into tissue.

The amplitude of a sound wave is defined as the maximum variation in pressure (Figure 1.1). With sound, pressure is perceived as *loudness* and, with clinical ultrasound, as *brightness*. The frequency (f) of a wave is the

Box 1.1 Some important facts

- The range of frequency (f) audible to humans is 20 Hz to 2 MHz.
- Echocardiography machines commonly operate between 2 MHz and 10 MHz— typically 5 MHz (5 cycles/μs).
- Some specialized instruments operate at higher frequencies (e.g. 30 MHz for intracoronary imaging).
- In soft tissues and blood, the average propagation speed of sound (c) ≈ 1540 m/s (1.54 mm/μs). By Equation 1.2, wavelength (λ) ≈ 0.3 mm:

  $$c = f\lambda$$

  $$\lambda = \frac{c}{f}$$

  $$\lambda = \frac{1.54\ \text{mm}/\mu\text{s}}{5\ \text{cycles}/\mu\text{s}} = 0.308\ \text{mm} \approx 0.3\ \text{mm}$$

  Doubling f to 10 MHz halves λ to 0.15 mm and improves axial resolution (≈λ), but reduces penetration.
- Sound travels faster in most tissues than in air, in which it travels at 330 m/s (0.330 mm/μs). This difference makes air/tissue interfaces very strong reflectors in echocardiography.

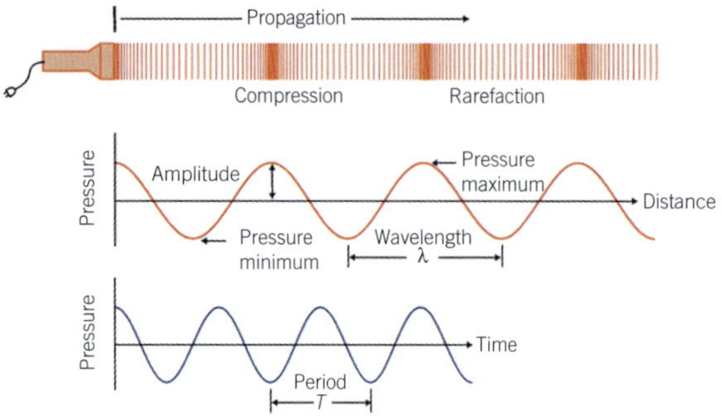

Figure 1.1 Diagram of the compression and rarefaction of a medium in which a sound wave generated by a transducer is travelling from left to right. The corresponding graph of the sinusoidal pressure wave versus distance, at some instant in time, is drawn on the same distance scale below this. The wavelength (λ) is indicated between successive pressure minima. Amplitude is also shown. The corresponding graph, also sinusoidal, of pressure versus time at some fixed point within the medium is shown next. The distance and time scales of the graphs are related by $\lambda = cT$ (from Equations 1.1 and 1.2) where c is the speed of propagation of sound in the particular medium and T is the period.

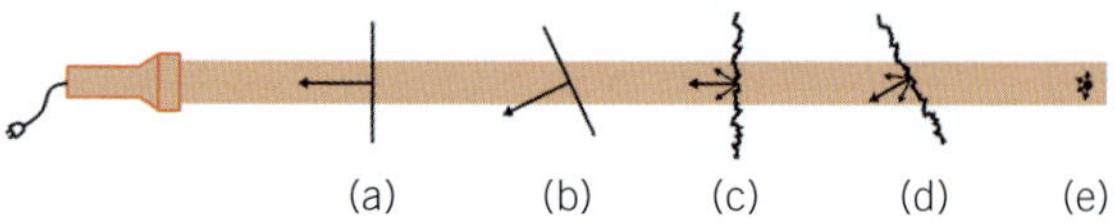

Figure 1.2 Schematic diagram of an ultrasound beam interacting with a series of interfaces. The strength of the returned echoes is indicated by the length of the arrows. (a) A perfectly specular reflector orientated perpendicularly to the incident beam gives a very strong reflection directly back to the transducer. (b) A perfectly specular reflector orientated obliquely to the beam causes all of the reflected energy to be directed away from the source and no image will be seen. Steel needles behave as nearly perfect specular reflectors and are very difficult to visualize with ultrasound. (c) A rough surface (more typical of tissue interfaces) orientated perpendicularly to the beam reflects most of the energy to the source, but a portion is backscattered in other directions. (d) When a rough surface is orientated obliquely to the beam, there is some loss of returned signal strength, but the target is visible unless the intercept angle is very acute. In (e), a target smaller than one wavelength scatters energy in tiny amounts and will not be visible.

number of peaks or troughs passing a given point per unit time. With sound, frequency is perceived as *pitch*. Frequency is the reciprocal of the period (T), which is the time taken for two successive corresponding reference points to pass a fixed position in space (Equation 1.1):

$$f = \frac{1}{T} \qquad \text{Equation 1.1}$$

Frequency is measured in cycles per second, or hertz (abbreviated Hz, after Heinrich Rudolf Hertz, a nineteenth-century German physicist). A kilohertz (kHz) is 10^3 Hz, and a megahertz (MHz) is 10^6 Hz. Period is measured in seconds (s) or milliseconds (ms). Thus, for a typical 5-MHz transducer:

$$5\ \text{MHz} = \frac{1\text{cycle}}{0.0000002\text{s}}$$

At any fixed time, wavelength (λ) is the distance between corresponding reference points on adjacent cycles of a sound wave. In 1 s, f waves of this length will be propagated. Thus, in 1 s, the front of the waveform will travel a distance of $f\lambda$ in the units of λ (typically in millimetres). Frequency and wavelength are related by the speed of sound (c) in the medium (Equation 1.2):

$$c = f\lambda \qquad \text{Equation 1.2}$$

As a sound wave passes from one medium into another, its frequency remains constant, but its speed of propagation changes. In general, the speed of propagation of sound is low in gases, higher in liquids, and highest in solids. Sound travels much faster in biological tissue (made mostly of water) than in air (Box 1.1).

Interaction of ultrasound with tissues

Ultrasound waves interact with tissues in several ways (Figure 1.2):

- **Reflection** at an acoustic interface
- **Refraction** at an acoustic interface
- **Scattering** by tiny reflectors within tissues
- **Absorption** by tissues.

Ultrasound images are formed by the **reflection** of some of the wave's energy at interfaces between media of different density. Two pieces of information contained within each returning ultrasound signal are used to generate an image: (1) the *time* taken to reach a structure and return to the transducer, which translates into how *far* the object is displayed from the transducer; and (2) the *strength* (amplitude) of the returning signal, which translates into how *bright* it will appear on the image.

The degree of reflection (and transmission) of an ultrasound wave at an interface between two tissues depends on their **acoustic impedance**. Acoustic impedance is defined as the product of the density of the medium and the propagation speed of sound within it. Propagation speed varies only slightly among soft biological tissues, so differences in acoustic impedance depend largely on differences in density. For example, there is a greater difference in density between blood and fat than between blood and muscle, so blood–fat interfaces produce stronger reflections (i.e. brighter interfaces) than blood–muscle interfaces. With very strong reflectors, the whole wave may be reflected, with no transmission beyond the interface (as in the case with ribs blocking imaging during transthoracic echocardiography (TTE)). Reflections are responsible for the major anatomic features seen on the image, whereas scattering produces image texture.

The angulation and structure of an interface influence the returned ultrasound signal (Figure 1.2). Large smooth interfaces (compared to the wavelength of the signal) produce *specular* (i.e. mirror-like) reflections, where the incident and reflected beams make the same angle with respect to a line perpendicular to the interface (Figure 1.3). If the incident beam is perpendicular to the specular reflector, it is reflected back along the same path, and the transducer receives a strong signal. If the specular reflector is oblique to the incident beam, the beam is reflected away from the transducer and (for a perfect specular reflector) no signal is received by the transducer, resulting in echo dropout. This phenomenon explains why in the transgastric mid-papillary short-axis view, image definition is best in the anterior and inferior walls where the beam intersects the cardiac tissues perpendicularly, and worst in the lateral and septal walls where the beam intersects the cardiac surfaces obliquely. However, cardiac surfaces are not perfect specular reflectors. With rough surfaces, the energy is reflected away in multiple directions, and the proportion that is perpendicular to the beam determines the strength of the returned signal. In general, reflections from rougher surfaces (e.g. endocardium) are less angle-dependent than reflections from smoother surfaces (e.g. epicardium). These phenomena are demonstrated in Figure 1.4.

When a beam passes from one medium to another with a different velocity of propagation, it *refracts* or bends (Figure 1.3). Some of the energy may also be reflected. The direction and extent of refraction depend on the relative speeds of propagation in the two media and the angle of incidence of the ultrasound beam. Refraction is greatest when the angle of incidence is low and the velocity difference in the two media (i.e. acoustic impedance) is high. Refraction does not occur when the incident beam is perpendicular to an interface, rather ultrasound energy is either reflected or transmitted with its direction unchanged.

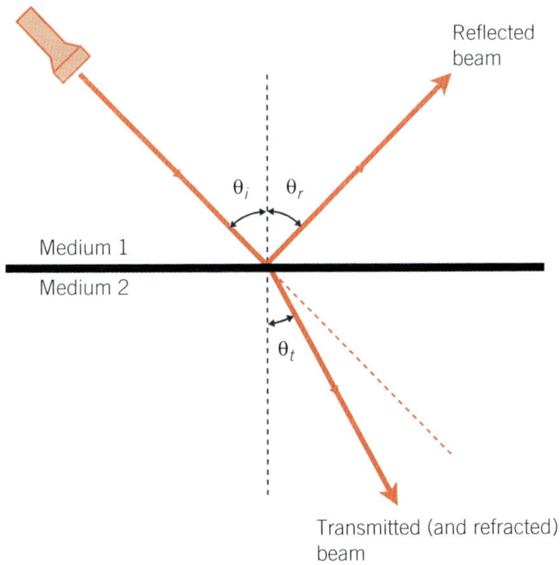

Figure 1.3 Ultrasound refraction. An incident beam is shown, directed obliquely at the interface between two media of different acoustic impedance. The angles of the incident beam (θ_i) and the reflected beam (θ_r) with respect to the perpendicular to the interface are equal. Whenever the propagation speeds of sound in the two media differ, the transmitted beam will be angled (refracted) with respect to the incident beam.

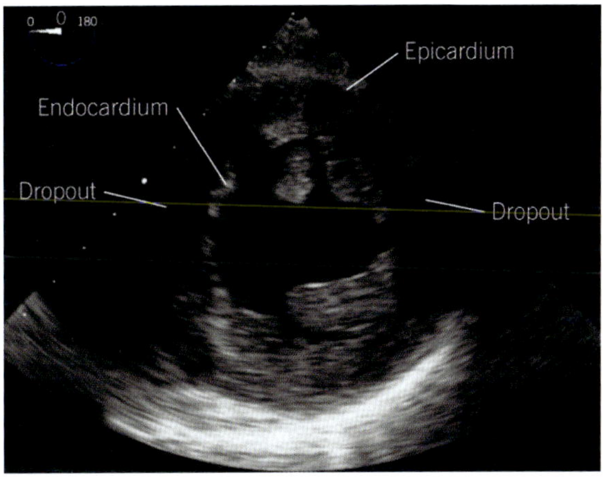

Figure 1.4 Echo dropout due to oblique imaging. The image is a transgastric mid-papillary short axis-view of the left ventricle. Image quality is best in the inferior and anterior walls (the 12 and 6 o'clock positions, respectively) where the ultrasound beam is perpendicular to the myocardium. Image quality is worst in the septal and lateral walls (the 9 and 3 o'clock positions, respectively) where the ultrasound beam is oblique to the myocardium. Specular reflectors that are perpendicular to the ultrasound beam reflect the beam back to the transducer, and specular reflectors that are oblique reflect the ultrasound beam away from the transducer, resulting in echo dropout. Because the endocardium is a 'rough' surface, it is less dependent on the angle of incidence than the 'smooth' epicardium. Thus, echo dropout is most apparent for the epicardium. Note that the endocardium is still well seen in the 9 and 3 o'clock positions.

Pulsed-wave versus continuous-wave ultrasound

Information on the structure or motion of tissues is obtained by using either continuous-wave (CW) or pulsed-wave (PW) ultrasound. CW ultrasound uses continuously generated signals, and in echocardiography, it is only used to measure peak velocities across orifices. However, for constructing 2D and 3D images, and for most Doppler applications, PW ultrasound is used.

PW uses brief bursts ('pulses') of ultrasound. Each burst lasts a short period of time (typically only a few cycles), followed by relatively long periods of silence, during which the ultrasound instrument 'listens' for returning signals. In addition to the frequency and amplitude of the underlying sound waves, pulses are characterized by their duration (in microseconds, μs) and their **pulse repetition frequency** (PRF, in Hz). The fraction of time the pulse is 'on' is called the duty cycle (which is relevant to dosimetry; see later).

The *time* taken for each pulse to reach a structure, be reflected, and return to the transducer allows the *depth* of that structure to be calculated. To avoid range ambiguity (i.e. uncertainty about the depth of a structure), a transducer element must receive reflected signals from only one ultrasonic pulse at a time. Thus, the next pulse cannot be sent until all reflected signals from the previous pulse have returned. Therefore, the maximum PRF that avoids range ambiguity is dependent on the *speed* of ultrasound in the medium and the scanning *depth*. To scan an area of space (called a 'sector'), multiple beams are fired in sequence. Thus, the time it takes to scan a sector is dependent on the speed of ultrasound in the tissue, the number of scan lines (beams), and the sector depth (Box 1.2).

The *strength* (amplitude) of pulses returning from a specific depth provides information on the *nature* of the reflector at that depth (density, size, etc.).

Power

Power (P) is defined as the amount of energy transferred per unit time and is measured in watts (W). Power is usually expressed as a ratio (relative power) in relation to a reference power (P_r), which is typically the maximum power output of the ultrasound machine (Equation 1.3):

$$\text{Relative power} = \frac{P}{P_r} \qquad \text{Equation 1.3}$$

Because useful ultrasonic power levels vary over several orders of magnitude, relative power is converted to a logarithmic sale and expressed in decibels (dB) (Table 1.1). Thus, relative power is usually expressed as:

$$\text{Relative power (dB)} = 10\log_{10}\left(\frac{P}{P_r}\right)$$

Or equivalently as (Equation 1.4):

$$\text{Relative power (dB)} = 10\log_{10}(P) - 10\log_{10}(P_r) \qquad \text{Equation 1.4}$$

Box 1.2 Pulse repetition frequency, viewing depth, and range ambiguity

- To avoid range ambiguity, any given pulse of ultrasound must complete the round trip to and from the structure of interest before the next pulse is transmitted.
- The average propagation speed of sound in tissue is 1.54 mm/μs (Box 1.1), so a pulse will travel 1 cm (10 mm) in 10 mm/1.54 mm/μs ≈ 6.5 μs.
- Therefore, 13.0 μs per cm of viewing depth is required for the round trip.
- Thus, for a viewing depth of 10 cm, the minimum time between transmitted pulses should be 130 μs (approximately). Equivalently, to avoid range ambiguity, the PRF must be no more than (1/130 μs) × 1 000 000 ≈ 7700 Hz = 7.7 kHz.
- It follows that *reducing depth allows the PRF to be increased.*

Table 1.1 Examples of power or intensity ratios and their decibel equivalents

Power ratio	Decibels
2:1	3
10:1	10
20:1	13
40:1	16
50:1	17
100:1	20
1000:1	30
100000:1	50
10000000:1	70

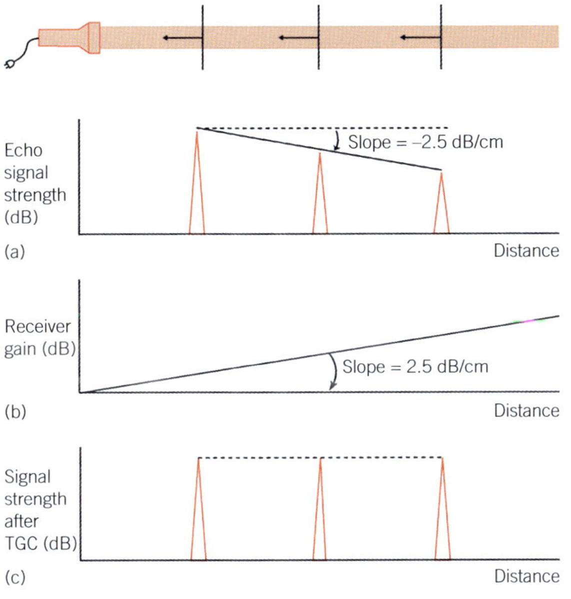

Figure 1.5 Ultrasound attenuation. (a) shows an ultrasound beam directed perpendicularly to interfaces between tissues of differing acoustic impedance. A proportion of the signal is reflected at each interface (as shown with arrows), and a proportion is absorbed as it passes through the tissues. Thus, the signal is progressively attenuated. (b) shows the returning signal amplitude plotted against distance (i.e. an A-mode image). For purposes of illustration, the strength of the successive returned echoes is assumed to diminish by 2.5 dB/cm of depth (for a typical 5-MHz probe, this would result in an attenuation coefficient of 0.5 dB/cm/MHz). The third graph shows the receiver gain per centimetre of depth, in decibels, needed to compensate for this. (c) shows the result of this adjustment to the returning signal. Most real-world situations are more complex and require a hand-tailored gain-versus-depth curve to produce the desired image.

Acoustic attenuation

As an ultrasound beam propagates through tissue, it loses energy through internal friction (which converts sound to heat), reflection, and scattering from inhomogeneities within the tissue. This energy loss manifests as a progressive reduction in signal amplitude (Figure 1.5) called **attenuation**. The reduction in power in watts of a signal is proportional to the exponent of the depth of penetration. As power is typically considered logarithmically, attenuation is measured in decibels. The reduction in power measured in decibels is therefore linearly proportional to the depth of penetration. The attenuation for each centimetre of sound travel is called the **attenuation coefficient** (in dB/cm/MHz).

Attenuation in soft solid tissue (e.g. muscle and organs) increases linearly with frequency, with a typical value of 0.5 dB/cm/MHz. A reduction of 3.0 dB (i.e. a halving of power) will therefore occur over 6 cm at 1 MHz, and one-fifth of this distance (i.e. 1.2 cm) at 5 MHz. The implication is that *increasing transmission frequency* (to reduce wavelength and improve resolution—see Chapter 2) *results in shallower tissue penetration*. Liquids (blood, water) cause much less attenuation than soft tissues. Solid tissues (bone, cartilage) and air produce very high attenuation.

Expert tip: In echocardiography, penetration and resolution are inversely proportional. High-resolution images can only be achieved at relatively shallow depths, and imaging deeper structures must be achieved at the cost of lower resolution.

To ensure tissue interfaces of the same reflectivity have the same appearance anywhere in the image, ultrasound machines use **time-gain compensation (TGC)**, in which the receiver gain is progressively increased for signals returning from deeper reflections. Slider controls that can be adjusted by the operator are superimposed on the inbuilt TGC for this purpose (see Chapter 2).

Ultrasound transducers

A **transducer** is a device that converts energy from one form into another. As explained earlier, ultrasonic transducers convert electrical energy (via mechanical energy) into acoustic energy when transmitting, and acoustic energy (via mechanical energy) into electrical energy when receiving.

When an ultrasonic crystal receives a pulse of electrical energy, it oscillates, much as a bell does, at a specific frequency called its **resonant frequency**.

Acoustic impedance is important in the design of transducers. There is a very large mismatch in impedance between the transducer material that produces the ultrasound signal and the tissue right in front of it. An impedance matching layer of intermediate material is placed between these two surfaces to facilitate the propagation of the signal from the transducer to the patient.

The size of the crystal and the structure of the transducer determine the characteristics of the ultrasound beam (see Chapter 2). Its resonant frequency depends upon the mechanical properties of the crystal. An ultrasound pulse typically contains a range of frequencies—the bandwidth. **Bandwidth** is analogous to variance around the central (and most powerful) frequency—the **operating frequency**. The simplest transducer consists of a single disc of lead zirconate titanate with a sound-absorbing (damping) layer on its back and an impedance-matching layer on its face. Electrical and acoustic lenses can be added to focus the beam.

A single-element transducer can only be used to make 2D images if its beam is swept back and forth over a region of interest by physically moving the transducer (think of primitive radars in old movies). Nowadays, scanning is achieved electronically. Electronic scanning requires *arrays* of closely placed transducer elements. Arrays can be either phased or linear.

In a **phased array**, adjacent groups of elements are fired with small time delays (Figure 1.6), to produce a beam angulated with respect to the face of the array. Repeated firing with different time delays generates a sequential series of beams, with each beam at a different angle to the face of the array, resulting in a 'sweep' of a *triangular* sector. Transoesophageal echocardiography (TOE) probes utilize phased array transducers.

In a **linear array**, several adjacent elements are fired simultaneously to form a beam perpendicular to the array face. Repeated firing with different subsets of adjacent elements generates a series of these beams to sweep a *rectangular* region of tissue (Figure 1.7). Linear arrays can image a relatively wide region of tissue close to the transducer and are used primarily for transcutaneous vascular and musculoskeletal imaging.

A standard phased array transducer used for TOE provides a 2D sector that is defined by its depth and width (azimuthal), both of which can be adjusted by the operator. However, 2D sectors also have a thickness (elevation height), which is determined by the dimensions of the transducer and cannot be adjusted by the operator (see discussion on resolution in Chapter 2). For 3D imaging, a **matrix array** transducer is used, in which several thousand individual piezoelectric crystals are arranged to allow a *pyramidal*-shaped volume of tissue to be imaged (see Figure 4.1). Sector width, depth, and elevation height can all be controlled to determine the volume of the 3D sector.

Imaging modes

There are various ways of displaying the information from reflected echo signals. The simplest one is the **amplitude mode** (A-mode), which is a plot of signal strength against time. Each peak on the image represents an interface between two tissues with different acoustic impedance (Figure 1.5). The horizontal scale can be calibrated in distance units calculated from the time the ultrasound pulse takes to make a round trip. The A-mode is no longer used in clinical practice.

The **motion mode** (M-mode) extends the A-mode by displaying the distance and signal strength over time. Repeated echo pulses are sent along the same path through the tissues, thousands of times per second, and

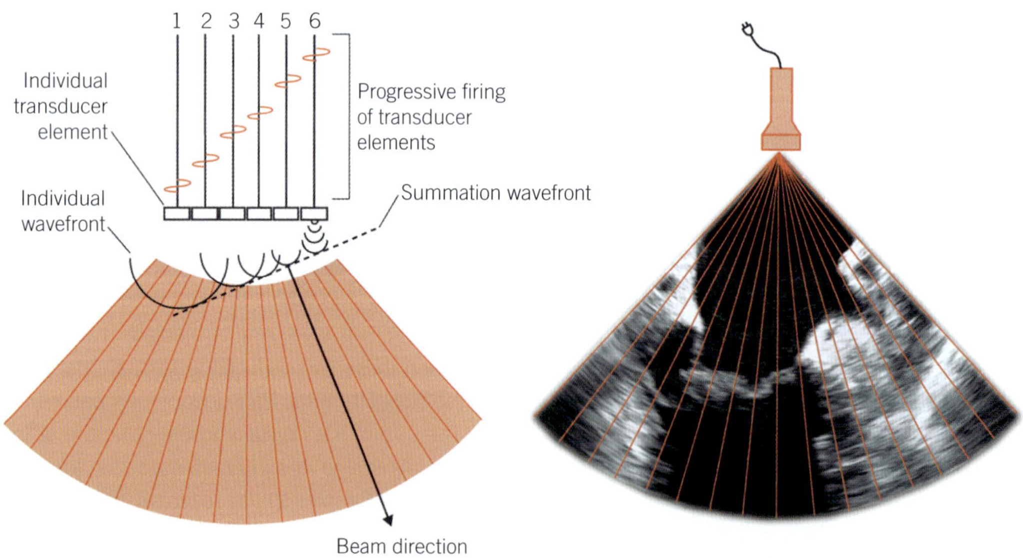

Figure 1.6 Scanning with a phased array. A sector is swept electronically by adjusting the timing of the firing of all the elements within the transducer. Each scan line within the sector is generated by firing the elements in a specific order. One such line directed laterally (depicted by the arrow) is generated by firing the elements in order from left to right (elements 1 to 6). The wavefronts from individual elements form arcs, but the summation wavefront, shown by the dashed line, appears as though it was coming from a virtual single-element transducer orientated perpendicular to the beam.

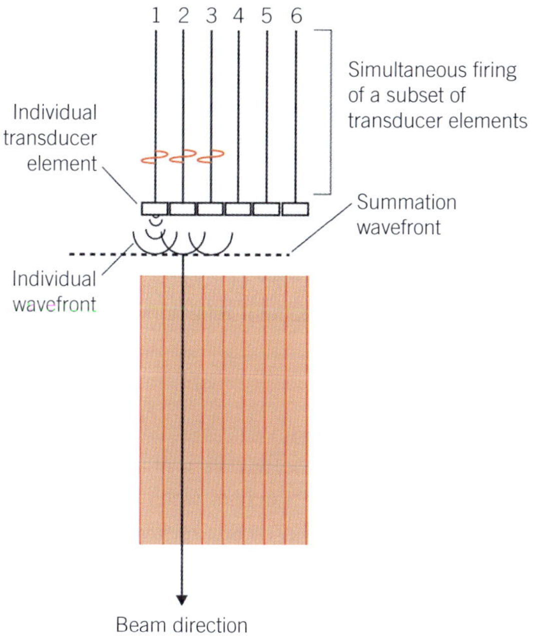

Figure 1.7 Scanning with a linear array. A rectangular region of tissue is scanned by simultaneously firing a subset of adjacent elements to generate a sequence of beams orientated perpendicular to the array. In this simplified illustration, elements numbered 1, 2, and 3 are fired to generate the left-hand scan line. Subsequent scan lines would then be generated by firing elements 2, 3, and 4, followed by elements 3, 4, and 5, etc.

the returning signals are represented by a raster of vertical lines, drawn from left to right at speeds that match the ECG recordings (signal strength on the *x*-axis vs time on the *y*-axis—see Figure 6.4 for an example). The brightness of each individual pixel represents the strength of the returned echo at that particular depth. Change over time is shown. Since there is no sector scan and only *one* scan line is displayed over time, the PRF is more than 100 times faster than with 2D imaging and temporal resolution is very high (see Chapter 2). M-mode imaging is ideal for measuring distances between two points along the path of the ultrasound beam. It is also well suited for observing rapidly moving structures (e.g. the fluttering of valve leaflets).

The **brightness mode** (B-mode) produces the familiar 2D ultrasound images that show the movement of structures in real time. Typically, 128 lines are scanned over a 90° sector with a phased array. As with the M-mode, the amplitude of the returned echoes is represented as pixel brightness. Each complete scan of the sector forms one *frame* of the image of a slice of tissue. Multiple frames are displayed sequentially to provide a moving 2D image.

For clinical purposes, it is assumed that all parts of a single frame are acquired at exactly the same time, but in fact a finite time is required to generate each frame of the moving image. This is the time (t) needed for a pulse of ultrasound to make n round trips, where n is the number of scan lines in the frame. If c is the speed of propagation in the tissue and d is the maximum depth of the sector, then (Equation 1.5):

$$t = \frac{2nd}{c} \qquad \text{Equation 1.5}$$

For example, creating a single frame composed of 128 scan lines to a depth of 10 cm requires 128 × 130 μs (Box 1.2) ≈ 17 ms. Therefore, to generate a moving image by displaying sequentially repeated frames, a maximal frame rate of 1000 ms/17 ms ≈ 60 frames per second (i.e. 60 Hz) can be achieved.

Note from Equation 1.5 that the operator can augment the frame rate by decreasing the maximum depth of the sector (d), but the number of scan lines (n) is a property of the transducer and the speed of propagation (c) is a property of the tissues being imaged.

With real-time 3D imaging, a 'stack' of multiple 2D sector slices are scanned back and forth to create a pyramidal scanning volume (Figure 1.8). A major limitation of 3D imaging is the time taken to scan a complete sector volume. Thus, if a thickness of 30 2D sectors are used, of the same depth and number of scan lines as in the example given in the previous paragraph, the time taken to scan for a single sector volume will be 30 × 17 ms = 510 ms, yielding a frame rate of less than two frames per second (<2 Hz!), which is insufficient to assess moving structures. The time taken to scan the sector volume can be reduced either by reducing the sector volume or by reducing the scan line density. Since scan line density influences spatial resolution and frame rate influences temporal resolution, there is an obvious trade-off between spatial resolution, temporal resolution, and sector volume. Spatial resolution and temporal resolution are discussed in more detail in Chapter 2.

To help overcome the interdependence of frame rate, image quality, and sector volume, **multi-beat acquisition** can be used, in which narrow volumes of data are acquired over several heartbeats and then electronically 'stitched' together to create a single data set, which is displayed as if acquired over a single heartbeat (Figure 1.8). Multi-beat acquisition is not real-time imaging and is subject to stitching artefacts (discussed in Chapter 2).

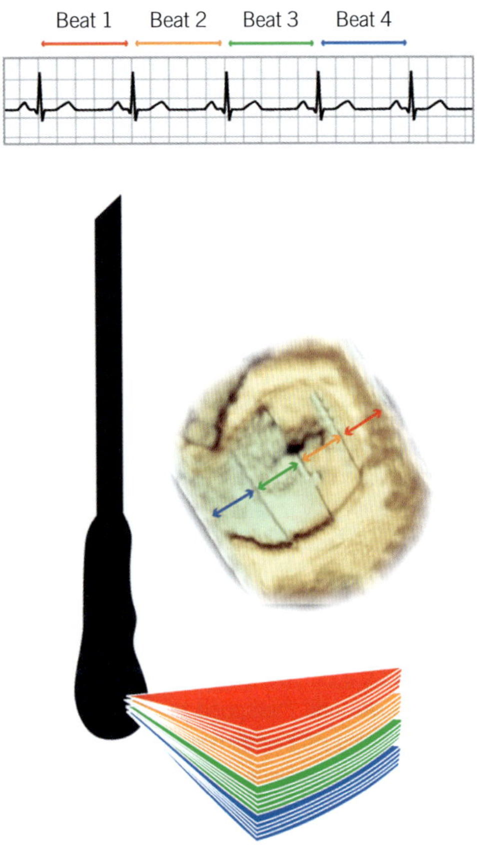

Figure 1.8 Multi-beat acquisition with a matrix array imaging transducer. This schematic demonstrates the acquisition of four sub-volumes of data over four cardiac cycles with a matrix array 3D transducer. The sub-volumes are electronically 'stitched' together to generate a full 3D data set. In this example, a 3D *en face* view of the mitral valve is shown. Once the 3D data set has been acquired, the entire view of the mitral valve is shown over a single cardiac cycle; however, data sets acquired in this way are not real-time imaging. Stitching artefact describes a situation where the junction between these sub-volumes becomes visible.

Principles of Doppler ultrasound

Doppler ultrasound uses the Doppler effect to obtain velocity information on moving blood cells or tissues. Most Doppler applications utilize PW ultrasound, although CW Doppler is also used. Doppler velocity data may be displayed using velocity–time curves (**spectral Doppler**) or as a colour map overlaid upon a conventional, 2D, 3D, or M-mode image (**colour Doppler**). While 2D and 3D imaging provides information about the physical structure of various cardiac elements, the main use of Doppler imaging is to obtain information on the *velocity* of blood flowing through the heart and great vessels. This velocity information can then be used to make calculations about pressure gradients and valve areas (see Chapter 3). Measuring the velocity of cardiac motion with *tissue Doppler imaging (TDI)* also has important clinical applications (see Chapters 2 and 6).

Because blood cells are much smaller than the wavelength of the ultrasound used in Doppler echocardiography, returned signals are generated only by **scattering**, not by reflection; hence, the blood cells themselves cannot be seen, but their velocity can be measured. Doppler signals are typically of the order of 100-fold (20 dB) weaker than the signals from specular reflectors in conventional ultrasound imaging.

The Doppler effect

The Doppler effect is the *apparent* change in the frequency of a wave, which occurs when the source and observer of a signal are in motion relative to each other. The observed frequency is higher than the source frequency when the source and observer are moving towards each other, and lower when they are moving apart (Box 1.3 and Figure 1.9).

Consider a source that is emitting sound with a constant wavelength λ_s and frequency f_s. Assume that the source is moving directly towards an observer at aconstant velocity *v*. The speed of propagation of sound in the medium will be a constant *c*. Assume $v<c$ (a supersonic

Box 1.3 More everyday examples of the Doppler effect

Consider a spectator at a Formula One race listening to the sound of a racing car as it approaches along a straight track, reaches the observer, and then races away into the distance. If the car is travelling at a constant velocity, the pitch of the sound heard by an observer on the side of the track would be constant while the car is approaching, and then would change abruptly to a lower, constant frequency as it moves away. Similarly, the high-pitched siren of an ambulance approaching an observer suddenly changes to a lower pitch as the ambulance moves away. The frequency of the emitted sound itself does not change, but the frequency of the sound *perceived* by the observer changes because of the direction of the movement.

The Doppler shift also affects light, which explains why far-away galaxies in the expanding universe appear red in our telescopes (the light they emitted is *shifted* to a lower frequency as they move away from us).

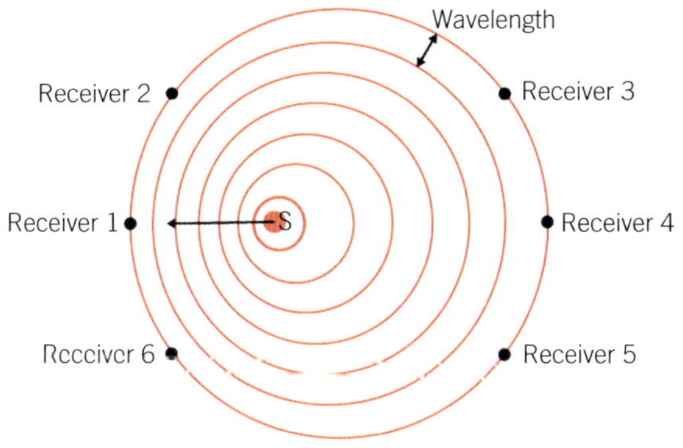

Figure 1.9 Doppler effect. A series of wavefronts emanating at a constant frequency and wavelength from a sound source S, which is moving from right to left. Receiver 1 will observe the highest frequency (and shortest wavelength) sound, while receiver 4 will observe the lowest frequency (and longest wavelength). Receivers 2 and 6 will observe an identical frequency, which will be higher than the source frequency and lower than the frequency observed by receiver 1; receivers 3 and 5 will observe an identical frequency, which will be lower than the source frequency, but higher than the frequency observed by receiver 4. The degree of shift of the wavefronts due to motion has been greatly exaggerated for purposes of illustration.

jet would reach the observer ahead of the noise from its engines; however, in echocardiography, *v* is always much less than *c*). During the time it takes to emit each successive sound wave, the leading edge of the waveform will have moved towards the observer by a distance λ_s, but the source will also have moved forward by a distance *s*. To the observer, the next wave emitted will therefore arrive sooner than if it had been sent from the original position of the source, because it will have less distance to travel. In effect, the wavelength will *appear* to have been shortened so that the observed wavelength λ_o will be $\lambda_s - s$. This process repeats itself as the source continues to travel towards the observer. Thus, it will seem to the observer as if the wavelength has been compressed and the observed frequency f_0 will be *higher* than the source frequency f_s (Figure 1.9). If the source moves away from the observer, the opposite will occur. During the time it takes to emit each successive sound wave, the source will have moved a constant distance away from the observer, so in this case the observed wavelength λ_0 will be $\lambda_s + s$ and f_o will be lower than f_s.

The *difference in frequency* between the signal transmitted from a moving source and the signal observed by a stationary observer is called the **Doppler shift** or **Doppler shift frequency**.

A common application of the Doppler shift in everyday life is a police officer measuring the speed of passing cars on a motorway—the radar device emits ultrasounds at a known frequency. These ultrasounds are reflected off the moving cars and return to the device. The returning signals are shifted to a higher frequency as the cars move towards the officer. The magnitude of the shift allows the device to calculate the car's velocity.

In clinical ultrasound, the source (the transducer) is stationary and the targets (moving blood cells or tissues) are moving. The targets (or scatterers) reflect part of the signal directly back to the transducer. It may be helpful to think of each scatterer as being like a boat travelling through ocean waves whose frequency is f_s. If the boat is travelling into the waves, the frequency with which it hits the waves will be higher than f_s. If it is travelling away from the waves, the frequency with which it hits the waves will be lower than f_s. If the boat creates a crashing sound every time it hits a wave, the frequency of the crashes will be the Doppler shift frequency.

Note that when a moving object (e.g. a police car) emits a sound, this creates *one* Doppler shift for the observer. However, when a signal is emitted from a fixed source and reflected back to that source by a moving object, a Doppler shift occurs *twice* because the moving object effectively acts as a receiver of the signal (accounting for one shift) and then effectively sends the signal back to the source (accounting for a second shift).

In clinical ultrasound, the Doppler shift f_Δ is defined by the Doppler equation (Equation 1.6):

$$f_\Delta = f_s\left(\frac{2V}{C-V}\right) \qquad \text{Equation 1.6}$$

where f_s is the source frequency, C is the speed of propagation of sound in the medium, and V is the velocity of the scatterer (e.g. a red blood cell) relative to the transducer. As explained, the factor '2' appears because the shift occurs twice.

Since in echocardiography, the speed of the scatterers is always much less than the speed of propagation of sound in tissue, *V* can be neglected in the denominator of Equation 1.6. This gives the approximate form of the **Doppler equation** that is shown in many textbooks (Equation 1.7):

$$f_\Delta = \frac{2f_sV}{C} \qquad \text{Equation 1.7}$$

Echocardiography machines use lower frequencies for Doppler measurements than for imaging, typically in the lower third of the useful bandwidth of the transducer. Using a lower frequency increases penetration, and therefore the strength, at any given depth of the reflected

Box 1.4 Everyday illustration of the cosine effect

If a sound emitter (perhaps a whistle) is attached to a piece of string and swung at a constant velocity around a person's head, that person will hear a constant pitch. A friend standing at one side will hear a constantly varying pitch, even though the sound and the speed of the source are constant. This is explained by the cosine effect, because the angle at which the sound approaches the observer will vary constantly. Using our previous example of a spectator at a Formula One race, the cosine effect also explains why spectators hear a constantly changing frequency of sounds as cars approach and move away, because they do not sit on the track, but in the stands, at a certain angle to the movement of the cars.

signal from weak scatterers such as blood cells. The use of lower transmission frequencies also reduces the Doppler shift frequency because, in Equation 1.7, $f_\Delta \propto f_s$.

Equations 1.6 and 1.7 are based upon the assumption that the scatterer is moving *directly* towards or away from the transducer. However, when the motion is at an angle θ to the path of the ultrasound beam, only the *component of velocity that is aligned with the path of the beam* will cause a Doppler shift. This component is determined by the ***cosine*** θ (Box 1.4 and Figure 1.10). Thus, Equation 1.7 becomes Equation 1.8:

$$f_\Delta = \frac{2f_s V\cos\theta}{C} \qquad \text{Equation 1.8}$$

This is extremely important in clinical practice. For any actual blood velocity, the measured Doppler shift (and hence the velocity calculated by the machine) will be modified by a factor between 0 and 1 (i.e. the cosine of the angle between the ultrasound beam and blood flow). The cosine of 0° is 1, so if θ is zero (i.e. the beam and flow are perfectly aligned), no correction is needed. In fact, the value of cosine θ only decreases to 0.94 as θ increases to 20° (a 6% error). Therefore, it is reasonable to ignore the correction if the angle of incidence between the Doppler beam and blood flow is <20°. It is important to remember that ignoring the cosine term can only *underestimate* the true velocity; therefore, the largest value of several measurements should be used.

It is important to remember that, because the cosine value of any angle can never be greater than 1, *Doppler can never overestimate the true value* of a velocity. It can only underestimate it if the angle is not zero (Figure 1.10).

Most echocardiography machines provide a steering control that will make the correction automatically if θ is entered. However, since the estimation of θ is approximate, the use of the automatic angle correction function in clinical practice is not recommended (see Chapter 2).

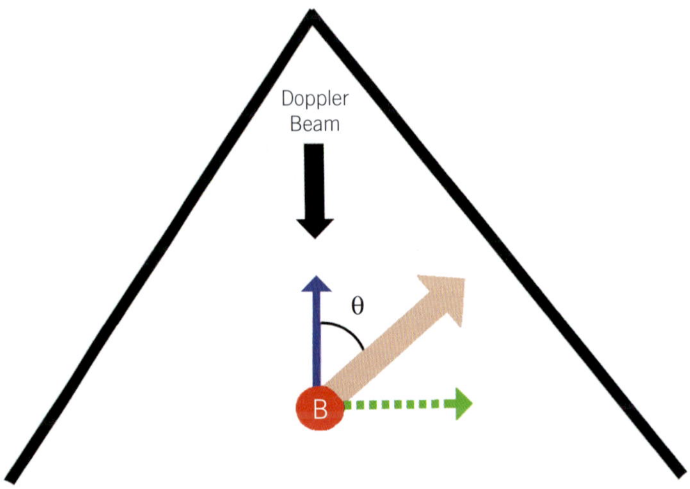

Figure 1.10 Graphic representation of the cosine effect using vectors. Imagine a blood cell 'B' travelling in the direction of the large brown arrow at an angle θ to the path of the Doppler beam, only the component of the velocity (or vector) that is *aligned* with the path of the beam (represented by the solid blue arrow) will cause a Doppler shift. This component is determined by the cosine of the angle θ. The component that is perpendicular to the beam (represented here by the dotted arrow) will not be detected. Since the blue arrow can never be longer than the brown arrow (it can only be equal at best, if the angle is 0° and the flow and Doppler beam are perfectly aligned), hence Doppler can never overestimate the true velocity of movement.

Spectral Doppler analysis and display

Spectral Doppler velocity–time curves are plots of velocity on the *y*-axis against time on the *x*-axis (Figures 1.11 and 1.12). A substantial amount of processing is required to extract velocity signals from the shifted ultrasounds returned from moving targets and to produce these deceptively simple displays. Sampling of the velocity spectrum of blood cells is performed by a **spectrum analyser** at discrete time points, depending on frequency and depth settings, using a process called **demodulation** and using mathematical algorithms called **fast-Fourier transform**, details of which are beyond the scope of this book. For each point in time on the *x*-axis, the height of the line on the *y*-axis represents the velocity and the brightness represents the signal strength associated with that velocity.

By convention, motion towards the transducer is displayed above the baseline (positive) and motion away from the transducer is displayed below the baseline (negative). Because strong signals from specular reflectors (e.g. myocardial wall) can overload the spectrum analyser and mask the fainter signals from blood cells, an adjustable low-frequency filter (wall filter) is used to block these signals (see Chapter 2). The wall filter may create a black band around the zero-velocity line on the spectral display (Figure 1.11).

Continuous-wave Doppler

As its name implies, CW Doppler requires the ultrasound beam to be continuously transmitted, received, and processed; therefore, it uses two separate transducers: one for continuous transmission and one for continuous reception. General-purpose phased array probes use two subsets of elements for transmission and reception of CW Doppler signals, and they can overlay a 2D image (and colour Doppler information) with a cursor representing the orientation of the CW beam (Figure 1.12). Overlaying 2D and CW Doppler information makes it easier for the operator to determine the source of the Doppler signals but reduces the quality of both the Doppler and the 2D information. For this reason, the 2D image is frozen or updated infrequently while CW is active.

With CW Doppler, velocities are sampled along the *entire path* of the Doppler signal. Thus, the sampled velocities range widely and the resulting display is a shaded area (Figure 1.12), with the outer edge of the envelope

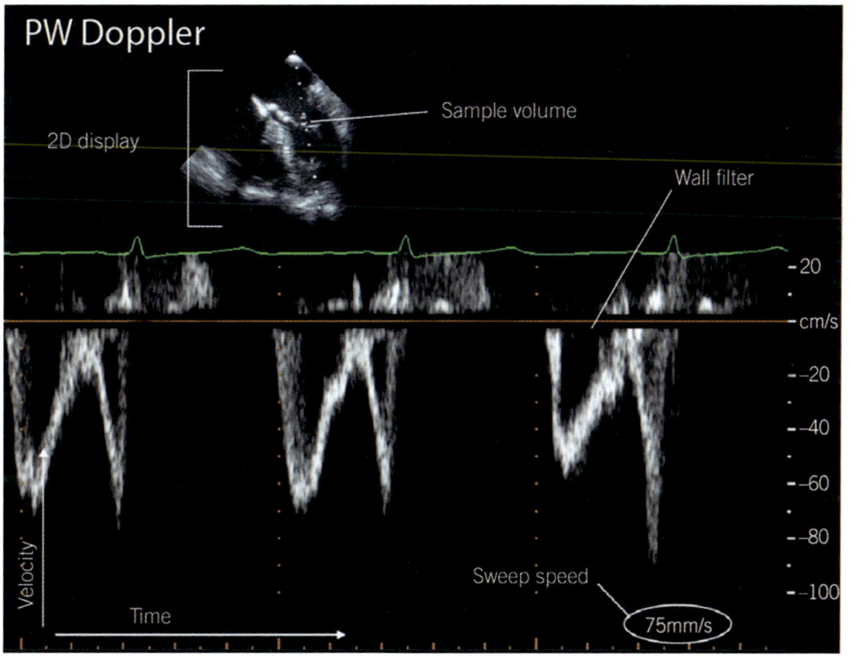

Figure 1.11 A PW Doppler display demonstrating normal mitral inflow. The baseline is set to show predominantly negative velocities (i.e. flow directed away from the transducer). Time is on the horizontal axis (*x*-axis). The sweep speed is 75 mm/s. The velocity scale (vertical axis, *y*-axis) is set to + 20 to −100 cm/s (compare this to the velocity range in Figure 1.12). The Doppler beam is directed across the MV, and the sample volume is located near the leaflet tips. Only velocity data from *within that sample volume* are shown on the spectral display (range specificity). Timing from the ECG indicates that all of the flow occurring during diastole is from the LA to the LV, with a biphasic pattern (see Chapter 4 for explanation of the waveform). The spectral signal is narrow, indicating laminar flow. The wall filter, set to eliminate very low-velocity signals, explains the black band surrounding the baseline.

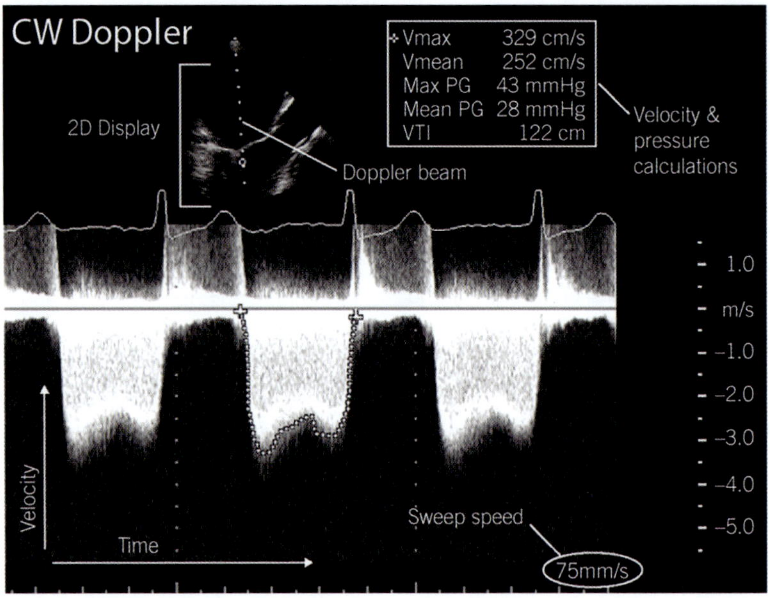

Figure 1.12 A CW Doppler display of mitral inflow in a patient with severe mitral stenosis. The baseline is set to show predominantly negative velocities. Time is on the horizontal axis (*x*-axis). The sweep speed is 75 mm/s. The velocity scale (vertical axis, *y*-axis) is set to +1 to −5 m/s (not cm/s; compare this to the velocity range in Figure 1.11). The Doppler beam is again directed across the mitral leaflets, but unlike Figure 1.11, *all* velocities along the *entire* length of the Doppler beam (from top of the LA to the LV) are shown on the spectral display (range ambiguity). As in Figure 1.11, timing from the ECG indicates that flow in diastole occurs predominantly from the LA to the LV and is of much higher velocity (peak velocity 3.29 m/s) than shown in Figure 1.11. The spectral waveform is filled in, indicating that at any given time, diastolic velocities ranging between 0 and 3.29 m/s are present somewhere along the Doppler beam. What makes this information useful is the fact that the velocity of interest is the *maximum* velocity, which can be assumed to originate from the *narrowest* point along the beam (presumably the stenosed MV). Additionally, some flow is seen to occur during systole, but in this example, the baseline is not set up to measure peak systolic flow. Additional velocity and pressure calculations can be obtained by tracing the velocity waveform (see Chapter 3 for details of those calculations). The bright horizontal band around the zero-velocity line represents vessel walls and other strong, slow-moving specular reflectors lying within the ultrasound beam. The use of CW, rather than PW, is necessary to obtain this particular measurement because the peak velocity (>3 m/s) exceeds the maximum unambiguous velocity for PW Doppler.

representing the maximum velocity detected along the entire beam at a given point in time.

The advantage of CW Doppler is that it can measure very high velocities unambiguously (up to several metres per second), such as occurs in valve stenosis. However, CW Doppler provides no information about the specific depth at which any particular velocity is measured, because the displayed spectrum represents the superposition of all velocities calculated from echoes returning from all depths along the ultrasound beam (**range ambiguity**).

Expert tip: CW Doppler is used to assess flow across orifices (e.g. ventricular septal defect (VSD) and valves), where the velocity is typically high, but where identifying the specific location of the highest velocity is not important, because it is assumed to originate from the narrowest point of that orifice or valve.

Pulsed-wave Doppler

As with 2D imaging, PW Doppler uses the same transducer crystal for both transmission and reception. Single pulses are repeatedly sent along the same path at a known PRF, and echoes returned from a specific depth along the scan line (**the sample volume**) are analysed. When flow is laminar, the signal on the spectral display is narrow (Figure 1.11). When flow is turbulent, and the range of velocities at the sample site is high, the line is wide (a process termed *spectral broadening*).

The operator controls the specific location and the size of the sample volume. A larger sample volume increases the range of velocities sampled and also results in spectral broadening. The operator should select the size of the sample volume on the basis of the clinical indication. In general, a small sample volume is preferred, as it provides a cleaner signal with less noise. However, when the precise location of the region of maximum flow is difficult to

Box 1.5 Water that flows upwards, stagecoach wheels, and aliasing

Suppose one were to make a movie of a stream of dripping water. Let the frame rate of the movie be one frame per second (for ease of illustration). If the drip rate is set to one drop per second, the drops will appear stationary on the movie, because during the time between frames, each drop will travel to exactly the position occupied by the drop below it when the previous frame was taken. If the drip rate is slightly slower than the frame rate, say one drop every 1.1 s, the drops will appear to flow upwards (defying gravity), because during the time between frames, each drop will travel to a position just *above* the location occupied by the drop below it when the previous frame was taken. Conversely, if the drip rate is slightly faster, say one drop every 0.9 s, the drops will appear to move downwards, but more slowly than they are actually falling.

Similarly, in old Western movies, the spokes of the stagecoach wheels that should be rotating forward rapidly often appear to rotate forward slowly, stand still, or rotate slowly backwards, depending on the movement of each spoke relative to each other, and relative to the camera's frame rate.

These strange illusions represent *under-sampling*. The cause of aliasing with PW Doppler is also under-sampling and, in these examples, the frame rate of the movie is analogous to the PRF of PW Doppler. The problem in movies only arises above a certain rate of wheel rotation or dripping water. Similarly, there is a maximum frequency of Doppler shift, called the *Nyquist limit*, that can be evaluated unambiguously with PW Doppler. To the extent possible, the primary solution to each of these problems when they occur is more frequent sampling (i.e. a faster movie frame rate or a higher PRF; Box 1.2).

anticipate (e.g. within a pulmonary vein), a larger sample volume is required to correctly determine the velocity.

The advantage of PW Doppler is the ability to determine the velocity of movement at a specific point in space (**range specificity**). The disadvantage is that only lower velocities can be measured unambiguously.

Nyquist limit and aliasing

To reconstruct a waveform accurately and unambiguously, it is necessary to sample it sufficiently often. If the sampling rate is at or below that value, then inaccurate or multiple solutions can be derived from the sampled data, a phenomenon known as **aliasing**. Box 1.5 shows a number of everyday examples of under-sampling and aliasing.

With PW Doppler, the sampling rate used to estimate velocity from the sine wave reflected by moving blood cells is the PRF. The PRF is limited by the speed of propagation of sound in the sampled medium (Box 1.2). This means that there will be a maximum frequency of Doppler shift (and a corresponding maximum velocity of blood cells), which can be measured *unambiguously*. This maximum frequency is called the *Nyquist limit* (after the physicist Harry Nyquist) and it is equal to PRF/2. At Doppler shift frequencies above the Nyquist limit, velocities will be displayed inaccurately, with the appearance of 'wrapping around' (i.e. aliasing) the spectral Doppler display, possibly with reversal of direction (Figure 1.13 and Box 1.6).

From the Nyquist criteria, the time to generate one scan, and the Doppler equation, one can obtain an equation for the maximum unambiguously displayed velocity v_{max} (Equation 1.9):

$$v_{\text{max}} = \frac{c^2}{8f_s d} \qquad \text{Equation 1.9}$$

where c is the propagation speed of ultrasounds, fs is the source frequency in MHz, and *d* is the depth setting on the machine. With a 5-MHz probe, a speed of sound of 1570 m/s in blood (in pure blood, it is slightly faster than in human tissue) and depth measured in metres, the maximum velocity in m/s is (approximately) given by (Equation 1.10):

$$v_{\text{max}} = \frac{0.06}{d} \qquad \text{Equation 1.10}$$

There are many situations where the velocity of blood flow exceeds v_{max} and cannot be unambiguously determined with PW Doppler. Within limits, adjusting the baseline and velocity scale may allow a complete PW Doppler waveform to be displayed without aliasing (Figure 1.13). However, adjusting these controls does not influence the Nyquist limit. Ways to increase the Nyquist limit and reduce aliasing are discussed in Box 1.6.

Some ultrasound machines have an operating mode called **high-PRF Doppler**, in which two or more sample

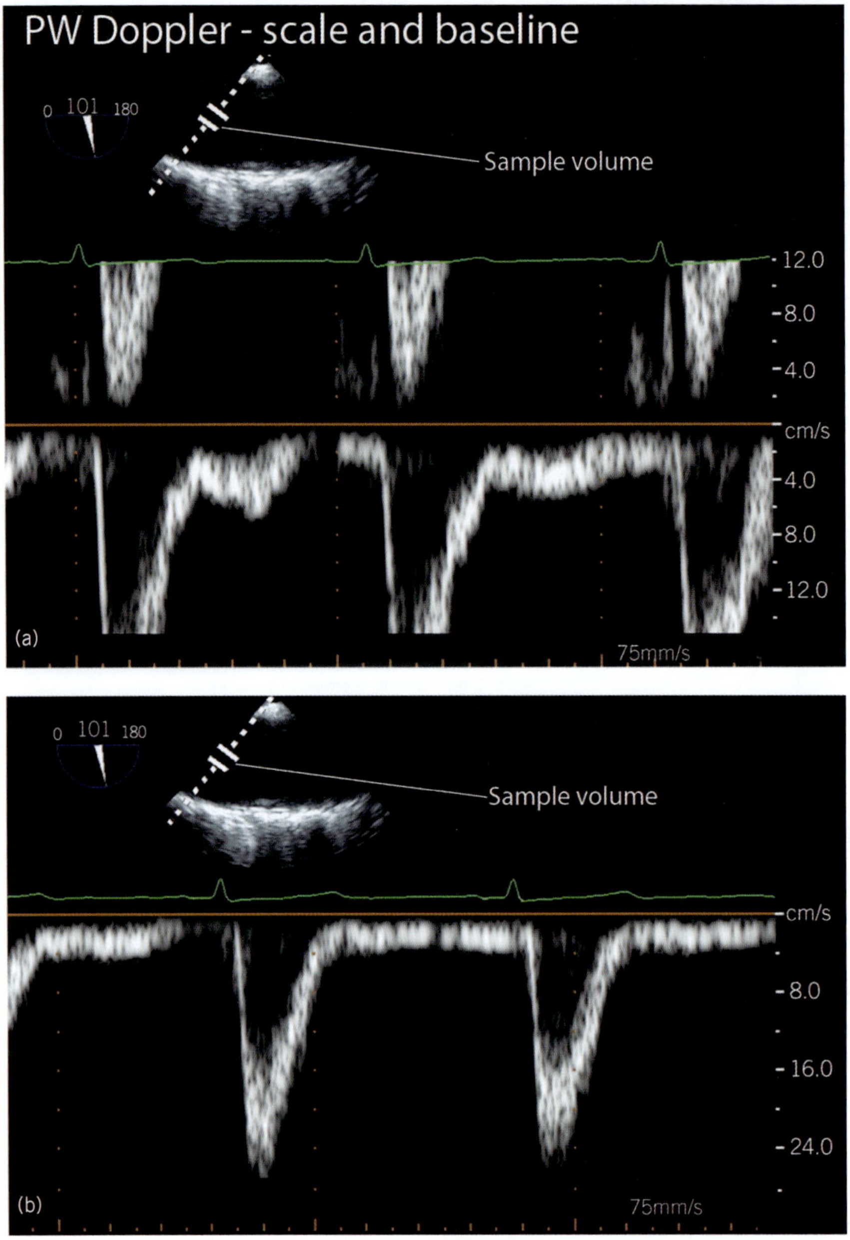

Figure 1.13 PW Doppler demonstrating aliasing in the descending thoracic aorta. The sample volume is positioned in the descending aorta. Flow at that location is away from the transducer, and therefore displayed below the baseline. In (a), the baseline is set near the centre of the display, with a measurable velocity of 12 cm/s above the baseline and about 16 cm/s below the baseline. With the peak velocity of blood cells at that location being >16 cm/s, aliasing is present, displayed as 'wrap around' of the signal (disappears at the bottom and reappears coming down from the top). In (b), the baseline is adjusted such that the maximum measurable velocity below the baseline is now 28 cm/s, with no velocity above the baseline (the range of measurable velocities in one direction was increased by sacrificing information in the other direction). This can be done because the flow of interest is known to be directed solely away from the transducer. The peak aortic velocity (approximately 24 cm/s) is now measurable unambiguously below the baseline, without aliasing. Note that the maximum setting on the velocity scale is limited by the Nyquist limit, and adjustments of the baseline can only compensate partially.

Box 1.6 Reducing aliasing with PW and colour Doppler

(Compare with Box 1.7.)

The relationship between the frame rate of a camera and the velocity of a turning wheel or drop of water explains the aliasing seen with cinematography in the examples given in Box 1.5, but the analogous factor in ultrasound to the frame rate in a movie is the **PRF** (*not* the frame rate) of the ultrasound device. Thus, with ultrasound, *aliasing depends on the relationship between two frequencies: the PRF (=the sampling rate) and the frequency of the Doppler shift (f_Δ), which reflect the velocity of the movement.* Ways to increase the maximum velocity that can be unambiguously displayed by PW Doppler and to avoid aliasing with PW Doppler and colour Doppler are:

1. ***Increasing the PRF by decreasing the depth of the 2D sector scan*** (for both PW and colour Doppler) ***and the depth of the colour box*** (for colour Doppler). Signals will have less distance to travel and will require less transit time, so a higher PRF will be possible. (Note that the *width* of the sector scan does not influence aliasing.)
2. ***Selecting a lower transducer frequency.*** This will decrease the Doppler shift frequency (f_Δ) for any given velocity (Equation 1.7)—many machines will select the lowest possible transducer frequency automatically and it may not be adjustable by the operator. Note that reducing the frequency also reduces the depth of penetration of the signal.
3. ***Adjusting the baseline of the spectral (or colour) display*** to provide the best match of the scale with the velocities in each direction (Figure 1.13).

If the velocity of interest still exceeds the limits of PW Doppler after optimizing these settings, it will be necessary to use CW Doppler.

volumes occur along the scan line. This technique multiplies the base PRF (and hence the Nyquist velocity limit) by the number of sample volumes, at the cost of introducing *some* range ambiguity. The 2D display at the top of the screen shows all the sample volumes along the beam, and the operator must decide which sample volume is the likely source of particular features in the spectral Doppler signal. In effect, CW Doppler is the extreme expression of high-PRF Doppler and has an infinite number of sampling volumes, and therefore no range resolution at all.

Colour Doppler

Colour Doppler imaging provides a dynamic representation of moving structures and flowing blood in real time. Information on blood velocity, represented on a selectable colour scale, is superimposed on a conventional 2D (Figure 3.1) or M-mode image (Figure 10.14). When colour Doppler is added to 2D images, the colour is shown in a sub-region of the image called the colour box, adjustable by the operator. With M-mode, the colour is integrated into the display automatically.

Colour Doppler is a pulsed technique that extends the concepts of PW Doppler to multiple points along multiple scan lines within a region of interest (Figure 1.14). The line density is lower (typically, one-half to one-quarter) than that of the underlying 2D image.

Packets of pulses are transmitted along each scan line and information is processed from between 100 and 400 sample volumes on each scan line, which requires an enormous amount of computation. Instead of the very demanding fast-Fourier transform employed in the spectrum analyser for CW and PW Doppler, simpler mathematical techniques are used in colour Doppler; thus, *one should not rely on colour imaging to measure specific*

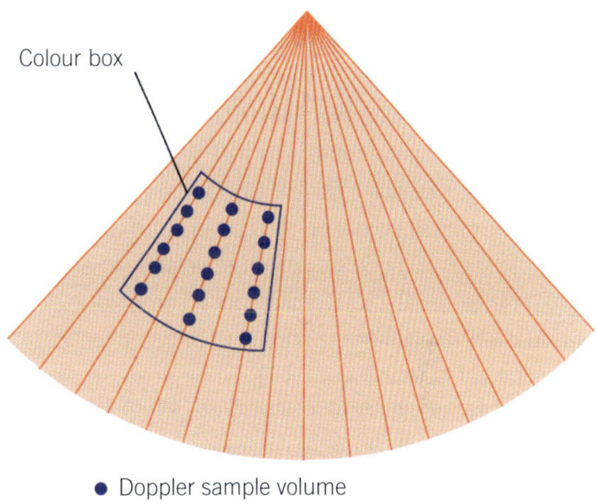

Figure 1.14 An ultrasonic sector with colour Doppler sampling. The scan lines of the sector and the locations of the sample volumes within the colour box are shown. The colour sampling lines (represented by the dots) are typically less dense than the 2D scan lines (represented by the solid lines). For each sample site along those lines, the computer displays a specific hue, luminescence, and saturation to reflect the direction and velocity of movement at that specific location, based on a selectable colour map. On the screen, colour is displayed overlying the 2D image.

velocities. As with PW Doppler, time is used to calculate the distance to the sample. The processor also yields the *direction* of the movement and the *strength* of the signal. These variables are rendered on a colour scale, using the hue, saturation, luminescence, and location of each pixel on the display, according to selectable **colour maps**. Each pixel displays only one colour at one level of luminescence. Hue is the perceived colour, ranging from dark red to dark blue, and it represents the direction and velocity of the movement. Luminescence is the brightness, and it represents the strength of the signal. White is a mixture of all the colours, and the addition of white reduces saturation.

In commonly used colour maps, the colours vary by convention, from saturated blue for maximal mean velocities away from the transducer to saturated red for maximal mean velocities towards the transducer (mnemonic: BART = blue away, red towards). Zero velocity is shown as black. **Variance** in velocity can also be displayed optionally, using shades of green. High variance usually indicates turbulent flow. Note that the conventional grey scale of 2D ultrasound is in effect a colour map, except that there is no hue and luminescence is used to represent the amplitude of the echo, with an appearance ranging from white to black.

Because colour Doppler uses pulses of ultrasound, it is subject to the same limitations as PW Doppler imaging (think of colour Doppler as PW Doppler applied simultaneously to multiple points on the colour window). Aliasing of the colour display occurs when the velocity in any sample volume exceeds the Nyquist limit. The colour of that individual sample volume abruptly changes from blue to red or vice versa (see Figure 3.1).

Since high-velocity flow is often associated with turbulence (i.e. blood cells travelling at many different velocities in many different directions), a *mosaic* of many different colours in a Doppler image typically indicates either turbulent flow or flow velocity that exceeds the Nyquist limit. When the variance option is activated, aliased signals often display a green hue, reflecting the high variance when the velocity exceeds the Nyquist threshold. As with PW Doppler, one can attempt to eliminate aliasing by: (1) adjusting the baseline of the colour scale (if the flow of interest is predominantly in one direction); (2) increasing the PRF by decreasing the depth of the colour box; or (3) decreasing the transmitted frequency (Box 1.6).

Overall resolution is lower with colour imaging than with conventional 2D imaging. Spatial resolution is limited by the reduced number of scan lines and the need for a discrete number of sample volumes along each line (2D echo does not have this requirement). There is little the operator can do to improve this. Temporal resolution is limited by the frame rate, and in colour Doppler, the frame rate is constrained by the need to acquire multiple scan lines with several pulses per line during the generation of each frame. Some adjustments by the operator can improve temporal resolution (Box 1.7).

Expert tip: Colour Doppler is a computer-generated representation of blood and tissue movement, based on multiple PW sample volumes, and using a large number of assumptions and calculations; though it is a very useful clinical tool, operators should be careful about relying on colour Doppler alone to make quantitative diagnoses.

As with other forms of Doppler imaging, if the beam is at an angle θ to the flow of blood or movement of a structure, the Doppler shift will reflect only the component of the

Box 1.7 Increasing temporal resolution with colour flow Doppler

(Compare with Box 1.6.)

Temporal resolution (in both echocardiography and cinematography) is dictated by the frame rate, which is the frequency with which the image is refreshed on the echo screen. The time needed to scan one line depends on its depth (Box 1.2).

The frame rate then depends on how many lines are scanned per frame and the depth of each of these lines. Thus, to increase the frame rate and temporal resolution with colour Doppler:

1. **Decrease the depth** of the overall sector scan and of the Doppler colour box to reduce the wait time for returning signals in each.
2. **Reduce the width** of the overall sector scan and of the Doppler colour box to reduce the number of scan lines in each (each line takes time to scan, and more computation time is required for more lines).

These adjustments obviously involve a trade-off with the field of view.

Note that transducer frequency and baseline position do not influence temporal resolution.

Because M-mode uses only one scan line, much higher frame rates (and therefore excellent temporal resolution) can be obtained with or without colour.

velocity (the vector) that is aligned with the beam, which is given by cosine θ (Equation 1.8). If the beam is perpendicular to the movement, cosine $90° = 0$, so the estimated velocity will be zero. This will typically be shown as *black* on the colour map. As an illustration of this, colour flow in a long-axis view of the descending aorta is typically red on one side of the sector, black in the centre, and blue on the other side, because the direction of flow in the vessel relative to the beam will be towards, then perpendicular, then away from the transducer (see Figure 12.4d)

It follows that alignment of the beam to the movement of interest must be taken into account when interpreting colour Doppler. As always, care should be taken to align the beam as closely as possible with the direction of movement of the target.

Effect of ultrasound on tissue

The biological effect of an ultrasound signal on tissue depends on the amount of energy transferred to it, and that amount of energy is greater if power is increased or time is increased. Intuitively, it seems prudent not to use more power or time than necessary, but the only known adverse effect of diagnostic ultrasound on human tissue is localized heating. Heating depends on the properties of the tissue and its perfusion, the properties of the transducer, and the intensity and time of exposure. The ALARA principle (As Low As Reasonably Achievable to obtain the necessary diagnostic information) is stressed by the American Institute of Ultrasound in Medicine.[1]

The transducer may cause oesophageal burn if it becomes hot. TOE probes have built-in thermometers that activate a safety shut-off of the echocardiography machine when the transducer temperature reaches approximately 40°C. However, it is still possible for burns to occur at lower temperatures than this, particularly when a patient is hypothermic or if the transducer is left in an unfavourable position for a prolonged time, which may also cause pressure necrosis.

It follows that acoustic transmission should be turned on only when images are being viewed. A simple way to turn off transmission is to *freeze the image*. The mechanical controls should also be left in an *unlocked* neutral position to prevent pressure injuries.

The electrical insulation of a transoesophageal probe can become damaged by repeated use and sterilization, and electric shock or electrocautery burns to the oesophagus can then occur. Probes should be inspected and tested for electrical leakage regularly, according to the manufacturer's instructions.

Acknowledgement

The authors wish to acknowledge Gerard Bashein and Paul R. Detmer for their contribution to prior editions of this book. While they did not contribute directly to this edition, the current authors used many of their ideas and concepts.

Multiple choice questions

Discover interactive multiple choice questions to test your knowledge on this chapter by searching for this book's title or ISBN (9780198873686) at **https://academic.oup.com/** and going to the online appendix at the end of the book. Use your scratch-off code on the inside cover to access the material.

Reference

1. Fowlkes JB. American Institute of Ultrasound in Medicine consensus report on potential bioeffects of diagnostic ultrasound: executive summary. *J Ultrasound Med.* 2008;**27**:503–15.

2

Resolution, instrument controls, and artefacts

For diagnostic accuracy and to avoid errors, it is essential to optimize image resolution and to recognize artefacts during TOE examinations. In this chapter, image resolution and the instrument controls that influence it are discussed, and important artefacts associated with echocardiography are reviewed. While general principles are discussed here, the knobology of specific machines (which varies across manufacturers) is beyond the scope of this chapter.

Resolution in two- and three-dimensional imaging

The resolution of an ultrasound system is its ability to distinguish echoes from different sources that are close to one another in space, time, or signal strength, known as spatial, temporal, and contrast resolution, respectively.

When it comes to ultrasound resolution, *closer is better.* The most important first step in optimizing resolution is to choose an image plane (i.e. a vantage point) that brings the structure(s) of interest as close to the transducer as possible. For instance, AV leaflets are better visualized in mid-oesophageal views (closer to the transducer) than in transgastric views (further from the transducer). Reducing the dimensions of the sector scan as much as possible is also of fundamental importance—this often allows for better resolution and never makes resolution worse.

Spatial resolution

Spatial resolution can be defined in relation to each of the three geometric dimensions of the ultrasound beam: axial, lateral, and elevational (Figure 2.1 and Box 2.1).

Axial resolution

Axial resolution is measured *parallel* to the beam, and it is the minimum separation (i.e. the difference in distance from the source) needed for a pair of reflectors along the path of the beam to produce separate echoes and appear as distinct objects.

As demonstrated in Figure 2.2, the receiver cannot distinguish targets located closer together than half the spatial pulse length. Thus, axial resolution is improved by shortening spatial pulse length by reducing pulse duration. In practice, the shortest spatial pulse length is two wavelengths (i.e. 2λ), so the highest achievable axial resolution is just over one wavelength (i.e. just over λ). It follows that *axial resolution is also improved by shortening the wavelength* (Box 2.2).

Wavelength is inversely related to the frequency of an ultrasound signal (see Equation 1.2). The wavelength for a typical 5-MHz probe is approximately 0.3 mm (Box 2.1), so this distance is the usual axial resolution of TOE in blood and soft tissue. That is, for two targets that lie on the path of the ultrasound beam to be distinguishable from each other, their separation (i.e. the difference in depth) must be at least 0.3 mm. Increasing the transducer frequency shortens λ, which improves axial resolution, but at the cost of more attenuation and less penetration, so there is a *trade-off between resolution and depth* (see Chapter 1). High frequencies are most useful for imaging structures that are close to the transducer.

Lateral resolution

Lateral resolution is measured perpendicular to the beam and parallel to the plane of the sector scan, and it is the minimum separation that is necessary for a pair of reflectors, located the same distance from the transducer (side-by-side), to produce separate echoes and appear as distinct objects. Lateral resolution depends on the width (azimuthal) of the ultrasound *beam* (not the sector), because two targets cannot be distinguished if they lie within the same beam (Figure 2.1). Thus, lateral resolution is improved if the beam is narrow at the depth of the target structure.

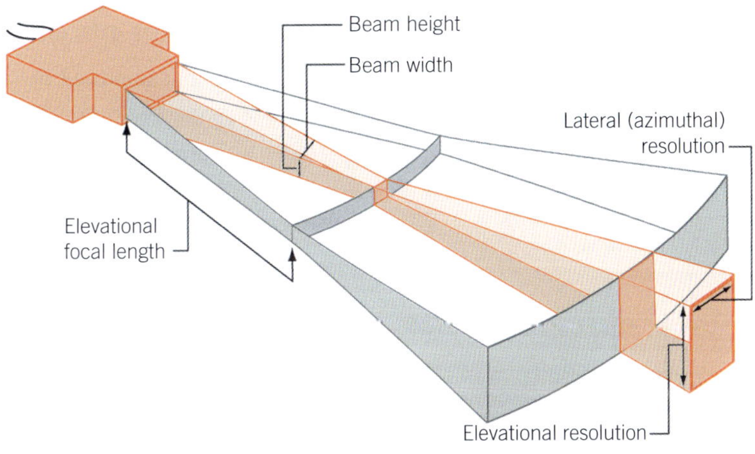

Figure 2.1 Ultrasound sector emitted by a phased-array transducer and a single scan line within it. The sector 'fan', shown in grey, has three dimensions: axial (its depth or *y*-axis, not labelled here), azimuthal (its width or *x*-axis), and elevational (its height or thickness or *z*-axis). Each scan line, shown in brown, has a height and a width, and it can be electronically focused at a specific point in space by firing the transducer elements in phase. Beyond the focal point, the beam diverges. With a single row of elements, electronic phasing is only possible in the azimuthal plane. With multiple rows of elements, it is possible to focus the elevational plane as well, but typically elevational focus is determined by the transducer design (its shape and lens) and is fixed. Transducer design and electronic focusing determine the azimuthal (i.e. lateral) resolution and azimuthal focal length, so these are adjustable. Azimuthal resolution is generally better than elevational resolution (see text). The best resolution occurs along the direction of the beam (axial resolution; not shown in this image) and is determined by the transmitted pulse duration (or length), not by the geometry of the transducer itself.

The edge of a sound beam is not perfectly abrupt, so beam width is customarily defined as the lateral distance between the points where the beam intensity diminishes by 3 dB (i.e. 50% power—see Box 1.3) from the intensity at the centre of the beam. Furthermore, the width of an ultrasound beam is not constant along its path—as the beam leaves the transducer, its width is approximately the same as the width of the transducer itself. In the absence of a lens, that width remains relatively constant for a certain distance from the face of the transducer. This part of the beam is known as the **near field**. Beyond that, the beam diverges into the **far field** and becomes progressively wider (Figure 2.3).

For an *unfocused* beam, the **near field length** is given by Equation 2.1:

$$\text{Near field length} = \frac{\text{Diameter}^2}{4\lambda} \qquad \text{Equation 2.1}$$

where diameter is the width of the transducer aperture and λ is the wavelength of the signal.

However, in clinical echocardiography, it is possible to *electronically focus* the beam of a phased array transducer in the lateral dimension, by changing the timing of the firing of the transducer elements (Figure 2.3). This is adjustable by the operator. Focusing changes the shape of the beam and narrows it down to a **focal point**, set by the operator, which is narrower than the narrowest part of the unfocused beam, and then diverges beyond that point, more markedly than does an unfocused beam. The best lateral resolution will be obtained by positioning the focal point *just beyond* the depth of the target structure on the screen. The width of the beam at the focal point is given by:

$$\text{Width at focal point} \approx \frac{\text{Focal length} \times \lambda}{\text{diameter}} \qquad \text{Equation 2.2}$$

Box 2.1 Spatial resolution in 2D imaging

The order in spatial resolution (from best to poorest resolution) is:

1. **Axial**—0.3 mm is achievable ($\approx \lambda$). This can be improved by increasing the frequency/decreasing the wavelength of the transducer
2. **Lateral** (rule of thumb: resolution = depth/50, so at a depth of 10 cm, a resolution of about 2 mm can be achieved). Can be improved with electronic focusing
3. **Elevational** (rule of thumb: resolution = depth/30, so at a depth of 10 cm, a resolution of about 3.3 mm can be achieved). Typically cannot be adjusted by the operator

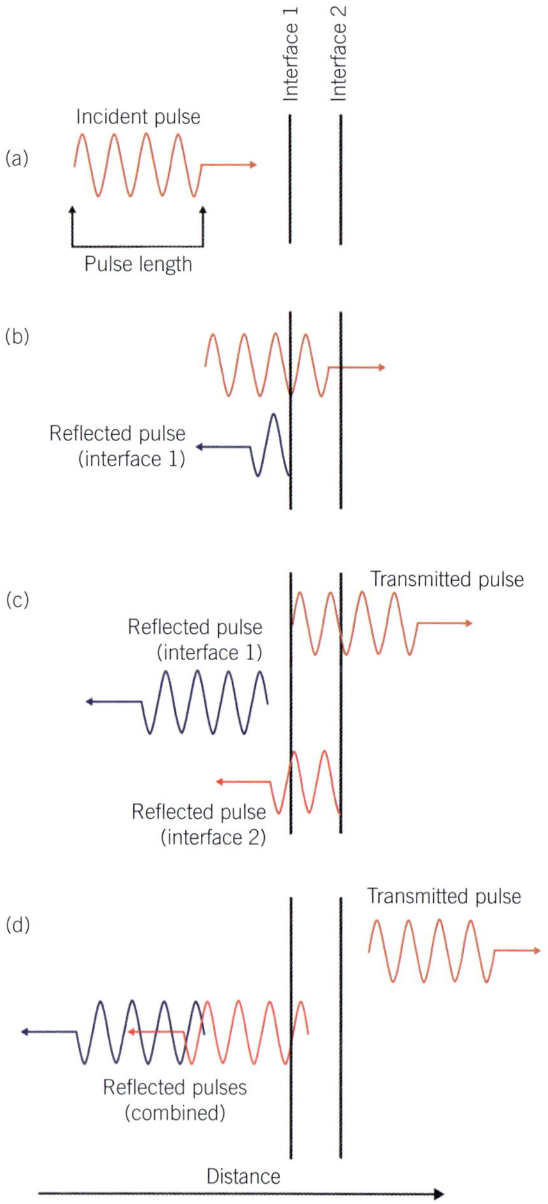

Figure 2.2 Ultrasonic pulse and its reflections, shown at four moments in time. (a) The incident pulse approaches a pair of interfaces. (b) The pulse hits the first interface and is reflected (blue wave). (c) A moment later, the incident pulse hits the second interface and is reflected (red wave). (d) Since less than half of the pulse length divides the two interfaces, the two reflected pulses (red and blue waves) merge, making the two targets indistinguishable in the final image. It can be readily appreciated that a difference in the distance between the two reflectors of slightly greater than half of the pulse length will result in separation of the two returning signals. It turns out that the best achievable axial resolution is *just over one wavelength* (i.e. just over 0.3 mm at 5 mHz; see text). Increasing the frequency reduces the wavelength and improves the axial resolution, at the cost of depth of penetration.

Box 2.2 Improving axial resolution in 2D imaging

Axial resolution is improved by:

- Increasing the frequency of the signal and thereby reducing its wavelength (at the cost of reduced penetration and reduced near field length)
- Reducing pulse duration

Equation 2.2 explains why increasing the frequency (which reduces λ) improves the lateral resolution *at the focal depth*—because the width at the focal point is decreased. A larger diameter of the aperture of the transducer increases the near field length of an unfocused beam (Equation 2.1), and it decreases the width at the focal point of a focused beam (Equation 2.2). Thus, the lateral resolution *at the focal depth* is improved with a larger transducer, a shorter focal length, and a higher frequency (Box 2.3). Note that while it may be possible to select a larger transducer in TTE, this is usually not possible in TOE.

Lateral resolution also depends on the number of beams within a sector—that is, how close each successive beam in a phased array is to the preceding one (without overlapping). This is called the **line density** or **beam density**. The beams fan out from the centre of the sector scan (see Figure 1.7). In addition, the beams themselves diverge in width beyond their focal point; thus, lateral resolution decreases as depth increases beyond the focal length. Increasing the line density also reduces the maximum achievable frame rate (see discussion of temporal resolution below), but reducing the depth and width of the sector scan will mitigate this.

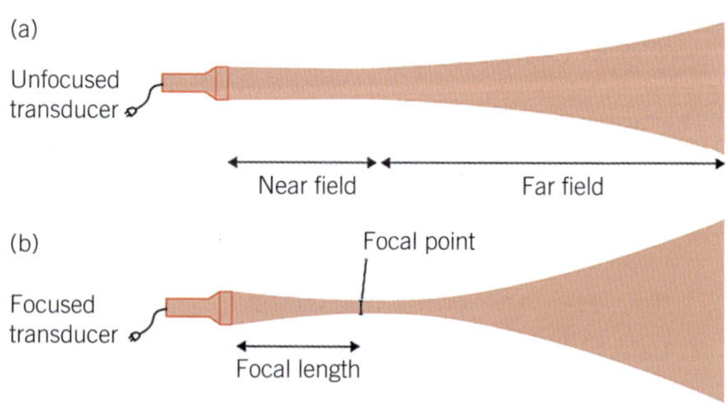

Figure 2.3 Main beam produced by (a) an unfocused single-element discoid transducer and (b) a focused transducer. The beam from a focused transducer is narrower at its focal depth than that of an unfocused transducer, at the expense of somewhat more rapid divergence in the far field.

Box 2.3 Improving lateral resolution in 2D imaging

Lateral resolution is improved by:

- **Increasing the size of the transducer aperture**, which narrows the beam at the focal point and reduces the focal length (selecting a transducer with a larger aperture is possible in TTE, but not in TOE)
- **Focusing the beam electronically** (adjustable by the operator—the focal point should be positioned just beyond the structure of interest)
- **Minimizing the depth from the transducer to the target** (by selecting an image plane closer to the target, e.g. imaging the MV from the transoesophageal vs transgastric view)
- **Increasing the frequency** because the frequency is inversely proportional to λ and λ is directly proportional to the beam width at the focal point (Equation 2.2). This is adjustable on some echocardiography machines
- **Increasing the beam density** (provided the beams do not overlap)

It is important to remember that:

- Beam divergence beyond the focal length will be increased by focusing and by shortening the focal length
- Minimizing the width of the sector scan will not in itself improve the lateral resolution, but it will facilitate an increase in beam density by mitigating its impact on the temporal resolution
- Minimizing the depth of the sector scan will also facilitate an increased beam density

Elevational resolution

The definition of elevational resolution is similar to that of lateral resolution, but the minimum separation is measured perpendicular to the beam and perpendicular to the plane of the sector scan (Figure 2.1). Elevational resolution depends on the height (or thickness) of the beam. In most respects, this is subject to the same considerations as its width (Box 2.4), with the following differences:

1. Focusing in the elevational dimension depends on the shape of the transducer and/or the presence of an acoustic lens, both of which are less effective than focusing electronically and cannot be adjusted by the operator.
2. The face of a transducer aperture is typically wider than it is thick. From Equation 2.2, it follows that the beam height at the focal point will exceed its width.
3. The operator adjusts the focal length in the lateral dimension to its optimal depth, and if this does not happen to coincide with the focal depth in the elevational dimension, further reduction in elevational resolution may result.

The bottomline of this discussion is that the worst spatial resolution tends to occur in the elevational dimension (Box 2.1).

In practice, elevational resolution is usually less critical than lateral resolution. The greatest relevance of poor elevational resolution is the potential for beam thickness artefacts (discussed later in this chapter).

Box 2.4 Improving elevational resolution with 2D imaging

Elevational resolution is improved by:

- Increasing the size of the transducer aperture to reduce the height of the beam at the focal point (not adjustable by the operator)
- Focusing the beam acoustically (not adjustable by the operator)
- Minimizing the depth from the transducer to the target (by selecting an image plane closer to the target)
- Increasing the frequency (at the expense of reduced penetration) because the frequency is inversely proportional to λ, and λ is directly proportional to the beam height at the focal point (Equation 2.2)

Temporal resolution

Temporal resolution is the ability to detect that an object has moved over time and to correctly ascertain the extent and direction of the movement. In practice, temporal resolution manifests as the smoothness or jerkiness of a moving image. The human eye perceives 25 frames per second (FPS) or more as smooth motion, and this is the minimum frame rate used for cinema, television, and most streaming videos. It is possible to store images digitally at a higher frame rate and play them back in slow motion. For example, if images are stored at 50 FPS and replayed at 25 FPS, the effective temporal resolution of the eye can be doubled.

In ultrasonography, temporal resolution depends entirely on the **frame rate**. Frame rate, in turn, depends on:

1. How long each ultrasound signal takes to reach its target and return to the transducer (see Box 1.2), which depends on the sector *depth*.
2. How many sequential beams are used to generate a single frame of the image, which depends on the *line density* and the sector *width*.

The speed of sound in a given medium is fixed, so, in standard 2D imaging, the frame rate can only be increased by reducing the depth and width of the sector scan (Box 2.5). In colour Doppler imaging, the frame rate depends both on the formation of the background 2D image (the above factors) and on the formation of the colour image, so increasing temporal resolution *also* requires reduction of the depth and size of the colour box.

Because M-mode (with or without colour) involves only one scan line, it has much higher temporal resolution than 2D (with or without colour Doppler).

Contrast resolution

With 2D imaging, the intensity or strength of a returning signal is usually represented on the screen by brightness, or shade of grey. The smallest difference in intensity or strength that can be distinguished between two signals is called *contrast resolution*. Clinically, contrast resolution may make the difference between identifying a thrombus in the LA or missing it because it merges with the surrounding structures.

Dynamic range is the ratio (in decibels) of the largest to the smallest power (or intensity) that an ultrasound system can handle (typically >100 dB for modern ultrasound machines). The dynamic range is divided equally between each available shade of grey in the image, from the darkest to the lightest. However, there are not enough shades of grey to provide one shade for every strength of signal. Thus, it is necessary to divide the dynamic range into segments (i.e. the assignment of the signal to successive shades of grey is stepped, rather than continuous). Each shade then represents one of these segments of the dynamic range. Increasing the number of bits per pixel increases the available number of shades of grey and therefore increases the potential contrast resolution. However, our eyes can only handle a dynamic range of brightness of about 20 dB, so computing power is not the only limitation to displaying the dynamic ranges associated with the signals received in echocardiography. As the human eye can distinguish more shades of colour than shades of grey, contrast resolution can sometimes be enhanced by adding colour.

Box 2.5 Improving temporal resolution in 2D imaging

Temporal resolution is improved by increasing the frame rate, which can be done by:

- Reducing the depth of the 2D sector scan
- Reducing the width of the 2D sector scan
- Reducing the depth of the colour box (if using colour)
- Reducing the size of the colour box (if using colour)
- Using M-mode (with or without colour)

Doppler imaging and resolution

The use of Doppler shift to measure the velocity of blood or moving structures is discussed in Chapter 1. Doppler shift varies continuously, so resolution itself (i.e. the ability to distinguish between two similar velocities) is never a problem and is not something that the operator can, or would seek to, adjust. On the other hand, the *range* of velocities that can be measured unambiguously with PW Doppler or colour Doppler is restricted by the **Nyquist limit**, and adjustments can be made in relation to this. Furthermore, the accuracy with which a *maximum* velocity can be measured also depends on alignment of the ultrasound beam with the direction of movement (see cosine effect in Chapter 1).

Although temporal resolution does not directly affect the ability to measure velocity per se, it may impact the evaluation of blood flow through structures (such as stenotic or regurgitant valves) using colour Doppler, in as much as the maximum velocity must be captured in the frame rate. These factors are discussed in Chapter 1 (see Boxes 1.8 and 1.9).

Finally, the use of colour Doppler reduces the temporal resolution of the underlying 2D or 3D image (by virtue of the fact that it reduces the frame rate of the whole image).

Resolution in 3D imaging

As with 2D ultrasound, with 3D imaging, there is interdependence between temporal resolution, spatial resolution, and sector dimensions. The main trade-off is between sector volume and temporal resolution. Increasing the sector volume while keeping the scan line density the same necessarily increases the time taken to acquire a single frame, and therefore reduces the number of times the image is refreshed on the screen. Conversely, if the scan line density remains the same, reducing the sector volume improves the frame rate at no cost to the lateral resolution.

Options to improve the temporal resolution include: (1) reducing the scan line density; (2) increasing the beam thickness; (3) reducing the sector volume; and (4) using ECG-gated multi-beat acquisition (see Chapter 1). Scan line density and beam thickness are adjusted automatically by the ultrasound system, depending on the 3D imaging mode, the sector volume, and the application of colour Doppler.

Three-dimensional imaging in narrow sector mode (aka 'live-3D') typically affords high spatial and temporal resolution (frame rate 20–30 Hz). By comparison, the frame rate with a focused wide sector using real-time imaging is typically in the range of 5–10 Hz and falls <5 Hz with the addition of colour Doppler imaging. Frame rate can be increased to 10–20 Hz by using ECG-gated multi-beat acquisition and choosing a smaller sector volume—to display only the structure of interest.

Instrument controls for 2D imaging

A number of controls influence the spatial and temporal resolution of the ultrasound image. These include sector width, sector depth, frequency, harmonic imaging, and focus. Other controls influence the appearance and contrast resolution of the image. These include receiver gain, time-gain compensation (TGC), compression, and reject.

Transmit power

The transmit power control determines the electrical energy applied to the ultrasound transducer, and therefore the amplitude ('loudness') of the transmitted ultrasound beam, which is measured in decibels. If the transmit power is too high, it makes certain artefacts (reverberation, secondary lobe) more common and it increases the risk of thermal injury to the patient; if the transmit power is too low, image quality is reduced. In practice, the power control rarely requires manual adjustment and the machine's default settings should be used.

Transmit frequency

Phased array ultrasound transducers operate across a range of frequencies, typically between 2 and 7 MHz. As explained previously, higher frequencies provide enhanced spatial (axial, lateral, and elevational) resolution at the focal point of the beam, at the cost of reduced tissue penetration; lower frequencies allow better tissue penetration, but reduced spatial resolution. Transmit frequency is usually adjusted automatically by the ultrasound system in response to changes in the depth of the sector, but can also be adjusted manually by the operator on some machines.

Focus

The focus control adjusts the focal zone of the ultrasound beam in its lateral dimension. This influences the *lateral resolution* but can adversely affect the elevational resolution (Boxes 2.3 and 2.4). In practice, lateral resolution is usually more important than elevational resolution, because TOE imaging is essentially tomographic (thin slice). For best effect, the focus should be positioned *slightly beyond* the region of interest.

Harmonic imaging

Conventional (or fundamental) ultrasound imaging involves transmitting a burst of sound at a certain frequency and listening for returned echoes at the same frequency (but at lower amplitude). As the transmitted ultrasound wave interacts with tissues, it becomes distorted, creating **harmonics**, which are multiples of the fundamental frequency. Harmonic imaging listens for returned echoes at twice the fundamental frequency. Harmonic imaging has the advantage of providing better lateral and elevational resolution and being less subject to artefacts and acoustic noise. On many modern echocardiography machines, harmonic imaging is on by default.

Receiver gain

Like the volume control on a radio, **receiver gain** adjusts the sensitivity to all received echoes. Increasing the receiver gain produces a uniformly brighter image (Figure 2.4). If the gain is too low, some signals may not be detected and the corresponding structures may not be visible. When it is too high, the differences in texture between structures with similar reflectance become difficult to perceive. Reducing the gain may improve visualization of strong reflectors, whereas increasing the gain may improve visualization of weak reflectors. Receiver gain should be set at a level that displays only a trace of electronic noise in echo-free regions of the image.

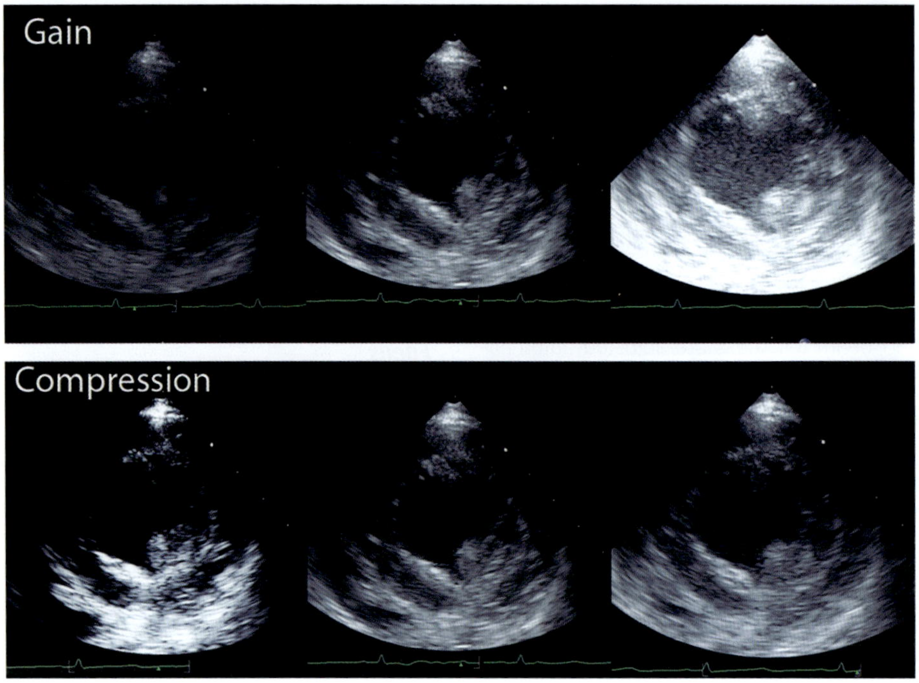

Figure 2.4 The effect of receiver gain and compression controls. The images are all short-axis views of the LV. The gain and compression settings have been gradually increased from left to right. See text for details.

Time-gain and lateral-gain compensation

As shown in Figure 1.6, ultrasound machines automatically increase the amplitude of signals returned from deeper structures. Additional selective manual adjustment of the gain is available on many machines in the form of **TGC slider controls**, allowing augmentation of echoes returned from different depths, to improve visualization. These adjust the relative sensitivity of the system to signals at specific depths—each control adjusts the gain from one particular band of depth—to 'fine-tune' the image quality (this is analogous to a sound equalizer on a stereo system). Some ultrasound systems also provide lateral-gain compensation (LGC) to adjust receiver sensitivity across the image from left to right.

Compression and reject

As explained previously, the dynamic range of modern ultrasound machines is typically >100dB, which is much greater than can be displayed by monitors or perceived by the human eye. Thus, to display 2D images on a video screen, the dynamic range must be reduced. On most modern ultrasound systems, the dynamic range itself is not under the direct control of the operator. Instead, the receiver gain, compression, and (sometimes) reject controls can be adjusted to map the returned echoes to the grey scale display.

Increasing **compression** enhances weaker signals and suppresses stronger signals. This has the effect of producing a smoother, softer image (Figure 2.4). Subtle variations between weaker echoes (e.g. when viewing a thrombus among trabeculae) are enhanced, but contrast resolution between stronger signals is reduced. Reducing compression increases contrast between black and white on the image. In general, compression should be reduced when image quality is poor.

Ultrasound machines also have built-in filters to automatically reject signals below a certain amplitude to remove background noise (e.g. electrical interference). On some ultrasound machines, a reject control is provided, which allows the operator to increase the default amplitude threshold for eliminating signals.

Lastly, many modern ultrasound machines have an automatic 'image optimization' button, which automatically sets the controls to what the machine believes is optimal for the current image.

Sector width and sector depth

On most echocardiography machines, the sector width can be adjusted between 15° and 90° and the depth from about 4 to 25 cm. At a constant line density, increasing the sector width and depth reduces the frame rate and therefore degrades the temporal resolution. For instance, at a sector width of 15° and a depth of 6 cm, a frame rate of approximately 150 Hz can be achieved for 2D imaging. The frame rate drops to approximately 50 Hz at a sector width of 90° and a depth of 20 cm.

Expert tip: In TOE imaging, the sector depth and width should always be large enough to demonstrate the structures of interest, but not too large in order to maximize the frame rate.

Zoom

The zoom function allows the user to choose and expand a region of interest when using 2D imaging. The operator controls both the size and location of the zoomed area. Two types of zoom function are available: transmit and receive. *Transmit* zoom is used during live imaging and is the equivalent of reducing the sector dimensions. Only reflected signals from the structure of interest are analysed, and spatial and temporal resolution is enhanced, compared to imaging with the full sector scan. *Receive* zoom is performed on stored images. Here, a region of interest is *magnified* for a better view, but spatial and temporal resolutions are not improved.

Freeze

Pressing the freeze control stops ultrasound transmission but retains in digital memory (buffer) a sequence of the immediately preceding image frames. The operator can then scroll through the stored frames to study evanescent phenomena, enter annotations, or acquire selected frames.

Colourization and grey scale

As explained previously, the human eye perceives colour better than shades of grey, and it can be difficult for the human eye to distinguish between the subtle shades of grey used to represent adjacent signals that are only slightly different in strength. With technological improvements providing more bits per pixel and higher processing speeds, it has become possible to map images in various ways to improve contrast resolution. The grey scale and colourization controls on some machines use various preselected maps to distribute the digitized image across the available display scale.

Instrument controls for Doppler imaging

Doppler receiver gain

The Doppler receiver gain (colour, PW or continuous wave (CW)) is equivalent to 2D echo receiver gain. It

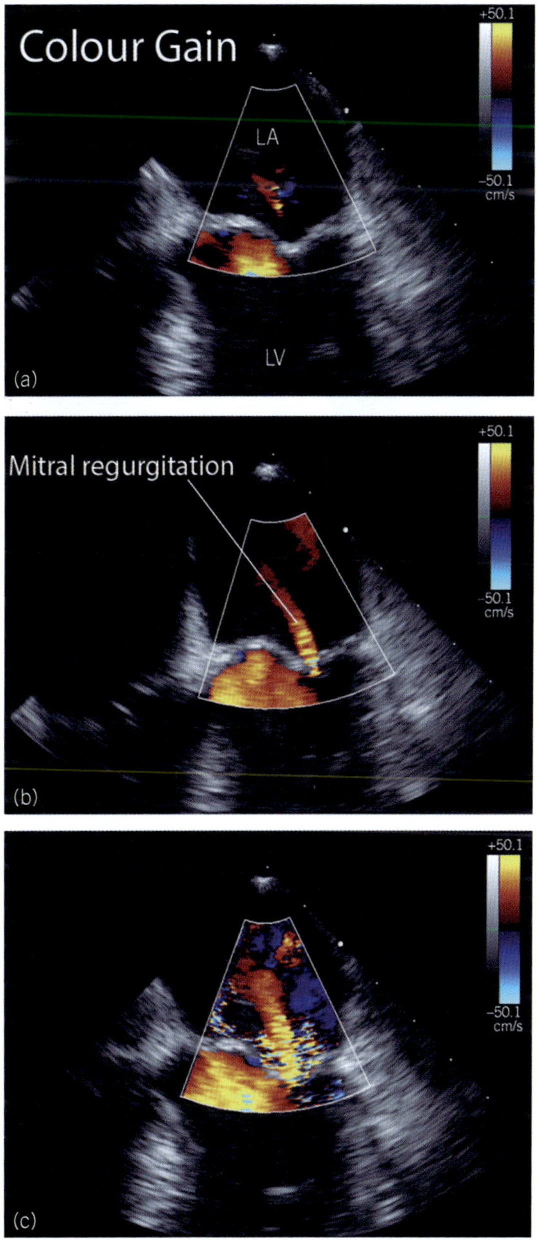

Figure 2.5 The effect of gradually increasing the colour gain control on a jet of mitral regurgitation. As described in the text, the colour gain should be set as high as possible, without displaying more than very slight background noise in the colour box (b). If the colour gain setting is much too low (a), the severity of mitral regurgitation can be underestimated; if the gain setting is much too high (c), the severity of the regurgitation can be overestimated

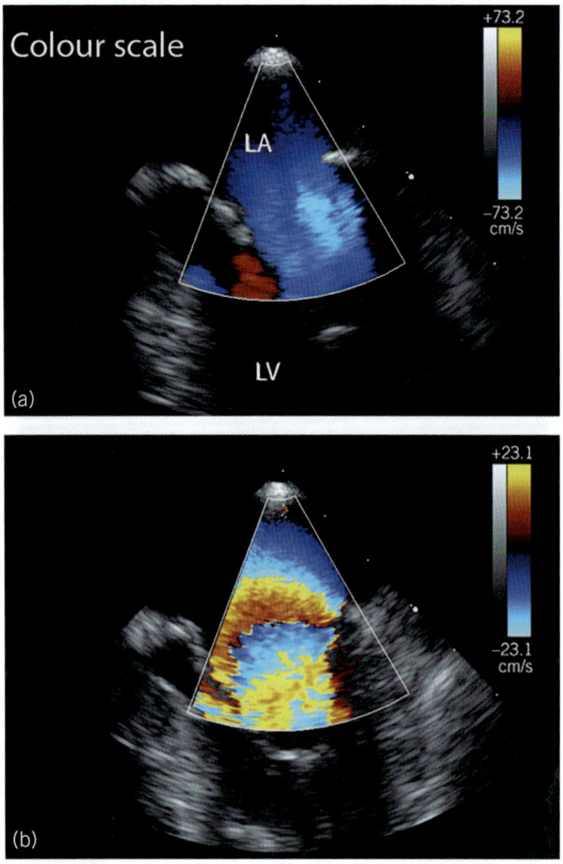

Figure 2.6 Changing the colour Doppler velocity scale. Frames (a) and (b) show normal diastolic flow across the *same* MV. In (a), the colour velocity scale is set to ±73.2 cm/s. Flow across the MV is blue (i.e. away from the transducer) and there is no colour aliasing. In (b), the colour velocity scale is set to ±23.1 cm/s, which is less than the normal peak diastolic trans-mitral velocity. Diastolic mitral inflow now shows aliasing (blue-to-yellow colour transition). This could give the operator the false impression that there is a problem with the MV.

should be set as high as possible, without displaying more than very slight background noise in the colour box or spectral display. Setting the colour gain too high can falsely enlarge the size of a flow jet and produce spurious signals, or display reverberation artefacts. Setting the colour gain too low can miss diagnostically important flow signals. The effect of altering the colour gain is shown in Figure 2.5.

Velocity scale and baseline

The velocity scale control adjusts the velocity range displayed for all Doppler modes. For colour Doppler, various colour maps may also be chosen by the operator to represent velocities in different directions (see Chapter 1).

As explained earlier, the maximum velocity setting for PW Doppler or colour imaging is the *Nyquist limit.* For PW Doppler, adjustment of the velocity scale and baseline settings can help prevent wrap-around of the Doppler waveform (see Figure 1.13).

Careful attention should be paid to the velocity scale in colour Doppler. As discussed in Chapter 1, the *maximum* achievable Nyquist limit is dependent on the pulse repetition frequency (PRF), and the operator cannot increase it beyond a certain point dictated by the laws of physics. However, the operator can set the Nyquist limit to a *lower* value, if desired. This may help visualization of low-velocity jets (e.g. slow flow across a patent foramen ovale). However, when the colour scale is set to a low value (<40 cm/s), aliasing will be displayed at lower velocities, and marked aliasing can occur across normal heart valves, giving the false impression of pathology (Figure 2.6).

Expert tip: In routine practice, the scale of the colour map (i.e. Nyquist limit) should always be set at the highest possible value, except in some specific circumstances (discussed in the text).

Sweep speed

The sweep speed control adjusts the rate at which information (i.e. the waveform) is displayed during spectral Doppler imaging. Sweep speed can typically be adjusted from 25 to 100 mm/s. Displaying more waveforms simultaneously is useful when comparing multiple waveforms (e.g. assessing signal variations over the respiratory cycle); displaying fewer waveforms makes analysing individual waveforms easier.

Sample volume

The sample volume control adjusts the size of the sample volume along the Doppler beam during PW Doppler imaging. A smaller sample volume restricts measurements to a very specific area in space, but it may also make it harder to pinpoint a region of peak flow and may miss the peak flow altogether. Conversely, a larger sample volume may unnecessarily 'pollute' a measurement with signals from adjacent areas. Increasing the sample volume can result in spectral broadening on the PW Doppler display (see Chapter 1).

Steering angle

The steering angle control allows the operator to specify the angle to be used by the ultrasound machine in the cosine correction (see Equation 1.8) during spectral Doppler imaging, when it is not physically possible to align the Doppler beam with blood flow. Correcting for the steering angle increases the value of the velocity calculated from any given Doppler shift, but it does not change the extent of the Doppler shift itself (in other words, it is a post-acquisition correction by the machine). Therefore, correcting for the steering angle has no effect on the Nyquist limit or the occurrence of aliasing. Because the steering angle is based on the 2D appearance on the screen of a jet that is, in fact, a 3D structure, it is highly prone to error, and *its use is not recommended during routine TOE examinations*. Steering angle correction can, however, be used effectively in vascular ultrasound.

Colour box size and position

The colour box size and position controls determine the region within which colour Doppler information is displayed on the 2D image. Reducing the depth of the colour box increases the Nyquist limit (see Box 1.8). Reducing its depth and width improves the temporal resolution (see Box 1.9).

Colour map and variance

As noted previously, different colour maps can be chosen to represent flow towards or away from the transducer. In addition, a **variance** function may be employed, in which a colour code is used to signify a high range of velocities within a sample. In laminar flow, where all the blood cells move in an orderly fashion, the range of velocities in a given area is low, and velocity can be adequately coded by using a standard red-blue map. Turbulent flow is associated with a high range of velocities within a sample and is commonly assigned the colour green. Application of the variance function reduces the resolution of the velocity display because some of the colour is used to represent variance.

Wall filter

Strong signals from large specular reflectors (e.g. myocardial walls) can overload the spectrum analyser and cover the weaker signals from small structures like blood cells (see Chapter 1). Therefore, an adjustable wall filter is commonly used. This is called a *high-pass* filter, meaning it eliminates frequencies below a set level, notably high-amplitude, low-velocity signals from slow-moving structures (e.g. ventricular or vessel walls or other tissue signals). This setting is a trade-off between eliminating signals from slow undesired objects and avoiding missing slow-moving blood flow. The wall filter may create an echo-free, black band around the zero-velocity line in the spectral display (see Figures 1.11 and 1.12).

Note that during **TDI**, a *low-pass* wall filter is used, which does the exact opposite—it displays the mean velocity of slower-moving tissue structures, such as ventricular walls, while excluding signals from faster-moving blood cells.

Artefacts

The term **artefact** (from Latin *arte*=by skill and *facere*=to make) describes any image that is not an accurate representation of reality. Generally speaking, artefacts can be:

- Objects that appear to be there when they are not
- Objects that do not appear to be there when they actually are
- Objects that appear different from their real appearance
- Objects that appear to be in a different location from where they really are.

Artefacts may arise from altered propagation of ultrasounds through tissue, from interactions between ultrasounds and various structures within the tissue, or from attenuation. Structures that appear consistently on multiple images are less likely to be artefactual, so the use of multiple views and multiple imaging modalities reduces the likelihood of misdiagnosis. Appropriate adjustment of imaging controls is also important (e.g. gain and Nyquist limit).

> ***Expert tip: As a rule of thumb, real structures are visible in multiple views; real structures are visible with multiple modalities (2D, 3D, Doppler); real structures respect anatomic boundaries; and real structures tend to make sense clinically. Any image that does not meet these criteria should raise the suspicion of being artefactual.***

Basic assumptions in ultrasound imaging

Ultrasound image interpretation is based on several basic assumptions by the imaging transducer about the propagation of ultrasounds through tissue: (1) the distance of a structure from the transducer can be calculated from the time taken for transmitted ultrasound pulses to reach that structure and return to the transducer; (2) all signals detected by the transducer have travelled in a *straight line* and were reflected by structures directly in the path of the

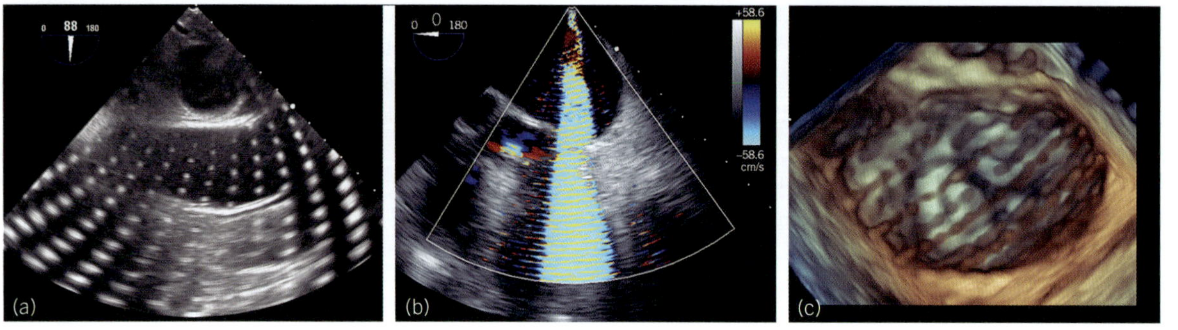

Figure 2.7 Electrical interference from surgical electrocautery/diathermy: on (a) a 2D image; (b) a colour Doppler image; and (c) a 3D zoom image.

main ultrasound beam; and (3) all signals detected by the transducer originate from the last transmitted ultrasound pulse. Artefacts arise when these assumptions are violated.

Artefacts can be broadly classified as originating from multiple reflections, misplaced reflections, or missing reflections. Surgical electrocautery/diathermy is also a common source of artefact, particularly during colour Doppler imaging (Figure 2.7).

Artefacts from multiple reflections

When a transmitted signal bounces back and forth between two or more strong reflectors in the tissues, and thus follows an artificially prolonged (and not necessarily straight) route back to the transducer, artefacts may be generated (Figure 2.8). Common examples include reverberation artefacts, comet tails, and mirror image artefacts.

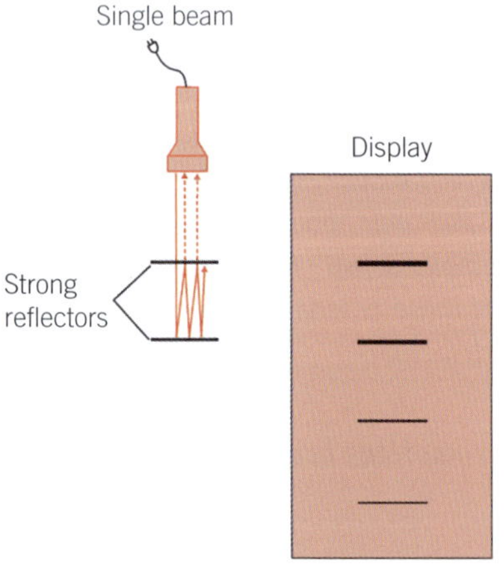

Figure 2.8 The generation of reverberation artefacts. The transmitted signal is reflected back and forth between two strong reflectors; much of the energy is reflected, but some passes through each reflector at each iteration. Signals of diminishing strength return to the transducer at equally spaced intervals of time and create an impression of multiple structures, giving the appearance of a stepladder with equally spaced 'steps'.

Reverberation artefacts occur when a reflected echo encounters a strong reflector on its way back to the transducer. The ultrasound beam may bounce back and forth between the two reflectors before returning to the

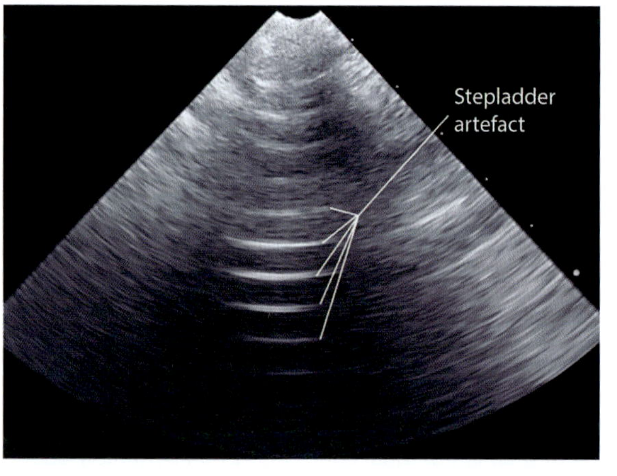

Figure 2.9 Stepladder artefact due to reverberations from tracheal rings during removal of a TOE probe from the oesophagus.

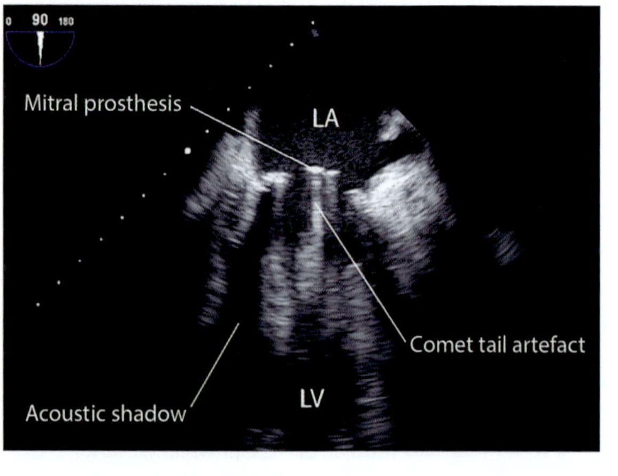

Figure 2.10 Comet tail artefacts and acoustic shadowing from an MV prosthesis.

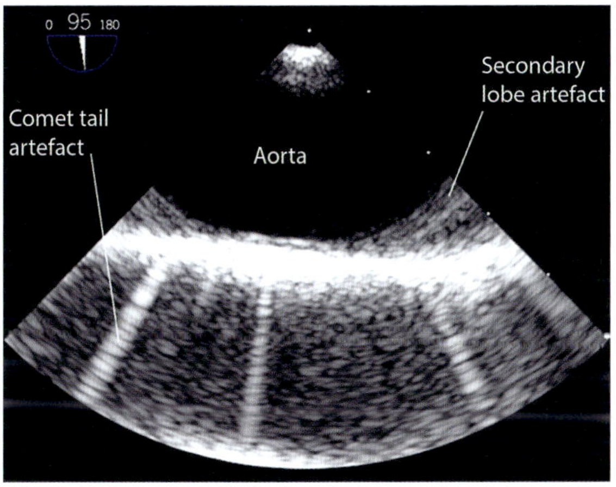

Figure 2.11 Comet tail and secondary lobe artefact in the descending thoracic aorta. The image is a descending aorta long-axis view. The distal aortic wall is thickened and acts as a strong reflector, which results in reverberations (comet tails) and secondary lobe artefacts.

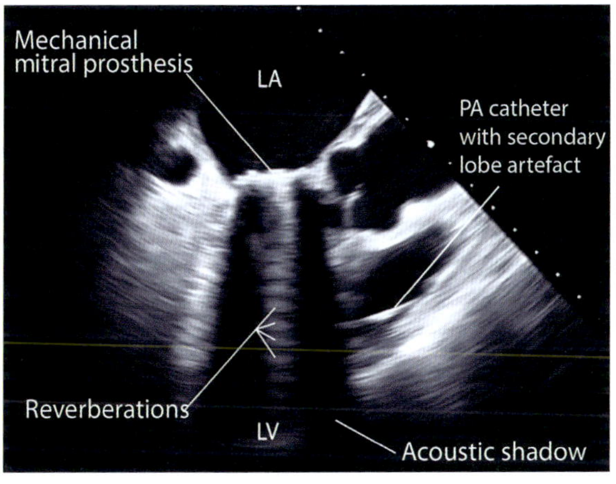

Figure 2.12 Reverberation artefacts and acoustic shadowing from a mitral prosthesis. In this example, the reverberation results in an artefact that resembles both a comet tail and a stepladder. Note also the secondary lobe artefact generated by the PA catheter in the RVOT.

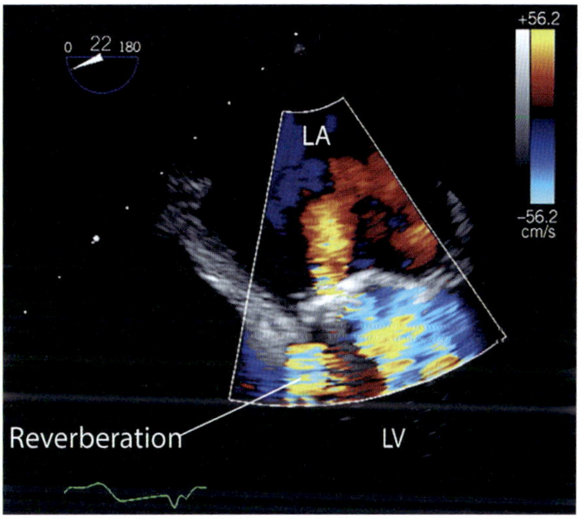

Figure 2.13 Colour reverberation artefact from a mitral prosthesis.

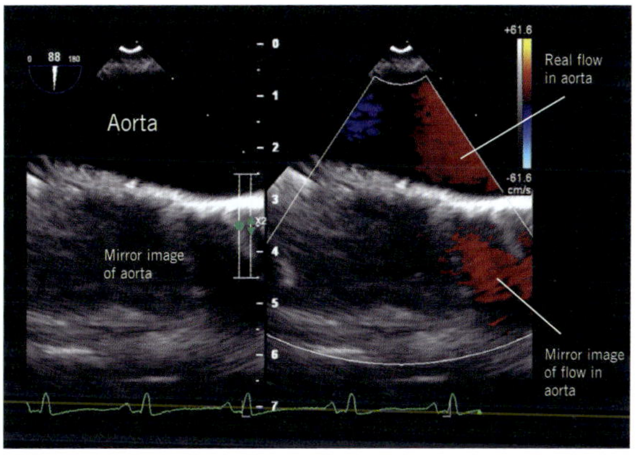

Figure 2.14 Double-barrelled aorta. The image is a descending aorta long-axis view. A mirror image artefact of the aorta can be seen at *twice* the distance from the transducer of the true aorta. This is because the bright aortic walls caused reverberation, and the returning signal made a second trip and took *twice* as long to return to the transducer. Note that the phenomenon also affects Doppler signals, and the 'false' aorta also appears to contain colour flow signals, which are also artefactual.

source, creating a series of parallel linear echoes (Figure 2.8). The distance between the successive echoes is equal, but their intensity decreases with increasing distance from the transducer. The classic example of a **stepladder reverberation** artefact can be seen from tracheal rings (Figure 2.9) during insertion or removal of the TOE probe. **Comet tails** are a specific example of a reverberation artefact that result from very closely spaced strong reflectors. Prosthetic valves (Figure 2.10), thickening of the aortic wall (Figure 2.11), aortic atheroma, and lung pleura are common causes of comet tail artefacts. The artefact from prosthetic valves can also resemble a stepladder (Figure 2.12), indicating that stepladder and comet tail artefacts are both variations of the same phenomenon. Reverberation artefacts can also occur with colour Doppler imaging, resulting in colour appearing in regions of the image where there is no flow (Figure 2.13). Reverberations can also create **mirror image** artefacts when the ultrasound beam bounces between two parallel strong reflectors. The bright walls of the thoracic aorta are particularly prone to mirror image artefacts; examples can include the false impression of a dissection flap created by linear artefacts within the

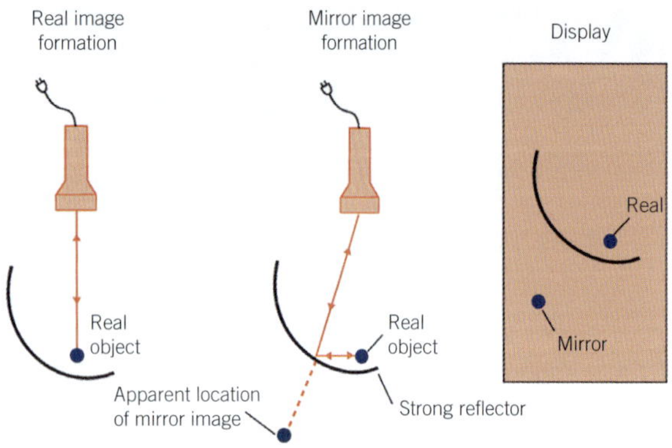

Figure 2.15 Mechanism of mirror image artefact due to deflection of the ultrasound beam from a curved strong reflector. A laterally positioned beam from a phased-array transducer encounters a curved strong reflector and deflects onto the structure of interest. The ultrasound beam is then reflected back to the transducer via the strong reflector. Because the time taken for the deflected beam to return to the transducer is prolonged (compared to the reflected beam from the true image), the ultrasound system interprets the returned signals as a second structure lying further than the true structure.

aorta and the double-barrelled aorta (Figure 2.14). Mirror image artefacts can also arise when an ultrasound beam is deflected from its original path by an adjacent curved reflector (e.g. the diaphragm or aortic wall), resulting in a circuitous journey between the transducer and the structure of interest (Figure 2.15).

Artefacts from misplaced reflections

An ultrasound beam consists of a strong primary beam and a series of weaker secondary beams, extending off to the sides, away from the primary beam. The reason is that longitudinal vibrations of the piezoelectric crystals within the transducer create the primary ultrasound beam, but piezoelectric crystals also vibrate from side to side, which generates side beams, lateral to the primary beam.

As stated before, reflections are assumed by the transducer to arise from the *primary* ultrasound beam. Strong reflectors located outside of the primary beam may reflect a secondary beam, and this reflection may erroneously be interpreted by the transducer as having arisen within the primary beam, resulting in an artefact. **Beam width artefacts** and **secondary lobe artefacts** (Figure 2.16) are examples of this phenomenon. There are two types of secondary lobe: **side lobes** and **grating lobes**.

With phased array transducers, where the beam is constantly moving from side to side, beam width and

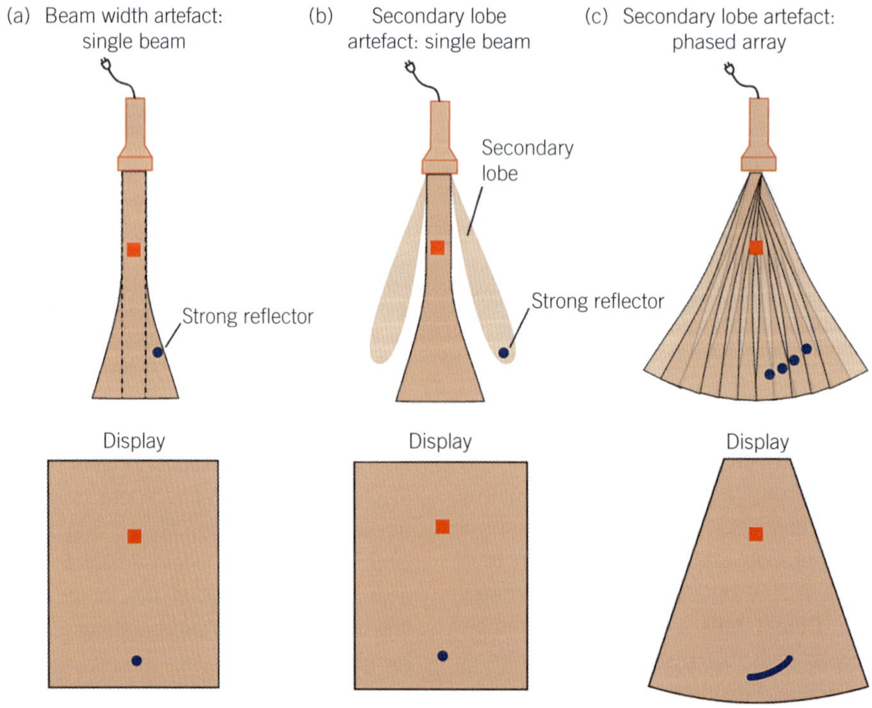

Figure 2.16 Mechanism of beam width and secondary lobe artefacts. (a) and (b) show the appearance of beam width and secondary lobe artefacts for single-beam transducers. (c) shows how overlapping secondary lobe artefacts in a phased-array transducer lead to the appearance of an arc-shaped, or 'smeared-out', structure. The squares represent the structure of interest.

secondary lobe artefacts result in strong reflectors being *smeared out* to form a line or an arc (Figure 2.16). Beam width and secondary lobe artefacts only occur with strong reflectors (dense fibrosis, calcium, metal), and they are common in the aortic arch (Figures 2.11 and 2.14) and around intravascular wires, catheters, and other artificial devices (see Chapter 20).

A similar principle to beam width artefacts explains **beam thickness artefacts**. As explained previously, 2D ultrasound beams have a certain thickness, or elevational width (Figure 2.1), which increases beyond the elevational focal zone. Strong reflectors above or below the scan plane can cause reflections that are interpreted by the transducer as coming from within the primary beam and displayed on the screen, even though the source itself is outside the plane of view.

Missing reflections

As an ultrasound signal passes through tissue, its strength is reduced by reflection or attenuation. Strong reflectors (e.g. prosthetic heart valve) or attenuators (e.g. calcium on a valve or a pulmonary artery catheter) may leave little or no energy to penetrate deeper structures, and thus create an **acoustic shadow** (Figures 2.10 and 2.12) distal to the structure. Severe shadowing is usually obvious, but more modest reductions in the energy of the signal may obscure important diagnostic features without creating a particularly noticeable shadow.

Enhancement is the opposite of acoustic shadowing. Enhancement occurs when there are only weak reflectors or weak attenuators in the signal path. As a result, returning echoes reflected from structures distal to the weak reflector/attenuator may have a higher amplitude than returning echoes from structures surrounding it. Such regions are incorrectly displayed as having increased echogenicity. The LV apex, at the boundary between the epicardium and the pericardium, is particularly prone to enhancement artefacts (Figure 2.17).

3D artefacts

The laws of physics apply equally to 2D and 3D echocardiography, and all artefacts discussed in this chapter affect both 2D and 3D imaging. As discussed, the amount of processing required to generate a 3D image is much

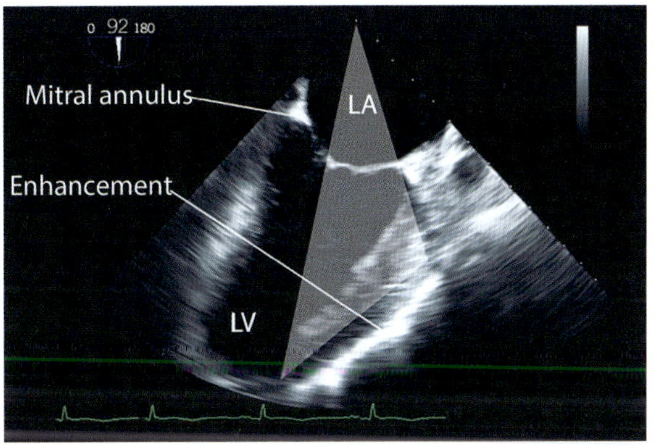

Figure 2.17 Enhancement artefact. The image is a mid-oesophageal two-chamber view. There is minimal reflection and attenuation of the ultrasound sector (shaded area) between the transducer and the region of enhancement. By contrast, reflection and attenuation of the signal from the mitral annulus weaken returning echoes from regions distal to the annulus. The ultrasound machine interprets the increased amplitude of reflections distal to the shaded region as the presence of strong reflectors, resulting in an enhancement artefact.

greater than that required for a 2D image and temporal resolution is always a challenge. Despite improvements in computer technology, the operator must always be cognizant of this fact, and limiting the size of the sample volume to the structure of interest remains important in 3D imaging. Also, as illustrated in Figure 1.8, the ECG-gated acquisition of multiple 'slices' to form a larger 3D image greatly improves 3D temporal resolution. This technique requires a regular heart rate and the absence of any external movement or electrical interference during the acquisition of multiple images. An irregular ECG signal (from atrial fibrillation or premature ventricular beats), electrocautery, and respiratory or physical movement of the patient during acquisition will result in imperfect 'stitching' and the junction between the various slices of the image will become visible. This is referred to as stitching artefact and it makes images difficult to interpret (Figure 2.18).

Expert tip: 3D echocardiography adds many diagnostic possibilities, but it uses the same ultrasounds as 2D echocardiography. One cannot change the laws of physics! Good-quality 2D images usually lead to good-quality 3D images, whereas poor 2D images usually result in poor 3D images (Figure 2.19)***.***

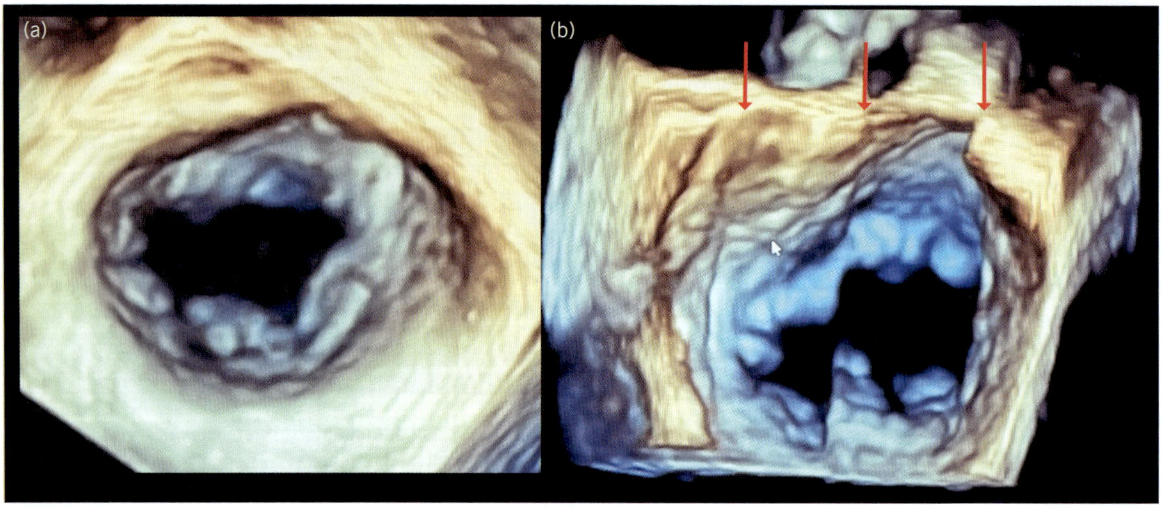

Figure 2.18 Stitch artefact. The images are 3D wide-sector *en face* views of the MV. (a) shows a normal view. In (b), a 4-beat ECG-gated acquisition demonstrates stitch artefacts. Note how the four slices of the image are not precisely joined (arrows), leading to a distorted image of the MV.

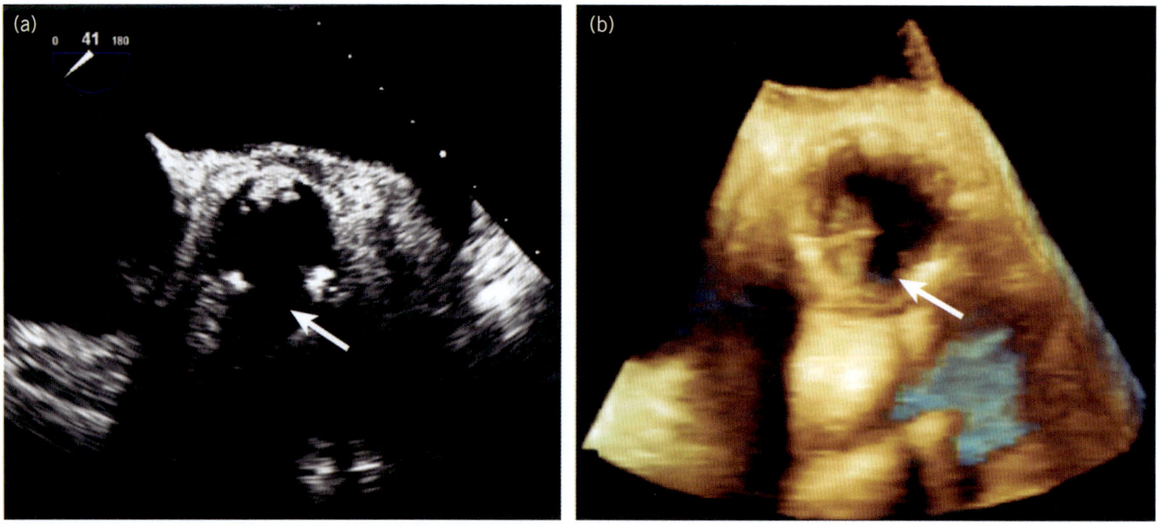

Figure 2.19 Acoustic shadow in 2D and 3D. (a) shows a 2D mid-oesophageal short-axis view of a bioprosthetic AV. Note the strong acoustic shadow produced by the posterior stent post (arrow). (b) shows a 3D *en face* view of the same valve. Note the same acoustic shadow (arrow) as the 2D image. Because the probe location is the same in the oesophagus (i.e. the same vantage point), 3D ultrasound is subjected to the same limitations as 2D ultrasound.

Multiple choice questions

Discover interactive multiple choice questions to test your knowledge on this chapter by searching for this book's title or ISBN (9780198873686) at **https://academic.oup.com/** and going to the online appendix at the end of the book. Use your scratch-off code on the inside cover to access the material.

3 Quantitative Doppler echocardiography

The aim in this chapter is to explain the theory underlying the quantitative methods used in perioperative TOE for calculating stroke volume, transvalvular pressure gradients, and valve areas, based on the measurement of blood velocity with Doppler imaging. The emphasis here is on the basic principles underlying each method. The practical application of these techniques is outlined in the appropriate chapters throughout the book.

Principles of quantitative Doppler echocardiography

Blood is a fluid. Fluids are capable of flowing from one place to another under the influence of a force. Force per unit area is pressure. Pressure and flow are integrally related, because fluids flow down pressure gradients.

Neither flow nor pressure can be measured directly with echocardiography, but the dimensions of a structure can be measured with 2D or 3D imaging and the velocity of blood flowing through it can be determined by using the Doppler effect (see Chapter 2), allowing flow to be calculated (described later).

The amount of blood that goes forward through a heart valve during one cardiac cycle is the stroke volume. The continuity principle states that, in the absence of an intracardiac shunt, net forward flow in different parts of the heart is equal over time. This principle allows the area of stenotic or regurgitant valves to be calculated from velocity data. The rate of change of velocity (i.e. deceleration) across a stenotic or regurgitant valve provides an alternative method of calculating the valve area. The Bernoulli equation allows the pressure gradient across a restrictive orifice to be estimated from the blood velocity. In this way, blood velocity data obtained with spectral Doppler imaging, in combination with simple 2D or 3D measurements, allow stroke volume, transvalvular pressure gradients, and valve areas to be calculated.

Jets

As blood flowing down a pressure gradient approaches a narrow orifice, it speeds up. When seen with colour Doppler imaging, the changes in blood velocity and flow characteristics (laminar vs turbulent) result in characteristic appearances proximal to, at, and distal to the orifice (Figure 3.1).

Proximal to the orifice, a zone of flow convergence may be seen, depending on the size of the orifice, the pressure gradient, and settings of the machine. As blood cells are forced into the orifice, they accelerate along a continuum of concentric hemispheric isovelocity 'shells', some of which are visible with colour Doppler. Specifically, when the

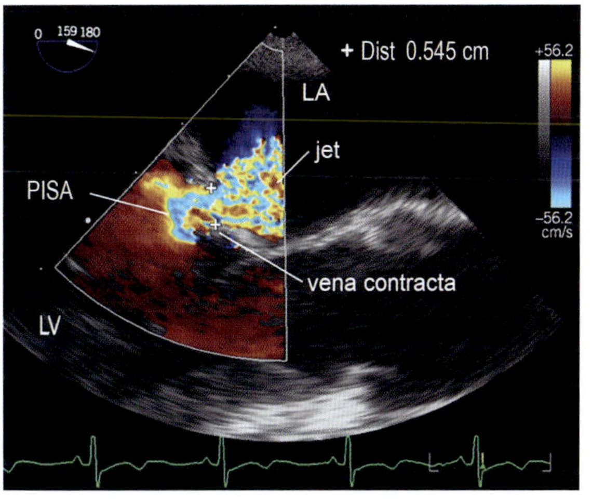

Figure 3.1 Appearances with colour Doppler imaging as blood flows towards and through a regurgitant mitral valve. Mid-oesophageal AV long-axis view in mid systole. A flow convergence zone can be seen on the LV side of the valve, and a regurgitant jet can be seen on the LA side of the valve. The narrowest part of the jet as it passes through the valve is termed the vena contracta, identified by the calliper marks (it measures 0.545 cm in this example). The first proximal isovelocity surface area (PISA) within the flow convergence zone is identified. The velocity at the first PISA is the Nyquist limit, which, in this example, is 56.2 cm/s.

velocity reaches the Nyquist limit, aliasing will occur (see Chapter 1) and the colour will abruptly change from a shade of red to a shade of blue, or vice versa, depending on the direction of flow. Visually, this creates layers within the flow convergence zone. Each layer represents a zone of equal velocity for all blood cells at the surface of that layer, called the **proximal isovelocity surface area (PISA)**. The dimensions of the PISA hemishells can be used to determine the size of the valvular orifice (discussed later). The narrowest point of flow occurs just distal to the orifice and is called the **vena contracta**. The width and area of the vena contracta are used to grade the severity of valvular regurgitation.

Distal to the vena contracta, a turbulent jet is formed. Blood velocity decreases, but in accordance with the principle of conservation of momentum, the jet entrains mass and its volume increases. The volume of the fully developed jet is a function of its kinetic energy. The area of a jet is often assumed to be proportional to its volume; however, in practice, a jet is three-dimensional and its cross-sectional area varies according to the 2D imaging plane in which it is visualized. Furthermore, the dimensions of a jet may be affected by the geometry of the orifice, and by other physiological, physical, and machine-related factors.

Jets may be free or confined. A free jet flows into the centre of a relatively stagnant chamber whose cross-sectional area is large in comparison with that of the jet. The geometry of a free jet is unaffected by the chamber boundaries, so jet size may be a relatively reliable indicator of a lesion's severity. Central MR into an enlarged LA is an example of a free jet (e.g. see Online appendix 6.3.4.3). By contrast, the presence of solid boundaries close to a jet modifies its geometry and confines its volume (e.g. see Online appendix 6.2.1.2). The **Coanda effect** is the tendency of a jet to follow and stay close to a surface, especially a convex surface. Jet size underestimates the lesion severity for confined jets. Aortic stenosis (AS) and eccentric mitral regurgitation are examples of confined jets. Jets may also be affected by interaction with other jets. Interaction will attenuate the size of the jet of interest if the second jet is in the opposite direction, and accentuate it if the second jet is in the same direction.

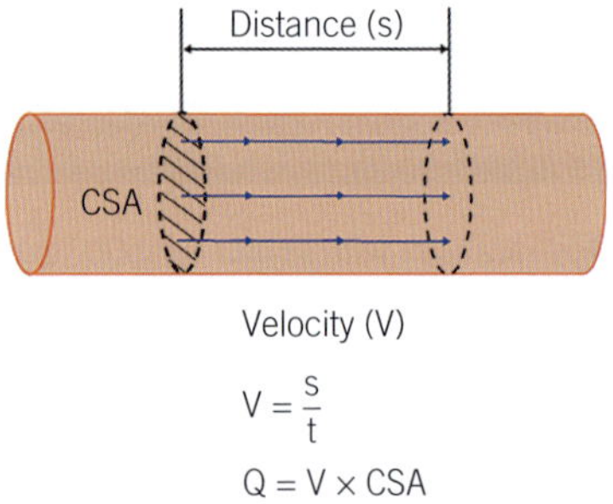

Figure 3.2 Schematic demonstration of liquid flowing through a rigid conduit at constant flow (Q). Over time (t), the liquid moves a distance (s). Flow is the product of velocity and the cross-sectional area (CSA) of the cylinder. If flow and CSA are constant, velocity is constant.

Using velocity to estimate flow and volume

Consider a rigid uniform cylinder, through which a liquid flows (Figure 3.2). Assume flow is constant. If the fluid moves a distance *s* over time *t*, then the velocity (*V*) is (Equation 3.1):

$$V = \frac{s}{t} \qquad \text{Equation 3.1}$$

Flow (*Q*) is the product of velocity (*V*) and the cross-sectional area (CSA) of the cylinder (Equation 3.2):

$$Q = V \times CSA \qquad \text{Equation 3.2}$$

If the cylinder is rigid and flow is constant, velocity is also constant. However, if the diameter of the cylinder changes, the *velocity* of the fluid changes to maintain constant *flow*, increasing as the CSA decreases, and vice versa (Figure 3.3). Alternatively, if flow changes, but the cylinder diameter is constant, velocity varies.

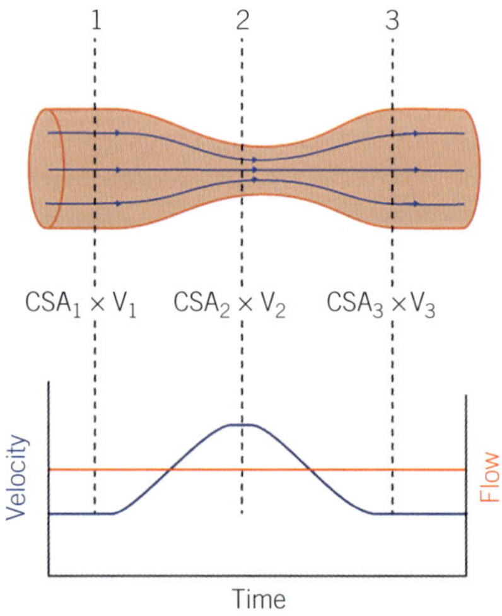

Figure 3.3 Schematic demonstration of constant flow through a rigid conduit of varying cross-sectional area (CSA). Since flow is constant, the product of CSA and velocity (V) must be the same throughout the cylinder. If CSA falls, velocity must proportionally increase, and vice versa. By contrast, in a pulsatile system, instantaneous flow (and velocity) is not constant but varies throughout the conduit. However, average flow—throughout a cardiac cycle—is constant. See text for details.

The principle outlined above can be applied to blood flow through the heart. However, unlike liquid flowing through a rigid tube, blood flow through the heart is pulsatile. Flow across normal valves is limited to systole or diastole, and does not remain constant but varies throughout the time the valve is open. Consequently, blood velocity also changes throughout the time the valve is open, varying from zero to a maximal value. Thus, *mean* values for velocity and flow must be used when applying Equations 3.1 and 3.2 to pulsatile flow through the heart. The time over which the mean velocity is calculated is one cardiac cycle.

Rearranging Equation 3.1 yields the distance travelled by blood over one pulse period (Equation 3.3):

$$s = V_{mean} \times t \qquad \text{Equation 3.3}$$

which can be expressed as the integral of instantaneous velocity with respect to time (Equation 3.4):

$$s = \int V.dt \qquad \text{Equation 3.4}$$

This distance (s) is the area under the spectral Doppler velocity–time curve and is known as the **velocity–time integral (VTI)**. Ultrasound machines automatically calculate the VTI once the outline of a spectral Doppler velocity–time curve is traced.

In the absence of regurgitation, the volume passing through a cardiac valve during one cardiac cycle represents the stroke volume (SV), and is represented by Equation 3.5:

$$SV = CSA \times VTI \qquad \text{Equation 3.5}$$

Because there are often difficulties in obtaining the CSA of a cardiac structure by planimetry, certain shapes are attributed to particular structures for the (approximate) calculation of their CSA by standard formulae using dimensions obtained with 2D imaging (Table 3.1). Note that the SV can be indexed by dividing it by the patient's body surface area (BSA) (**stroke volume index (SVI)**).

***Expert tip: Equation 3.5 can be used to calculate the SV at several intracardiac sites. The left ventricular outflow tract (LVOT) is the most widely used and reliable site (see Online appendix 1.6.12). The technique is described in* Chapter 21.**

Cardiac output (CO) is calculated from the SV and heart rate (HR), and cardiac index (CI) is obtained by dividing CO by BSA (Equations 3.6 and 3.7):

$$CO = SV \times HR \qquad \text{Equation 3.6}$$

$$CI = \frac{CO}{BSA} \qquad \text{Equation 3.7}$$

Note that in the presence of significant valve regurgitation, net forward SV must be used to calculate CO. Net forward SV is the difference between total SV and regurgitant volume (RV) (Equation 3.8):

$$SV_{net} = SV_{total} - RV \qquad \text{Equation 3.8}$$

Units of measurement are critically important and should be included in each step of any haemodynamic calculation. Distance is measured in metres (m) or centimetres (cm), velocity in centimetres per second (cm/s)

Table 3.1 Approximate cross-sectional shapes attributed to various cardiac structures, and the formula for calculating the area in each case

Structure	Assumed cross-sectional shape	Formula
LVOT (or RVOT)	Circle	πr^2
Aortic valve (or PV)	Equilateral triangle	$\frac{\sqrt{3}}{4}s^2$ (or $0.433s^2$)
Mitral valve	Ellipse	$\pi r_1 r_2$
PISA	Hemisphere	$2\pi r^2$

Where r is the radius of a circle or hemisphere, or the major (r_1) and minor (r_2) axes of an ellipse, and s is the side of an equilateral triangle.

or metres per second (m/s), CSA in square centimetres (cm^2), and flow in millilitres per second (mL/s) or litres per minute (L/min). Note that VTI is a *distance* (the distance '*s*' travelled by an average blood cell in that column of blood during a given time, shown in Figure 3.2) and is therefore measured in metres or centimetres.

The continuity principle

By the principle of continuity of flow, on average, in the absence of intracardiac shunts and under conditions of cardiovascular stability, net forward SV through any one part of the heart must equal net forward SV at any other part. The continuity principle can be used clinically to measure the areas of stenotic or regurgitant valves. Thus, for two sites within the heart (Equation 3.9):

$$CSA_1 \times VTI_1 = CSA_2 \times VTI_2 \qquad \text{Equation 3.9}$$

Equation 3.9 is commonly termed the **continuity equation**. If all but one of the variables can be measured, the remaining unknown variable (typically a stenotic or regurgitant orifice area) can be calculated. Different forms of the continuity equation can be written containing more than four variables, but the same principle applies: measurement of all but one variable is performed to obtain an unknown valve area.

Quantification of valvular stenosis

Clinically, the most widely used application of the continuity equation is to measure the valve area in patients with AS. During systole, forward flow (i.e. SV) through the LVOT is the same as forward flow across the stenotic aortic valve (AV). Thus (Equation 3.10):

$$CSA_{LVOT} \times VTI_{LVOT} = CSA_{AV} \times VTI_{AV} \qquad \text{Equation 3.10}$$

where CSA_{AV} is AV area, the unknown quantity (Equation 3.11):

$$CSA_{AV} = \frac{CSA_{LVOT} \times VTI_{LVOT}}{VTI_{AV}} \qquad \text{Equation 3.11}$$

The VTIs across the LVOT and AV can be measured with PW and CW Doppler, respectively, and the CSA of the LVOT can be calculated by measuring its diameter (e.g. see Online appendices 7.2.7 and 7.3.13). Because the LVOT and AV are adjacent structures, total forward flow is the same across both structures, even in the presence of aortic regurgitation (AR). Thus, in this application of the continuity equation, regurgitant flow can be ignored. Details of the practical application and limitations of using the continuity equation for measuring the AV area in AS are outlined in Chapter 10.

In a steady state, the flow into and out of a cardiac chamber, or the heart as a whole, must be the same. Therefore, the continuity equation can be applied to non-adjacent structures on the same side of the heart (e.g. the mitral valve (MV) and the LVOT) and even structures on the opposite side of the heart (e.g. the AV and the pulmonary valve (PV)). However, for non-adjacent structures, the presence of valvular regurgitation must be considered, and for structures on opposite sides of the heart, the presence of intracardiac shunting must be considered.

Thus, the continuity equation can be used to work out valve areas in patients with mitral stenosis (MS) by comparing the SV across the MV in diastole and across the LVOT in systole, in which case Equation 3.9 becomes Equation 3.12:

$$\begin{aligned} &CSA_{LVOT\,(systole)} \times VTI_{LVOT\,(systole)} \\ &= CSA_{MV\,(diastole)} \times VTI_{MV\,(diastole)} \end{aligned} \qquad \text{Equation 3.12}$$

Note that Equation 3.12 is not valid in the presence of MR or AR. In practice, the continuity equation is rarely used to measure the valve area for MS, as the pressure half-time (PHT) method (described later) is simpler.

Quantification of valvular regurgitation

The continuity equation can be modified to determine the severity of valvular regurgitation. Three indices of severity may be calculated: regurgitant volume, regurgitant orifice area (ROA), and regurgitant fraction (RF). From Equation 3.8, it can be seen that regurgitant volume is the difference between total SV and net forward SV, and from Equation 3.5, it follows that regurgitant volume is the product of ROA and the VTI of the regurgitant jet ($VTI_{regurgitation}$). Thus (Equations 3.13 and 3.14):

$$RV = SV_{total} - SV_{net} \qquad \text{Equation 3.13}$$

$$RV = ROA \times VTI_{regurgitation} \qquad \text{Equation 3.14}$$

RF is the regurgitant volume divided by the total forward SV (Equation 3.15):

$$\mathrm{RF} = \frac{\mathrm{RV}}{\mathrm{SV_{total}}} \qquad \text{Equation 3.15}$$

Taking the example of a regurgitant MV and a competent AV, net forward SV in systole across the LVOT is equal to net forward SV in diastole across the MV. Thus (Equation 3.16):

$$SV_{LVOT} = SV_{MV\,(total)} - RV_{MV} \qquad \text{Equation 3.16}$$

Expanding and rearranging Equation 3.16 yields Equation 3.17:

$$RV_{MV} = CSA_{MV\,(diastole)} VTI_{MV\,(diastole)} - CSA_{LVOT\,(systole)} VTI_{LVOT\,(systole)} \qquad \text{Equation 3.17}$$

which can be further expanded and solved for the mitral ROA (Equation 3.18):

$$ROA_{MV\,(systole)} = \frac{CSA_{MV\,(diastole)} \times VTI_{MV\,(diastole)} - CSA_{LVOT\,(systole)} \times VTI_{LVOT\,(systole)}}{VTI_{MR\,jet\,(systole)}} \qquad \text{Equation 3.18}$$

where VTI_{MRjet} is the VTI of the mitral regurgitant jet.

Theoretically, all of the variables on the right of the equals sign in Equation 3.18 can be measured with echocardiography: the cross-sectional areas of the MV and LVOT can be measured with 2D or 3D imaging; the VTIs of the MV in diastole and of the LVOT in systole can be measured with PW Doppler; and the VTI of the mitral regurgitant jet can be measured with CW Doppler. However, in practice, this calculation is unwieldy and prone to error. Also, measurement of the diastolic mitral annular area is problematic; measuring the major and minor axes of the annulus assumes the MV is a planar ellipse, which is not accurate (see Chapter 8). For these reasons, quantitative measurement of MR severity is usually performed by the flow convergence (PISA) method (described later).

Shunt fraction

In the presence of a left-to-right intracardiac shunt, the pulmonary-to-systemic flow ratio (Q_p/Q_s) can be quantified by measuring SV separately for the right heart and for the left heart (Equation 3.19):

$$\frac{Q_p}{Q_s} = \frac{SV_{right\ heart}}{SV_{left\ heart}} \qquad \text{Equation 3.19}$$

Right heart SV can be measured from the right ventricular outflow tract (RVOT) or PV, and left heart SV can be measured from the LVOT or AV. CSA is calculated by measuring the diameters of the outflow tracts (LVOT, RVOT) or the sides of the equilateral triangle of the open valves (AV, PV) (Table 3.1). The tricuspid valve (TV) and MV are generally considered unsuitable sites of measurement due to the high incidence of physiological regurgitation and difficulties in measuring the valve dimensions. In practice, shunt fraction is difficult to quantify accurately with TOE because of problems with obtaining accurate measurements of CSA and VTI across the RVOT and TV. It is necessary to take an average of 5–10 measurements of flow to allow for left-to-right respiratory variation in SV.

The flow convergence (PISA) method

As explained earlier, when blood flow converges towards a narrow orifice, it accelerates along a continuum of concentric isovelocity hemispheres. At any distance (*r*) from the centre of the orifice, the velocity (*V*) will be constant. For an infinite series of hemispheres centred on the orifice, the velocity at all points on the surface of any given hemisphere is constant. Each of these surfaces is called a proximal isovelocity surface area (PISA). A PISA becomes visible with colour Doppler imaging at every point where the velocity reaches the Nyquist limit (or a multiple thereof) and aliasing occurs, which is represented by an abrupt colour change (from red to blue or blue to red—see Chapter 1).

Using the continuity principle, (instantaneous) flow at any PISA hemisphere (Q_{PISA}) is the same as (instantaneous) flow (Q_{valve}) at the valve orifice (Equation 3.20):

$$Q_{PISA} = Q_{valve} \qquad \text{Equation 3.20}$$

This application of the continuity principle, termed the flow convergence method, can be used to calculate the valve area of stenotic and regurgitant valves.

It is usually possible to adjust the Nyquist limit, so that a particular PISA assumes the contour of a hemisphere (Figure 3.1). In this circumstance, and assuming the base of the hemisphere is flat, the surface area of the PISA is given by Equation 3.21:

$$Area_{PISA} = 2\pi r^2 \qquad \text{Equation 3.21}$$

(Note that the surface area of a complete sphere is $4\pi r^2$).

The flow convergence method has many limitations: any situation where a PISA hemishell is not a *true hemisphere* will lead to inaccurate measurements. For example, if adjustment of the Nyquist limit produces a PISA whose shape is too flat, Equation 3.21 overestimates the surface area; if its shape is too tall, the surface area is underestimated. The shape of the regurgitant orifice itself and the morphology of the valve on which the PISA is formed can also alter the shape of the PISA. For example, a regurgitant MV will be closed in systole at the time of PISA formation, so the base of the PISA will (theoretically)

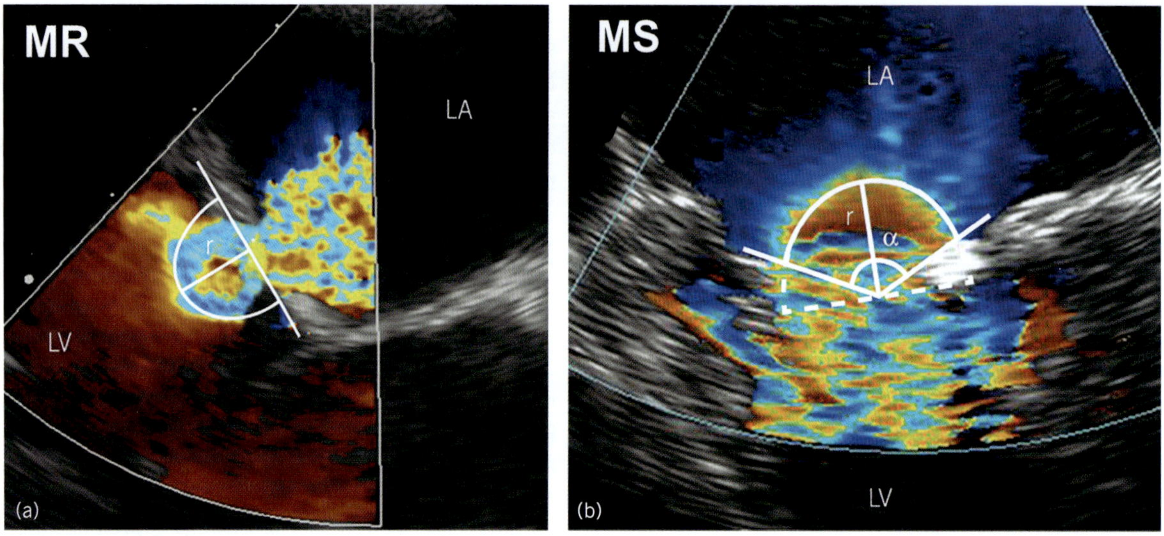

Figure 3.4 Proximal isovelocity surface area (PISA) in MR and MS. (a) shows a PISA hemisphere of radius r in MR. (b) shows the same in MS. Note how with MR, the closed MV leaflets form a flat base to the hemisphere. Here, the surface area of the PISA is $2\pi r^2$. With MS, however, the open mitral leaflets form a funnel. In this case, the surface area of the PISA is $2\pi r^2 \times \alpha/180$, where α is the angle between the two cusps.

be flat, whereas a stenotic MV will be partially open in diastole and the base of the PISA will be cone-shaped (Figure 3.4). Hence, with MS, one must correct Equation 3.21 to account for this fact (Equation 3.22; see discussion in Chapter 8):

$$\text{Surface Area}_{\text{PISA}} = 2\pi r^2 \times \frac{\alpha}{180} \qquad \text{Equation 3.22}$$

where α is the angle (in degrees) between the two cusps (Figure 3.4).

The velocity at the PISA hemisphere is the Nyquist limit (NL), which is under the control of the operator, and therefore known. Flow across this PISA is the product of velocity and surface area (Equation 3.23):

$$Q_{PISA} = 2\pi r^2 \times \frac{\alpha}{180} \times \text{NL} \qquad \text{Equation 3.23}$$

This is equal to the flow through the stenotic or regurgitant valve, which is the product of velocity and valve area, the unknown quantity (Equation 3.24):

$$Q_{valve} = \text{CSA}_{\text{valve}} \times V_{\max(valve)} \qquad \text{Equation 3.24}$$

Peak instantaneous velocity through the valve can be measured with CW Doppler imaging. Combining Equations 3.23 and 3.24 and rearranging yields Equation 3.25:

$$\text{CSA}_{\text{valve}} = \frac{2\pi r^2 \dfrac{\alpha}{180} \times \text{NL}}{V_{\max(valve)}} \qquad \text{Equation 3.25}$$

Theoretically, the flow convergence method can be used for measuring the orifice area for any regurgitant or stenotic valve. In practice, the technique is most commonly used for assessing the severity of MR (see Chapter 8), in which case the $\alpha/180$ correction can usually be ignored (see Online appendices 6.2.2.2 and 6.5.1.3).

Because the flow convergence method is essentially an application of the continuity principle for adjacent structures, it applies equally well for mixed (regurgitant and stenotic) lesions. As the PISA radius is squared in the calculation, any errors in measurement are magnified.

Expert tip: Because the flow convergence method is based on instantaneous flow (rather than on averaged flow throughout the pulse period), it is important that the PISA radius (colour Doppler) and maximal regurgitant velocity (CW Doppler) be measured at the same time in the cardiac cycle. Using the frame in which the PISA radius is maximal and recording the maximal regurgitant velocity satisfy this criterion.

Using velocity to estimate pressure

The pressure gradient across a stenotic valve is commonly used to quantify severity. Pressure is force per unit area. Pressure cannot be measured directly with echocardiography, but the Bernoulli equation allows the transvalvular pressure gradient to be estimated from the spectral Doppler velocity waveform.

The pressure gradient across a valve ($\Delta P = P_1 - P_2$) is proportional to the flow (Q) through the valve and the resistance (R) across the valve (Equation 3.26):

$$P_1 - P_2 = QR \qquad \text{Equation 3.26}$$

At any point in time, resistance is constant (it will increase gradually if stenosis progresses). Across an open normal valve, resistance is effectively zero, so $P_1 = P_2$. Thus, in the absence of stenosis, pressures in the LV and aorta are equal during systole, and pressures in the LA and LV are equal during diastole. The resistance across a stenotic valve is greater than zero, so the pressure gradient varies with CO.

The Bernoulli equation

The Bernoulli equation is based on the principle of conservation of energy, during movement of a given volume of a non-compressible fluid down a pressure gradient from one point to another along a rigid pipe. Relevant factors include: (1) the work done in overcoming viscous resistance; (2) the change in potential energy and in kinetic energy (which is proportional to the mass and the square of the velocity of the fluid at each point); and (3) acceleration.

For short orifices, viscous resistance and the change in potential energy are negligible. Also, at the point of maximum velocity in systole or diastole, acceleration becomes zero as it changes from positive to negative, and thus can be ignored. A shortened form of the Bernoulli equation therefore applies (Equation 3.27):

$$P_1 - P_2 \cong \frac{1}{2}\rho\left(V_2^2 - V_1^2\right) \qquad \text{Equation 3.27}$$

where P_1 and P_2 are the proximal and distal pressures, respectively; V_1 and V_2 are the proximal and distal velocities, respectively; and ρ is the density (mass per unit volume) of the fluid. The density of blood can be taken as 1 mg/mL, and ignored.

For maximum velocities, with a conversion factor for measuring velocity in m/s and pressure in mmHg, the equation can be approximated to (Equation 3.28):

$$\Delta P \cong 4(V_2^2 - V_1^2) \qquad \text{Equation 3.28}$$

If the proximal velocity is much smaller than the distal velocity, it too can be ignored. Thus, a (highly) simplified form of the Bernoulli equation, suitable for most clinical purposes is (Equation 3.29):

$$\Delta P \cong 4V^2 \qquad \text{Equation 3.29}$$

The constant is related to the units used in the simplified Bernoulli equation. Therefore, velocity must be in m/s and pressure must be in mmHg. It is safe to use the simplified form of the Bernoulli equation (Equation 3.29) when the proximal velocity is <1 m/s (because squaring a number less than 1 reduces it), and reasonable accuracy can be expected provided V_1 <1.5 m/s. However, *when V1 >1.5 m/s Equation 3.28 should be used.*

The simplified Bernoulli equation applies to mean velocities as well as to maximum velocities. Mean pressure is obtained from the mean of the squared velocities, not the square of the mean velocity (Equation 3.30):

$$\Delta P_{mean} = \frac{\left(4V_1^2 + 4V_2^2 + \ldots + 4V_n^2\right)}{n} \qquad \text{Equation 3.30}$$

In practice, machine software automatically calculates the maximum and mean pressure gradients when the transvalvular VTI is traced (see Figure 10.11f and Online appendices 6.3.1.4 and 7.2.8 for examples). Box 3.1 presents some clinical applications of the simplified Bernouilli equation.

Considerations when using the simplified Bernoulli equation

Strictly speaking, the Bernoulli equation is not applicable to pulsatile blood flow through compliant vessels and chambers, but in practice, it has been found to give accurate estimations of pressure gradients in various clinical situations. However, the Bernoulli equation is not well suited to normal valves (where resistance is effectively zero) or to long tubular stenoses and extreme pinpoint stenoses (because viscous friction then becomes significant). In severe anaemia, reduced blood viscosity

Box 3.1 Practical applications of the simplified Bernouilli equation

Whenever there is flow between two cardiac chambers, the gradient driving that flow can be calculated by using Doppler. If the pressure in one of the two chambers is known, then one can use the gradient to calculate the pressure in the other chamber. Here are a few examples:

- Calculating the RV (and PA) systolic pressure from the TR jet and the RA pressure
- Calculating the LA pressure from the MR jet and the systolic blood pressure
- Calculating the RV (and PA) systolic pressure from a VSD jet and the systolic blood pressure

may also result in overestimation of pressure gradient. With prosthetic valves, there may be some resistance to valve opening and acceleration may be significant. With two stenoses in series (e.g. subvalvular and valvular AS) and with certain prosthetic valves, *distal pressure recovery* may occur (see Chapter 13).

Changes in CO affect the gradient across a stenotic valve. The orifice area is independent of flow and is therefore preferable to pressure gradient for evaluating the severity of a stenotic lesion. However, the continuity equation involves several measurements and is more technically demanding. If valvular regurgitation is present, total forward flow through a valve is increased, and this increases the pressure gradient for any given degree of stenosis. The continuity equation is also unreliable in this situation, except when applied to two adjacent structures (discussed earlier).

> ***Expert tip: When using Equation 3.28, care should be taken to perform the calculation correctly. It is a common error (and a common incorrect option in MCQs!) to calculate Equation 3.28 as 4(V2 – V1)2 rather than correctly as 4(V22 – V12). Thus, in a patient with valvular AS and a sub-aortic membrane, in which valvular velocity (V2) is 5 m/s and LVOT velocity (V1) is 2 m/s, the correct value for ΔP is 4(25 – 4) = 84 mmHg (rather than incorrectly as ΔP being 4(5 – 2)2 = 36 mmHg).***

It is important to remember that the peak pressure gradient calculated by echocardiography is based on the peak *instantaneous* velocity, whereas the peak pressure gradient measured by angiography is *peak-to-peak* (Figure 3.5). These two numbers can differ due to the phenomenon of pressure recovery, which is explained in more detail in Chapter 13 (see Figure 13.9). Pressure recovery explains why Doppler-derived pressure gradients tend to be higher than catheter-derived gradients.

The Venturi effect

It follows from the full Bernoulli equation that high kinetic energy is associated with low pressure. Thus, the fast-moving air over an airplane wing is associated with low pressure, which creates lift, and the passage of fluid through a Venturi (a narrowed orifice) generates suction. This is the mechanism of systolic anterior motion of the anterior mitral leaflet in hypertrophic cardiomyopathy (see Chapter 6). When blood passes through a stenotic valve, the kinetic energy is highest and the pressure is lowest at the narrowest part of the stenosis.

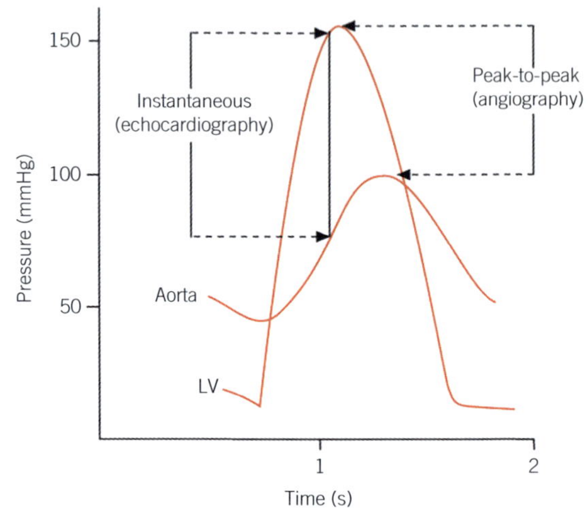

Figure 3.5 Echocardiographic versus angiographic measurements of AV gradient in AS. As blood flows through a stenotic valve, its velocity increases. Due to the principle of conservation of energy, an increase in velocity (kinetic energy) is associated with a fall in pressure (potential energy). This drop in pressure is maximal at the narrowest part of the valve (see Figure 13.11). Distal to the valve, some of the pressure recovers as kinetic energy is converted back to potential energy. However, as mechanical energy is lost (mainly due to friction and turbulent flow), pressure recovery is incomplete. With Doppler echocardiography, peak instantaneous pressure gradient across the valve is measured, before pressure recovery has occurred. By contrast, with angiography, the peak pressures proximal (in the LV) and distal (in the aorta) to the valve are measured separately. The distal pressure in the aorta is measured after pressure recovery has occurred. For this reason, peak instantaneous measurements (echocardiography) tend to be higher than peak-to-peak (angiography) measurements.

Applications of the Bernoulli equation

The two main applications of the simplified Bernoulli equation are: (1) estimating transvalvular pressure gradients in the assessment of stenotic heart valves (most commonly AS; see Chapter 10); and (2) estimating unknown pressures in cardiac chambers separated by regurgitant jets from adjacent cardiac chambers in which the pressure is known. For the second of these applications, the simplified Bernoulli equation is written as Equation 3.31:

$$P_1 - P_2 = 4V^2 \qquad \text{Equation 3.31}$$

Pulmonary artery (PA) systolic pressure can be estimated in this way. Right ventricular (RV) systolic pressure is estimated first, from right atrial (RA) pressure (measured by a central venous catheter if available, or estimated if not) and the gradient across the TV (a small degree of tricuspid regurgitation (TR) is very common in normal patients). The velocity of the TR jet (V_{TR}) is determined by the pressure difference in systole between the RV ($P_{RV(systolic)}$) and the RA (P_{RA}) (Equation 3.32):

$$P_{RV(systolic)} - P_{RA} = 4V_{TR}^2 \quad \text{Equation 3.32}$$

Or (Equation 3.33):

$$P_{RV(systolic)} = 4V_{TR}^2 + P_{RA} \quad \text{Equation 3.33}$$

Assuming the PV is not stenotic, at end-systole, when the PV is open and no flow is occurring, the PA systolic pressure $P_{PA(sys)}$ equals the RV systolic pressure, so (Equation 3.34):

$$P_{PA(systolic)} = 4V_{TR}^2 + P_{RA} \quad \text{Equation 3.34}$$

Similar reasoning can be used to estimate the LA pressure from the aortic diastolic pressure, which is assumed to equal the diastolic blood pressure ($P_{BP(diastolic)}$) and the velocity of an AR jet (V_{AR}), if present. Equation 3.31 is first used to calculate the LV diastolic pressure ($P_{LV(diastolic)}$) (Equation 3.35):

$$P_{BP(diastolic)} - P_{LV(diastolic)} = 4V_{AR}^2 \quad \text{Equation 3.35}$$

At end-diastole, when the MV is fully open and no flow occurs, LV diastolic pressure equals LA pressure (P_{LA}); thus (Equation 3.36):

$$P_{LA} = P_{BP(diastolic)} - 4V_{AR}^2 \quad \text{Equation 3.36}$$

Similarly, LA pressure (in systole) can be estimated from the velocity of an MR jet (V_{MR}) and systolic arterial pressure ($P_{BP(systolic)}$) (Equation 3.37):

$$P_{LA} = P_{BP(systolic)} - 4V_{MR}^2 \quad \text{Equation 3.37}$$

In practice, it is common and clinically useful to use the simplified Bernoulli equation to estimate the PA systolic pressure (see Chapter 21); however, the LA pressure is rarely estimated from a jet of MR or AR, particularly with TOE. Obtaining a reliable estimate of velocity for AR is difficult with TOE (see Chapter 4). Also, Equations 3.36 and 3.37 involve subtracting two large numbers from each other to obtain a small number, which is very prone to error.

Using velocity to measure pressure deceleration

The rate of fall of the pressure gradient (i.e. pressure deceleration) across a valve during diastole is the basis of the **pressure half-time** (PHT) method of estimating the valve orifice area in MS and AR.

During diastole, the rate of decrease in the pressure gradient between the LA and the LV (in MS), or between the aorta and the LV (in AR), is related to the severity of the valve lesion. This deceleration is quantified by the PHT, which is the time, in milliseconds, for the peak transvalvular pressure gradient (not the velocity!) to fall to half of its maximal value.

PHT is inversely related to the orifice size: the smaller the valve area, the longer it takes for the pressure to equalize across the valve, and therefore the longer the PHT. For MS, more severe disease (i.e. a smaller valve area) is associated with a longer PHT, whereas for AR, more severe disease (i.e. a larger ROA) is associated with a shorter PHT.

Velocity is related to pressure by the simplified Bernoulli equation (Equation 3.27). Pressure is proportional to the square of velocity, so the velocity associated with half the peak pressure is the peak velocity divided by $\sqrt{2}$ (or multiplied by 0.7, the reciprocal of $\sqrt{2}$). Thus, if the velocity associated with the maximal transvalvular pressure gradient is V_p and the velocity associated with half the maximal pressure gradient is $V_p/\sqrt{2}$ (Equation 3.38):

$$V_p/\sqrt{2} = 0.7V_P \quad \text{Equation 3.38}$$

Thus, the PHT is the time required for the transvalvular velocity to fall to 70% of its maximal value. In practice, the echocardiography machine automatically calculates the PHT when the relevant two calliper points are placed on the slope of the spectral Doppler velocity waveform (Figure 3.6).

The use of PHT in the evaluation of MS is discussed in detail in Chapter 8. PHT in the evaluation of AR is discussed in detail in Chapter 10.

Technical considerations

For all measurements, data from three to five cardiac cycles (more in the presence of atrial fibrillation) and from more than one view should be obtained. For a 2D measurement (e.g. length), the *average* should be taken. When measuring velocity with spectral Doppler, the ultrasound beam should be as close as possible to parallel with the direction of blood flow, so more than one view should be examined, and the view providing the *highest* velocity used (see cosine effect in Chapter 1). For calculations using the simplified Bernoulli equation, any errors in estimating velocity will be squared.

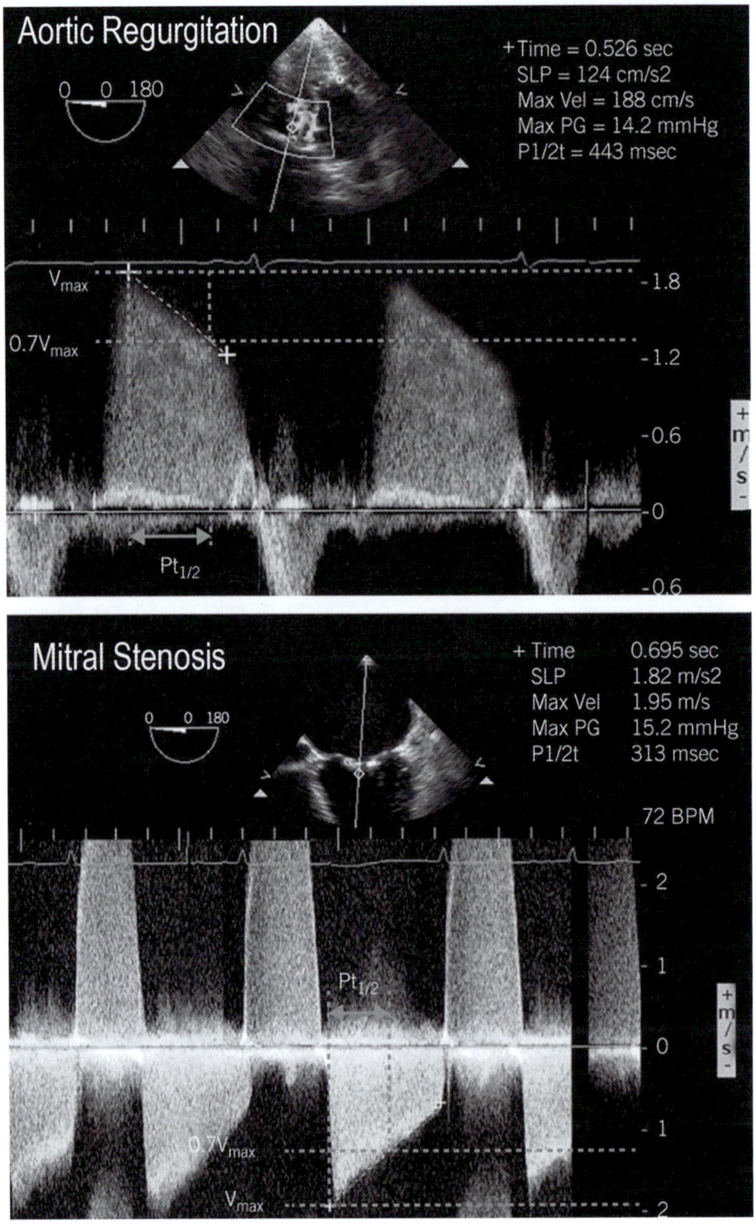

Figure 3.6 Pressure half-time measurements in AR and MS with CW Doppler imaging. The pressure half-time is the time taken for the transvalvular *pressure gradient* to fall to half of its maximal value, which corresponds to the time for the transvalvular *velocity* to fall to 70% of its maximal value (V_{max}). See text for details.

> ***Expert tip:** With PW Doppler, the outer edge of the most dense or brightest portion of the tracing (the modal velocity—the velocity of most of the red cells) should be used. With CW Doppler, the outer edge of the envelope should be used.*

With 2D imaging, it is ideal for the ultrasound plane to be orthogonal to the structure being measured, and to pass through its centre. Any error in measurement of the dimensions of a structure will be magnified when squared during calculation of an area.

The dimensions of cardiac structures vary with the cardiac cycle, so spectral Doppler and 2D measurements used in the continuity equation need to be made at the *same phase* of the cardiac cycle, as well as at the same *anatomical location*. Ideally, end-diastole is defined as the frame after MV closure, and end-systole as the frame after AV closure (see Chapter 6). If the MV is not visible, the R-wave on the electrocardiogram (ECG) can be used to define end-diastole. If the AV is not visible, the smallest visible ventricular size may be used to define end-systole. For determining SV, the LVOT should be measured in early systole just proximal to the AV, and the MV annulus in mid to late diastole.

Multiple choice questions

Discover interactive multiple choice questions to test your knowledge on this chapter by searching for this book's title or ISBN (9780198873686) at **https://academic.oup.com/** and going to the online appendix at the end of the book. Use your scratch-off code on the inside cover to access the material.

4 Standard views

To maximize the diagnostic yield from TOE, it is essential to have a detailed knowledge of the standard echocardiographic views and anatomic–echocardiographic relationships. To avoid misdiagnosis, a structured comprehensive TOE examination should be performed in all patients. In time-critical situations, it may be appropriate to initially perform an abbreviated examination, focusing on the structure(s) of interest. However, a complete examination should be completed once the clinical situation permits.

Probe insertion

Image quality with TOE is generally very good, but it is rare for every view in an individual patient to be of high quality. If image quality is poor, it may be helpful to remove the probe and suction air from the stomach with an orogastric tube before reinserting the probe. After thorough suctioning, all indwelling naso-/orogastric tubes should be removed, as they may prevent adequate contact between the transducer and the oesophageal wall. Transgastric views may be impossible to obtain in patients with a hiatal hernia. Surgical diathermy interferes with image quality, particularly for colour Doppler imaging. Therefore, it is preferable to complete the pre-cardiopulmonary bypass (CPB) study prior to surgical incision.

Anatomic considerations

Because of the relationship of the oesophagus and trachea with cardiac structures, some regions are difficult or impossible to image with TOE. The distal ascending aorta and proximal aortic arch may not be seen at all because the air-filled trachea lies between these structures and the oesophagus (remember that ultrasounds are poorly transmitted in air); also, transgastric visualization of the LV apex is often unreliable. Rarely, depending on the rotation of the heart, it may also be difficult to adequately align a CW Doppler signal across the LVOT/AV.

Indications and contraindications

Indications and contraindications for perioperative TOE examination are listed in Boxes 4.1 and 4.2, respectively.[1,2] The American Society of Echocardiography (ASE)/Society of Cardiovascular Anesthesiologists (SCA) guidelines recommend considering the use of TOE in all coronary artery bypass graft (CABG) surgeries.[3] A recent retrospective analysis of 1.3 million isolated CABG patients from the Society of Thoracic Surgeons Adult Cardiac Surgery Database demonstrated a lower risk of operative mortality for patients who received intraoperative TOE compared with those who did not (odds ratio (OR) 0.95, confidence interval (CI) 0.91–0.99—for patients with available data). After multivariable adjustment and matching, the effect

Box 4.1 Indications for perioperative TOE

- All open heart procedures (valvular, thoracic aortic procedures)
- High-risk coronary artery bypass graft surgeries (see text)
- Non-cardiac surgery when patients have known or suspected cardiovascular pathology that may impact clinical management or perioperative course
- Guidance of catheter-based intracardiac procedures
- Critically ill patients where TTE alone cannot provide diagnostic information expected to impact management

Box 4.2 Absolute and relative contraindications to TOE

Absolute

- Perforated viscus
- Oesophageal stricture
- Oesophageal tumour
- Oesophageal perforation or laceration
- Oesophageal diverticulum
- Active upper gastrointestinal bleeding

Relative

- History of radiation to neck and mediastinum
- History of upper gastrointestinal surgery
- Recent upper gastrointestinal bleeding
- Barrett's oesophagus
- Restriction of neck movement (severe cervical arthritis, atlantoaxial joint disease)
- Symptomatic hiatal hernia
- Oesophageal varices
- Coagulopathy, thrombocytopenia
- Active oesophagitis
- Active peptic ulcer disease

was most significant for intermediate-risk (OR 0.93) and high-risk (OR 0.89) patients. Of CABG patients undergoing TOE, 0.49% had an unplanned valve procedure compared with 0.09% of those not undergoing TOE. The authors concluded that their findings '*supported the use of TOE for isolated CABG to improve outcomes in the highest-risk patients and could possibly be deferred safely in patients at low risk*'.[4]

Expert tip: The rotation of the transducer can be reproduced by placing the right hand in front of you and supinating it from palm down (= 0°) to palm up (= 180°).

Movements of the probe and transducer

The probe and transducer can be manipulated in several ways (Figure 4.1). The probe may be **advanced** or

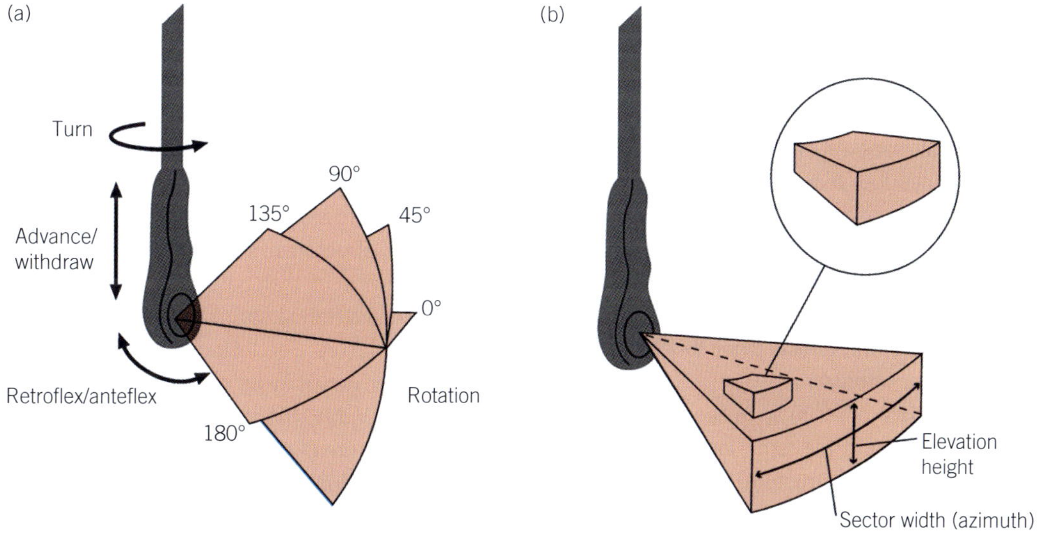

Figure 4.1 Multi-plane 2D and matrix array 3D TOE probes. (a) shows a standard multi-plane probe for 2D imaging, with movements of the probe and multi-plane sector. (b) shows a matrix array 3D probe. The size of the 2D sector is determined by the sector width and depth; the volume of the 3D sector is determined by the sector width, sector depth, and elevation height. The azimuth is the angle formed by the sector width.

withdrawn, and **turned right** (clockwise) or **turned left** (anticlockwise). Turning the large control wheel on the handle moves the tip of the probe anteriorly (**anteflexion**) or posteriorly (**retroflexion**). Turning the small control wheel moves the tip of the probe laterally (**flexion to the right**, **flexion to the left**). Finally, the small control buttons on the handle electronically rotate the transducer imaging plane between 0° and 180°. Moving the image plane towards 180° is termed **forward rotation**; moving the image plane towards 0° is termed **backwards rotation**. At 0°, the scan plane is in the horizontal (transverse) plane and lies perpendicular to the probe. At 90°, the scan plane is in the vertical (longitudinal) plane and lies parallel to the probe. The view at 180° is a mirror image of the view at 0°.

Adjustments of a matrix array sector for 3D imaging are discussed later, under '3D imaging'.

Expert tip: If TOE is deemed critical to the surgical intervention in the setting of a contraindication, consultation with gastroenterology colleagues and/or preoperative gastroscopy may be of benefit. Epicardial echocardiography can also be considered (for such cases, the reader is referred to the ASE/SCA guidelines on the use of epicardial echocardiography).5

Sector display

The apex of the sector scan is shown at the top of the screen and displays structures closest to the oesophagus. The base of the sector is at the bottom of the screen and displays anterior structures (remember the oesophagus is a posterior mediastinal structure). In the transverse plane (0°), the left of the image is towards the patient's right and the right of the image is towards the patient's left. In the vertical plane (90°), the left of the image is towards the patient's feet (caudad) and the right of the image is towards the patient's head (cephalad; Figure 4.2). **Centering on a structure** means positioning it in the middle of the display. To centre a structure in the transverse image plane (0°), the probe is turned left or right. To centre a structure in the vertical plane (90°), the transducer is advanced or withdrawn.

The term '**short axis**' refers to an image plane *perpendicular* to a structure, and the term '**long axis**' refers to an image plane *parallel* to a structure. With respect to the LV, the term 'long axis' has a specific meaning—it refers to an image plane in which both the AV and MV are seen simultaneously. Because of the orientation of the heart, many structures are seen in short axis in (or close to) the transverse (0°) plane, and in long axis in (or close to) the

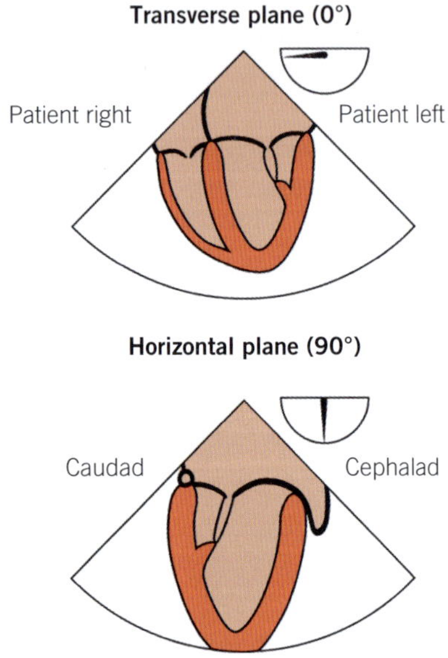

Figure 4.2 The standard sector display.

longitudinal (90°) plane. However, this is not always the case—notably for the aortic arch.

A systematic approach to imaging

Guidelines for performing a comprehensive TOE examination have been developed by the ASE and SCA. Initially published in 1999, these guidelines were updated in 2013.[1,3] The updated ASE/SCA guidelines describe 28 standard views that form the basis of a comprehensive TOE examination. The probe position and sector scan angles for obtaining the standard views should be viewed as a guide only because variability in the size, shape, and orientation of the heart (especially in pathologic conditions) can result in standard views being visible in non-standard probe positions or not at all.

While a standard view often provides information on several cardiac structures, it may be necessary to acquire several versions of that particular standard view, each focusing on a different structure, to obtain all the appropriate information. For instance, the mid-oesophageal four-chamber view may be obtained multiple times when imaging the LV, MV, RV, and TV, each time focusing on a different structure of interest (Figure 4.3). Note that there is significant redundancy in the 28 views.

The novice operator will find that following the basic 28 views helps to ensure that the TOE examination is comprehensive and covers the entire heart. With experience, it may be more clinically useful to take a 'structure-based' approach to performing a comprehensive examination, rather than a

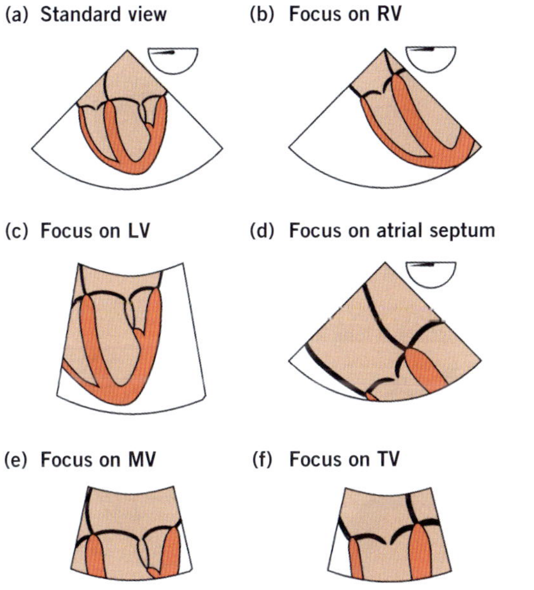

Figure 4.3 Multiple versions of a single view. From a standard mid-oesophageal four-chamber view, the probe may be turned, and the depth and zoom functions used to focus on different structures of interest. (a) Standard view; (b) Focus on RV; (c) Focus on LV; (d) Focus on atrial septum; (e) Focus on MV; (f) Focus on TV.

step-by-step progression through the standard views. This means focusing on one cardiac structure at a time (e.g. obtaining all LV views, followed by all RV views, AV views, MV views, etc.). This may result in more probe movements but may facilitate diagnosis and reporting. A structure-based approach also provides the flexibility to perform a detailed assessment of the primary structure(s) of interest first (e.g. the MV during MV repair surgery) followed by the remainder of the systematic TOE examination. Ultimately, every operator may develop their own preferred approach as long as all cardiac structures are imaged.

Before starting an examination, the patient's identifiers should be entered in the system; ECG input should be connected, and controls adjusted for image optimization (see Chapter 2). Sector depth should be initially set to 15cm and then adjusted to display the structures of interest. The focus should be initially set to the midpoint of the sector depth, and then adjusted to a depth just beyond the structure of interest.

Mid-oesophageal views

(See Figure 4.4 and Online appendix 1.1.) The mid-oesophageal five-chamber view is a useful starting point. The five-chamber view is easily recognized, typically comes into view as the probe is advanced into the oesophagus, and logically leads to the interrogation of other structures at the mid-oesophageal level.

Mid-oesophageal five-chamber view (0°)

With the sector scan at 0°, the probe is advanced into the oesophagus 35–40cm until the AV and LVOT come into view. The five 'chambers' are the RA, RV, LA, LV, and LVOT/proximal aorta. The heart is usually significantly foreshortened, and gentle retroflexion of the probe may be necessary to visualize the ventricles. Even when the probe is retroflexed, the apex of the heart is frequently not demonstrated.

Mid-oesophageal four-chamber view (0–15°)

From the five-chamber view, the probe is advanced slightly until the AV and LVOT disappear from the screen and the four-chamber view is seen. It may be necessary to forward-rotate the transducer to 10–15° to exclude the AV.

The four-chamber view is useful in assessing the LV and RV, the inter-atrial septum, and the inter-ventricular septum. When assessing the LV, the image should be centred on the left heart, and gentle retroflexion of the probe applied to visualize as much of the LV apex as possible. The inferoseptal LV wall is on the left, and the anterolateral wall on the right. The anterolateral papillary muscle is usually seen. The longer anterior mitral leaflet is on the left, and the shorter posterior mitral leaflet is on the right. To assess the RV and TV, the probe is turned to the right to centre the image on the right heart.

Advancing (or retroflexing) the probe from the standard position brings the coronary sinus (in long axis) into view, as it runs along the posterior atrioventricular groove. Visualizing the coronary sinus is important when checking the position of a retrograde cardioplegia catheter.

Mid-oesophageal mitral commissural view (50–70°)

From the four-chamber view, with the image centred on the MV, the transducer is rotated forward to 50–70° until the mitral commissural view is seen. The image plane runs along the inter-commissural line of the MV, cutting the posterior leaflet twice. A portion of the anterior mitral leaflet appears to float in the centre of the LV inflow, between two scallops of the posterior mitral leaflet. The posteromedial papillary muscle is seen on the left of the image, and the anterolateral papillary muscle on the right. The mitral commissural view is important when assessing the MV (see Chapter 8).

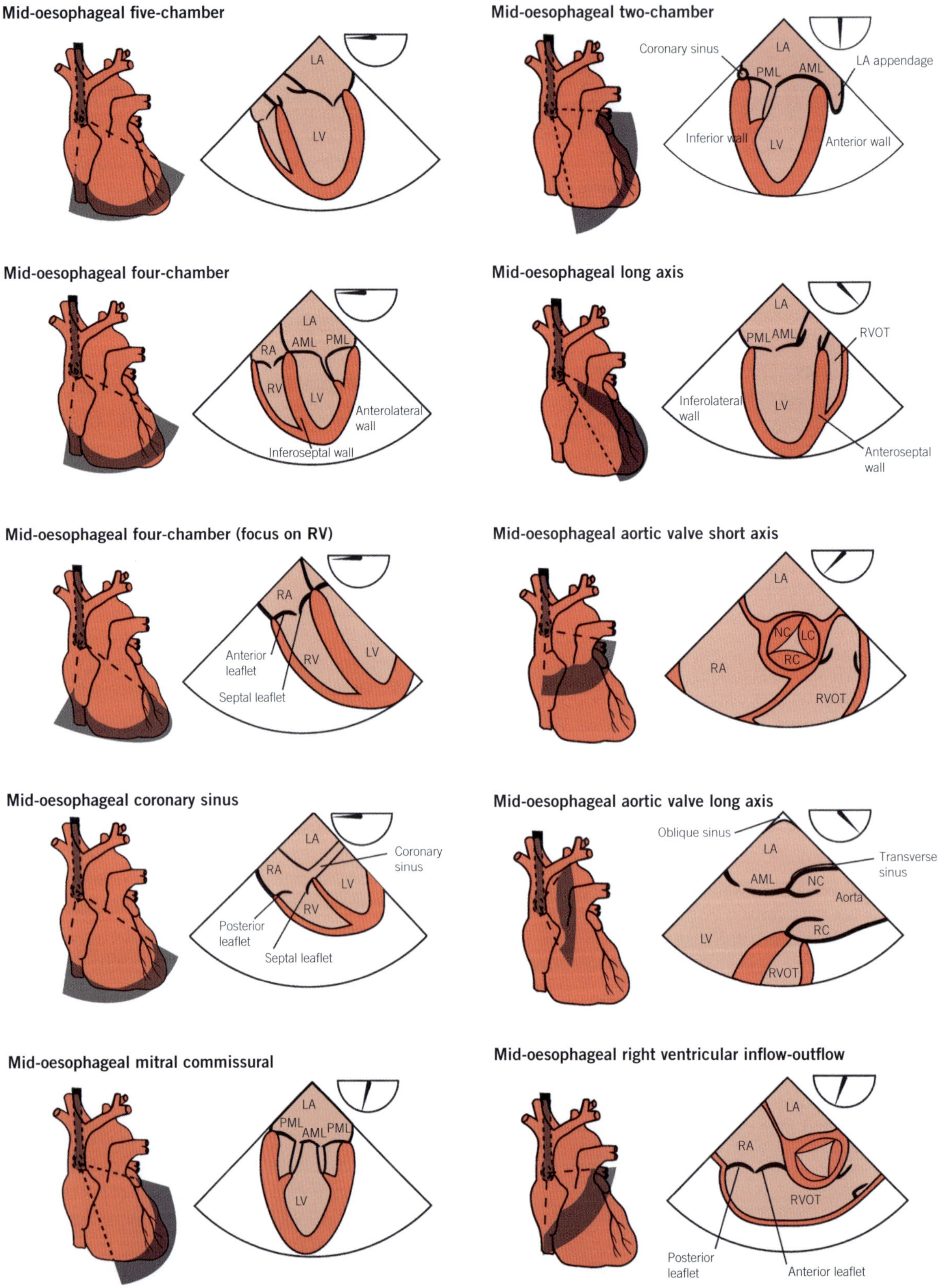

Figure 4.4 Standard mid-oesophageal views. AML, anterior mitral leaflet; PML, posterior mitral leaflet; NC, non-coronary cusp; LC, left coronary cusp; RC, right coronary cusp; MPA, main pulmonary artery; RPA, right pulmonary artery. See Online appendix 1.1.

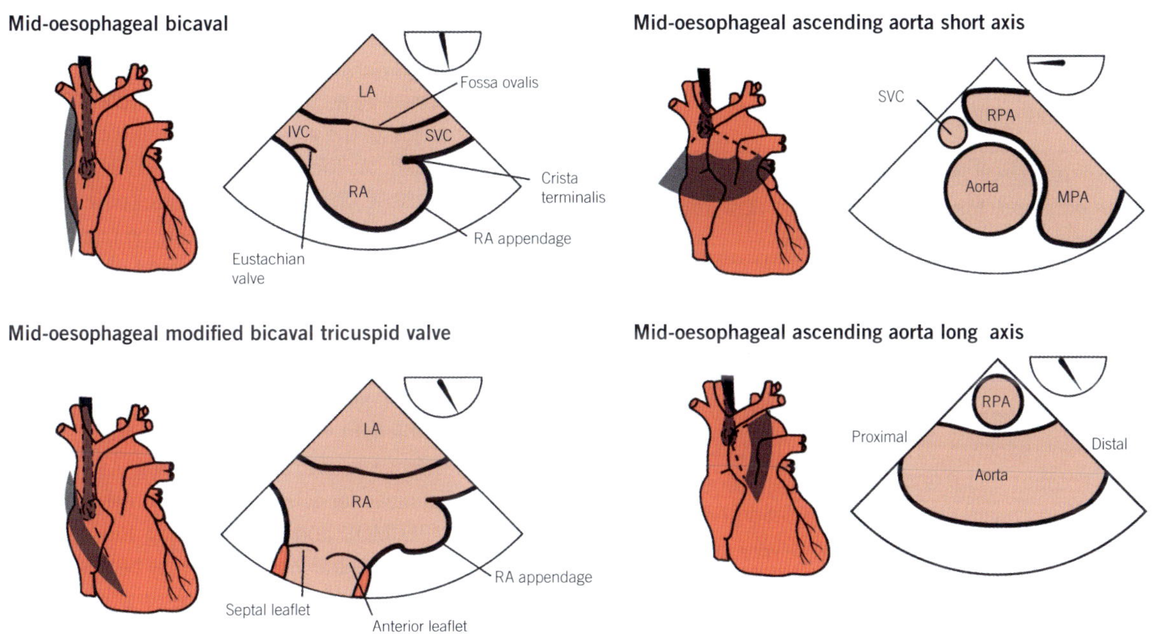

Figure 4.4 *Continued*

Mid-oesophageal two-chamber view (80–100°)

From the commissural view, the transducer is rotated forward to 80–100° until the two-chamber view is seen. The two-chamber view is identified by the appearance of the coronary sinus (in short axis) on the left of the screen and the LA appendage on the right. The appearance of the LVOT indicates the scan plane has been forward-rotated too far. The posterior mitral leaflet now appears on the left, and the longer anterior mitral leaflet on the right. The inferior LV wall is seen on the left of the image, and the anterior LV wall on the right. The posteromedial papillary muscle is typically seen arising from the inferior LV wall.

Apparent lengthening of the LV during forward rotation of the transducer indicates that the apex was not adequately visualized in the four-chamber view. A clue to the presence of LV foreshortening is excessive motion of the apparent apex (see Figure 6.1). The two-chamber view is useful for assessing LV and MV function, and it is the best view for visualizing the LV apex.

Mid-oesophageal long-axis view (120–140°)

From the two-chamber view, the transducer is rotated forward to 120–140° until the MV, AV, and LVOT are simultaneously visualized. No papillary muscles should be visible when the view is correctly obtained.

The inferolateral (posterior) LV wall is on the left, and the anteroseptal wall on the right. The posterior mitral leaflet is seen on the left, and the anterior mitral leaflet, which forms the roof of the LVOT, on the right of the image. The chamber on the lower right of the screen is the RVOT. Turning the probe to the left brings the PV into view.

The long-axis view is used when assessing LV and MV function. Because the image plane cuts the mid section of the MV, perpendicular to the valve coaptation line, this view is particularly important when assessing the MV (see Chapter 8).

Mid-oesophageal AV short-axis view (30–50°)

Starting at the mid-oesophageal five-chamber view, with the image centred on the AV, the probe is withdrawn slightly and the transducer rotated forward to 30–50° until the characteristic three leaflets of the AV are seen in short axis. The non-coronary cusp lies adjacent to the atrial septum (on the left of the display); the right coronary cusp is the most anterior, and therefore the lowermost on the display, and the left coronary cusp is seen on the right of the display. The probe may be withdrawn slightly to visualize the origins of the coronary arteries. The left main coronary artery is commonly seen arising above the left coronary cusp; the right coronary artery is less commonly seen. The probe may be advanced to visualize the LVOT in short axis, which is useful when assessing AR (see Chapter 10).

Mid-oesophageal AV long-axis view (120–140°)

From the AV short-axis view, the transducer is forward-rotated to about 120–140° to obtain a long-axis view of the LVOT and aortic root.

> ***Expert tip: Once an optimal AV short-axis view has been obtained, the best AV long-axis view should be 90° from the best AV short-axis view.***

The probe should be turned right and left until the largest aortic diameter is identified and the leaflet excursion can be clearly seen. The right coronary cusp of the AV is the most anterior and is therefore seen lowermost on the display, adjacent to the RVOT. The cusp adjacent to the anterior mitral leaflet is either the non-coronary or the left coronary cusp. The association between the anterior mitral leaflet and the AV is very useful when identifying which mitral leaflet is seen in a particular view.

Fluid in the transverse pericardial sinus is sometimes seen as an echo-free space between the posterior wall of the ascending aorta and the LA. If fluid has collected behind the heart, the oblique pericardial sinus may be also seen from any mid-oesophageal view between the posterior wall of the LA and the oesophagus.

The AV long-axis view is useful for assessing the AV and for measuring the dimensions of the aortic root and proximal ascending aorta (see Chapter 10).

Mid-oesophageal RV inflow–outflow view (50–70°)

From the mid-oesophageal five-chamber view, the probe is turned slightly to the left and the transducer forward-rotated to 50–70° until the TV and PV can be seen wrapping around the AV. The probe position is similar to that used to obtain the AV short-axis view, but with further forward rotation of the transducer.

The RV inferior free wall is seen on the left, and the RVOT on the right of the display. If a PA catheter is *in situ*, it can be seen passing through the RA, TV, and RVOT. The posterior leaflet of the TV appears on the left, and the anterior leaflet on the right, adjacent to the AV.

The RV inflow–outflow view is used for assessing TV and PV function, and usually provides reasonable alignment between a CW Doppler signal and a jet of TR for measuring jet velocity (see Chapters 14 and 15).

Mid-oesophageal bicaval view (90–120°)

From the mid-oesophageal five-chamber view, the probe is advanced slightly—until the AV disappears– and turned to the right (clockwise) to centre on the inter-atrial septum. The transducer is then forward-rotated to 90–110° until the vena cavae come into view.

In the bicaval view, the superior vena cava (SVC) is seen on the right of the image, and the inferior vena cava (IVC) on the left. At the junction of the IVC and RA, a small flap of tissue (the Eustachian valve) or a long filamentous structure (Chiari network) may be present. The RA appendage may be seen on the right of the image. The thickening at the origin of the SVC is known as the crista terminalis and is the line of union between the RA and the RA appendage. Forward-rotating the transducer to about 120° or turning the probe further to the right often reveals the right-sided pulmonary veins.

The bicaval view is used when assessing the position of wires and cannulae for CPB or extracorporeal membrane oxygenation (ECMO), and for evaluating the inter-atrial septum. The thin central fossa ovalis may be interrogated with colour Doppler for the presence of a patent foramen ovale.

Mid-oesophageal modified bicaval tricuspid valve view (110–130°)

From the standard bicaval view, the probe is turned to the left and the transducer is forward-rotated to about 120° until the TV comes into view. The septal leaflet of the TV is seen on the left of the image, and the anterior leaflet on the right. As the name suggests, the modified bicaval TV view is used for assessing the TV and often provides excellent alignment of a Doppler beam with a jet of TR when measuring jet velocity. The RA appendage is usually seen on the right of the image.

Mid-oesophageal ascending aorta short-axis or 'great vessel' view (10–30°)

From the mid-oesophageal five-chamber view, the probe is withdrawn and the sector scan forward-rotated to 10–30° until a short-axis view of the ascending aorta is seen. This view shows the proximal ascending aorta, main PA, right PA, and SVC. As the probe is progressively withdrawn from the five-chamber view, the main PA, which initially appears circular, becomes oval-shaped as it passes posteriorly (i.e. towards the transducer) before branching into the left and right PAs. Turning the probe to the right displays more of the right PA; turning the probe to the left images displays more of the PA bifurcation. The ascending aorta short-axis view may be difficult to visualize due to interposition of the airways between the oesophagus and the vascular structures. In particular, the left PA is rarely seen due to interposition of the left main bronchus.

The ascending aorta short-axis view is useful for assessing aortic atheroma or calcification, aortic dissections, and/or the presence of thrombus in the PA.

Mid-oesophageal ascending aorta long-axis view (110–140°)

From the ascending aorta short-axis view, the transducer is forward-rotated to about 130° to show the ascending aorta in long axis. The right PA is now seen in short axis. As with the ascending aorta short-axis view, interposition of the airways frequently obscures this view.

Mid-oesophageal views of the pulmonary veins and LA appendage

(See Figure 4.5 and Online appendix 1.5.)[6] The LA appendage and each of the four pulmonary veins are imaged at the mid-oesophageal level. There is significant individual variability in the best image plane to visualize the pulmonary veins. Colour Doppler often helps to identify them.

Starting from the five-chamber view, turning the probe to the left typically brings the left upper pulmonary vein (LUPV) and the LA appendage into view (Figure 4.5a). Slow forward rotation of the sector scan towards 90° may improve visualization of the LUPV. Blood flow in the LUPV is typically well aligned with the ultrasound beam and is therefore suitable for interrogation with spectral Doppler. Advancing the probe may bring the left lower pulmonary vein (LLPV) into view (Figure 4.5b), which typically lies perpendicular to the ultrasound beam and is therefore poorly suited to Doppler interrogation. Forward rotation of the sector scan to about 100–120° typically improves visualization of the LA appendage (Figure 4.5c).

Returning to the five-chamber view, and with the sector scan at 0°, turning the probe to the right typically demonstrates the right upper (RUPV) and lower (RLPV) pulmonary veins (Figures 4.5d and 4.5e). Advancing and withdrawing the probe may be necessary to distinguish the upper and lower veins. Blood flow in the RUPV is typically well aligned with the ultrasound beam, and therefore suitable for spectral Doppler interrogation. The RUPV may also be imaged from a modified mid-oesophageal bicaval view. From a standard bicaval view, slight forward rotation of the sector scan or rightward turn of the probe brings the RUPV (and less frequently the RLPV) into view (Figure 4.5f).

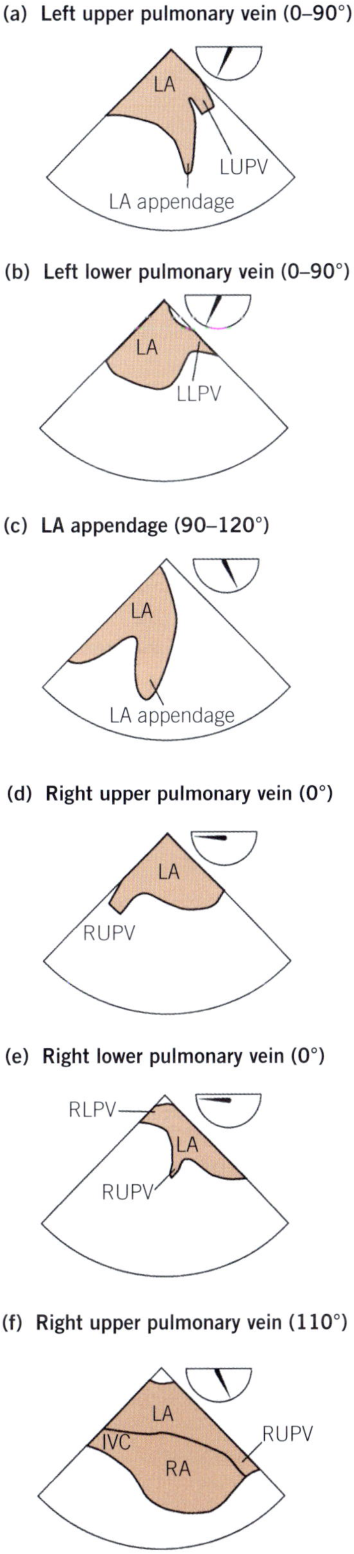

Figure 4.5 Mid-oesophageal views of the pulmonary veins and LA appendage. (a) LUPV, left upper pulmonary vein; (b) LLPV, left lower pulmonary vein; (c) LA appendage; (d) RUPV, right upper pulmonary vein; (e) RLPV, right lower pulmonary vein; (f) RUPV, Right upper pulmonary vein (1100). See Online appendix 1.5.

Transgastric views

(See Figure 4.6 and Online appendix 1.2.)

Transgastric basal short-axis view (0–15°)

From the mid-oesophageal five-chamber view, the probe is advanced into the stomach and anteflexed until the characteristic 'fish-mouth' view of the MV is seen. Care must be taken in interpreting motion of the ventricular septum at this level. If the cut is oblique or too high, the septum will seem thinned and appear to move abnormally as a result of scanning across the LVOT. The basal short-axis view is useful for assessing LV function and the MV.

Transgastric mid-papillary and apical short-axis views (0–15°)

From the basal short-axis view, the probe is advanced slightly and then anteflexed (to maintain apposition to the diaphragmatic surface of the stomach) to obtain the transgastric mid-papillary short-axis view. Gentle flexion and forward rotation of up to 10–15° may be helpful to avoid oblique imaging (indicated by an oval LV shape). The posteromedial papillary muscle is seen at 1 o'clock, and the anterolateral papillary muscle at 5 o'clock. The mid-papillary short-axis view is useful for monitoring preload and global and regional LV function.

From the mid-papillary short-axis view, the probe is further advanced and anteflexed to image the LV apex. The apical view may not be obtainable in all patients.

Transgastric two-chamber view (80–100°)

From the mid-papillary short-axis view, the sector scan is forward-rotated to 80–100° to obtain the transgastric two-chamber view. The inferior wall of the LV is seen at the top of the screen and the anterior wall at the bottom. This view is useful for assessing LV function and the mitral subvalvular apparatus.

Transgastric long-axis view (120–140°)

From the two-chamber view, the sector scan is forward-rotated to 120–140° until the AV is visualized. Turning the probe clockwise to the right or decreasing the scanning angle to between 100° and 110° may improve visualization of the LVOT and AV. This view cannot be obtained in all

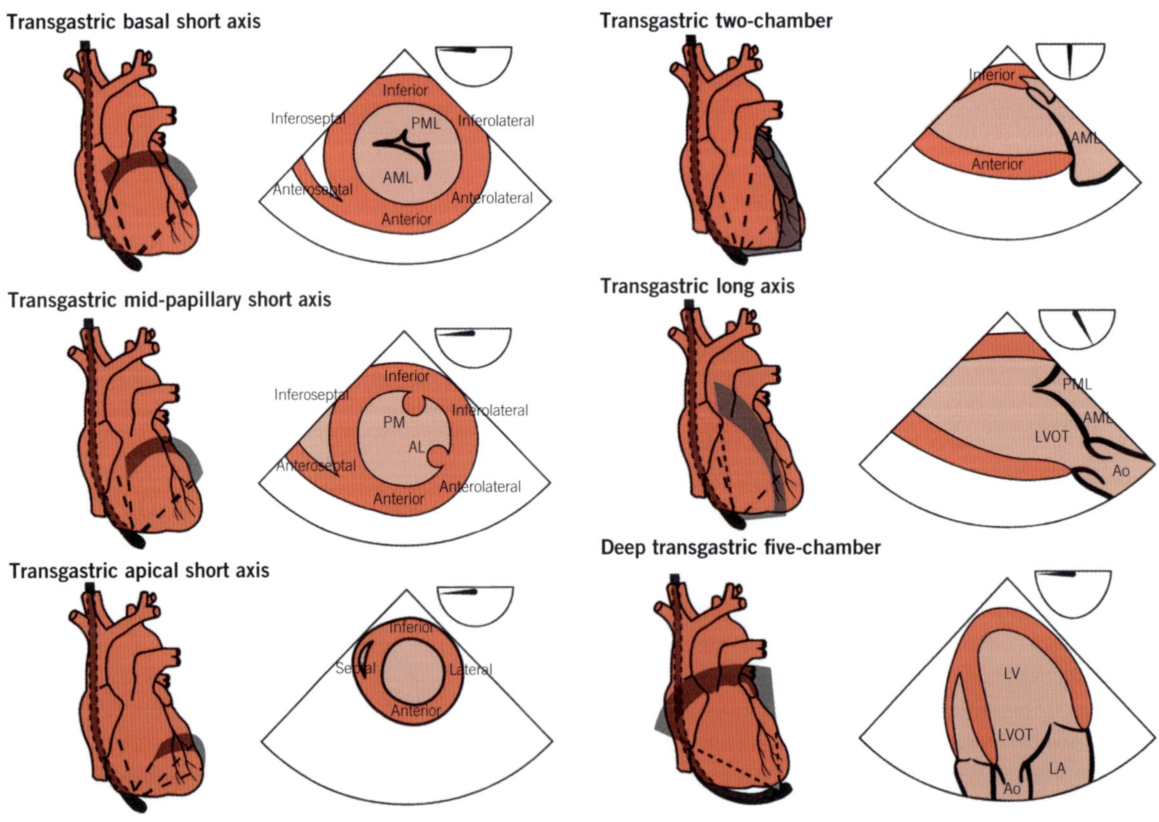

Figure 4.6 **Transgastric views of left heart structures.**

patients. However, if visualized, blood flow in the LVOT and AV is typically well aligned with the ultrasound beam, and therefore suitable for interrogation with spectral Doppler.

Deep transgastric five-chamber view

From the transgastric mid-papillary short-axis view, the probe is advanced further into the stomach and then slowly withdrawn, while maintaining sharp anteflexion until the deep transgastric five-chamber view is seen. In this view, the tip of the probe is positioned towards the apex of the heart, producing a view similar to an upside-down mid-oesophageal five-chamber view. The deep transgastric five-chamber view is an alternative to the transgastric long-axis view for Doppler interrogation of blood flow through the LVOT. This view was previously called the **deep transgastric long-axis view**.

Transgastric views of right heart structures

(See Figure 4.7.)[7] From the transgastric basal short-axis view, turning the probe to the right and slightly forward-rotating the sector scan display the **transgastric RV basal short-axis view**, in which an *en face* view of the TV is seen. From the transgastric RV basal short-axis view, sharp right flexion of the tip of the probe reveals the **transgastric RV inflow–outflow view**, in which the TV and PV can be seen simultaneously.

From the transgastric mid-papillary short-axis view of the LV, turning the probe to the right reveals the **transgastric RV mid-short-axis view**. In a true short-axis view, the RV is crescent-shaped. It is often necessary to advance the probe beyond the depth at which the mid-papillary short-axis view of the LV is obtained. RV papillary muscles cannot be reliably identified.

From the transgastric two-chamber view, turning the probe to the right demonstrates the **transgastric RV inflow view**. Alternatively, this view can be obtained by starting from the transgastric mid-papillary short-axis view, centering the image on the RV, and forward-rotating the sector scan to about 90°. Forward-rotating the sector scan further to about 130° and turning the probe slightly leftwards may bring the PV into view. The view at 130°

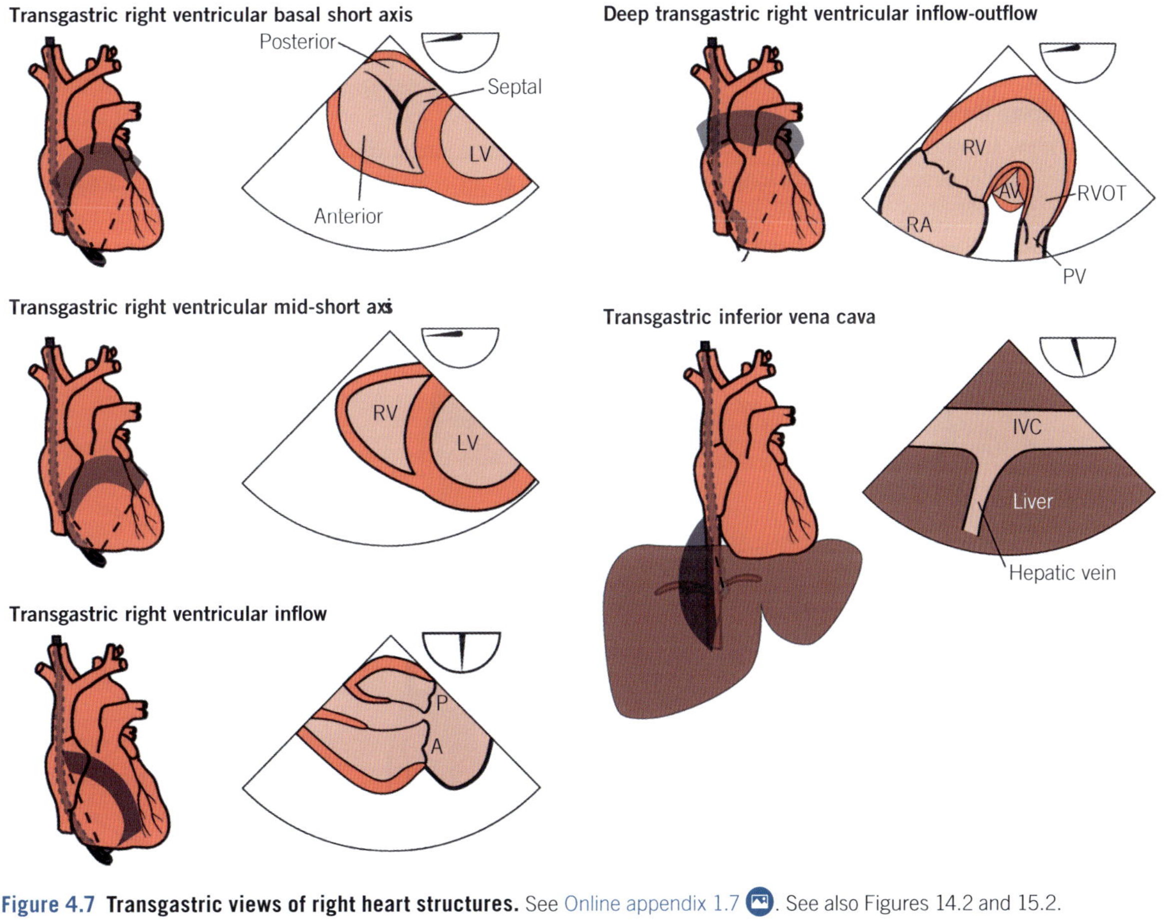

Figure 4.7 Transgastric views of right heart structures. See Online appendix 1.7. See also Figures 14.2 and 15.2.

provides an alternative to the transgastric RV inflow–outflow view described previously.

From a transgastric RV basal short-axis view, the probe is advanced and turned clockwise to the right until the liver comes into view. The sector scan is forward-rotated to 90–110° until the IVC and one of the hepatic veins are seen, developing the **transgastric inferior vena cava view**. Three hepatic (right, middle, and left) veins arise at approximately the same level, 5–10 cm below the IVC–RA junction. The most anterior is the middle hepatic vein, and this is the most frequently imaged hepatic vein. This view is useful for determining the position of cannulae in the IVC and for assessing hepatic venous flow.

Additional views of the RV and TV are provided in Chapters 14 and 15, respectively.

Thoracic aorta and pleural views

(See Figures 4.8 and 4.9 and Online appendices 1.3 and 4.2.)

From the mid-oesophageal five-chamber view, the probe is turned to the left, beyond the heart, to display the **descending aorta short-axis view**. The sector depth should be reduced to about 6 cm. With the aorta centred on the screen, the probe is withdrawn and advanced to image the entire descending thoracic aorta. From the short-axis view, forward rotation of the sector scan to 80–100° reveals the **descending aorta long-axis view**.

From the descending aorta short-axis view, withdrawing the probe to the upper oesophagus and turning clockwise bring the curved walls of the distal aortic arch into view—the **upper oesophageal aortic arch long-axis view**. Forward-rotating the sector scan to about 90° demonstrates the distal arch in short axis—the **upper oesophageal aortic arch short-axis view**. The origin of the left subclavian artery may be seen in the short-axis view, but other arch vessels cannot typically be visualized. The RVOT and main PA may also be seen in this view. Note that because of the orientation of the aortic arch, the usual arrangement of seeing a structure in short axis in the transverse plane (0°) and in long axis in the longitudinal plane (90°) is reversed. In addition, the distal ascending aorta, proximal aortic arch, and—in some patients—distal aortic arch cannot be visualized with TOE.

Normal lung tissue is poorly visualized because well-aerated alveoli do not conduct ultrasounds. However, atelectatic lung and pleural fluid collections are readily identified—liquid effusions appear black; atelectatic lung and clotted blood appear white, and pleural exudates light grey. The left pleural space is seen deep to the aorta in the descending aorta short-axis view. A left pleural effusion is seen as an echo-free space shaped like a tiger claw, pointing to the left of the screen. The probe should be advanced and withdrawn to visualize the entire thoracic space. To search for a right pleural fluid collection, the probe should be turned to the right from the mid-oesophageal five-chamber view to the point where the heart is no longer visible. A right pleural effusion is identified as an echo-free space in the shape of a tiger claw pointing to the right of the screen. Advancing the probe eventually brings the diaphragm and liver into view.

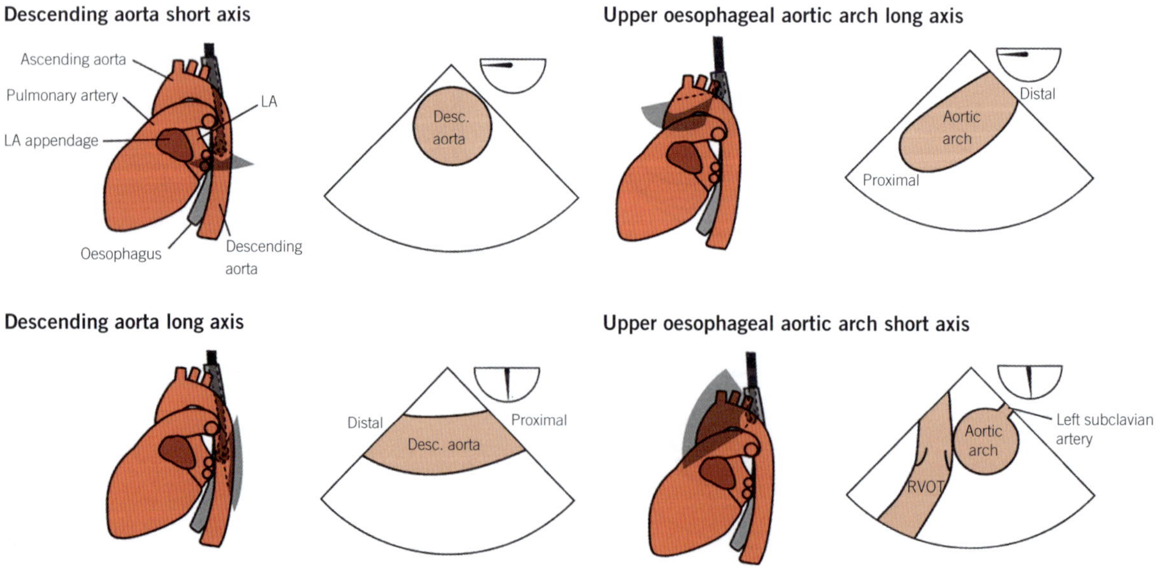

Figure 4.8 Views of the aortic arch and descending thoracic aorta. See Online appendix 1.3.

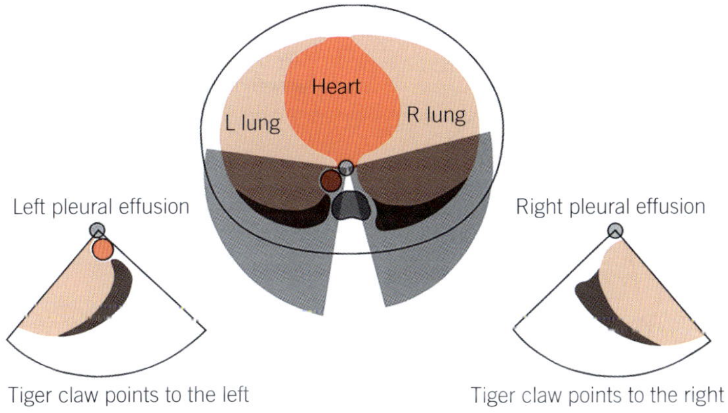

Figure 4.9 Views of the pleura. See Online appendix 4.2.

> ***Expert tip: The volume of a pleural effusion can be estimated using the Balik formula by measuring the distance between the chest wall and the lung at the midpoint of the effusion in centimetres and multiplying by 200 mL. For example, an effusion measuring 5 cm at its midpoint would give an estimated volume of approximately 1000 mL of pleural fluid.8 This formula was developed for surface pleural ultrasound, but it can be applied to TOE.***

Doppler imaging

A comprehensive TOE examination includes colour and spectral Doppler analysis of blood flow through the heart valves, LVOT, pulmonary and hepatic veins, and descending aorta, along with TDI assessment of mitral and tricuspid annular motion.

Colour Doppler

When colour Doppler mode is activated, an adjustable colour box is superimposed on the 2D (or 3D) sector display, and a colour scale is displayed on the side of the image. The operator can adjust the size and position (and the volume in 3D mode) of the colour box. Care should be taken to use the smallest colour box necessary to evaluate the structure of interest, in order to maximize the pulse repetition frequency (PRF) and frame rate (see Chapters 1 and 2).

The colour scale shows the colour baseline, aliasing velocity, and directional colour codes. Flow towards the transducer is coded red, and flow away is coded blue. Turbulent flow is displayed as a speckled pattern or coded with green for 'variance'. By default, the colour baseline is set to zero, meaning the aliasing velocity is the same for blood moving towards and away from the transducer. The baseline may be adjusted up or down to increase the aliasing velocity in one particular direction. The colour scale can be increased up to a maximum determined by the Nyquist limit. Colour gain should be adjusted to a level where spontaneous colour speckling is barely visible in the background, then turned down *just below* that level.

Blood velocity through normal valves is about the same as, or slightly higher than, the maximal aliasing velocity that can be achieved by adjusting the colour settings (approximately 50–100 cm/s). Thus, when imaging normal heart valves with colour Doppler, there is typically little or no aliasing. The exception is the AV, in which maximal normal blood velocity may be up to 1.5 m/s. Thus, colour imaging through a normal AV, particularly if displayed in the far field of a transgastric view, may show some aliasing. Much higher velocities (up to 7 m/s) occur through stenotic or regurgitant valves, resulting in intense aliasing or speckling due to turbulent flow.

Spectral Doppler imaging

(See Figure 4.10.) Spectral Doppler imaging includes PW, CW, and TDI. Prior to activating a spectral Doppler mode, the Doppler cursor should be positioned through the structure of interest, with the sample volume set to the appropriate depth for PW and TDI. It is helpful to use colour Doppler imaging to help position the spectral Doppler beam and sample volume.

When a spectral Doppler mode is activated, a small 2D sector is displayed at the top of the screen to indicate the position of the Doppler beam and sample volume. The lower part of the display shows a velocity–time plot. By convention, flow away from the transducer is displayed below the baseline, and flow towards the transducer above the baseline. Adjustments to the velocity

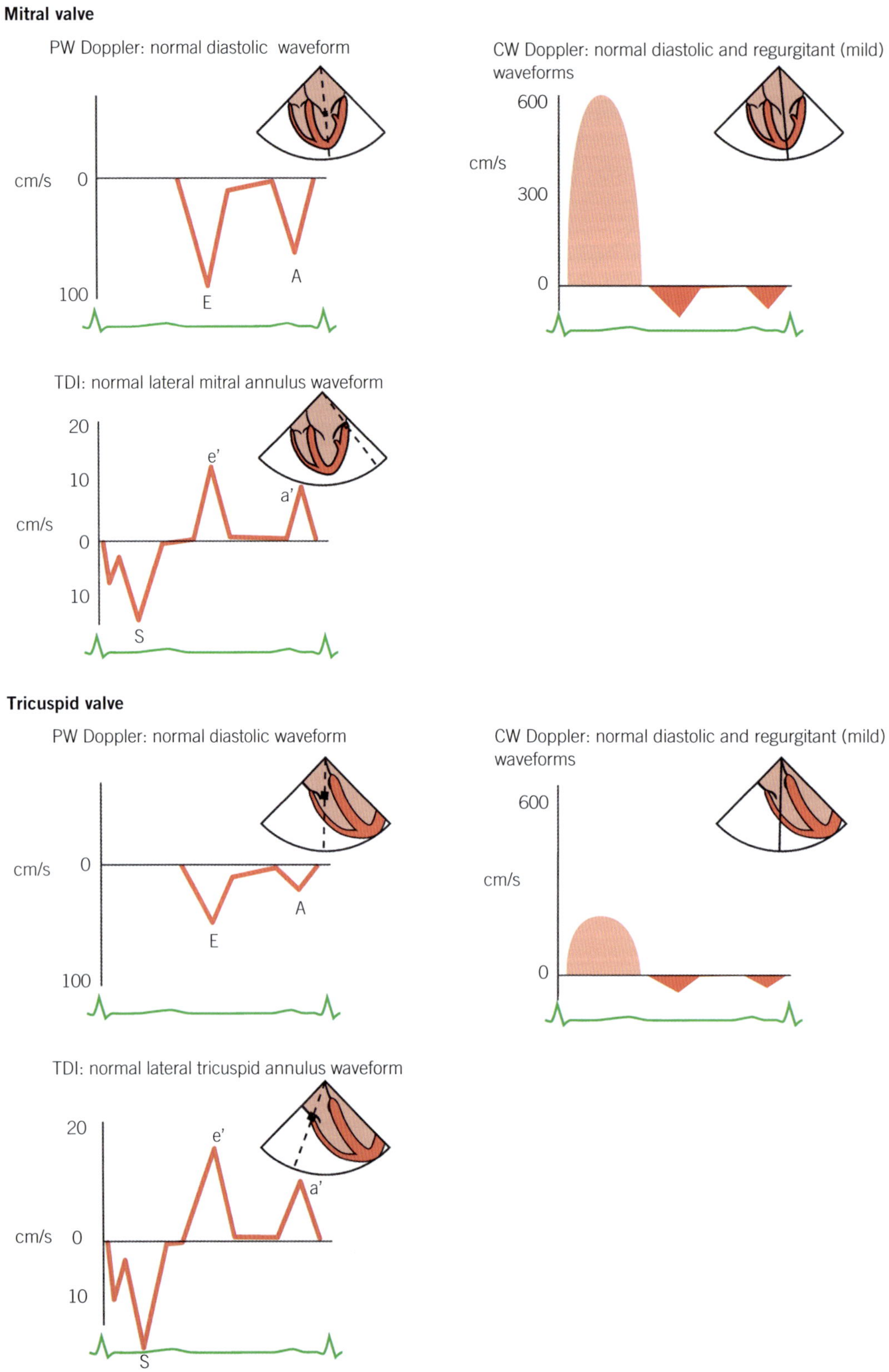

Figure 4.10 Spectral Doppler waveforms. See also the relevant subsections in Online appendices 1 and 5.

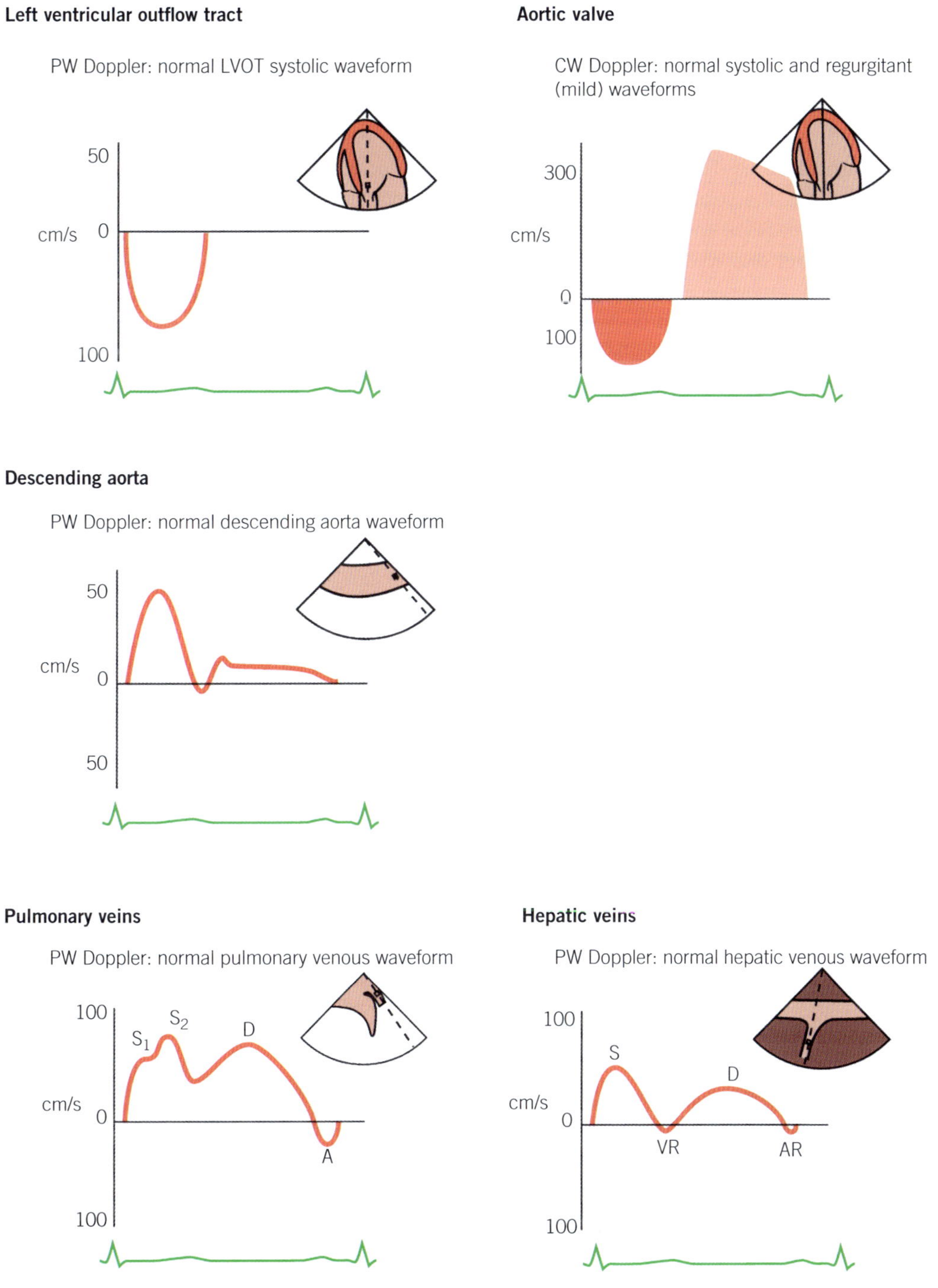

Figure 4.10 *Continued*

scale and baseline should be made to display a complete Doppler waveform without aliasing (see Chapter 1). The spectral Doppler gain should be adjusted until background 'noise' in the display is minimal or absent. The timescale can also be adjusted to optimize the shape of the waveform.

Mitral valve

All three spectral Doppler modes are used to evaluate the MV. PW Doppler is used for assessing diastolic trans-mitral blood flow. CW Doppler is used for assessing systolic flow (i.e. MR) and diastolic flow when velocities are abnormally high (i.e. MS). TDI of the mitral annulus provides information on LV systolic and diastolic function.[9]

PW Doppler evaluation of diastolic flow can be performed in any mid-oesophageal view of the MV. The sample volume should be positioned at the tips of the leaflets in diastole, and the velocity scale adjusted to the maximum allowable. Since flow into the LV is away from the transducer and displayed below the baseline, the baseline should be positioned at the top of the spectral display. The sweep speed should be initially set to 25–50 mm/s to assess for respiratory variation in velocity and then adjusted to 100 mm/s to evaluate individual waveforms. Ideally, measurements should be made at *end-expiration*.

Diastolic trans-mitral flow is normally biphasic, with a large peak in early diastole (**E-wave**) caused by rapid diastolic filling, and a smaller peak in late diastole (**A-wave**) due to atrial systole (e.g. see Online appendix 1.1.14). Peak E-wave velocity is normally 0.5–1.0 m/s, and E- and A-wave patterns provide information on diastolic LV function (see Chapter 7).

Trans-mitral flow in systole indicates valvular regurgitation (see example in Online appendix 6.2.2.2). Peak regurgitant velocity is determined by the pressure difference between the LV and the LA, typically 5–6 m/s. The intensity of the CW Doppler signal is determined by the severity of the MR and the Doppler gain setting.

TDI evaluation of lateral mitral annular motion should be performed in the mid-oesophageal four-chamber view. Typically, the medial mitral annulus is poorly aligned with the Doppler beam and is therefore unsuitable for analysis. The sample volume should be positioned 2–3 mm into the myocardium to ensure it remains within cardiac tissue as the annulus descends towards the apex during systole. The velocity scale should be set 15–20 cm/s above and below the zero-velocity baseline, and the sweep speed set to 50–100 mm/s. Ideally, measurements should be obtained at *end-expiration*. Lateral annular velocity is normally slightly higher than septal velocity; however, with basal segmental wall motion abnormalities (SWMAs), marked differences in velocity may exist. In this circumstance, the average of the lateral and septal velocities should be reported,[9] although this may not be feasible with TOE.

Expert tip: Using colour TDI to identify the moving myocardium helps in positioning the TDI-PW sample volume.

The TDI signal has systolic and diastolic components (see Online appendix 5.3.9). The systolic (**s**) wave normally has an early biphasic component during isovolumetric contraction and a larger monophasic wave during systolic ejection. Motion during systole is away from the transducer and therefore displayed below the baseline. The diastolic component is biphasic, with early (**e'**) and atrial (**a'**) waves analogous to the trans-mitral E- and A-waves. Motion during diastole is towards the transducer and therefore displayed above the baseline. Peak systolic and diastolic velocities are normally 8–12 cm/s (approximately one-tenth of the trans-mitral blood velocity). Abnormalities of mitral annular waveforms provide information on LV systolic and diastolic function (see Chapters 6 and 7). The presence of mitral annular calcification, an MV prosthesis, and/or MS reduces e'-wave velocity, adversely affecting its interpretation with respect to diastolic function.

Tricuspid valve

As with the MV, all three spectral Doppler modes are used to evaluate the TV (see Chapter 15). Similar systolic and diastolic waveforms are seen to those obtained from the MV, but with different reference values. Spectral Doppler imaging of the TV may be performed in one of several mid-oesophageal views.

Peak diastolic trans-tricuspid flow is normally 0.3–0.7 cm/s. Tricuspid stenosis causes higher diastolic velocities and may require assessment with CW Doppler. Trans-tricuspid flow in systole indicates valvular regurgitation. Peak regurgitant velocity is determined by the pressure difference between the RA and the RV, and is normally <2.5 m/s, with higher values indicative of pulmonary hypertension. The intensity of the systolic Doppler signal is determined by the severity of the regurgitation and the Doppler gain setting.

TDI evaluation of lateral tricuspid annular motion is used for assessing RV systolic function. Peak tricuspid annular **s'**-wave velocity is normally 10–15 cm/s (i.e. slightly higher than the mitral s'-wave), with lower values indicative of RV dysfunction (see Chapter 14).

Aortic valve and LVOT

Spectral Doppler assessment of systolic flow in the LVOT and across the AV is used to measure stroke volume (see Chapters 3 and 21) and to evaluate gradients across native and prosthetic AVs; spectral Doppler assessment of diastolic flow is used to evaluate AR (see Chapter 10).

In transgastric views, systolic flow is away from the transducer and displayed below the baseline. The highest velocity across the LVOT/AV normally occurs at the level of the valve and should be assessed with CW Doppler. Peak AV velocity is normally 1–1.5 m/s (see Online appendix 1.6.11) but may be as high as 6 m/s in the presence of severe AS. Peak LVOT velocity is normally 0.5–1 m/s and should be assessed with PW Doppler (see Online appendix 1.6.11). The sample volume should be placed in the centre of the LVOT approximately 5 mm from the AV. However, in the presence of AS, flow acceleration in the distal LVOT may require the sample volume to be moved proximally into a zone of laminar flow. Colour Doppler imaging aids in positioning the sample volume in a region of laminar flow.

Diastolic flow in the LVOT indicates AR (e.g. see Online appendix 7.5.6). The peak velocity of the diastolic waveform is determined by the pressure difference between the LV and the aorta, and is typically 3–5 m/s. The density of the diastolic waveform is determined by the severity of the regurgitation and the Doppler gain setting.

Descending aorta

Flow in the descending aorta is normally antegrade throughout the cardiac cycle and has a biphasic pattern, with a larger peak in systole and a smaller peak in diastole (e.g. see Online appendix 1.3.3). There may be a brief reversal of flow at end-systole. In the descending aorta long-axis view, with the sample volume placed proximally in the aorta, flow is towards the transducer (displayed above the baseline). Severe AR causes flow reversal (i.e. retrograde flow) in the descending aorta in diastole (see Chapter 10).

Pulmonary veins

Blood flow in both upper pulmonary veins is usually well aligned with the Doppler signal, and therefore suitable for Doppler interrogation. The sample volume should be placed centrally, 0.5–1 cm inside the vein. A sample volume of 2–3 mm is appropriate, and the sweep speed should be set to 50–100 mm/s. Flow is towards the transducer throughout most of the cardiac cycle and displayed above the baseline. There are two distinct peaks, one in systole (**S-wave**, which may be biphasic) and one in diastole (**D-wave**), with a brief reversal at end-diastole due to atrial systole (**A-wave**) (e.g. see Online appendix 1.5.7). In early systole, atrial relaxation promotes atrial filling and causes the first systolic peak (**S1**). In mid systole, ventricular contraction causes descent of the mitral annulus, further augmenting atrial filling and causing the second systolic peak (**S2**). In early diastole, ventricular relaxation causes the annulus to move away from the apex; LV pressure falls and the MV opens, causing blood to enter the LA, producing the pulmonary venous D-wave. In late diastole, atrial contraction increases atrial pressure and causes blood to reflux back into the pulmonary veins, resulting in the A-wave. Normally, the S-wave is slightly larger than the D-wave. Peak velocity in the pulmonary veins is normally <0.8 m/s. Abnormalities of pulmonary venous flow occur with MR (see Chapter 8) and LV diastolic dysfunction (see Chapter 7).

Hepatic veins

Flow in the hepatic veins is normally predominantly antegrade, towards the transducer, with a larger velocity peak in systole (S-wave) and a smaller velocity peak in diastole (D-wave) (e.g. see Online appendix 1.7.22). There may be two brief reversals of flow: at end-systole (ventricular reversal, V-wave) and at end-diastole (atrial reversal, A-wave). Peak velocity is typically <0.5 m/s. Abnormalities of hepatic venous flow occur with RV failure and TR (see Chapters 14 and 15).

3D imaging

Guidelines for 3D image acquisition and display have been published by the European Association of Echocardiography and the ASE,[10] and are also incorporated into the latest ASE/SCA guidelines.[1]

Matrix array transducers

Matrix array transducers contain thousands of individual transducer elements arranged in a block (matrix), allowing the transducer to function as a 'shower head' giving a pyramidal-shaped 3D block of ultrasound (Figure 4.1). Sector depth and the dimensions of the sector in the azimuthal (lateral) and elevation planes define the sector volume. The operator can adjust the volume and size of the 3D sector. When using zoom, a sub-region of interest can be defined (Figure 4.1). As discussed in Chapter 2, changing the volume of the 3D sector has a major impact on temporal resolution.

Acquiring 3D data sets

3D data sets may be acquired over a single heartbeat (real-time imaging) or over several heartbeats (multi-beat acquisition) using ECG triggering (see Chapter 1).

As previously discussed, multi-beat acquisition improves temporal resolution but is subject to stitching artefacts. Multi-beat acquisition is not true real-time imaging.

Imaging modes

Several imaging modes may be used to acquire and display 3D data sets. Rapid developments in software and hardware technology have blurred the distinctions between these different modalities. Colour Doppler imaging can be used with all 3D imaging modes. **Simultaneous multi-plane imaging** (also termed **biplane imaging** or **x-plane**) displays two 2D images side by side in a dual-screen display (Figure 4.11). The left of the screen shows the starting (reference) image, and the right of the screen displays an orthogonal (i.e. 90° forward-rotated) image, which can be adjusted in several ways from the standard orthogonal position (Figure 4.12). It can be forward- or backward-rotated; it can be adjusted in the elevation plane, and it can be swept from side to side across the reference image. Orthogonal imaging is very useful for measuring the dimensions of cardiac structures (like the MV or AV annulus) simultaneously along two axes (Figure 4.11). Sweeping the orthogonal view from side to side is useful for imaging LV segments (see Figure 6.13).

Narrow-sector mode (also termed **live**) shows a 'narrow' 3D sector in real time (Figure 4.13). Previously, this mode was limited to a maximum sector dimension of 60° by 30° (hence the name narrow sector). Current software versions provide sector dimensions of 90° in both planes, and the term 'narrow' sector is no longer appropriate.

Focused wide-sector mode (also termed **zoom**) displays a user-defined wedge of 3D data (Figure 4.14). Activating zoom mode displays two orthogonal 2D images (similar to biplane mode), with superimposed adjustable sector boxes. The lateral plane is defined on the left-hand image, and the elevation plane is defined on the right-hand image. Once the sample boxes have been defined, the 3D data set is acquired (either in real time or with multi-beat acquisition) and then cropped and orientated on the screen to display the structure(s) of interest. The main limitation of 3D zoom is low temporal resolution, which is improved by limiting the sector scan to the minimum required to display the structure(s) of interest and/or by using multi-beat acquisition. Multi-beat acquisition over 4–6 heartbeats should be used whenever 3D colour Doppler imaging is used.

Wide-sector mode (also termed **full volume**) displays a pyramid-shaped 3D data set, with maximal sector angles >90° in both the lateral and elevational planes. Given the large dimensions of the 3D sector, multi-beat acquisition

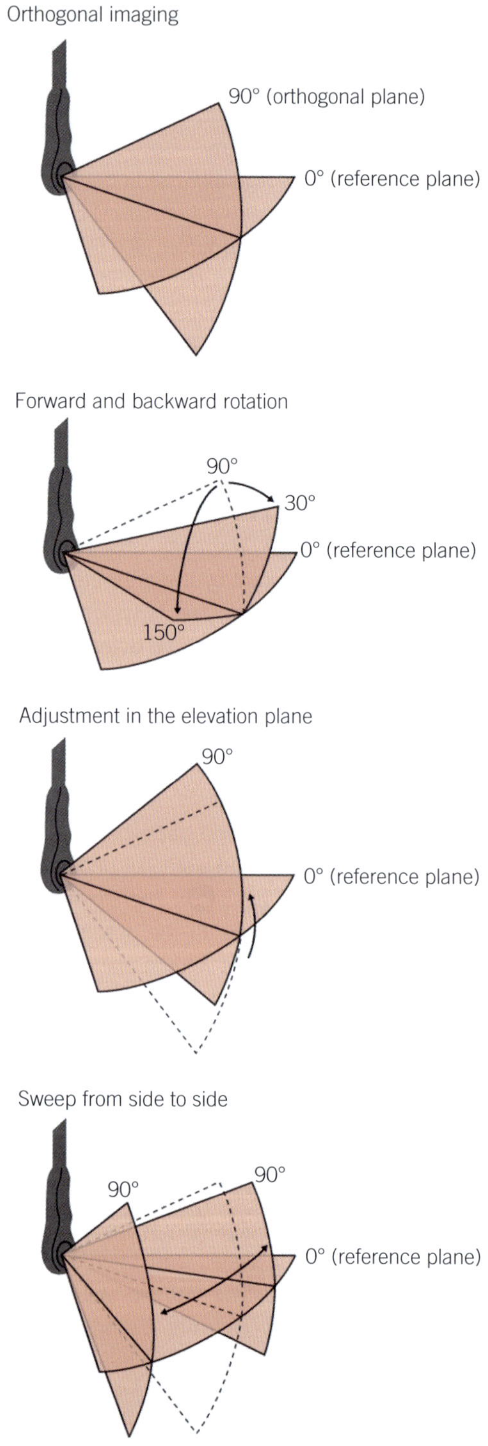

Figure 4.11 Movements of the sector scan with simultaneous biplane imaging. Activating the mode displays two orthogonal views. If the first (reference) image is at 0°, the second image is at 90°. From the standard orthogonal position, the second image can be forward- or backward-rotated, adjusted in the elevation plane, and swept from side to side. Note that in the schematic showing forward and backward rotation, for simplicity, only the top part of the sector scans is shown.

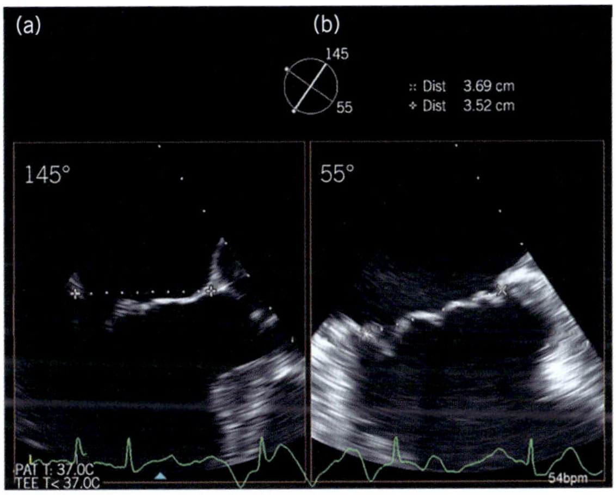

Figure 4.12 Simultaneous biplane imaging of the mitral annulus. The image shows orthogonal mid-oesophageal views of the MV. In this example, the reference image in (a) is the long-axis view at 145°. The image in (b) is forward-rotated by 90° from the reference image and shows the mid-oesophageal commissural view at 55°. Measurements of the mitral annulus in the long-axis and commissural orientations are shown.

over 4–6 beats is required if colour Doppler is used. The 3D data set can be displayed in full or with the autocrop function active (Figure 4.15), which allows cardiac structures to be more easily recognized. Once acquired, the data set can be manually cropped and reorientated on the screen to display the structure(s) of interest.

Display formats

3D data sets may be displayed using volume rendering or surface rendering, or as 2D tomographic slices. For routine qualitative use, **volume rendering** is the most intuitive method of display and the method used to display most 3D images in this book. With volume rendering, the 3D data set is mapped to a 2D display, with different colours applied to the **voxels** (3D pixels) to illustrate the depth and texture of the cardiac tissues. The data set can then be cropped and orientated on the screen to display the structure of interest.

2D tomographic imaging is used for quantitative assessments of 3D data sets, using a technique termed **multi-planar reconstruction** (MPR). MPR displays the 3D data set as three simultaneous, adjustable orthogonal 2D planes (coronal, sagittal, and transverse). Adjusting the three orthogonal planes allows the structure of interest to be interrogated. MPR is used for quantitative measurements (e.g. regurgitant orifice area) and detailed examination of cardiac structures (especially the MV and AV). Examples of MPR mode are shown in Figures 8.11, 8.24, and 10.6.

Acquisition and display of 3D data sets of the heart valves

Mitral valve

Focused wide sector is the most useful 3D modality for assessing the MV. The starting image should be the mid-oesophageal long-axis view. The sector boxes should be adjusted to the minimum necessary to display the entire mitral annulus and both leaflets. Including the AV and LA appendage helps to orientate the data set. Real-time (i.e.

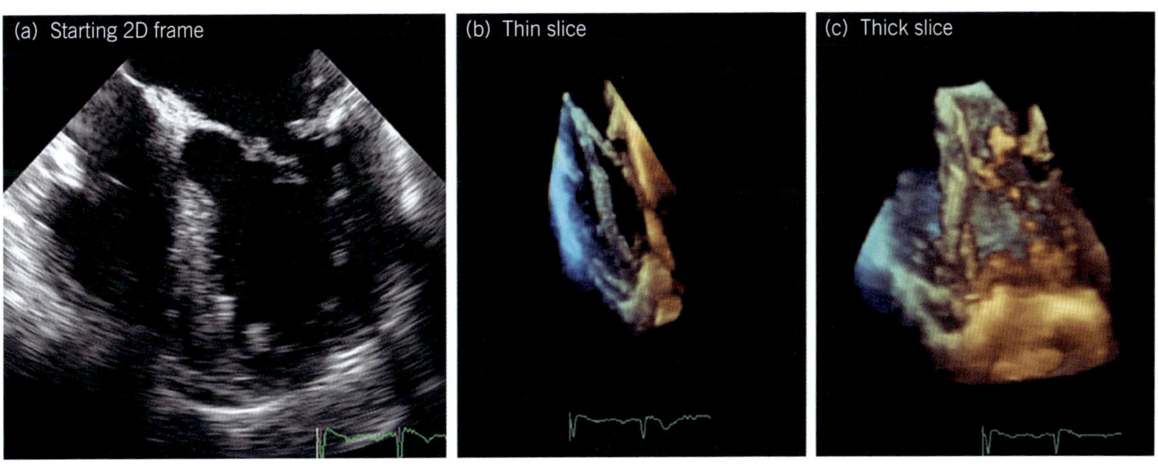

Figure 4.13 3D imaging in narrow sector mode. (a) shows the starting mid-oesophageal four-chamber view. (b) shows a thin slice, with the elevation height set at 5°. (c) shows a thick slice, with the elevation height set to 30°.

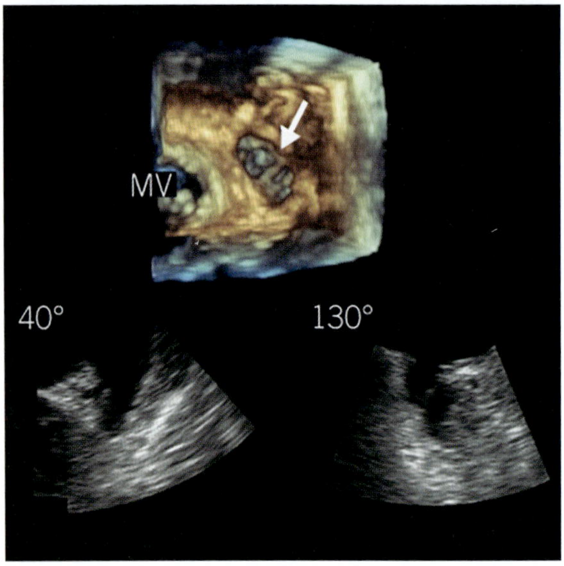

Figure 4.14 3D imaging in focused wide sector mode. The image shows a 3D zoom view of the LA appendage (arrow) and part of the MV from the LA aspect. The two orthogonal 2D views from which the 3D sector is derived are shown at the bottom of the screen. The starting view was a mid-oesophageal view of the LA appendage at 40°. The sector width (azimuth) and depth of the sector were defined from this view. The elevation width of the sector was defined in the orthogonal view at 130°. Note the image is orientated such that the LA appendage is to the right of the MV, which is the opposite orientation to the surgeon's view (compare to Figure 4.16).

single-beat) imaging is usually adequate; however, multi-beat acquisition should be used for colour Doppler imaging. The volume-rendered image should be orientated to show the MV in the *surgical view* (i.e. from the atrial side, with the AV at the top of the screen in the 12 o'clock position; Figure 4.16). (See also Online appendices 1.4 and 6.1.)

Aortic valve

The AV can be visualized by using either narrow sector or focused wide sector modes. Narrow sector is the most intuitive mode to acquire and orientate images of the AV. The starting image should be the mid-oesophageal AV short-axis view. The data set should be orientated to display the right coronary cusp at the bottom of the screen in the 6 o'clock position (i.e. the same leaflet orientation as the AV short-axis view). The valve can be displayed from both the aortic (Figure 4.17) and LVOT aspects. (See also Online appendix 1.6.)

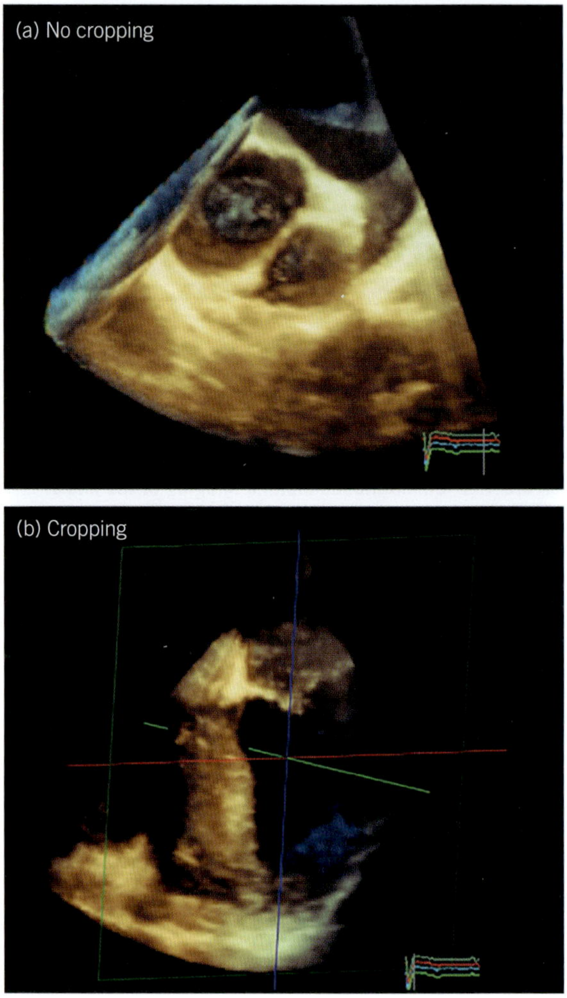

Figure 4.15 3D imaging in wide sector mode. The data set has been acquired over four heartbeats. (a) shows the full-volume 3D sector without any cropping ('blob' mode). (b) shows the 3D sector with the autocrop function activated. The three orthogonal cropping planes (blue, red, green) are shown.

Tricuspid valve

The TV may be imaged with wide sector or focused wide sector modes. Focused wide sector mode has the advantage of being able to limit the data set to just the tricuspid annulus and leaflets. Image quality is usually less than that achieved with 3D imaging of the MV and AV. The starting image should be the mid-oesophageal four-chamber view, with the image centred on the TV. The sector boxes should be adjusted to the minimum necessary to display the entire annulus and leaflet excursion. Including some of the atrial and ventricular septa helps to orientate the data set. Figure 4.18 shows a 3D data set of both the MV and TV from the atrial perspective.

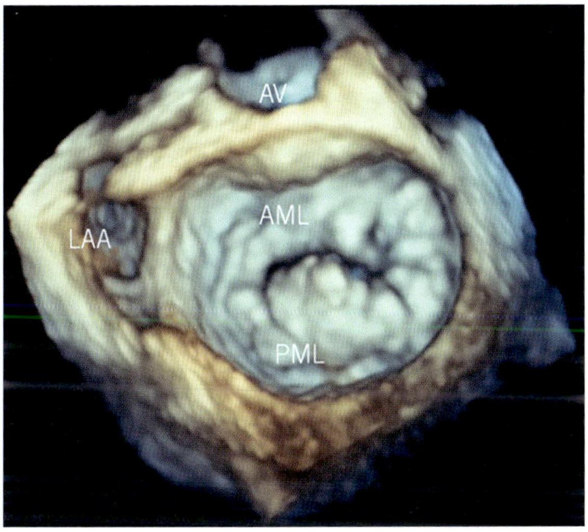

Figure 4.16 3D view of the MV in the standard orientation. The data set was acquired over a single heartbeat, using the focused wide sector mode, and orientated to display the MV from the LA aspect in the surgical orientation (with the AV in the 12 o'clock position). The AV and LA appendage (LAA) are included in the data set to help with orientation. The anterior (AML) and posterior (PML) leaflets are shown. Prolapse of the middle segment of the posterior leaflet can be seen. See also Online appendices 1.4 and 6.1.

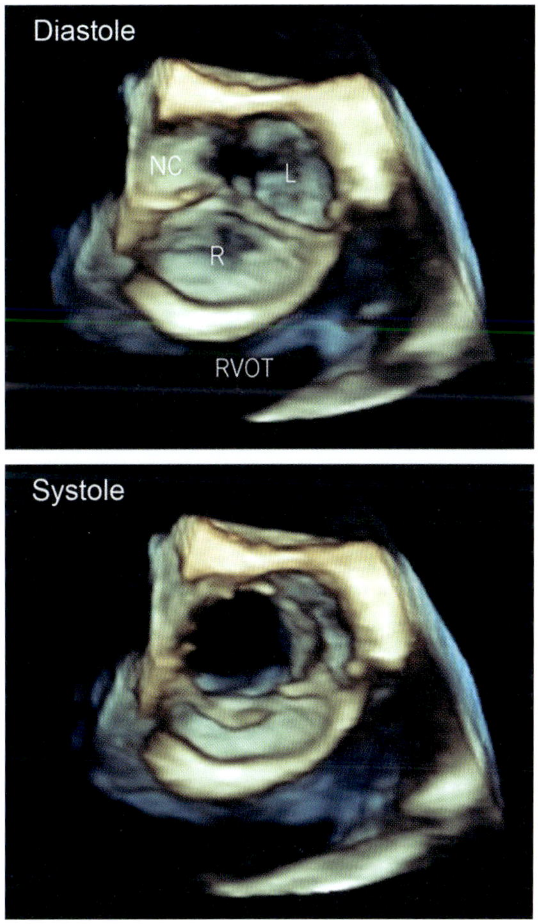

Figure 4.17 3D view of the AV in the standard orientation. The data set was acquired over a single heartbeat, using the narrow sector mode, and orientated to display the right coronary cusp at the bottom of the screen. The AV is shown from the aortic aspect in systole and diastole in this example. L, left coronary cusp; R, right coronary cusp; NC, non-coronary cusp. See also Online appendix 1.6.

The expert consensus in recent years has been to display 3D data sets of the isolated TV from the atrial side, with the AV in the 5 o'clock position and the septal leaflet between 12 and 5 o'clock (see Chapter 15 for details and Figure 15.5 for an example).

Pulmonary valve

3D imaging of the PV is rarely indicated, and image quality is often poor due to its location in the far field

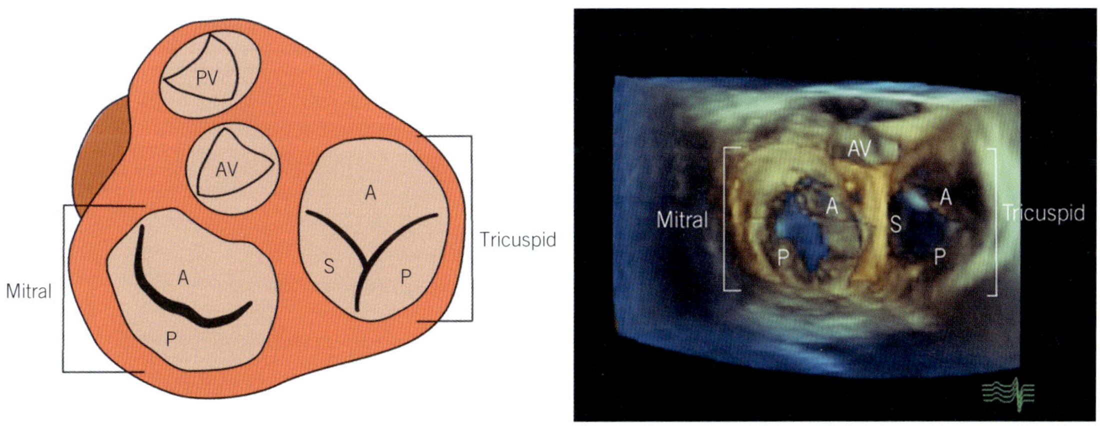

Figure 4.18 3D view of the base of the heart, showing the MV and TV from the atrial perspective. The data set was acquired over four heartbeats using the wide sector mode, and was orientated to show the TV in the same orientation as the MV. However, the recent expert consensus for 3D imaging of the isolated TV usually displays it in a different orientation (see text in Chapter 15 and Figure 15.5).

and echo dropout from the thin leaflets. Narrow sector is the most useful mode. The starting view should be a modified mid-oesophageal RV inflow–outflow view or a modified mid-oesophageal long-axis view. The probe is then withdrawn and turned to the left to bring the PV into view.

Multiple choice questions

Discover interactive multiple choice questions to test your knowledge on this chapter by searching for this book's title or ISBN (9780198873686) at **https://academic.oup.com/** and going to the online appendix at the end of the book. Use your scratch-off code on the inside cover to access the material.

References

1. Hahn RT, Abraham T, Adams MS, *et al.* Guidelines for performing a comprehensive transesophageal echocardiographic examination: recommendations from the American Society of Echocardiography and the Society of Cardiovascular Anesthesiologists. *J Am Soc Echocardiogr.* 2013;**26**:921–64.
2. American Society of Anesthesiologists and Society of Cardiovascular Anesthesiologists Task Force on Transesophageal Echocardiography. Practice guidelines for perioperative transesophageal echocardiography. An updated report by the American Society of Anesthesiologists and the Society of Cardiovascular Anesthesiologists Task Force on Transesophageal Echocardiography. *Anesthesiology.* 2010;**112**:1084–96.
3. Shanewise JS, Cheung AT, Aronson S, *et al.* ASE/SCA guidelines for performing a comprehensive intraoperative multiplane transesophageal echocardiography examination: recommendations of the American Society of Echocardiography Council for Intraoperative Echocardiography and the Society of Cardiovascular Anesthesiologists Task Force for Certification in Perioperative Transesophageal Echocardiography. *Anesth Analg.* 1999;**89**:870–84.
4. Metkus T, Thibault D, Grant M, *et al.* Transesophageal echocardiography in patients undergoing coronary artery bypass graft surgery. *J Am Coll Cardiol.* 2021;**78**:112–22.
5. Reeves ST, Glas KE, Eltzschig H, *et al.* Guidelines for performing a comprehensive epicardial echocardiography examination: recommendations of the American Society of Echocardiography and the Society of Cardiovascular Anesthesiologists. *J Am Soc Echocardiogr.* 2007;**20**:427–37.
6. Cartwright BL, Jackson A, Cooper J. Intraoperative pulmonary vein examination by transesophageal echocardiography: an anatomic update and review of utility. *J Cardiothorac Vasc Anesth.* 2013;**27**:111–20.
7. Tan CO, Harley I. Perioperative transesophageal echocardiographic assessment of the right heart and associated structures: a comprehensive update and technical report. *J Cardiothorac Vasc Anesth.* 2014;**28**:1112–33.
8. Wibowo A, Elhidsi M, Susanto AD. Calculation of pleural fluid estimation using ultrasonography. *Respir Sci.* 2022;**2**:156–64.
9. Nagueh SF, Appleton CP, Gillebert TC, *et al.* Recommendations for the evaluation of left ventricular diastolic function by echocardiography. *Eur J Echocardiogr.* 2009;**10**:165–93.
10. Lang RM, Badano LP, Tsang W, *et al.* EAE/ASE recommendations for image acquisition and display using three-dimensional echocardiography. *J Am Soc Echocardiogr.* 2012;**25**:3–46.

5

Anatomical variants and cardiac masses

The echocardiographic appearance of normal cardiac structures is variable. Differentiating between normal anatomical variations, echocardiographic artefacts (see Chapter 2), and masses is essential to avoid misdiagnosis. Echocardiography has limited ability to discriminate between tissue types, so the diagnosis of cardiac masses requires the assessment of location, appearance, attachment, mobility, and associated abnormalities. The echo reflectance of various tissues can be helpful in making a diagnosis. Soft tissue (myocardium, thrombus, vegetations) typically appears grey, whereas connective tissue (heart valves, valve strands, fibroelastomas) is more echo-reflective and appears white.

This chapter is divided into two sections: (1) normal anatomical variants, grouped by location, commencing in the right atrium and progressing through the atrial septum, LA, RV, LV, heart valves, and pericardium; and (2) cardiac masses and abnormal spaces, including thrombi, vegetations, and tumours.

Anatomical variants

Right atrium

The RA contains many embryological remnants;[1] the most common are depicted in Figure 5.1.

Crista terminalis

The **crista terminalis** is seen as a small ridge near the junction of the SVC and the RA. It separates the smooth wall of the SVC from the rough surface of the pectinate muscles of the RA. The crista terminalis is best seen in the mid-oesophageal bicaval view (Figure 5.2).

Eustachian valve

In utero, the **Eustachian valve** directs oxygenated blood from the IVC across the foramen ovale into the LA. The Eustachian valve is a membranous structure originating

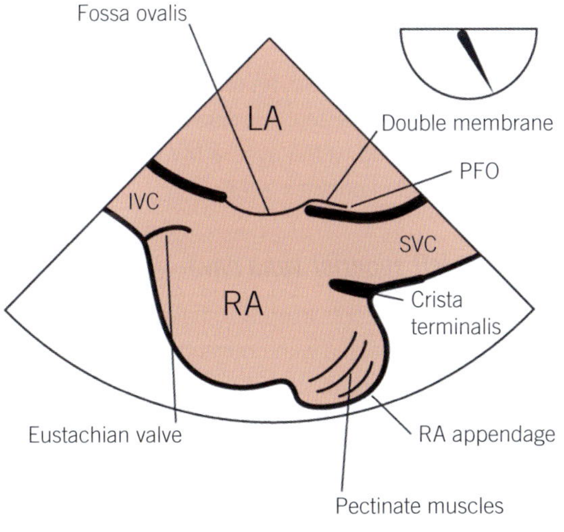

Figure 5.1 Schematic representation of normal structures within the RA, as seen in the mid-oesophageal bicaval view. PFO, patent foramen ovale.

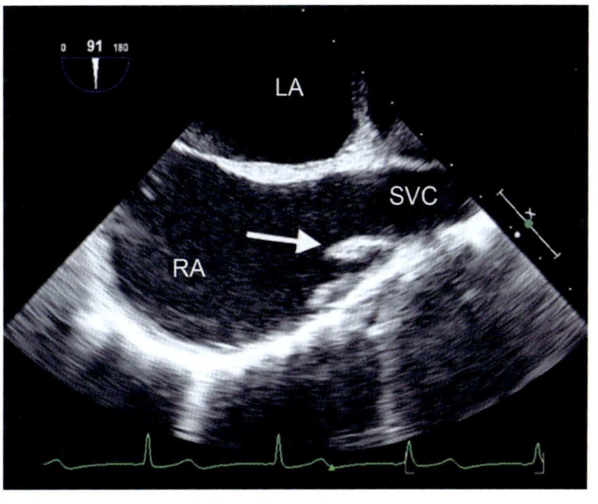

Figure 5.2 Crista terminalis. In this mid-oesophageal bicaval view, the crista terminalis (arrow) is seen as a prominent ridge at the junction of the SVC and RA. See Online appendix 2.2b S.

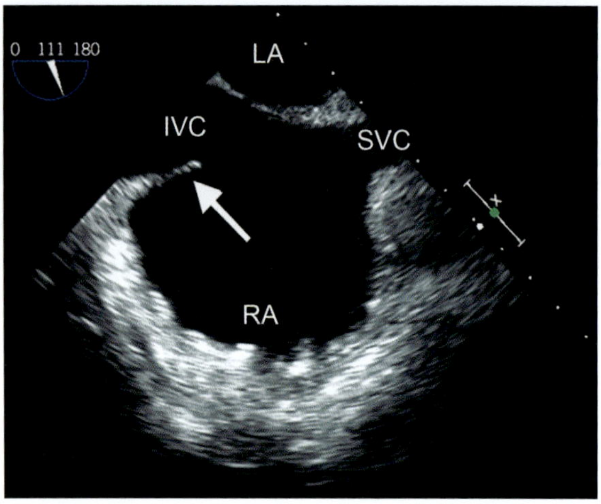

Figure 5.3 Eustachian valve. In this mid-oesophageal bicaval view, the Eustachian valve (arrow) is visible as a flap of tissue at the junction of the RA and IVC. See Online appendix 2.2a.

from the junction of the IVC and the RA, extending a variable distance across the LA towards the interatrial septum (Figure 5.3). A large Eustachian valve may sometimes interfere with the insertion of an IVC venous cannula before CPB.[2]

Thebesian valve

The **Thebesian valve** is a small endocardial fold at the origin of the coronary sinus (CS). This is rarely identified on TOE. However, if very prominent, it may obstruct the passage of a retrograde cardioplegia cannula (Figure 5.4; see Online appendix 2.15).[3]

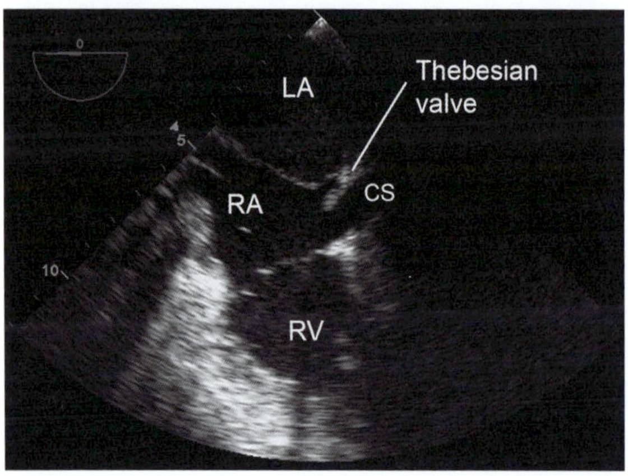

Figure 5.4 Thebesian valve. In this mid-oesophageal coronary sinus view, a Thebesian valve is demonstrated. See Online appendix 2.15.

Chiari network

A **Chiari network** is a thin, mobile, lace-like structure originating from the Eustachian and/or Thebesian valves, and present in approximately 2% of people (see Online appendix 2.17). A Chiari network has variable attachments to the RA free wall and atrial septum, which differentiate it from a large fenestrated Eustachian valve. The motion of Chiari network filaments appears random and unrelated to valve opening and closing. Chiari networks have been implicated in thromboembolism and endocarditis, and may cause obstruction or entrapment of vascular catheters. A Chiari network may be difficult to differentiate from thrombus or vegetations when seen in association with vascular access catheters or pacing wires.

Right atrial appendage

The RA appendage is a broad-based structure near the junction of the SVC and RA, best seen in the mid-oesophageal bicaval or modified bicaval view (Figure 5.1). As with the LA, the pectinate muscles are usually visible within the appendage; however, they may extend beyond the appendage, giving the wall of the RA a roughened, irregular appearance, particularly in RA hypertrophy. Due to its broad base, formation of significant thrombus in the RA appendage is uncommon.[4]

Enlarged coronary sinus

The CS opens into the RA at the floor of the interatrial septum. Normally approximately 1 cm in diameter, the CS is best seen in long axis in the mid-oesophageal CS view (Figure 5.5), and in short axis in the mid-oesophageal two-chamber view posterior to the MV annulus. An enlarged CS may be associated with an anomalous connection to a pulmonary vein, an unroofed CS in the LA, or the presence of a persistent left-sided SVC.[5] An enlarged CS may be confused with a cyst, a MV annular abscess, or an aneurysmal circumflex artery.

Persistent left superior vena cava

A **left-sided SVC** persists in approximately 0.5% of people and in 3–10% of people with congenital heart disease. It is due to the failed regression of the embryonic left superior cardinal vein, and it most often drains into the RA via the CS, which becomes dilated because of the additional blood flow (Figure 5.5). It is often asymptomatic, but if a dilated CS is identified in the operating room, a left-sided SVC should be actively sought, as it may compromise the delivery of retrograde cardioplegia. A left-sided

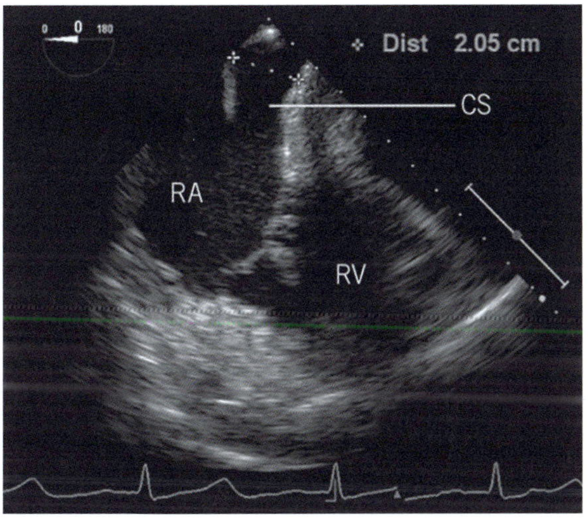

Figure 5.5 Enlarged coronary sinus. In this mid-oesophageal coronary sinus view, an enlarged coronary sinus (CS) (2.05 cm in diameter) can be seen entering the RA, adjacent to the septal leaflet of the TV. The cause of the enlarged coronary sinus was a persistent left-sided SVC. See Online appendix 2.4.

SVC is often visualized directly between the left upper pulmonary vein and the LA appendage (Figure 5.6). Flow between the left-sided SVC and the CS may be seen with 2D and colour flow Doppler imaging in the modified mid-oesophageal two-chamber view. Injection of agitated saline into a left neck or left arm vein may rapidly confirm the diagnosis, as the CS and then the RA rapidly opacify, before the right-sided SVC.[5]

Catheters and wires

Central venous catheters, PA catheters, pacing wires, and cannulae for CPB or extracorporeal membrane oxygenation (ECMO) may be present in the RA and venae cavae. These are usually easy to differentiate from native structures. Thrombi can be occasionally seen forming on these devices.

Left atrium

Warfarin ridge

The **warfarin (or Coumadin) ridge** refers to the tissue between the LA appendage and the left upper pulmonary vein (LUPV) (Figure 5.7). It got its name from the early days of echocardiography, when it being mistaken for LA thrombus led to patients being put on anticoagulants. The free edge of this ridge can accumulate fat, appearing as a mass with a thin proximal attachment to the atrial wall. Imaging in the orthogonal plane will reveal continuity with the atrial wall, and Doppler interrogation of the structure behind the ridge will be consistent with pulmonary vein flow.

Cor triatriatum

Cor triatriatum is a congenital condition comprising 0.1% of congenital heart conditions. It consists of a thin membrane separating either the LA (cortriatriatum *sinistrum*, more common) or the RA (cortriatriatum *dextrum*, less common) into two chambers, resulting in the appearance of three atrial chambers. This is strongly associated with other congenital cardiac defects, which are found in 50% of these individuals. In cortriatriatum sinistrum, there is typically a proximal chamber into which the pulmonary veins drain and a true atrial chamber which supplies the MV (Figure 5.8).

Expert tip: a similar appearance to cortriatriatum may be seen following heart transplantation, due to the suture line between the native and the transplanted LA, although the apparent 'membrane' is much thicker with heart transplantation.

Left atrial appendage

The LA appendage is a blind-ended structure lined with pectinate muscles, and is of variable size and shape. The use of 3D imaging, including biplane imaging, facilitates thorough evaluation of the LA appendage and is helpful to identify the presence of thrombus (see Online appendix 1.5).

Pectinate muscles

The normal LA appendage is lined with pectinate muscles. These are ridge-like projections into the appendage that can make identification of thrombus difficult (Figure 5.9). Examination of the pectinate muscles in orthogonal planes reveals them to be band-like structures forming the wall of the atrium, which move in synchrony with the atrial wall.

Shape variants

A number of complex morphological LA appendage variants have been described based on appearance such as 'chicken wing', 'cauliflower', 'windsock', and 'cactus' (see Chapter 17). LA appendage morphology is associated with differential stroke risk in patients with

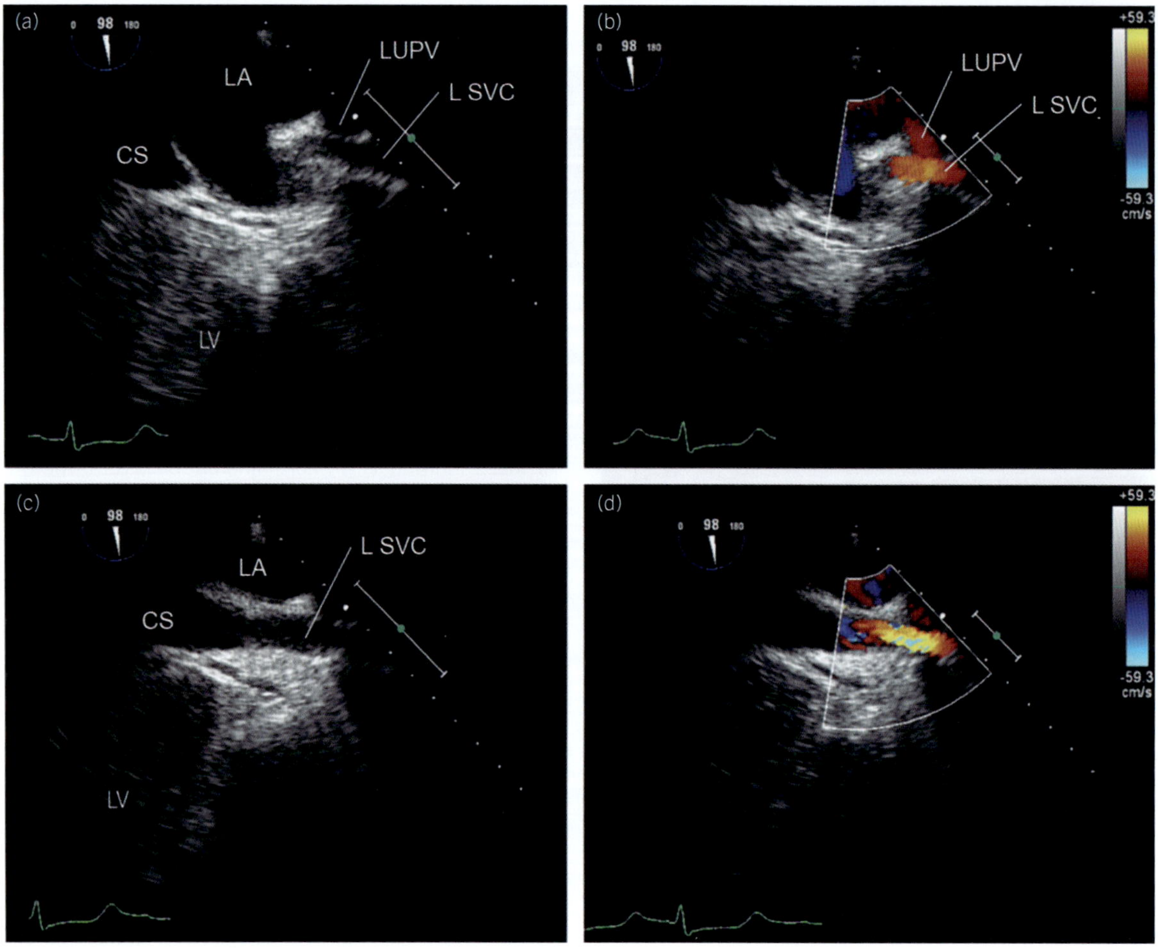

Figure 5.6 Persistent left-sided SVC. Frames (a) to (d) were obtained in a modified mid-oesophageal two-chamber view. The probe was advanced from the standard position to image the posterior LA, close to the posterior atrioventricular groove, such that the lower part of the images passes through the inferolateral (posterior) wall of the LV, not the LV cavity. The enlarged coronary sinus (CS) is shown on the left of each frame, and the left upper pulmonary vein (LUPV) and the left SVC (LSVC) on the right. Frames (a) and (b) were obtained in early diastole, with and without colour Doppler, and the relationship between the LUPV and the LSVC can be appreciated. Frames (c) and (d) were obtained in late diastole, with and without colour Doppler. The connection between the CS and the LSVC can now be appreciated. See Online appendices 2.5–2.8.

atrial fibrillation, with chicken wing conveying the lowest stroke risk.[6,7]

Stapled-off left atrial appendage

The LA appendage may be stapled off during cardiac surgery in some circumstances (e.g. in a patient with atrial fibrillation). A stapled-off appendage may appear as a cavity where the appendage would normally be seen. Residual flow may be seen into the space with colour Doppler imaging if the appendage is not completely isolated.

Inverted left atrial appendage

This may occasionally present after manipulation during cardiac surgery, as a new mass arising from the normal position of the LA appendage. In such cases, the LA appendage is no longer visible. The apparent mass is homogenous and freely mobile, and may prolapse through the MV. Surgical inspection and remanipulation are indicated if suspected during surgery. If identified post-operatively, there is controversy as to whether reoperation is indicated, as the condition may resolve spontaneously or, rarely, cause complications (thrombus, necrosis, MV obstruction).

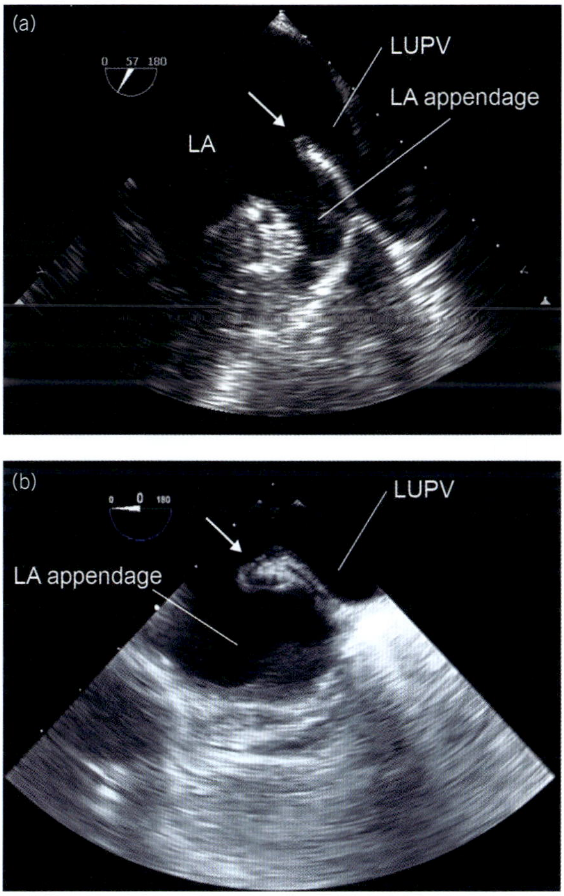

Figure 5.7 Two views of the warfarin ridge. In these mid-oesophageal views, (a) the image plane and sector rotation were adjusted to display the LA appendage and left upper pulmonary vein (LUPV). The warfarin ridge (arrows) is the fold of atrial tissue separating the two structures. In (b), the distal end of the ridge appears bulbous, probably due to the accumulation of fat within the tissue fold. See Online appendix 2.3.

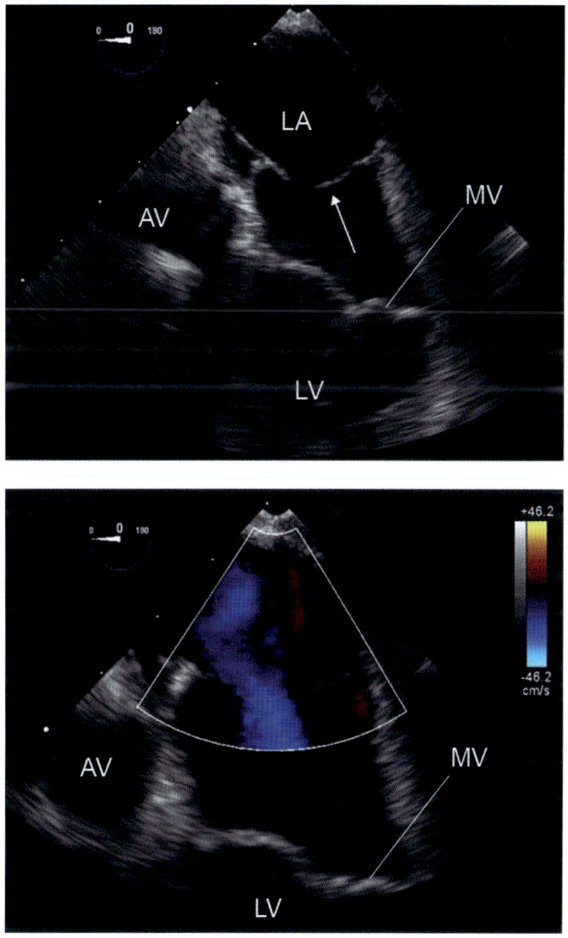

Figure 5.8 Cor triatrium. In these mid-oesophageal five-chamber views, a membrane (arrow) can be seen in the LA superior to the MV. Laminar flow across the membrane suggests there is no obstruction to flow. See Online appendices 2.12 and 2.13.

Atrial septum

Double membrane of the fossa ovalis

The postero-superior margin of the fossa ovalis membrane overlaps the superior limbus of the inter-atrial septum (IAS), which may create the appearance of a double membrane or even a cavity when viewed in the mid-oesophageal bicaval view (see Online appendix 2.1).

Lipomatous hypertrophy of the inter-atrial septum

Lipomatous hypertrophy of the IAS occurs due to infiltration of the superior and inferior portions of the IAS by unencapsulated lipomatous tissue, with sparing of the fossa ovalis (Figures 5.10 and 17.1a). A dumbbell-shaped appearance of the septum on 2D imaging results, with the IAS being >2cm in thickness. Lipomatous hypertrophy is present in 2–8% of normal individuals and is usually asymptomatic. In extreme cases, hypertrophy may extend into the RA and cause SVC obstruction. The differential diagnosis is septal infiltration by a tumour, which typically shows variable echogenicity and is often associated with pericardial effusion. Benign tumours such as lipomas tend to be encapsulated.

Atrial septal aneurysm

Atrial septal aneurysm is a localized elongation of thin, mobile redundant tissue of the fossa ovalis (Figure 5.10). The tissue is excessively mobile throughout the cardiac cycle. The IAS is defined as aneurysmal when the basal width is >15mm and the excursion is >10mm from the midposition

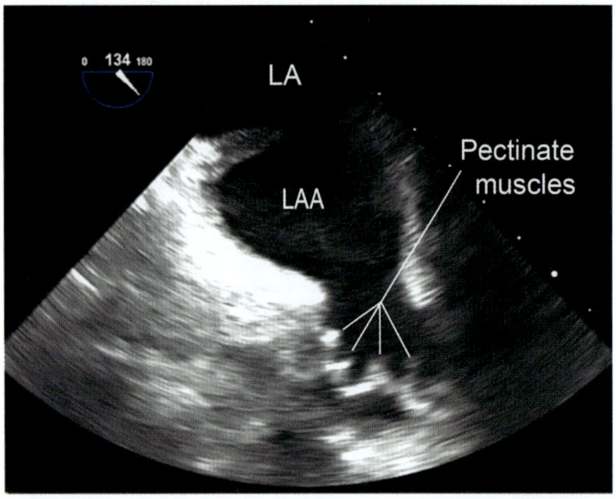

Figure 5.9 Pectinate muscles (lines) in the LA appendage (LAA).

into either or both atria. The incidence of this condition is 1%, whereas 50% of people with this condition also have a patent foramen ovale (PFO). Atrial septal aneurysm with PFO is associated with an increased risk of embolic stroke.[7,8]

Right ventricle

Trabeculae

Trabeculae are muscular ridges formed on the endocardial surface of the RV. They become more prominent in patients with RV hypertrophy.

Moderator band

The **moderator band** (also known as the septo-marginal trabecula) is a prominent trabecula, which extends from the septum to the anterolateral wall in the apical third of the RV (Figure 5.11). The anterior papillary muscle supporting the TV arises at the junction of the moderator band and the free wall of the ventricle. The moderator band is thought to be important in facilitating function of the anterior papillary muscle.[9]

Papillary muscles

Up to three papillary muscles (anterior, posterior, and septal) arise from the RV walls and support the TV (see Chapter 15). All three are present in approximately 25% of hearts. The anterior papillary muscle is usually present, arising at the point of insertion of the moderator band with the anterolateral wall of the RV. The posterior and septal papillary muscles have variable positions and may be absent. Papillary muscles are identified by the insertion of chordae attached to the TV leaflets.[10]

Left ventricle

Trabeculae

The LV has much less prominent trabeculae than the RV.

False tendons

These are fine, filamentous, fibro-muscular structures traversing the LV cavity, connected to the free wall, septum, or papillary muscles. They are considered a normal variant (see Online appendix 2.16).

Mitral subvalvular apparatus

Lobulated or bifid papillary muscles occur rarely and may resemble small masses attached to the LV wall. Thrombi

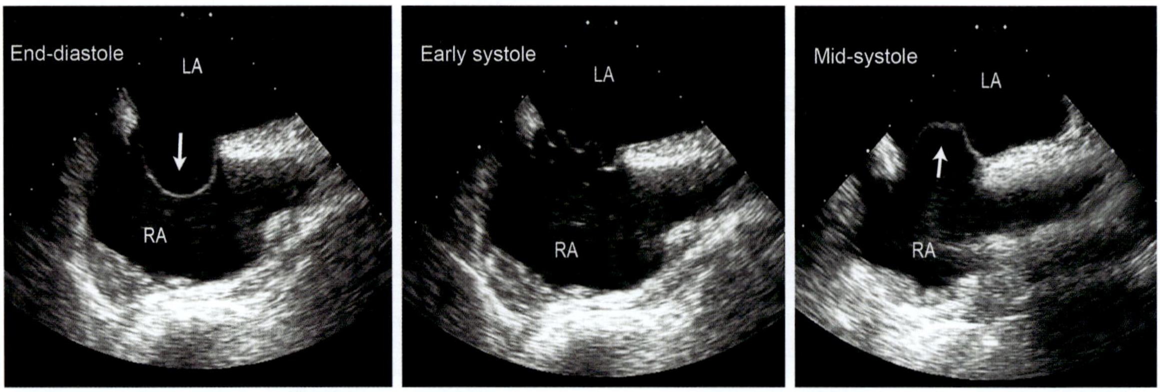

Figure 5.10 Atrial septal aneurysm. These mid-oesophageal bicaval views were taken sequentially during the cardiac cycle, and the atrial septum appears to be highly mobile. Under normal conditions, the inter-atrial septum bows towards the right throughout the cardiac cycle, reflecting the higher pressure in the LA compared to the RA, with a brief reversal in mid systole. Note the thick upper and lower portions of the septum, consistent with lipomatous hypertrophy of the septum.

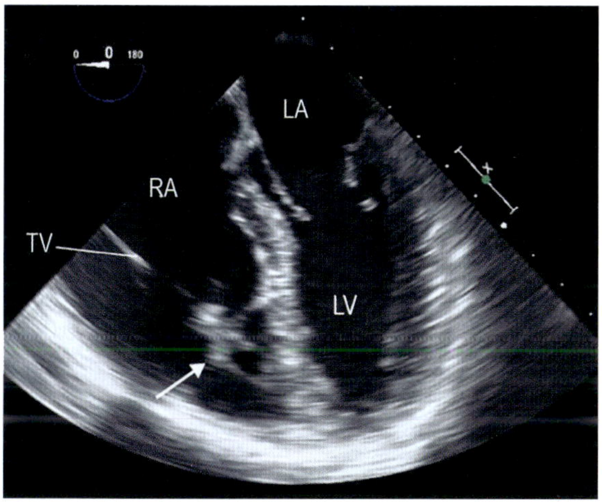

Figure 5.11 Moderator band. In this mid-oesophageal four-chamber view, a prominent moderator band (arrow) can be seen in the apical third of the RV. The anterior leaflet of the TV can also be seen. See Online appendix 2.11.

are typically associated with regional wall motion abnormalities (RWMAs). The continuation with MV chordae may distinguish variant papillary muscles from thrombi. Thickening and calcification of the subvalvular mitral apparatus may occur in rheumatic heart disease or renal failure.

Heart valves

Valve strands

Valve strands (**Lambl excrescences**) are thin (<2 mm), mobile structures up to 10 mm long, attached to valve leaflets. They can occur on any native or prosthetic valve, but they are most common on the AV (Figure 5.12; see Online appendices 3.2.3 and 3.2.4). They are common and their incidence increases with age. On native valves, strands are typically attached near the coaptation line. With prosthetic valves, they can attach to the

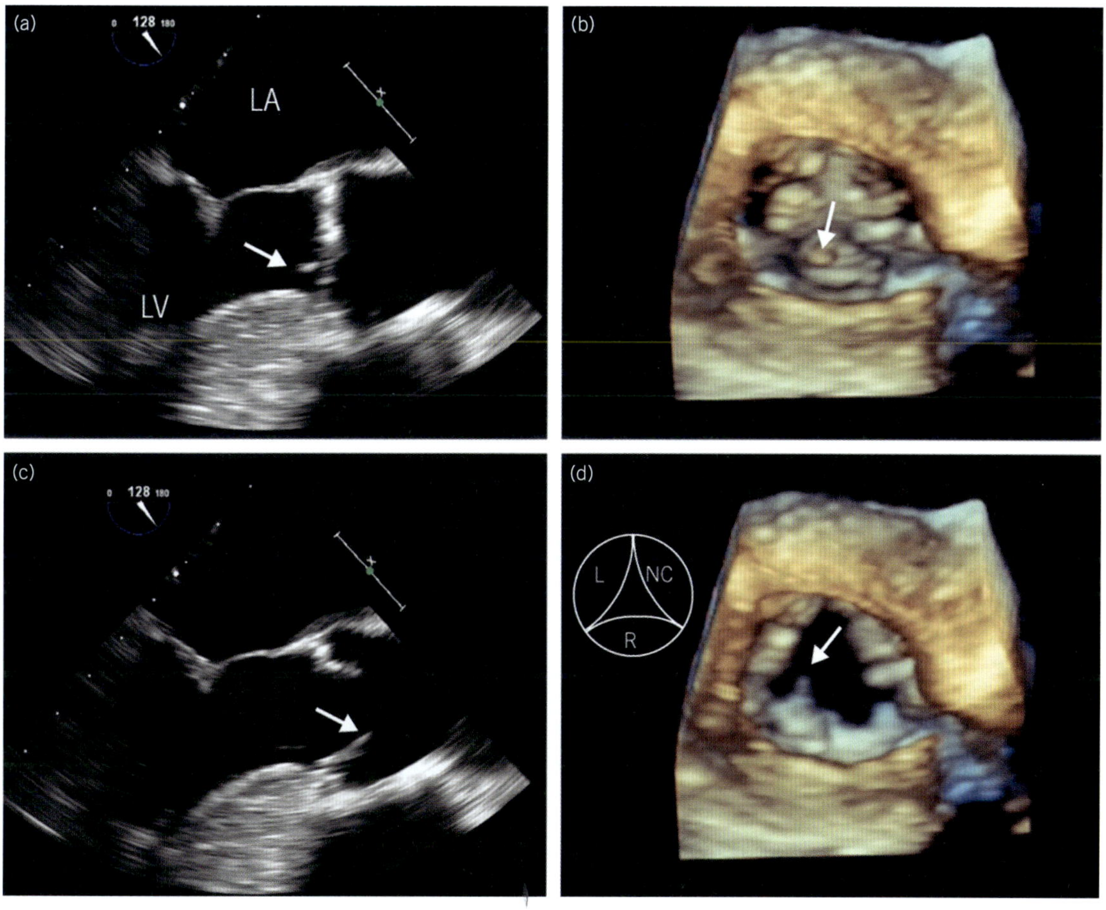

Figure 5.12 Valve strands attached to the right cusp of the AV. Frames (a) and (b) are in diastole, and frames (c) and (d) are in systole. (a) and (c) demonstrate the mid-oesophageal AV long-axis view; (b) and (d) are 3D *en face* views of the AV from the LVOT aspect. The orientation of the AV leaflets in the 3D views is demonstrated in the schematic. A small strand (arrows) can be seen attached to the right cusp of the AV. The strand prolapses into the LVOT in diastole and moves into the aortic root in systole. L, left coronary cusp; R, right coronary cusp; NC, non-coronary cusp.

sewing ring, struts, or hinge points and can be mistaken for sutures. Usually an incidental finding, their presence has been associated with an increased risk of embolic events.[11] However, detection is not independently associated with future embolic events.[12] Other differential diagnoses include thrombi, infective vegetations, and cardiac neoplasms.

Mitral annular calcification

Mitral annular calcification (MAC) is age-related deposition of calcium and lipid within the mitral annulus (see Online appendix 2.14) and occurs in approximately 10% of older adults. MAC causes acoustic shadowing, which impairs visualization of far-field structures. For instance, posterior MAC can make it difficult to assess RWMAs involving the basal inferolateral wall. The presence of MAC can make MV replacement or repair difficult, so detection of MAC is important in surgical planning. Involvement of the atrioventricular node can lead to heart block. When assessing MAC, attention must be paid to the presence of tissue density mobile masses (thrombus and vegetation), as MAC is a potential site for infective endocarditis. MAC is associated with the development of calcific AS, coronary artery disease, and stroke.

Rarely, caseous calcification of the mitral annulus can occur in patients with MAC. Fat and calcium accumulate in the posterior mitral annulus, resulting in a smooth, round, echo-dense mass with a central echolucent area. The differential diagnosis includes tumour, thrombus, or abscess.[13]

Lipomatous hypertrophy of the tricuspid annulus

Fat can accumulate in the tricuspid annulus, producing an echogenic mass in the right atrioventricular groove (Figure 5.13; see Online appendix 2.10). The lesion rarely has functional consequences but can make tricuspid annular dimension measurements challenging.

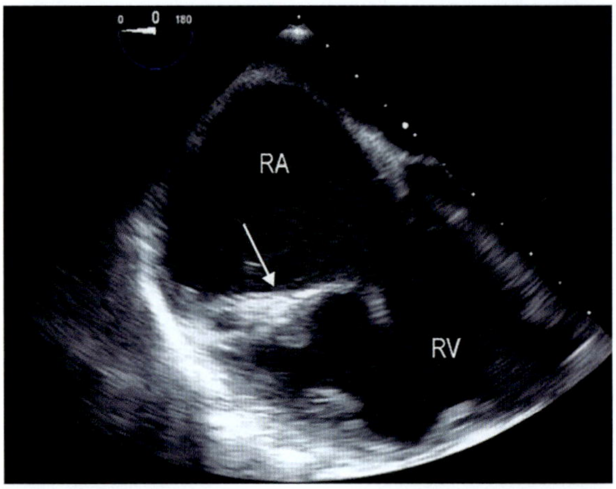

Figure 5.13 Hypertrophy of the tricuspid annulus. In this mid-oesophageal four-chamber view focused on the RV, marked hypertrophy (arrow) can be seen in the posterior tricuspid annulus. See Online appendix 2.10.

Pericardium

Transverse sinus

The transverse sinus is a fold of pericardium lying between the aorta and the pulmonary trunk anteriorly and the LA posteriorly. In the presence of pericardial fluid, it appears as an echolucent space adjacent to the aorta in the mid-oesophageal AV views (Figure 5.14; see Online appendix 2.9).[14] Fluid in the transverse sinus may be misinterpreted as a cyst, an abscess cavity, or an anomalous vessel. The absence of flow within the structure on colour Doppler imaging helps to distinguish it from the LA or LA appendage.

Oblique sinus

The oblique sinus is a fold of pericardium between the pulmonary veins and the posterior wall of the LA. This is a common site for blood to accumulate following cardiac surgery. Blood appears as either an echo-free (unclotted) or echo-dense (clotted) space between the LA and the oesophagus. Fluid in the oblique sinus must be differentiated from a pericardial cyst, which can occur in the same location.

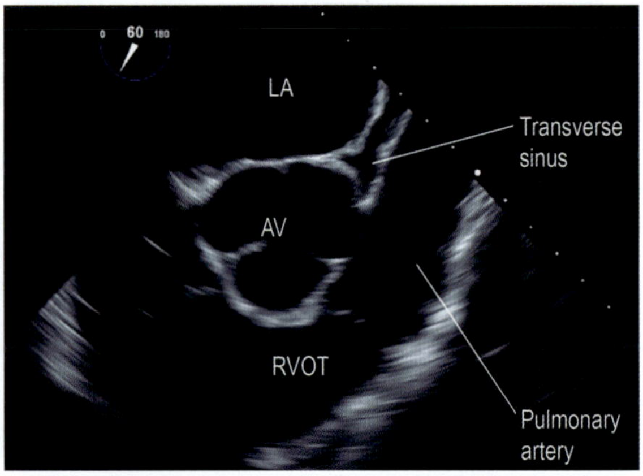

Figure 5.14 Transverse pericardial sinus. In this mid-oesophageal AV short-axis view, the transverse sinus can be seen between the LA, AV, and pulmonary artery. See Online appendix 2.9.

Cardiac masses and spaces

TOE is useful for detection of cardiac masses, including thrombi, vegetations, abscesses, tumours, cysts, and vascular abnormalities. Whilst TOE is useful for assessing the functional consequences of these lesions, it does not provide tissue diagnosis.

Expert tip: Echocardiographic characterization of a mass requires assessment of its size, attachment, and associated features, motion relative to adjacent structures, echogenicity, and other echo abnormalities. Soft tissue (myocardium, thrombi, and vegetations) typically appears grey (soft tissue reflectance), whereas connective tissue (chordae, heart valves, valve strands, fibroelastomas) typically appears white (connective tissue reflectance).

Thrombi

Left ventricular thrombi

LV thrombi usually form at the apex or apical segments of the LV (Figure 5.15) in association with RWMAs and/or low flow states, often associated with **spontaneous echo contrast (SEC)**. TOE has lower sensitivity than TTE for detection of LV apical thrombus due to the relatively greater distance between the echo probe and the LV apex, together with a propensity for the LV to be foreshortened in some TOE views. The LV apex is best seen in the mid-oesophageal two-chamber or long-axis view, with gentle retroflexion of the probe to reduce LV foreshortening. Selecting a lowerprobe frequency and carefully adjusting the contrast and focus settings can improve visualization of the apex.

LV thrombus may be mural, protruding, or mobile, and may be regular or irregular. *Mural* thrombus is seen adherent to the LV wall, with only one surface exposed to the LV cavity. *Protruding* thrombus is seen extending from the LV wall into the LV cavity. *Mobile* thrombus protrudes from the LV wall and displays independent motion. LV thrombi are typically homogenous and demonstrate soft tissue reflectance. Hence, thrombi may be hard to differentiate from the myocardium, normal trabeculations, and papillary muscles, particularly if small. The risk of embolization is highest with mobile thrombus, and lowest with mural thrombus; however, LV thrombus morphology frequently changes, particularly within the first months after formation. Options for management of LV thrombus include surgical removal, post-operative anticoagulation, or observation. If not removed at operation, surgical manipulation of the area should be minimized as much as possible, and insertion of devices such as LV vents or wires should be avoided. The region should be carefully inspected post-CPB to ensure that the thrombus has not changed or disappeared.

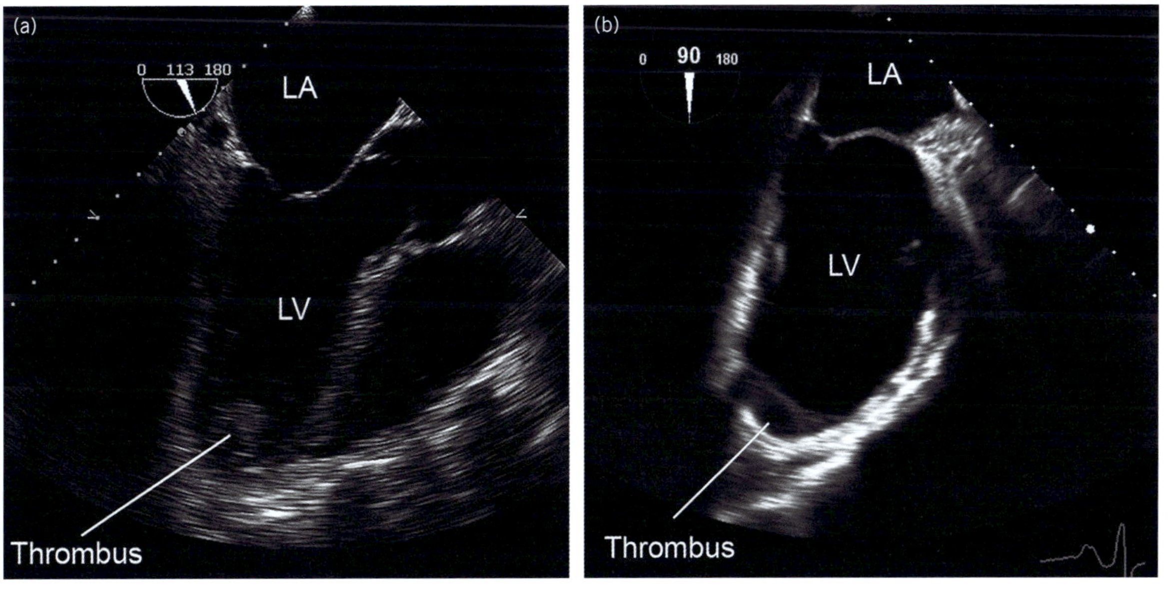

Figure 5.15 LV thrombi. Frame (a) is a mid-oesophageal long-axis view of a protruding thrombus at the LV apex. Frame (b) is a mid-oesophageal two-chamber view of a mural thrombus at the LV apex. Note the grey soft tissue appearance of the mass. See Online appendices 3.1.10 and 3.1.11.

> ***Expert tip: Thrombus formation is made possible by relative stasis of blood inside the heart. Consequently, it is rare for an LV thrombus to occur without an associated RWMA, usually an akinetic or aneurysmal myocardial segment.***

Left atrial thrombi

LA thrombus most commonly forms in the LA appendage. The development of LA thrombus is associated with LA chamber enlargement, and with blood stasis within the LA. Hence, atrial fibrillation and MS are strongly associated with LA thrombi (Figure 5.16; see Online appendices 3.1.5–3.1.9). Thrombus forms along a continuum, starting with SEC, progressing to *sludge* and finally to frank thrombus formation. The presence of dense SEC and peak flow velocities of <27 cm/s inside the LA appendage confer an increased risk of thromboembolic events. Risk of thromboembolism is also related to the shape of the LA appendage (Figure 17.10), with a chicken wing-shaped appendage having a lower risk than cactus, cauliflower, or windsock morphologies.[15,16]

The presence of pectinate muscles within the LA appendage can make identification of LA appendage thrombus challenging. Thrombi tend to be larger, rounder, and less regular than pectinate muscles. Pectinate muscles display continuity with, and similar echogenicity to, the appendage wall and lack the independent motion of a thrombus. 3D imaging, particularly simultaneous orthogonal plane imaging, is useful for differentiating pectinate muscles from thrombi. M-mode imaging is useful to identify independent motion of thrombus relative to atrial structures. Although rarely used in the perioperative context, intravenous echo contrast can help to differentiate between normal muscle and thrombus.

Right heart thrombi

Thrombi in the RA most commonly develop in the RA appendage, and contributing factors include atrial enlargement and low-flow states such as tricuspid stenosis. RA thrombus can also occur on vascular catheters, pacing wires, and ECMO cannulae (see Online appendices 3.1.1, 3.1.2, and 11.3.6). Uncommonly, thrombi in transit are seen in the right heart, having originated in the deep veins of the pelvis and extremities. In patients with a PFO and elevated right heart pressures, paradoxical passage of thrombus across the atrial septum is occasionally seen (Figure 5.17, see Online appendix 3.1.3). With large pulmonary embolism, TOE may detect significant thrombi in the main or right PAs (see Online appendix 8.8).

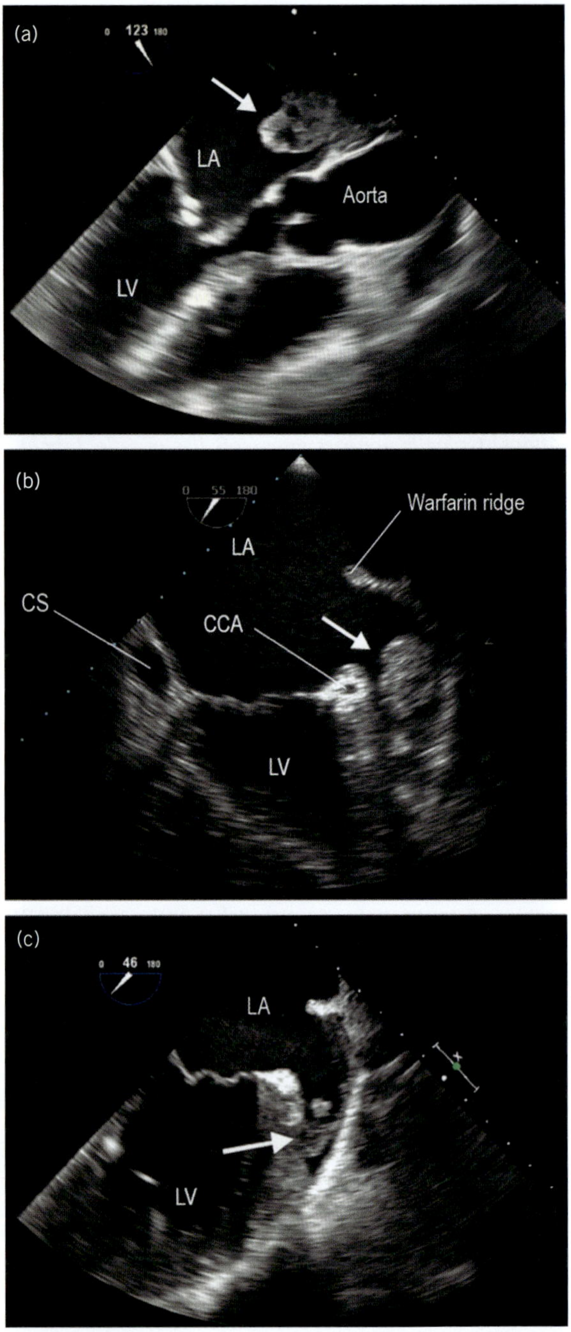

Figure 5.16 LA thrombi. Frame (a) is a mid-oesophageal long-axis view showing a thrombus (arrow) within the LA. Frames (b) and (c) are modified mid-oesophageal commissural views demonstrating thrombi (arrows) in the LA appendage. Frame (a) is from a patient with severe MS (note the thickened MV leaflets). Frames (b) and (c) are from patients with chronic atrial fibrillation. An incidental note is made of the coronary sinus (CS) and circumflex coronary artery (CCA).

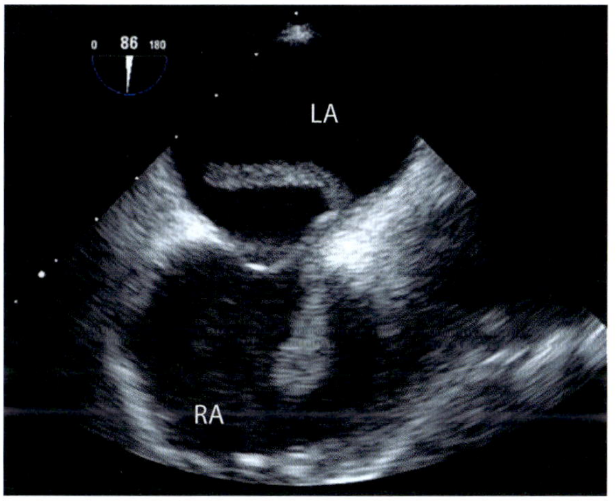

Figure 5.17 Thrombus in transit. A mid-oesophageal bicaval view showing a thrombus traversing the atrial septum across a patent foramen ovale. See Online appendices 3.1.3 and 3.1.4.

Vegetations

Vegetations are pathological masses of platelets, fibrin, and infected debris, arising from infective endocarditis. Typically, vegetations are adherent to valvular structures but may also be present on indwelling catheters and wires, at the site of atrial septal defects (ASDs) or VSDs, and in other congenital abnormalities. Abnormal native valves (such as bicuspid AV or prolapsed MV) and prosthetic valves are more susceptible to infection. Right-sided vegetations are commonly associated with intravenous drug use and indwelling lines. Infective vegetations are typically adherent to the *upstream* (low-velocity) aspect of heart valves (i.e. the LA side of the MV or the LV side of the AV). Vegetations are often irregular, with variable sizes from 0.1 to 3 cm in diameter, and have chaotic motion influenced by the cardiac cycle. 2D measurements often underestimate vegetation size compared with 3D measurements. 3D imaging is also useful to determine the site(s) of attachment and the presence of complications (perforation, abscess, fistulae) (Figure 5.18).

Native valve findings that may be misdiagnosed as infective endocarditis include valvular strands, papillary fibroelastoma, degenerative MV disease (e.g. myxomatous degeneration), MAC with mobile components, redundant chordae, healed vegetations, and non-bacterial thrombotic endocarditis. Prosthetic findings that may be confused with endocarditis include valve strands, thrombi, mitral subvalvular tissue remnants, and microcavitations. Vegetations and thrombi display soft tissue reflectance, whereas the other structures display connective tissue reflectance; thus, the distinction is usually between vegetations and thrombi. Unlike thrombi, vegetations can also cause valvular regurgitation, leaflet perforation, cardiac abscess or fistula, and, in the case of prosthetic valves, partial dehiscence resulting in new paravalvular regurgitation and rocking motion of the prosthesis.

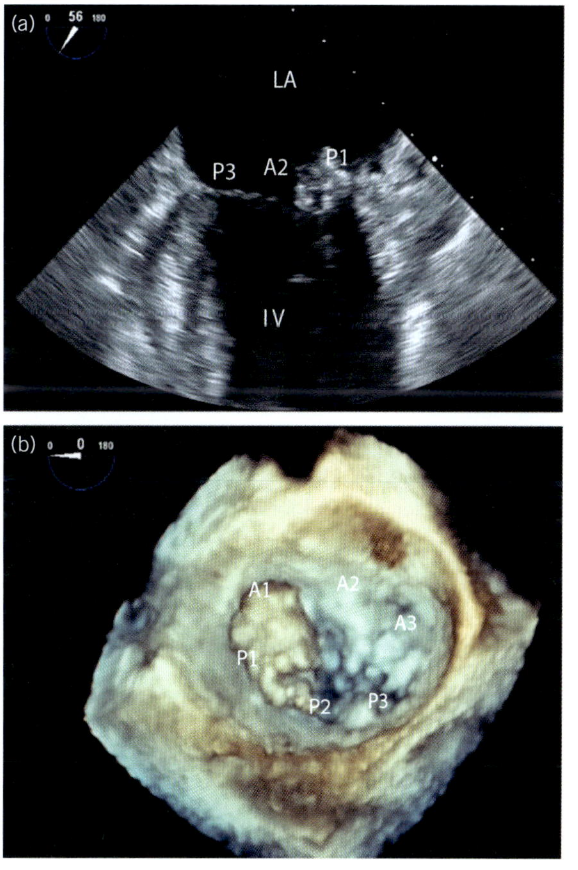

Figure 5.18 MV vegetation. (a) is a mid-oesophageal commissural view, and (b) is a 3D *en face* view of the MV from the atrial aspect in the surgical orientation. The mitral segments are indicated. A large vegetation can be seen in the A1/P1 region of the MV. See Online appendix 6.4.

Vegetations may embolize. Predictors for systemic embolism include vegetation size of >10 mm, highly mobile vegetations (prolapse across the coaptation plane of the valve during the cardiac cycle), abscess formation, MV endocarditis, and multiple valve involvement. Vegetation size of > 15 mm has been associated with increased mortality.[17,18]

TOE is superior to TTE for diagnosing endocarditis. However, it may still fail to detect small vegetations. If a high index of suspicion for endocarditis remains despite a negative study, the TOE examination should be repeated after several days.

Tumours

Cardiac tumours may be primary or secondary. Secondary tumours are more common than primary tumours, and spread to the heart from distant sites, extension via the IVC, or direct extension from the primary site. Most primary cardiac tumours are benign but can be clinically significant due to mass effect or embolic potential. Both 2D and 3D echocardiography are useful in the evaluation of cardiac tumours to establish the location, size, appearance, attachment, and mobility of a mass. Doppler is useful for evaluating haemodynamic consequences such as valve stenosis or regurgitation associated with the mass.

Benign primary cardiac tumours

Myxoma

Myxomas are the most common primary cardiac tumour, accounting for 25% of primary cardiac neoplasms and 50% of all primary benign tumours. In >75% of cases, myxomas arise in the LA, predominantly from the IAS (Figure 5.19; see Online appendices 3.2.7 and 3.2.8), with 5–20% of myxomas occurring in the RA. In 5% of cases, multiple synchronous cardiac myxomas are identified. Myxomas usually appear as large-diameter (1–15 cm) polypoid masses with soft tissue reflectance, attached to the wall by a stalk. The surface frequently has villous projections and may have adherent thrombus. Embolization is common and has been reported to occur in up to 30% of cases. Myxomas have variable vascularity and may contain focal calcification, areas of necrosis, or cystic lucency, features that can be useful to distinguish myxomas from a thrombus (avascular) or secondary tumour (highly vascular). Myxomas should be removed due to the embolic potential and risk of atrioventricular valve obstruction or leaflet damage. They may recur after incomplete resection, but recurrence is rare after complete resection. TOE is useful to establish the attachment point, to facilitate and document complete removal. Post-resection, TOE should also assess the absence of inadvertent damage to the atrial septum and/or relevant atrioventricular valve.

Papillary fibroelastoma

Papillary fibroelastomas are the second most common primary cardiac tumour in adults. Fibroelastomas are small (<1 cm diameter), 'pom-pom'-like pedunculated mobile masses, with a dense stalk and frond-like extensions of varying size (from several millimetres to several centimetres in diameter). They are usually attached to heart valves (most frequently left-sided valves) but can occur on any endocardial surface (Figure 5.20). The differential diagnosis includes valve strands, vegetations, thrombi, and myxomas. Fibroelastomas usually develop on the downstream side of the valve, in contrast to infective vegetations, and

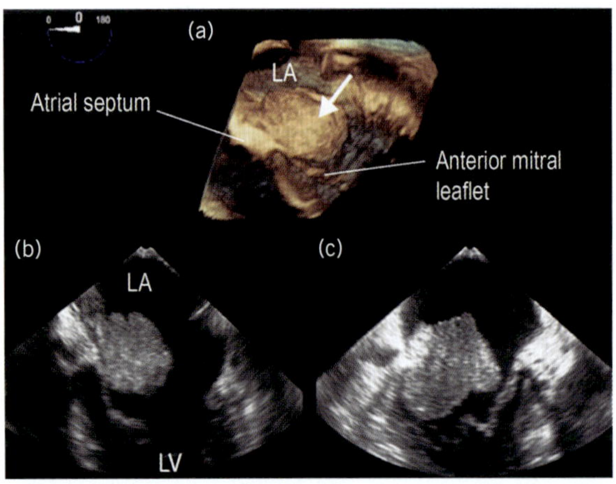

Figure 5.19 LA myxoma. (a) is a 3D zoomed view of the LA and MV, showing a large mass attached to the inter-atrial septum (arrow), consistent with myxoma. (b) and (c) are orthogonal views of the LA and MV obtained with biplane imaging, again showing the mass in the LA. The mass appears to be attached to the inter-atrial septum, although it is difficult to be certain in these still frames. See Online appendix 3.2.8.

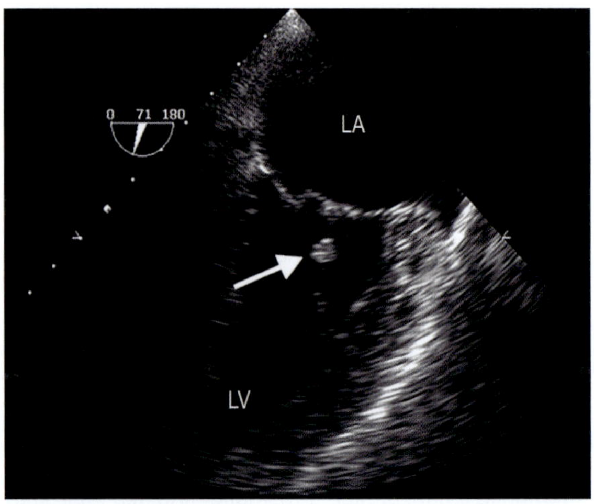

Figure 5.20 Papillary fibroelastoma. In this mid-oesophageal two-chamber view, a round mass (arrow), consistent with a papillary fibroelastoma, is attached to the subvalvular apparatus of the MV. See Online appendices 3.2.5 and 3.2.6.

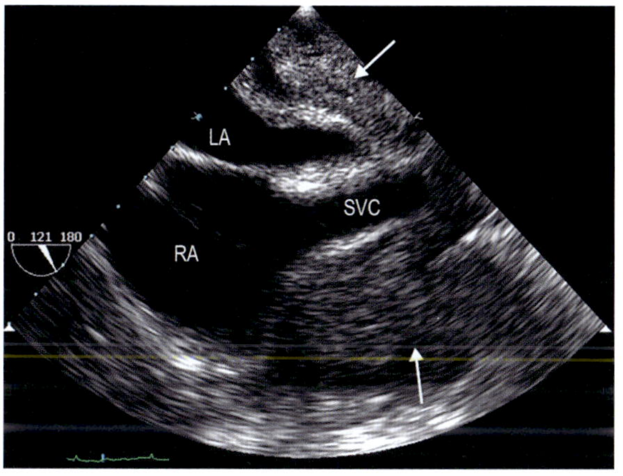

Figure 5.21 Angiosarcoma. In this mid-oesophageal bicaval view, two large masses are seen (arrows) compressing the LA and RA. The patient presented with clinical features of cardiac tamponade.

display connective tissue reflectance; these features, along with site, can aid in diagnosis. Platelet and fibrin aggregation may occur on fibroelastomas and cause embolization. Large, left-sided, and mobile papillary fibroelastomas present the highest risk. Fibroelastomas should therefore be surgically removed in patients with a history of embolization. Small tumours in asymptomatic patients may be observed.[19,20] Fibroelastomas do not recur following resection.

Other benign cardiac tumours

Lipomas and fibrolipomas are benign tumours of adipocytes that can occur anywhere in the heart or pericardium. These tumours tend to progressively enlarge and, if symptomatic, require excision. Lipomas and fibrolipomas are usually homogenous and encapsulated—differentiating them from lipomatous hypertrophy.

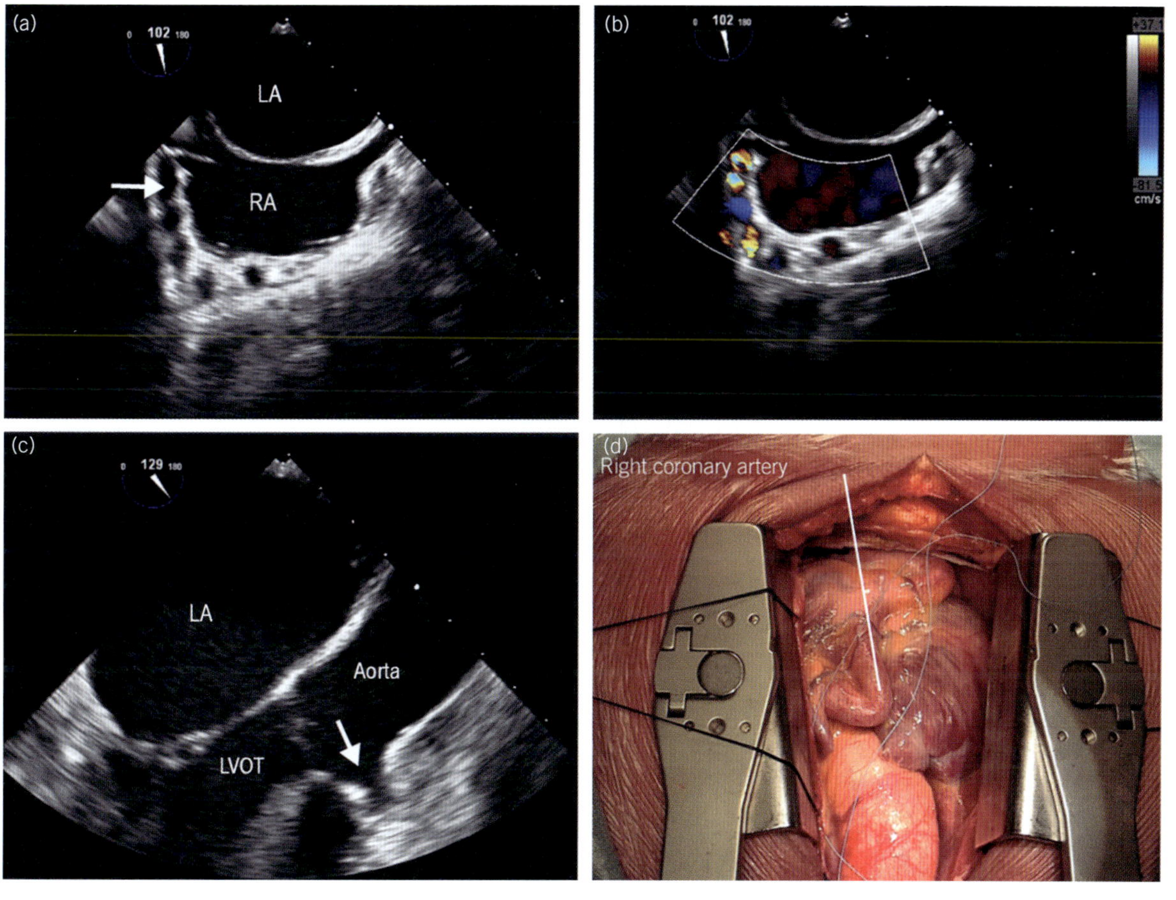

Figure 5.22 Right coronary artery aneurysm. (a) and (b) are mid-oesophageal bicaval views. Multiple cystic spaces can be seen around the inferior wall of the RA. With colour Doppler imaging, flow can be seen in the cystic spaces. (c) is a mid-oesophageal AV long-axis view, showing a wide orifice (arrow) to the right coronary artery. (d) At surgery, aneurysmal dilatation of the right coronary artery was identified. See Online appendix 3.3.

Table 5.1 Differentiating masses adherent to valves

	Reflectance	Location	Where on valve	Appearance	Mobility	Associated abnormalities
Lambl excrescence	Connective tissue (bright)	AV/MV > TV/PV	Coaptation line (native valves) Upstream side (atrial side of MV, LV side of AV)	Thin (<2 mm), 3–10 mm length	Undulating	None
Acute thrombus	Soft tissue (grey)	Mechanical > bioprosthetic >> nativeTV > AV	Upstream side most common	Variable size May be layered on leaflet in bioprosthesis	Moderate (usually less mobile than vegetations)	Subtherapeutic anticoagulation, valvular stenosis
Chronic thrombus	Connective tissue(bright)	Mechanical > bioprosthetic >> nativeTV> AV	Upstream side most common	Variable size (1–15 mm) May be layered on leaflets in bioprosthesis	Variable (may be immobile)	Valvular dysfunction
Infective vegetation	Soft tissue(grey)	All valves	Upstream side most common	Variable size Shaggy, lobulated	Variable, chaotic motion	Valvular dysfunction and destruction, abscess cavity, prosthetic valve dehiscence
Healed vegetation	Connective tissue(bright)	All valves	Upstream > downstream	Small, echogenic Often calcified	Less mobile	History of endocarditis Valvular dysfunction or destruction
Papillary fibroelastoma	Connective tissue(bright)	AV > MV > endocardial tissue	Downstream	2 mm to 2 cm in diameter Stalk attachment	Mobile	No valvular dysfunction

Rhabdomyomas are the most common benign cardiac tumours in children and usually involve the ventricles. They are usually multiple, homogenous, and hyperechoic, and may be intramural or extend into the cavity.

Malignant primary cardiac tumours

Only 25% of primary cardiac tumours are malignant, and almost all are sarcomas (angiosarcoma, rhabdosarcoma, fibrosarcoma). Malignant sarcomas are typically rapidly progressive, and infiltrate and disrupt adjacent cardiac anatomy (Figure 5.21). Usually, sarcomas are poorly demarcated and immobile. Pericardial effusion is common, and tumour extension into the IVC can occur.

Non-primary cardiac tumours

Non-primary tumours are much more common than primary cardiac tumours. They involve the heart by direct extension from adjacent structures or metastatic spread from distant sites. They are rarely seen as intracardiac masses, usually involving the pericardium rather than the heart itself, and often present with a pericardial effusion. The most common tumours to spread in this way are lung, lymphoma, breast, stomach, melanoma, liver, and colon cancers. Renal cell cancer can extend proximally inside the IVC.

Extracardiac masses

TOE may detect mediastinal tumours, pericardial cysts, and aneurysms or pseudoaneurysms of cardiovascular structures.

Pericardial cysts

Pericardial cysts appear as localized, discrete, fluid-filled structures overlying the heart. They are discussed in Chapter 16.

Coronary artery aneurysm

Coronary artery aneurysm may be congenital or acquired (e.g. Kawasaki disease), and may involve one or more coronary arteries. Typically tortuous, they are highly variable in size, length, and position. Congenital aneurysms may be associated with anomalous connections. On TOE, coronary artery aneurysms appear as echolucent spaces surrounding the heart, with flow evident on colour Doppler imaging. An aneurysmal orifice to the origin of one of the coronary arteries will confirm the diagnosis (Figure 5.22).

Table 5.1 summarizes the main characteristics of some of the most common masses that can be seen adherent to cardiac valves.

Multiple choice questions

Discover interactive multiple choice questions to test your knowledge on this chapter by searching for this book's title or ISBN (9780198873686) at **https://academic.oup.com** and going to the online appendix at the end of the book. Use your scratch-off code on the inside cover to access the material.

References

1. Faletra FF, Muzzarelli S, Dequarti MC, Murzilli R, BelluR, HoSY. Imaging-based right-atrial anatomy by computed tomography, magnetic resonance imaging, and three-dimensional transoesophageal echocardiography: correlations with anatomic specimens. *Eur Heart J Cardiovasc Imaging*2013;**14**:1123–31.
2. Schmid E, Scheule A, Locke A, Rosenberger P. Echocardiographic-guided placement of venous cannula due to inferior vena cava obstruction through a large Eustachian valve. *Anesth Analg*2010;**111**:76–8.
3. Kuroda M, Takahashi T, Mita N, Kagaya S, Miyoshi S, SaitoS. Difficult cannulation of the coronary sinus due to a large Thebesian valve. *Anesth Analg*2013;**116**:563–6.
4. Bonnin T, Roumegou P, Sridi S, *et al.* Prevalence and risk factors of cardiac thrombus prior to ventricular tachycardia catheter ablation in structural heart disease. *Europace*2023;**25**:487–95.
5. Gonzalez-Juanatey C, Testa A, Vidan J, *et al.* Persistent left superior vena cava draining into the coronary sinus: report of 10 cases and literature review: persistent left superior vena cava. *Clin Cardio*2004;**27**:515–18.
6. Suwa Y, Miyasaka Y, Taniguchi N, *et al.* Atrial fibrillation and stroke: importance of left atrium as assessed by echocardiography. *J Echocardiogr*2022;**20**:69–76.
7. Kim S, Liu H. Impairment of venous drainage due to atrial septal aneurysm during open-heart surgery. *J Cardiothorac Vasc Anesth*2013;**27**:1339–42.
8. Rigatelli G, Zuin M, Bilato C. Atrial septal aneurysm contribution to the risk of cryptogenic stroke in patients with patent foramen ovale: a brief updated systematic review and meta-analysis. *Trends Cardiovasc Med*2022;**33**:329–33.
9. Lee JY, Hur MS. Morphological classification of the moderator band and its relationship with the anterior papillary muscle. *Anat Cell Biol*2019;**52**:38–42.
10. Saha A, Roy S. Papillary muscles of right ventricle—morphological variations and its clinical relevance. *Cardiovasc Pathol*2018;**34**:22–7.
11. Leitman M, Tyomkin V, Peleg E, Shmueli R, Krakover R, Vered Z. Clinical significance and prevalence of valvular strands during routine echo examinations. *Eur Heart J Cardiovasc Imaging*2014;**15**:1226–30.

12. Saric M, Armour AC, Arnaout MS, *et al.* Guidelines for the use of echocardiography in the evaluation of a cardiac source of embolism. *J Am Soc Echocardiogr*2016;**29**:1–42.
13. Deluca G, Correale M, Ieva R, DelSalvatore B, GramenziS, DiBiaseetM. The incidence and clinical course of caseous calcification of the mitral annulus: a prospective echocardiographic study. *J Am Soc Echocardiogr*2008;**21**:828–33.
14. Rodriguez ER, Tan CD. Structure and anatomy of the human pericardium. *Prog Cardiovasc Dis*2017;**59**:327–40.
15. Di Biase L, Santangeli P, Anselmino M, *et al.* Does the left atrial appendage morphology correlate with the risk of stroke in patients with atrial fibrillation?*J Am Coll Cardiol*2012;**60**:531–8.
16. Yaghi S, Chang A, Ignacio G, *et al.* Left atrial appendage morphology improves prediction of stagnant flow and stroke risk in atrial fibrillation. *Circ Arrhythm Electrophysiol*2020;**13**:e008074.
17. Mohananey D, Mohadjer A, Pettersson G, *et al.* Association of vegetation size with embolic risk in patients with infective endocarditis: asystematic review and meta-analysis. *JAMA Intern Med*2018;**178**:502.
18. Yang A, Tan C, Daneman N, *et al.* Clinical and echocardiographic predictors of embolism in infective endocarditis: systematic review and meta-analysis. *Clin Microbiol Infect*2019;**25**:178–87.
19. Barbarossa A, Coraducci F, Cipolletta L, Guerra F, Dello RussoA. Very mobile left ventricular outflow tract papillary fibroelastoma presenting with multiple ischemic strokes: acase report and brief review of the literature. *J Cardiovasc Echogr*2022;**32**:222.
20. Pilato G, Argirò A, Barletta G, Del Bene MR. Papillary fibroelastoma of the right atrial appendage: is it that rare?*Ech ocardiography*2020;**37**:1308–11.

6 Left ventricular systolic function

Assessment of systolic LV function is an important component of every TOE examination performed in cardiac surgical patients. Prior to surgery, evaluation of LV function helps with risk stratification and identifies patients likely to have difficulty in separating from CPB or to need mechanical cardiovascular support.[1] Assessment of LV function in patients with haemodynamic instability guides fluid and inotropic therapy, and it identifies mechanical complications.

This chapter is divided into three sections: (1) assessment of global systolic function; (2) assessment of regional systolic function; and (3) cardiomyopathies. TOE-derived normal values for LV systolic function have not been published, and the guideline values provided in this chapter are derived from TTE studies (Table 6.1). Important discrepancies between values obtained from TTE and TOE are highlighted in the text.

Global LV systolic function

LV systolic dysfunction derives from one of three primary mechanisms: (1) impaired myocardial contractility; (2) volume overload; or (3) pressure overload. Impaired contractility may be due to insufficient coronary arterial flow or cardiomyopathy. Coronary insufficiency results in regional wall motion abnormalities (RWMAs), which, when extensive, lead to global LV dysfunction. LV volume overload results from MR or AR, or from intracardiac shunting (e.g. large VSD). Pressure overload exists when there is an obstruction to LV ejection, which may be mechanical (e.g. AS, aortic coarctation) or functional (hypertensive heart disease). In addition to these three primary mechanisms, LV function may be compromised by external compression (cardiac tamponade, constrictive pericarditis, tumours) or by RV dilation.

Table 6.1 Normal values for echocardiographic measures of LV function

Parameter	Male	Female
Internal dimension (mm)		
EDD	50 (42–58)	45 (38–52)
ESD	32 (25–40)	28 (22–35)
LV volume (biplane) (ml/m²)		
EDV	54 (34–74)	45 (29–61)
ESV	21 (11–31)	16 (8–24)
LV ejection fraction (%)	62 (52–72)	64 (54–74)
Wall thickness (mm)		
Septal wall (end-diastole)	6–10	6–9
Inferolateral wall (end-diastole)	6–10	6–10

Values are shown as mean and normal range. Data are derived from TTE measurements.

EDD, end-diastolic dimension; ESD, end-systolic dimension; EDV, end-diastolic volume; ESV, end-systolic volume.

Data are derived from TTE measurements; Lang RM, Badano LP, Mor-Avi V, Afilalo J, Armstrong A, Ernande L, *et al.*, Recommendations for cardiac chamber quantification by echocardiography in adults: an update from the American Society of Echocardiography and the European Association of Cardiovascular Imaging. *J Am Soc Echocardiogr.* 2015;28:1–39 e14.

There is significant overlap between LV systolic dysfunction and the clinical syndrome of heart failure. However, heart failure may occur without LV systolic dysfunction, for example in cases of RV dysfunction, LV diastolic dysfunction, or pericardial disease. Conversely, it is possible to have severe LV dysfunction and not exhibit clinical features of heart failure.

Preload, afterload, contractility, stroke volume, and left ventricular ejection fraction

Stroke volume is determined by contractility, preload, afterload, and ventricular geometry. **Contractility** is the intrinsic contractile strength of the ventricles and can be defined as the amount of work the heart can perform under constant loading conditions (i.e. constant preload and afterload). **Preload** is the myocardial fibre stretch immediately prior to the onset of contraction, which corresponds to LV end-diastolic volume (LVEDV). **Afterload** is ventricular wall stress (σ or 'T' in some physiology books) at the onset of systolic contraction and can be expressed by using the Laplace equation (Equation 6.1):

$$\sigma \alpha \frac{\Delta Pr}{w} \qquad \text{Equation 6.1}$$

where ΔP is the transmural pressure gradient across the LV wall, r is the radius of the LV cavity, and w is the wall thickness.

Thus, high intracavity pressure (e.g. arterial hypertension, AS) and ventricular dilation (e.g. chronic AR) increase LV afterload, whereas LV hypertrophy and raised intrathoracic pressure (e.g. positive pressure ventilation) reduce afterload. By the Frank–Starling mechanism, increasing preload proportionally increases stroke volume (SV) over the working range of the LV (see Chapter 21). An abrupt increase in afterload immediately reduces SV. Over the next few heartbeats, SV gradually recovers due to increased preload (secondary to ongoing systemic venous return). However, patients with impaired LV systolic function who are operating at the peak of their Starling curve are unable to increase SV. Such patients are said to have reduced preload reserve, and their SV is exquisitely sensitive to changes in afterload. Whilst preload is relatively simple to measure with echocardiography (as LVEDV), afterload and contractility cannot be as easily assessed.

SV can be calculated as the difference between LVEDV and LV end-systolic volume (LVESV), as (Equation 6.2):

$$SV = LVEDV - LVESV \qquad \text{Equation 6.2}$$

By extension, LVEF can be calculated by dividing SV by LVEDV (Equation 6.3):

$$LVEF = \frac{LVEDV - LVESV}{LVEDV} \qquad \text{Equation 6.3}$$

LVEDV and LVESV can be estimated from the mid-oesophageal four- and two-chamber views by using the method of discs (described later).

In patients with cardiac disease, LVEF is important prognostically, whereas SV and cardiac output are key factors that determine tissue oxygen delivery. As LVEF and SV are related by LVEDV, they do not always change in parallel (Equation 6.8). For instance, chronic heart failure is associated with low LVEF, but SV may be normal (if afterload is kept low) as LVEDV is high. By contrast, acute heart failure tends to reduce both LVEF and SV (as LVEDV is normal). Thus, if reduced LVEF is identified, it is important to determine whether cardiac output is also reduced. Because of ventricular foreshortening (Figure 6.1), SV tends to be underestimated by the volumetric technique and is best assessed by using Doppler techniques, outlined in Chapter 21.

3D TOE may improve the accuracy of SV assessment with both volumetric and Doppler methods. Volumetric methods improve because foreshortening is eliminated. With Doppler methods, the LVOT area is measured more precisely with 3D-guided measurements. Indeed, the LVOT is oval in >96% of patients, and thus 2D assumptions of a round orifice lead to systematic underestimation of the effective area.[2] The LVOT area can be measured using 3D multi-plane imaging by tracing the true cross-sectional area in short-axis views, as demonstrated in Figure 10.7.

Left ventricular size and wall thickness

LV systolic dysfunction is associated with abnormalities of ventricular size, shape, and wall thickness (Figure 6.2). Chamber size is typically normal or reduced with LV pressure overload, hypertrophic cardiomyopathy (HCM), and restrictive cardiomyopathy (RCM). LV enlargement is a feature of dilated cardiomyopathy (DCM), ischaemic cardiomyopathy, and chronic volume overload. LV enlargement also results in altered LV geometry. As the LV shape transitions from cylindrical to spherical, systolic tethering of the mitral leaflets and secondary MR may occur (see Chapter 8). Localized myocardial infarction (particularly anterior wall infarction) can result in LV remodelling and global LV dilation.

Left ventricular hypertrophy (LVH) is a condition in which there is an increase in LV mass. Two types of LVH

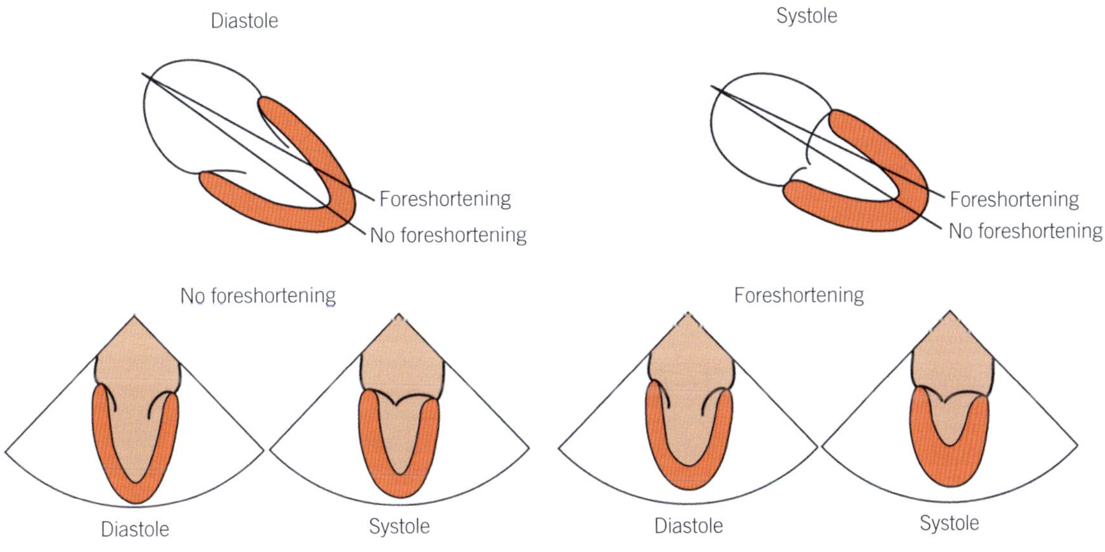

Figure 6.1 Ventricular foreshortening. Ventricular foreshortening reduces both LVEDV and LVESV; however, LVESV is disproportionately affected. Therefore, foreshortening leads to overestimated LVEF.

can be associated with LV systolic dysfunction: concentric and eccentric. Chronic pressure overload (see Online appendix 5.3.1) and HCM (see Online appendix 5.3.4) result in concentric hypertrophy where wall thickness is increased despite a normal chamber size. Concentric hypertrophy may be asymmetric, particularly with HCM. Chronic volume overload causes eccentric hypertrophy, as

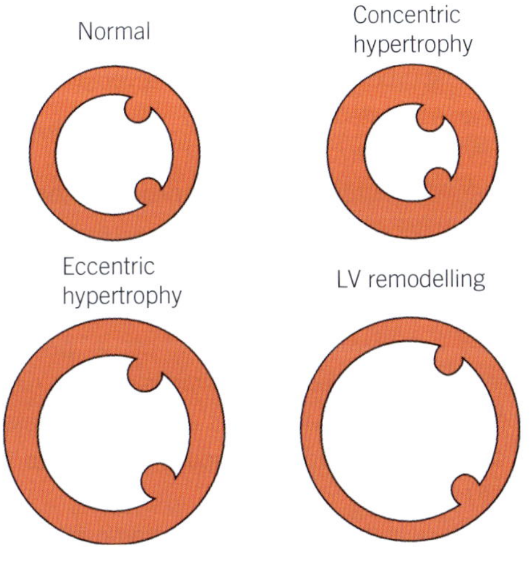

Figure 6.2 Abnormalities of LV size and wall thickness. With concentric hypertrophy, wall thickness is increased and chamber size is normal or reduced. With eccentric hypertrophy, wall thickness is normal or mildly increased and chamber size is increased. With LV remodelling, wall thickness is normal or reduced and chamber size is increased. See Online appendix 5.3.

wall thickness is increased in proportion to an increased chamber size. With DCM (see Online appendix 5.3.6) and post-myocardial infarction remodelling, LV wall thickness is typically reduced.

Two-dimensional echocardiography

2D parameters used for evaluating LV size include internal chamber dimensions, LV area, and LV volume.

TTE guidelines recommend measuring internal chamber dimensions and wall thickness in the parasternal long-axis view.[3] TOE guidelines recommend measuring chamber dimensions with M-mode or 2D imaging in the *transgastric mid-papillary short-axis view* (Figure 6.3).[4] Foreshortening or oblique imaging (suggested by an oval-shaped LV) can result in wall thickness and chamber dimensions being overestimated. TOE measurements are made at the *mid-anterior* and *mid-inferior* walls (see Online appendix 5.1.1), whereas TTE measurements are made at the basal anteroseptal and inferolateral walls.[3] Note that wall thickness should be measured at *end-diastole*.

One tool to help distinguish between concentric and eccentric hypertrophy is to measure *relative wall thickness* (RWT), which is defined as (Equation 6.4):

$$RWT = \frac{2PWT_d}{LVEDD} \qquad \text{Equation 6.4}$$

where PWT_d is the posterior (inferolateral) wall thickness at end-diastole and LVEDD is LV end-diastolic dimension.

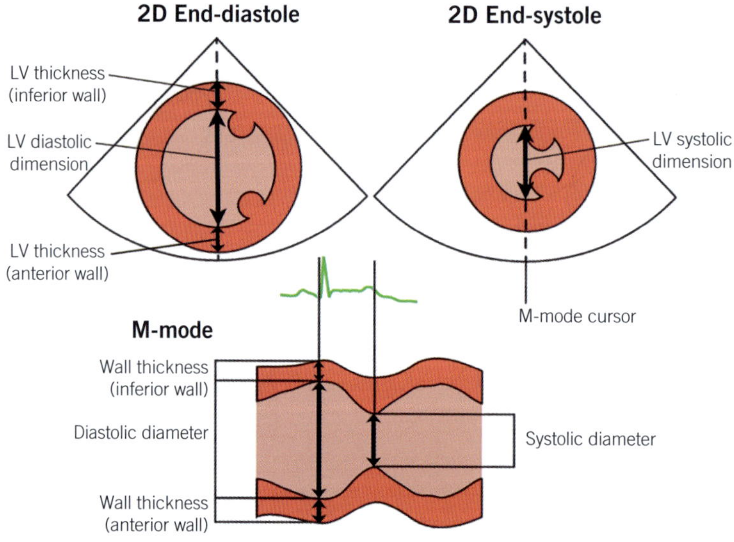

Figure 6.3 Measurement of wall thickness and internal chamber dimensions. Measurements should be made in the transgastric mid-papillary short-axis view at end-diastole (largest chamber size) and end-systole (smallest chamber size) using 2D or M-mode imaging. Wall thickness should be measured at end-diastole. See Online appendices 5.1.1 and 5.1.2.

An RWT >0.42 suggests concentric hypertrophy, whereas normal wall thickness and eccentric hypertrophy are associated with an RWT <0.42.[3] Note that this TTE concept has not been formally validated by TOE but may be helpful in some cases.

Three-dimensional echocardiography

3D echocardiography transcends 2D geometrical assumptions, provides more precise measurements of LV dimensions and volumes, and correlates better with cardiac magnetic resonance imaging (MRI) than 2D echocardiography, despite limitations in spatial resolution. Underestimation of volume and overestimation of LVEF with 3D echocardiography may still occur in patients with decreased LVEF, because trabecular abnormalities may impair automated endocardial border detection.[5] Endocardial detection is improved by manually correcting the cavity border to include trabeculations rather than the endocardium, and by increasing temporal and spatial resolution using multi-beat acquisition. 3D-derived LV mass evaluation has remained challenging for similar reasons but correlates more closely with MRI despite lower values than 2D echocardiography.[6] 3D LV volume and mass measurements correlates better with prognostic data in non-cardiac surgical applications, and this may eventually translate to the preferential use of 3D assessment during cardiac surgery.[7]

Although there are no official guideline reference ranges for normal LV volumes and mass by 3D echocardiography, European Association of Cardiovascular Imaging (EACVI) Normal Reference Ranges for Echocardiography (NORRE) and the World Alliance Societies of Echocardiography Normal Value studies provide high-quality data with age and gender differences for readers to refer to.[6,8]

Global left ventricular systolic function

LV systolic function is assessed qualitatively or quantitatively. For qualitative assessment, the echocardiographer visually estimates global systolic function by using a severity rating (from hyperdynamic to severely depressed) or within an estimated range of LVEF values (e.g. >70% to <20–25%). Qualitative assessment is a reliable method, compared with automated 2D bi-plane methods, with good inter-observer correlation but requires training and experience.[9,10]

Most quantitative techniques calculate the fractional change of a parameter expressed as a percentage. Parameters include short-axis dimensions (to calculate **fractional shortening**), short-axis area (to calculate **fractional area change**), and ventricular volume (to calculate **LVEF**).

End-diastole is defined as the first frame after MV closure or, alternatively, when the LV dimension is largest. End-systole is defined as the frame after AV closure or, alternatively, when the LV dimension is smallest.[3] Timing end-diastole to the R-wave of the ECG is not recommended due to the time delay between the electrical activity and the mechanical activity of the heart.

Fractional shortening

Fractional shortening (FS) is defined as (Equation 6.5):

$$FS = \frac{LVEDD - LVESD}{LVEDD} \quad \text{Equation 6.5}$$

FS is measured in the transgastric mid-papillary short-axis view with 2D or M-mode imaging (Figure 6.3). It is important to centre the M-mode beam *perpendicularly* to avoid overestimation from oblique imaging, and *centrally* through the short axis of the LV to avoid underestimation.

Despite good correlation between FS and LVEF, FS is unreliable in the presence of RWMAs. RWMAs at the site of interrogation (mid-anterior and mid-inferior walls) lead to underestimation of LV function and overestimation when RWMAs are distant from the site of interrogation (e.g. akinetic LV apex).

Mitral annular plane systolic excursion

During systole, the mitral annulus moves towards the relatively stationary apex, shortening the long axis of the LV. In the mid-oesophageal four-chamber view, mitral annular plane systolic excursion (MAPSE) is measured at the lateral mitral annulus with the M-mode cursor placed parallel to the longitudinal motion of the heart (Figure 6.4). MAPSE provides a measure of global LV function that is useful when endocardial definition is poor. The technique has been validated with TTE, rather than with TOE, with values of ≥13 mm for men and ≥11 mm for women defined as normal LV function, and a value <6 mm indicative of severely reduced LVEF.[11]

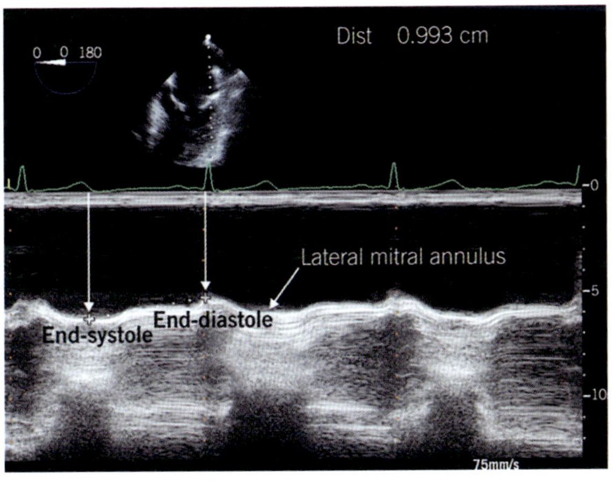

Figure 6.4 Mitral annular plane systolic excursion (MAPSE). In this mid-oesophageal four-chamber view, the M-mode cursor was placed across the lateral mitral annulus. The difference in position of the mitral annulus between end-diastole and end-systole is measured, which, in this example, is 0.993 cm.

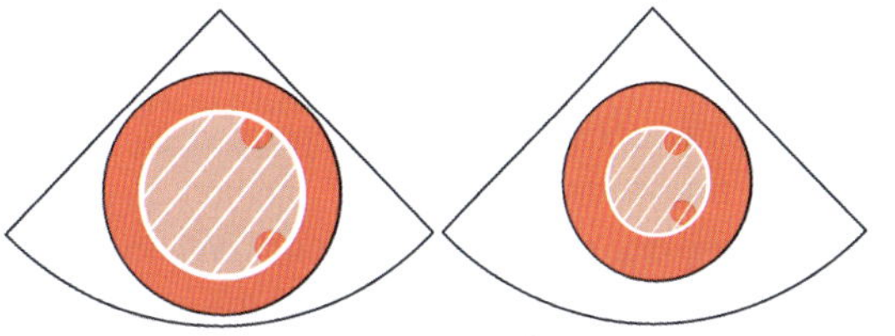

Figure 6.5 Measurement of FAC. End-diastolic (largest chamber size) and end-systolic (smallest chamber size) frames are identified in the transgastric mid-papillary short-axis view. The tracing goes around the papillary muscles (i.e. they are included in the LV volume). Hypothetical normal values are shown. LVEDA, LV end-diastolic area; LVESA, LV end-systolic area. See also Online appendix 5.1.2.

Fractional area change

Fractional area change (FAC) is defined as (Equation 6.6):

$$FAC = \frac{LVEDA - LVESA}{LVEDA} \quad \text{Equation 6.6}$$

where LVESA is LV end-systolic area and LVEDA is LV end-diastolic area.

FAC is measured in the transgastric mid-papillary short-axis view (Figure 6.5; see Online appendix 5.1.2). The 'blood pool' is included in the measurement, meaning the trace should go around the papillary muscles (Figure 6.5). The endocardial borders of the septum and the lateral walls are often poorly visualized, as they lie parallel to the echo beam. In such instances, the trace should be extrapolated to form a smooth curve.

Perioperatively, FAC is often used to assess global LV systolic function as it requires only a single view and is not influenced by ventricular foreshortening. FAC is measured in the same view used for monitoring preload (changes in LVEDA; see Chapter 21) and myocardial ischaemia. FAC may overestimate LVEF in the presence of basal or apical aneurysms. Reference values for FAC and LV short-axis areas are not well defined, but as a rule of thumb, FAC is approximately 10% less than LVEF.[12]

Ejection fraction

LVEF is defined as (Equation 6.7):

$$LVEF = \frac{LVEDV - LVESV}{LVEDV} \quad \text{Equation 6.7}$$

Or as (Equation 6.8):

$$LVEF = \frac{SV}{LVEDV} \quad \text{Equation 6.8}$$

The mathematical model recommended by the ASE/EACVI is the modified Simpson's method (method of discs, biplane disc summation method).[3] With the method of discs, LV volume (*V*) is calculated as the summation of the volume of a stack of 20 discs, as (Equation 6.9):

$$V = (\pi/4)\sum_{i=1}^{20} a_1 b_1 \times (L/20) \quad \text{Equation 6.9}$$

where *L* is the long axis length of the LV, $\sum_{i=1}^{20} a_1 b_1$ is the sum of areas of 20 discs (i_1 to i_{20}) of diameters *a* and *b* obtained from two orthogonal TOE views—the mid-oesophageal four-chamber and two-chamber views (Figure 6.6).

The main pitfall in the TOE assessment of ventricular volumes and LVEF is the underestimation of ventricular volumes due to ventricular foreshortening. This is particularly true in the four-chamber view where foreshortening can be minimized by gentle retroflection of the probe to demonstrate the true apex. As LVEF is based on volume *ratios*, rather than on absolute values, it is less impacted by foreshortening than by ventricular volumes. However, since foreshortening disproportionately affects LVESV, compared with LVEDV, foreshortening tends to overestimate LVEF (Figure 6.1; see Online appendices 5.1.3 and 5.1.4).

The main advantage of the method of discs over other techniques like FS or FAC is that there are few geometric assumptions and shape distortion is accounted for as long as the distortions are visualized.

3D imaging allows accurate imaging of ventricular volumes, LVEF, and SV, and the issue of foreshortening is largely eliminated. Perioperative data are limited, but 3D TOE appears to show similar feasibility and reproducibility, compared with 2D-TOE. It has not been directly compared with MRI.[13]

Semi-automated 3D LV volume quantitation begins with 2D mid-oesophageal four-chamber imaging, including the apex, LVOT, and MV apparatus, to allow proper landmarking (Figure 6.7; see Online appendix 5.1.5). Full-volume acquisition can be performed via two methods: real-time (live) imaging and multi-beat ECG-gated imaging. Real-time imaging provides single-beat acquisition but suffers from decreased spatial resolution, given the high number of scan lines that must be obtained to

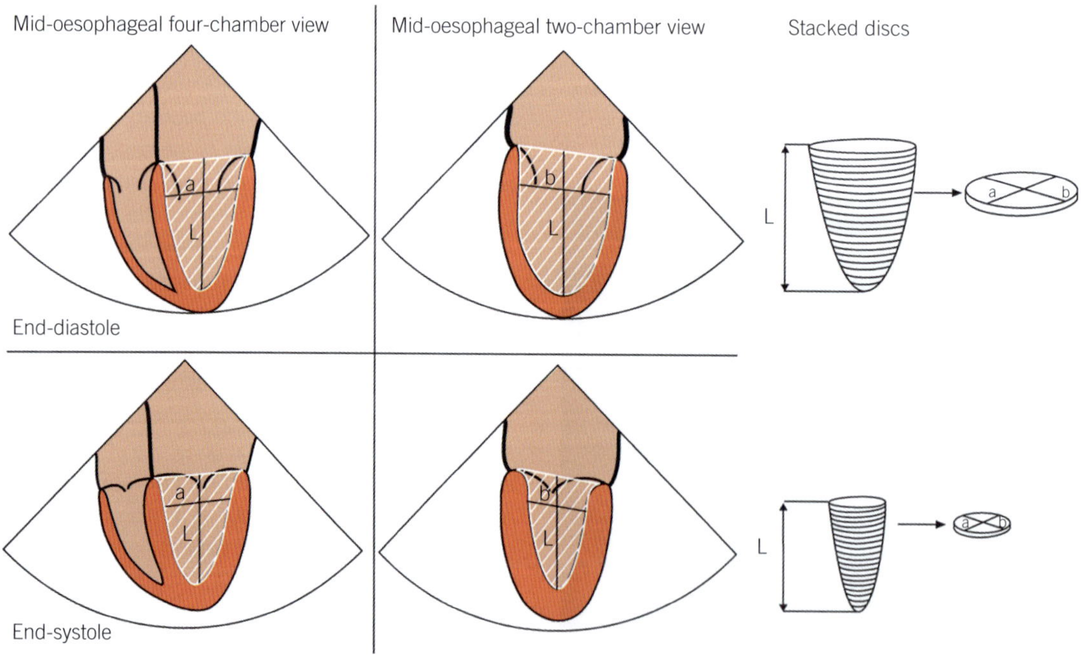

Figure 6.6 Measurement of LVEF using the method of discs (modified Simpson's method). End-diastolic and end-systolic frames are identified in the mid-oesophageal four-chamber and two-chamber views. The areas are traced, and the long-axis marker is placed through the apex to provide the length (L) of the LV. Diameter *a* is obtained from the four-chamber view, and diameter *b* from the two-chamber view, and the machine software automatically calculates LVESV and LVEDV based on 20 stacked discs. Using Equation 6.7, the machine then calculates the LVEF. See also Online appendices 5.1.3 and 5.1.4.

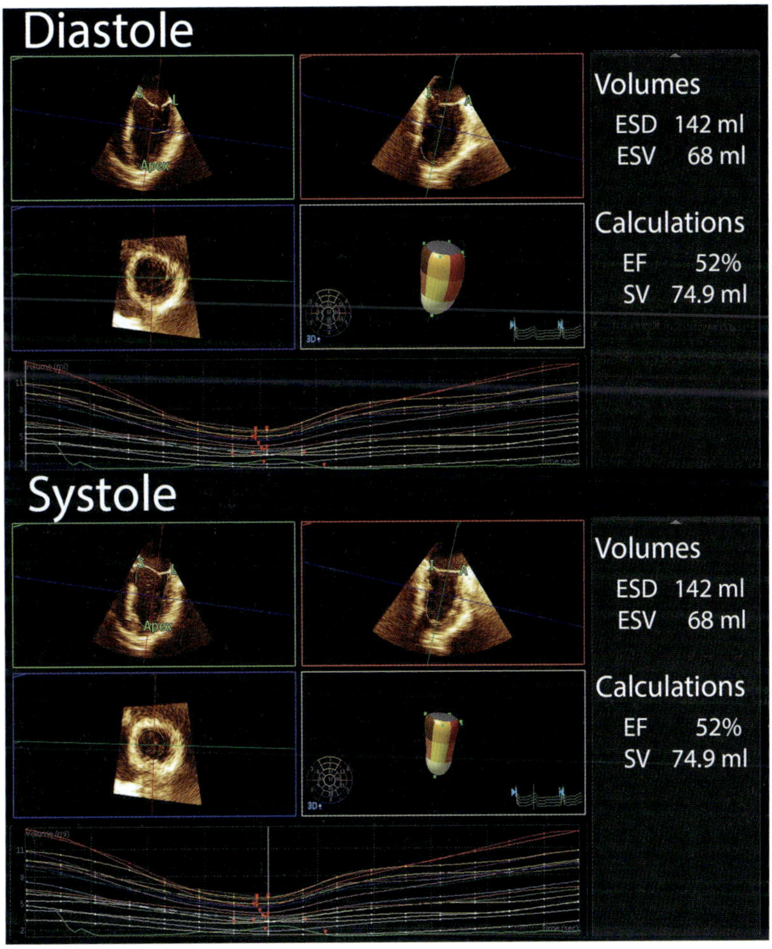

Figure 6.7 3D assessment of LV volumes, LVEF, and SV using multi-planar reconstruction. Measurements are made at end-diastole and end-systole in two orthogonal views. The operator manually marks the mitral annulus and the LV apex, then the machine software automatically identifies the endocardial surface and calculates the LVEDV, LVESV, LVEF, and SV. See text for details, and Online appendices 5.1.5 and 5.1.6.

complete a volume. Multi-beat imaging compensates for this problem by acquiring sequential portions of the full volume over multiple beats and creating an aggregate image. This method provides increased spatial resolution, whilst maintaining temporal resolution, but can suffer from stitching artefacts (see Chapter 2). Respiration causing heart displacement is a major cause of stitching artefact, and this is corrected in an anaesthetized patient by pausing the ventilator. Arrhythmias and electrocautery causing irregular R-R interval or poor-quality ECG tracing are also frequent causes of stitching artefacts.

Most software currently employs a semi-automated process, for which the apex and mitral annulus will be marked by the operator in at least two perpendicular views. An automatic delineation of the endocardial border is performed and displayed for manual correction. The system software then makes volume calculations. Automated software has two limitations: it cannot compensate for dropout or a significant trabecular burden. Like for FAC, trabeculations should be included as *part of the cavity*, rather than the wall, to minimize the risk of volume underestimation.

Optimization begins with good -quality 2D imaging, free of significant areas of dropout or uneven power signal. Temporal resolution is improved by minimizing the capture volume or decreasing the line density, although this comes at the expense of spatial resolution. Gain must be adjusted during initial capture, as post-processing cannot compensate for areas of dropout or decreased resolution. The operator should aim for even gain levels across the whole ventricle, using time-gain compensation (TGC) rather than overall power gain (see Chapter 1). Dropout areas may be related to poor windows or undergaining, which may be resolved by adjusting gain, TGC, compression, and dynamic range.

Using ASE/EACVI guidelines, LVEF may be classified as normal (52–72%), mildly depressed (41–51%), moderately depressed (30–40%), or severely depressed (<30%).[3]

Myocardial velocity, strain, and strain rate

Two techniques have become widely used for assessing systolic ventricular function in echocardiography laboratories: TDI and speckle tracking.[14] Both techniques allow myocardial velocity, strain, and strain rate (SR) to be measured, and provide information on global and regional myocardial function.

Tissue Doppler imaging

TDI measures myocardial velocity and may be used in PW or colour modes. Myocardial tissue velocities are much lower (<15 cm/s) than blood velocities through cardiac valves (>50 cm/s). PW-TDI measures *peak instantaneous velocity*, whereas colour TDI measures *mean velocity*, which is about 20% lower. PW-TDI data are displayed as a standard velocity–time curve (Figure 6.8) and cannot be subjected to further processing. By contrast, colour-coded TDI data can undergo offline post-processing to generate strain and SR curves (explained later).

In general, reduced myocardial velocity is indicative of impaired systolic function. However, interpretation of myocardial velocity waveforms is subject to several

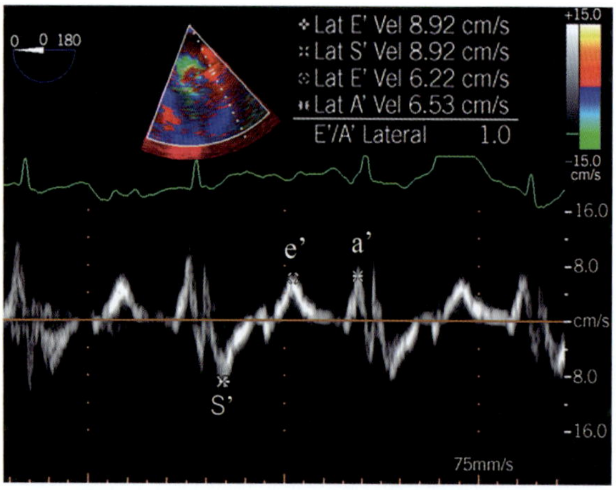

Figure 6.8 Normal PW-TDI waveform obtained from the septal and lateral mitral annulus. Systolic (S'), early diastolic (e'), and late diastolic (a') waveforms are shown. Because the mitral annulus moves away from the transducer towards the apex in systole, the S' wave is displayed below the baseline. The diastolic waves are discussed in Chapter 7.

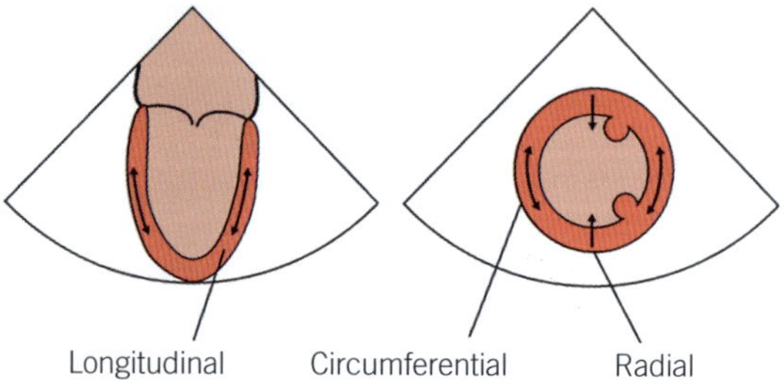

Figure 6.9 Directions of myocardial fibre shortening during systole.

confounding factors. Systolic motion is complex and involves longitudinal, circumferential, and radial contraction (Figure 6.9). TDI techniques measure only a single component of the velocity vector. Furthermore, velocity varies throughout the LV, being lower in the apical than in basal segments and lower in the anterior than in the inferolateral wall. To avoid underestimating velocity, the TDI signal must be well aligned with the velocity vector, which may be difficult with TOE. Finally, TDI signals do not distinguish between active myocardial contraction and myocardial motion due to tethering.

Speckle tracking imaging

Speckle tracking is a technique for measuring myocardial velocity, strain, and SR, based on tracking the movement of speckles seen on grey scale 2D images (Figure 6.10). *Angle independence* is the main advantage of speckle tracking over PW or colour-coded TDI for measuring strain and SR. Speckle tracking is performed online or offline on stored 2D images.

Strain and strain rate

Strain is the fractional change in length of a myocardial segment. Strain is dimensionless and usually expressed as a positive or negative percentage change. Thus, stretching a rubber band from 10 to 15 cm equates to a strain of +50%. **Strain rate (SR)** is the rate of change of strain and has units of s^{-1}.

SR is calculated as the difference in velocity (v) at two sample points divided by the distance between them (d), as (Equation 6.10):

$$SR = \frac{v_1 - v_2}{d} \qquad \text{Equation 6.10}$$

Strain (e) is then calculated as the integral of SR with respect to time, as (Equation 6.11):

$$e = \int SR.dt \qquad \text{Equation 6.11}$$

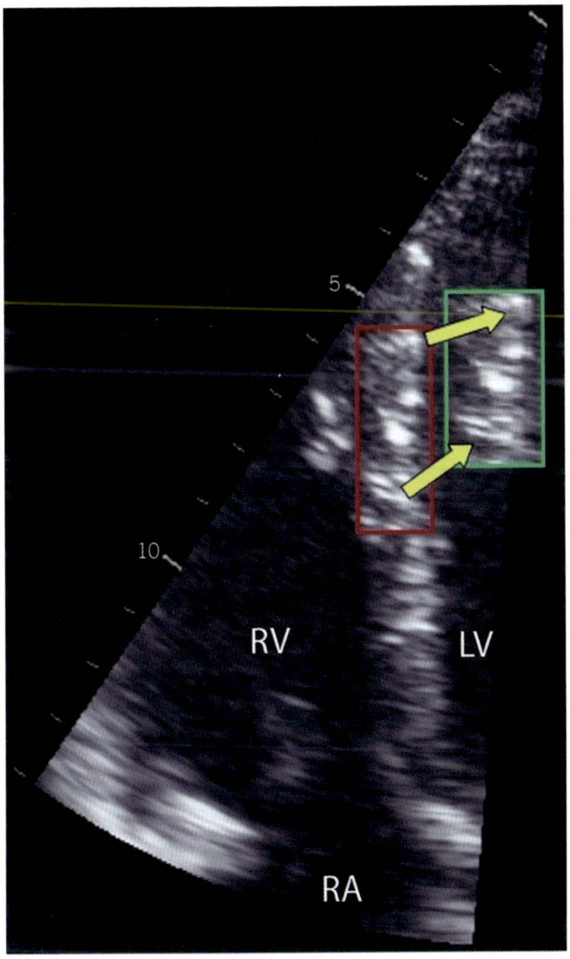

Figure 6.10 Speckle tracking. The red square represents the location of the speckles at end-diastole, and the green square the location of the speckles at end-systole. Note that both longitudinal shortening and radial thickening of the green square affect the change in distance between the speckles due to myocardial deformation.

Reproduced with permission from Teske AJ, De Boeck BWL, Melman PG *et al.*, Echocardiographic quantification of myocardial function using tissue deformation imaging, a guide to image acquisition and analysis using tissue Doppler and speckle tracking, *Cardiovascular Ultrasound*, 2007, 5, 27, Figure 8. © Teske *et al*; licensee BioMed Central Ltd. 2007. This article is published under license to BioMed Central Ltd. This is an Open Access article distributed under the terms of the Creative Commons Attribution License (http://creativecommons.org/licenses/by/2.0), which permits unrestricted use, distribution, and reproduction in any medium, provided the original work is properly cited.

Strain is *negative* when the myocardium *shortens* and, by convention, displayed below the baseline on a strain–time curve (Figure 6.11). SR is the *slope of the strain curve* (Figure 6.11). The steeper the strain curve, the more positive the SR curve. Strain and SR curves can be generated for each of the velocity vectors (longitudinal, circumferential, and radial). Strain may be calculated for an entire myocardial wall (global strain) or for an individual myocardial segment (regional strain). In general, reduced strain and SR indicate myocardial dysfunction. The main advantage of strain and SR over velocity measures is that the former can distinguish active contraction from passive movement, which is of particular use in ischaemic-induced hypokinesia.

Assessment of global left ventricular function by tissue Doppler and speckle tracking

Speckle tracking echocardiography (STE) has, for the most part, completely replaced colour and PW-TDI for myocardial assessment in TTE, with the exception of diastology. TOE-derived STE strain and SR measurements are feasible in the operating room, but less widely used than in diagnostic laboratory TTE. Both modalities correlate well, with a non-significant trend towards less negative values in TOE.[15] Data for TTE strain and SR measurements have shown prognostic capabilities for a large range of conditions, including chemotherapy-induced cardiomyopathy, AS, and ischaemic cardiomyopathy.

Strain analysis

Strain can be measured in different vectors and in different parts of the cardiac cycle. Most of current STE research involves peak systolic strain, with emerging data on diastolic STE. Peak systolic strain can be analysed per segment, providing a map of regional strain and SR, or as a global measure, providing a mean peak systolic strain for all segments.[16] Regional STE is helpful for analysis of RWMAs that can identify early ischaemia and specific cardiomyopathies such as HCM. Global STE provides a numerical value that can track temporal changes in global cardiomyopathies such as in chemotherapy-related cardiomyopathy.

Strain vectors are related to the direction of deformation of specific muscle fibres during cardiac contraction, as depicted in Figure 6.9. **Longitudinal strain**, or myocardial shortening from base to apex, predominantly reflects the function of longitudinal subendocardial fibres in providing the bulk of contraction and this is most prone to ischaemic insults. Global longitudinal strain (GLS) is derived from the mean of the peak systolic strain of all longitudinal segments and is the commonly reported value. **Circumferential strain** measures short-axis systolic shortening and myocardial wall shortening in this axis. It is best obtained in the transgastric mid-papillary short-axis view. **Radial strain** represents mostly subepicardial and subendocardial transmural deformations and myocardial thickening from the endocardium to the epicardium, as there are no radial fibres. Circumferential and radial strain have been studied but currently lack prognostic data in TTE and TOE applications.

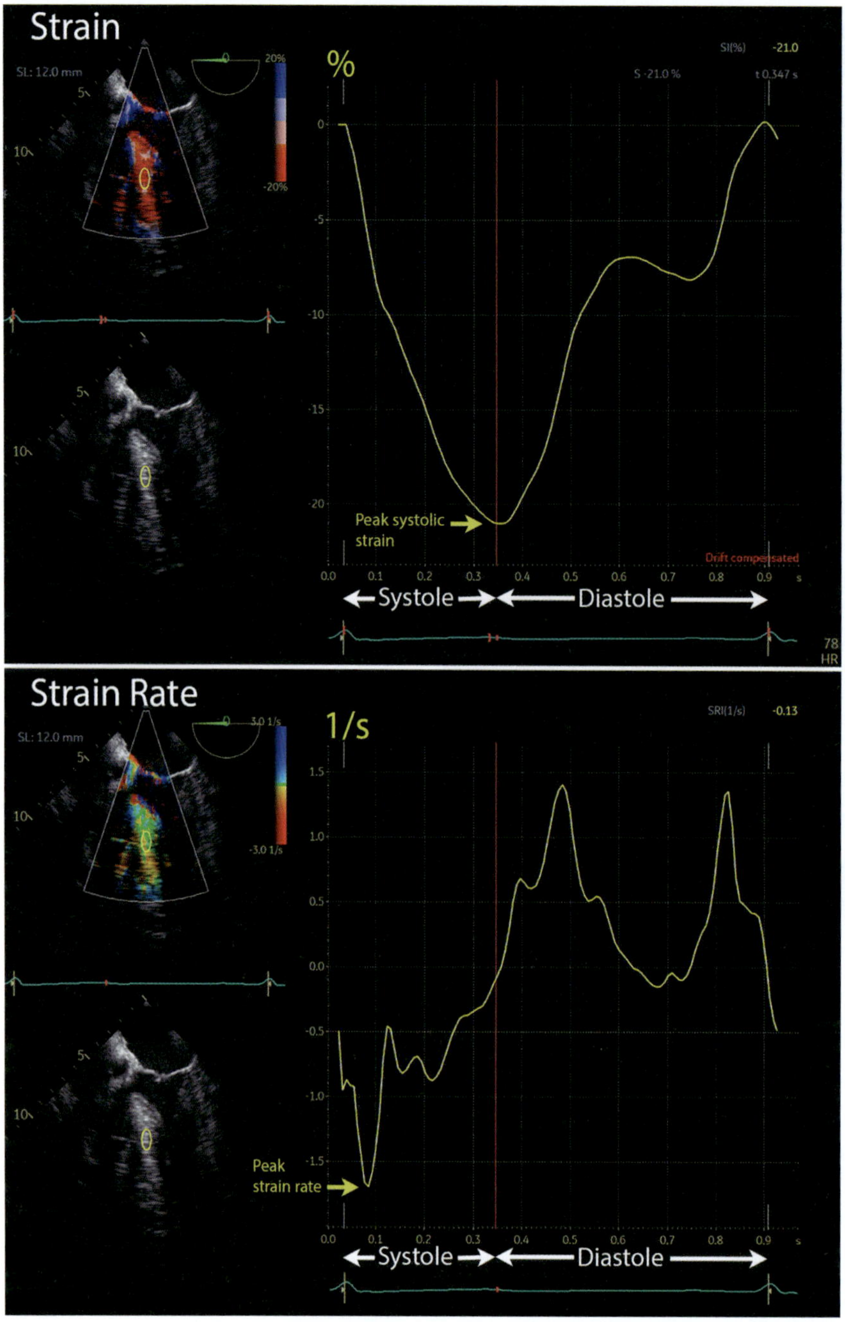

Figure 6.11 Tissue Doppler-derived longitudinal strain and strain rate curves from the ventricular septum of a patient using TOE. The vertical axes represent strain (%) and strain rate (s^{-1}), and the horizontal axis represents time (one cardiac cycle). During systole, the myocardium shortens longitudinally, which is displayed as negative strain; during diastole, the myocardium lengthens longitudinally, returning to baseline. Strain rate is derived from velocity gradients using tissue Doppler. The integration of strain rate over time results in strain.
Courtesy Dr. C. Tousignant.

Technical considerations for speckle tracking echocardiography

STE strain can be obtained from standard 2D echocardiography, including offline post-acquisition analysis, assuming adequate image quality. TDI-based analysis requires independent data acquisition from each myocardial segment and is angle-dependent. The significant expertise needed for acquisition and interpretation has decreased its use in favour of STE strain. STE acquisition should aim at maximizing image quality and maintaining a high frame rate (50–80 frames per second). Whilst less angle-dependent, speckles are better visualized when parallel to ultrasound beams, and the strain vector being analysed should be optimally aligned. With TOE acquisitions, mid-oesophageal views are preferred to deep transgastric views because of better image quality and temporal resolution.

Confounders mostly relate to asynchronous contraction patterns. Bundle branch blocks result in depressed GLS, as peak systolic strain of all segments is not simultaneous. Other septal abnormalities related to RV failure or constrictive pericardial disease may also lead to inaccurate GLS measurements.

Standardized measurements

There are currently no guideline recommendations for normal strain values by TOE. However, multiple studies have demonstrated that a reduction in intraoperative strain assessed with TOE is an independent predictor of complications during cardiac surgery.[17] Guidelines for TTE recommend using GLS in apical views by speckle tracking as a measure of global LV function. In general, values in excess of negative 20% should be expected in healthy adults, with negative 16% generally as the lower limit of normal (2 standard deviations).[3] Strain is influenced by preload, afterload, and heart rate, but SR appears to be less load-dependent. Normal resting longitudinal SR varies from 1.0/s to 1.4/s (standard deviation: 0.5–0.6/s).

Regional left ventricular systolic function

Myocardial ischaemia and infarction rapidly result in RWMAs in the distribution of the affected coronary artery (see Online appendix 5.4). RWMAs are characterized with respect to their anatomical location and severity. Additionally, distinguishing non-ischaemic from ischaemic wall motion abnormalities is a critical part of the assessment.

Segmental analysis of the left ventricle

Depending on the clinical situation, ASE/EACVI guidelines recommend using a 16- or 17-segment model of the LV (Figure 6.12).[3] The LV is divided into three equal thirds: basal; mid; and apical. The basal and mid levels are each divided into six segments: anterior; anteroseptal; inferoseptal; inferior; inferolateral (formerly called posterior); and anterolateral. The apex is divided into four segments: anterior; septal; inferior; and lateral. The final (17th) segment is the apex, which is the myocardium beyond the LV cavity. For perioperative TOE, the 17-segment model should be used.[3]

Segmental blood supply follows a predictable pattern (Figure 6.12), particularly when the dominant coronary artery is known. The artery supplying the atrioventricular node or the posterior descending artery (PDA) is the dominant artery. The PDA supplies the inferior and inferoseptal walls at the basal and mid levels. In >80% of patients, the right coronary artery (RCA) is dominant. In left coronary artery dominance, the PDA is supplied by the circumflex coronary artery (Cx), and hence the LV septum is entirely supplied by the left main coronary artery.

All segments can potentially be visualized in either a mid-oesophageal or transgastric window, although the apical segments are the most difficult to visualize from both perspectives.

> ***Expert tip: A handy way to rapidly assess segmental LV function is with simultaneous biplane imaging. Starting from the transgastric two-chamber view, moving the cursor from right to left on the reference image displays the LV in short axis from base to apex on the right-hand image (Figure 6.13; see Online appendices 1.2.4 and 1.2.5).***

Wall motion

Wall motion consists of endocardial movement and wall thickening. Wall motion may be graded semi-quantitatively as normal or as hyperkinetic, hypokinetic (reduced thickening), akinetic (minimal or absent thickening), or dyskinetic (systolic *thinning* or stretching).[3] Wall thickening is a more reliable sign than endocardial movement, as akinetic segments may move because of tethering from adjacent segments. In mid-oesophageal views, foreshortening normally causes the apical segments to appear hyperdynamic. Thus, in the presence of foreshortening, hypokinetic or akinetic apical motion may appear 'normal'.

Aetiology of wall motion abnormalities

RWMAs can result from a number of ischaemic and non-ischaemic causes (Box 6.1).

Ischaemic

Ischaemic RWMAs include acute ischaemia, myocardial stunning, hibernating myocardium, and myocardial infarction. **Stunning** refers to post-reperfusion myocardial dysfunction (i.e. RWMA despite adequate blood flow). Stunning may occur following CPB and

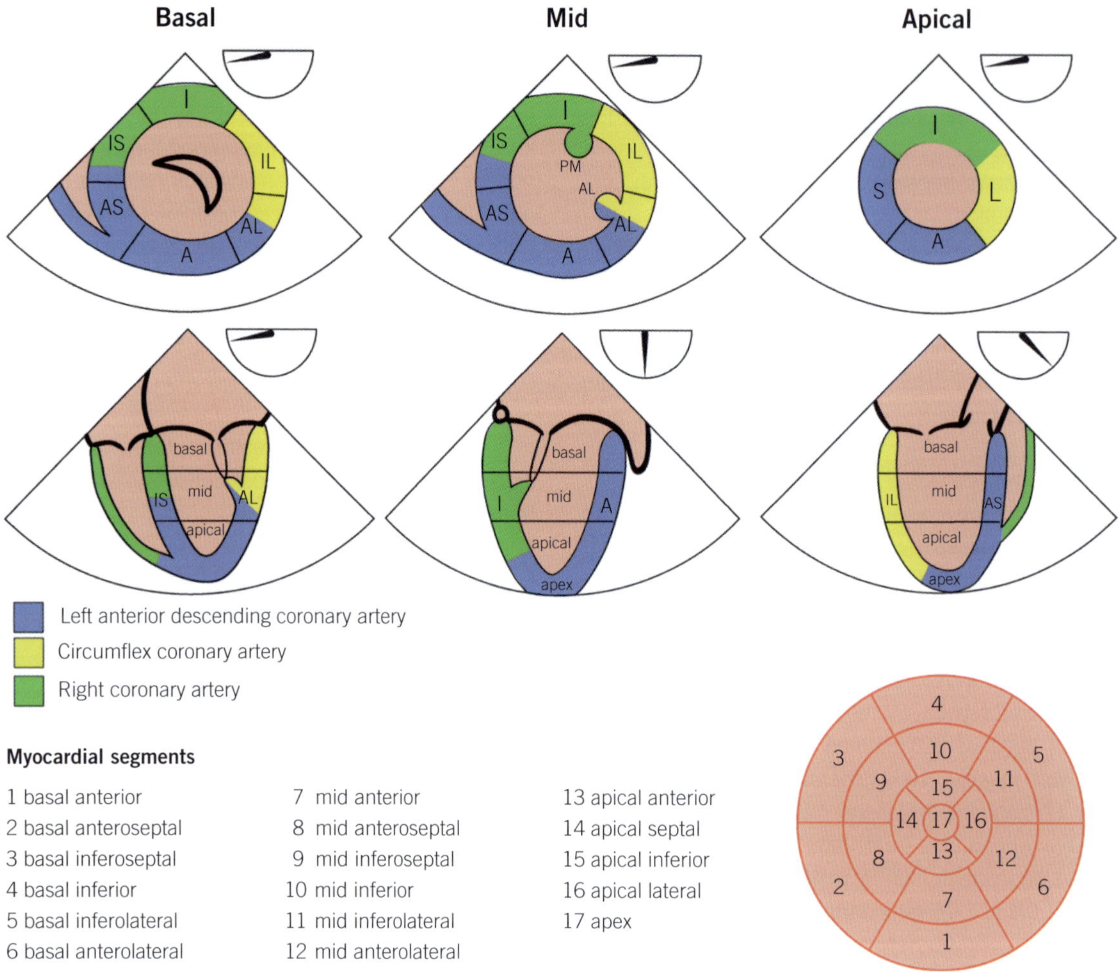

Figure 6.12 Myocardial segments and their coronary blood supply. I, inferior; IL, inferolateral; AL, anterolateral; A, anterior; AS, anteroseptal; IS, inferoseptal; S, septal; L, lateral.

resolves spontaneously over hours to days. **Hibernating** myocardium refers to ischaemic dysfunction due to chronically reduced blood flow. Hibernating myocardium typically persists for days to weeks following revascularization. Collectively, acute ischaemia, stunning, and hibernating myocardium represent viable myocardium.

Viable myocardium appears hypokinetic or akinetic, whereas infarcted myocardium appears akinetic or dyskinetic. However, in practice, viable and (acutely) infarcted myocardium are difficult to differentiate. Chronic infarction is associated with myocardial thinning and chamber dilatation, which distinguishes it from viable myocardium or acute infarction. LV thrombus and aneurysm formation are associated with infarction, but not with ischaemia.

New RWMAs that appear following CPB represent stunning or acute ischaemia. Stunned myocardium causes hypokinesis and improves gradually over time and with inotropic support. By contrast, acute ischaemia causes akinesis and typically deteriorates with inotropic support.[18] Hibernating myocardium is usually present prior to, and following, CPB, appears hypokinetic, and is associated with a biphasic response to inotropic support.

Coronary air embolism

Air embolism to the coronary arteries causes acute, transient myocardial ischaemia and may occur following separation from CPB. Gas collections inside the heart usually appear on TOE as intense regions of bright echoes, often causing acoustic shadowing, most commonly in the pulmonary veins, LA and LA appendage, overlying the anteroseptal wall, and at the LV apex (remember that air rises *anteriorly* in a supine patient, and this is displayed at the *bottom* of the TOE screen). Air embolism most frequently occurs with open-cavity procedures (e.g. valve

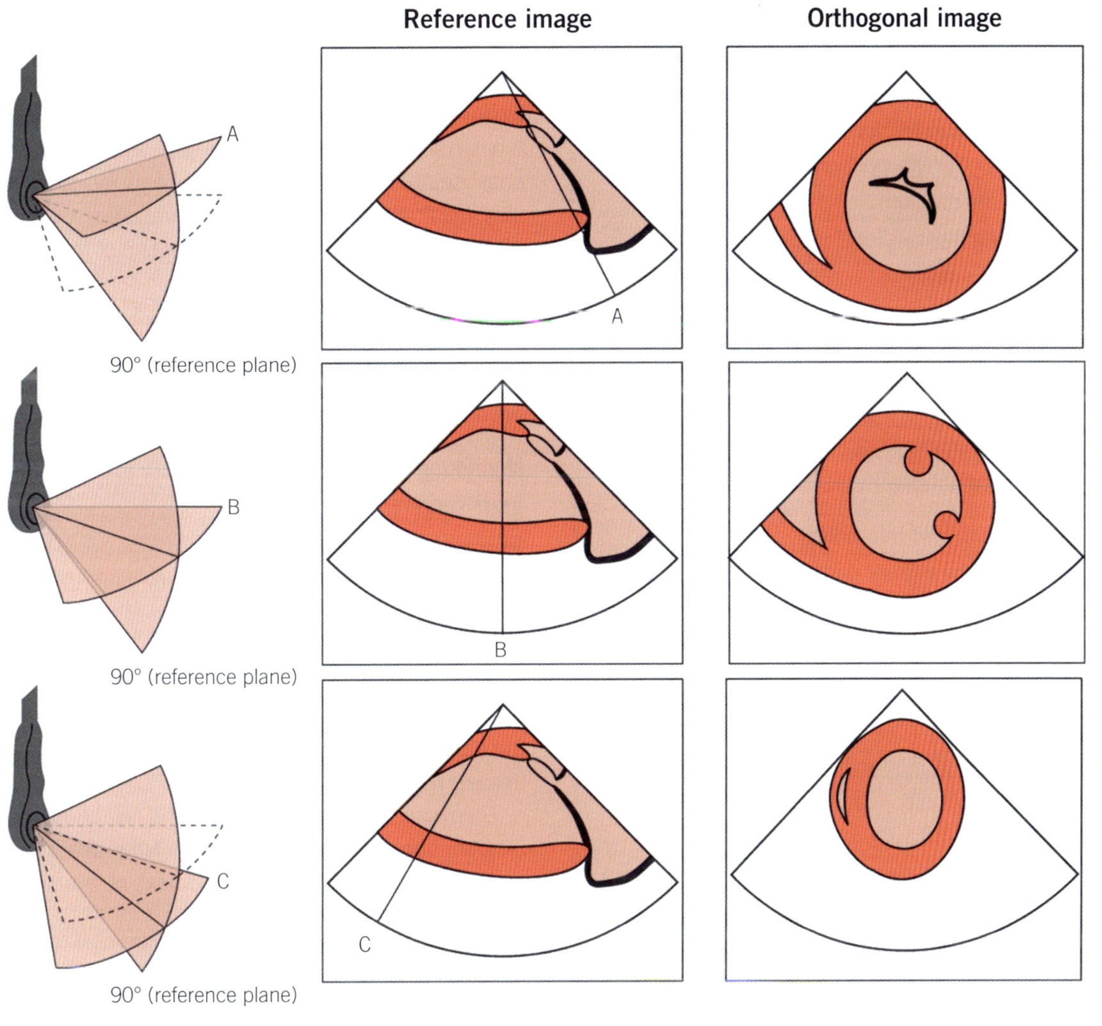

Figure 6.13 Assessment of LV segments using simultaneous multi-plane imaging. The starting (reference) image is the transgastric two-chamber view. The orthogonal image displayed on the right is a transgastric short-axis view of the LV. By moving the cursor on the reference image from right to left (positions A–C), the orthogonal image is swept across the reference sector from the base to the apex of the LV. See also Online appendices 1.2.4 and 1.2.5.

replacement surgery), but it can also occur in coronary bypass procedures, especially in the presence of a patent foramen ovale. Air embolism preferentially affects the RCA due to its anteriorly positioned ostium.

> ***Expert tip:** After coronary bypass surgery, because air rises to the front of a supine patient, air embolism can affect any coronary graft attached to the anterior wall of the aorta, not only the RCA.*

Embolism to the RCA usually manifests as acute RV dysfunction/distension or as a RWMA of the LV inferior wall. Air embolism also causes increased echogenicity of the affected myocardial segments. RWMAs usually spontaneously resolve over 5–10 minutes, although inotropic support and/or return to CPB may be necessary during this period (Figure 6.14; see Online appendices 5.4.20 and 5.4.21).

Direct coronary occlusion

RWMAs due to mechanical obstruction of a coronary artery tend to be seen after specific cardiac operations: (1) following AV replacement due to occlusion of a coronary ostium; (2) aortic root replacement involving coronary artery reimplantation; and (3) MV surgery with injury to the Cx. Such events typically cause hypo-/akinesis of the affected segments and haemodynamic instability.

Non-ischaemic wall motion abnormalities

RWMAs can occur in the absence of myocardial ischaemia/infarction. Non-ischaemic RWMAs may be due to

Box 6.1 Aetiology of wall motion abnormalities

Ischaemic

- Acute ischaemia (includes coronary air embolism and direct coronary occlusion)
- Stunned myocardium
- Hibernating myocardium
- Myocardial infarction

Non- ischaemic

- Hypovolaemia
- Acute myocarditis
- Takotsubo cardiomyopathy
- Dilated cardiomyopathy

Apparent (i.e. no wall thickening)

- Mitral stenosis (due to tethering of basal segments)
- Imaging through the membranous ventricular septum
- Post-operative state
- Paradoxical motion of the ventricular septum

myocarditis and stress-induced (Takotsubo) cardiomyopathy. Severe hypovolaemia is another common cause of transient RWMAs during separation from CPB. Following cardiac surgery, it is also common to see inferoseptal hypokinesis, which may persist for several months. The cause is poorly understood.

Several abnormalities of wall motion are not associated with abnormal thickening and are termed 'apparent' RWMAs. In the transgastric basal short-axis view, the sector scan may pass through the membranous ventricular septum, resulting in an apparent RWMA of the basal septum. Severe MS or mitral annular calcification may result in tethering of the LV, impeding contraction of the basal segments. Abnormal motion of the ventricular septum may be also mistaken for septal dyskinesis. This has a variety of causes (see Chapter 21) and it can be distinguished from true dyskinesis in that the septum *thickens* in systole, but there is outward motion. This is not a true RWMA.

Monitoring ischaemia during coronary artery bypass graft surgery

Prior to initiating CPB, all myocardial segments should be examined and loops recorded for later comparison. The transgastric mid-papillary short-axis view is commonly used for continuous monitoring for ischaemia, as segments supplied by all three coronary arteries are visible in one plane. Note that only six LV segments are visualized in the transgastric mid-papillary short-axis view and RWMAs in other regions may be missed.

Following separation from CPB, a complete LV examination should be repeated. New abnormalities should be interpreted in the context of the following questions:

- Is the heart adequately filled?
- Is air trapped within the heart?

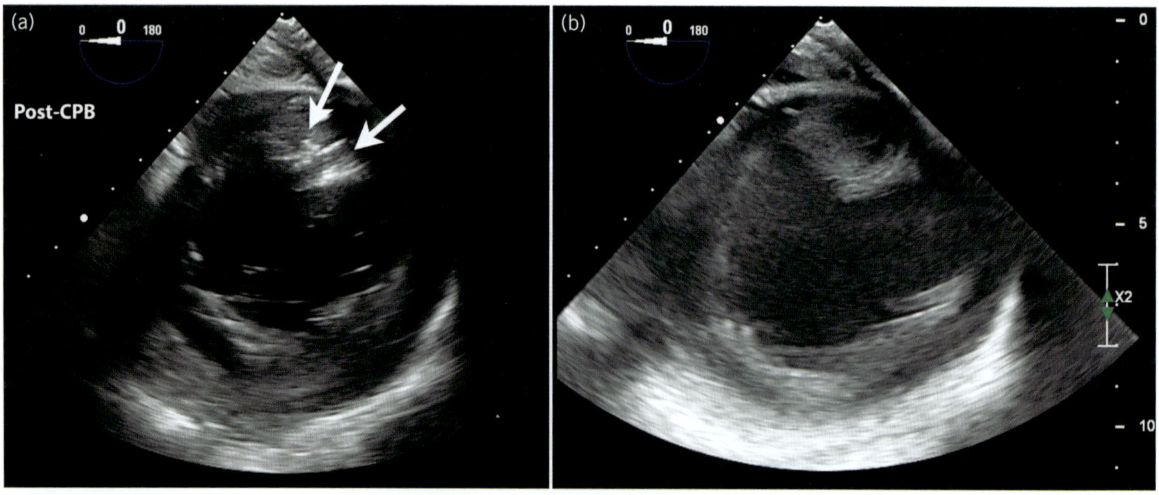

Figure 6.14 Intramyocardial air. Frame (a) is a mid-papillary short-axis view of a patient who sustained air embolism to the RCA immediately after separation from CPB. Note the bright echogenicity in the inferior wall and inferior papillary muscle (arrows), representing intramyocardial air. Note also the residual intracavitary air ('fireflies'). Frame (b) shows the same patient 10 minutes later, after the air has cleared from the myocardium. See also Online appendices 5.4.20 and 5.4.21.

- Is the RWMA significantly different from that before CPB?
- How does the RWMA change over time or in response to inotropic support?
- Is the RWMA commensurate with any surgical concern regarding non-revascularized myocardium or marginal graft function?
- Is the segment akinetic, suggesting ischaemia rather than stunning?
- Is the patient haemodynamically unstable, suggesting ischaemia?
- Are there associated signs of ischaemia such as worse MR?

A new RWMA that develops well after separating from CPB suggests acute thrombosis or kinking of a graft (e.g. with sternal closure).

Three-dimensional echocardiography and speckle tracking strain

Three-dimensional echocardiography is validated against MRI for reliable assessment of RMWAs in ischaemic and non-ischaemic cardiomyopathy, including low LVEF states.[19] RWMAs can be assessed in 3D, using global and regional LV volume and wall motion time curves (Figure 6.15) for easier, and potentially automated, identification and quantification of hypokinesis. It improves on 2D by rapid acquisition and avoiding LV foreshortening.[20] Speckle tracking strain and SR demonstrate benefit for identifying RWMAs during acute myocardial infarction and chronic ischaemic disease when added to visual assessment (Figure 6.16).[21,22] It also provides benefit comparable to MRI for prediction of global myocardial viability.[23]

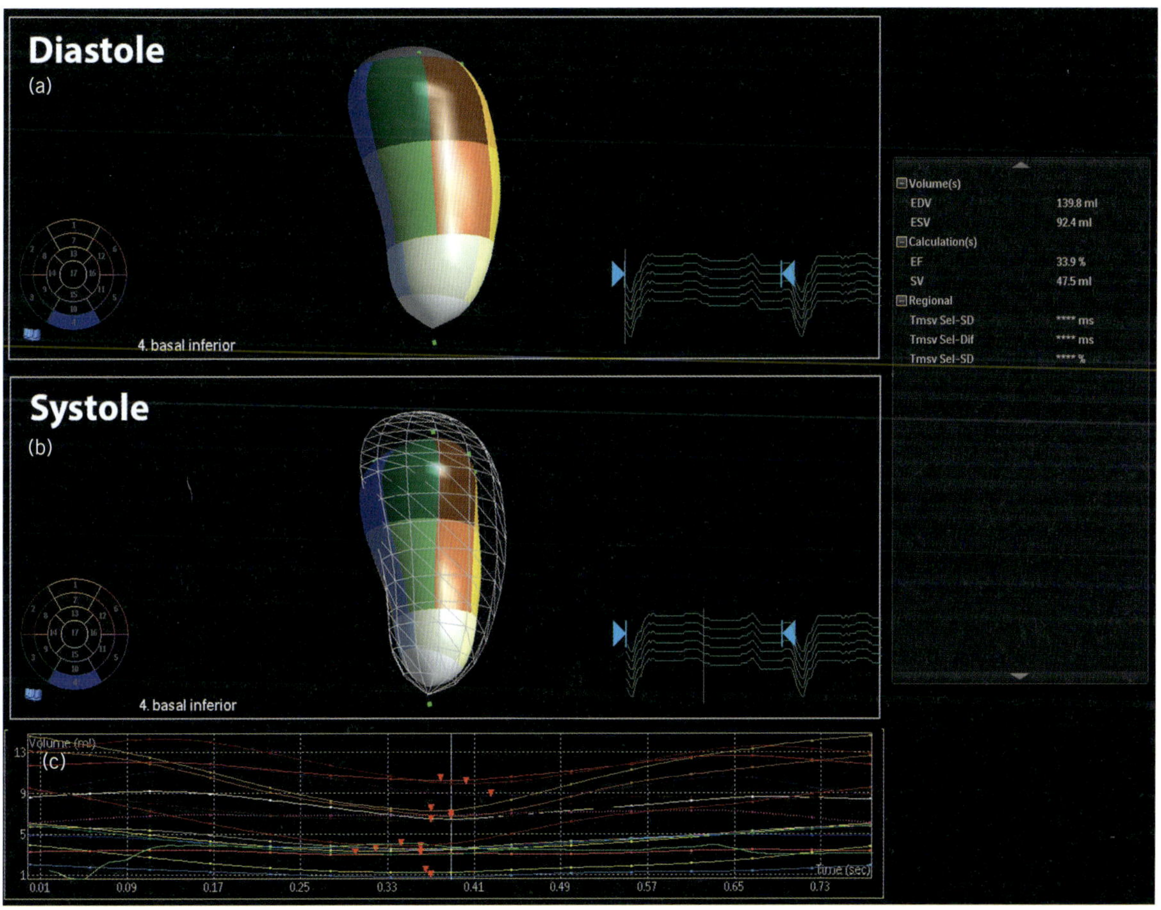

Figure 6.15 3D assessment of LV volumes, EF, and SV using multi-plane reconstruction. A full-volume data set of the LV is obtained. Measurements are made at (a) end-diastole and (b) end-systole in two orthogonal views. The operator manually identifies the MV annulus and LV apex. The machine software automatically identifies the endocardium and calculates LVEDV, LVESV, LVEF, and SV. Individual segments are colour-coded, and hypokinetic/akinetic segments can be visually identified. (c) Segmental motion is also plotted over time by the software, which helps to identify hypo-/akinetic LV segments.

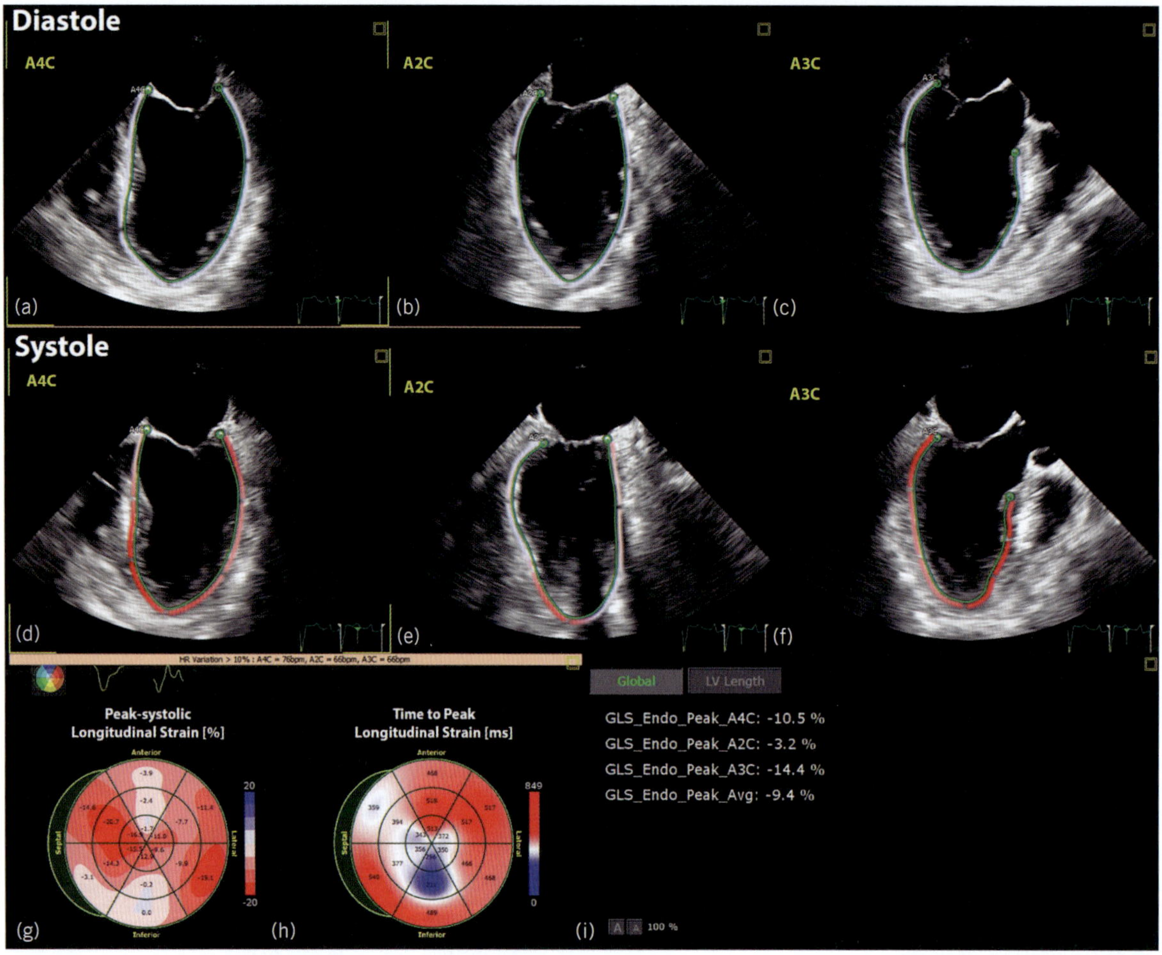

Figure 6.16 Regional wall motion assessment by speckle tracking strain. (a), (b), and (c) show the LV segments at end-diastole. (d), (e), and (f) show the same LV segments in systole, with superimposed colour-coded speckle tracking strain. (g), (h), and (i) show the machine-generated colour-coded representation of systolic strain across the entire LV. Note the reduced strain in the basal-to-mid inferior segments demonstrating a regional wall motion abnormality.

Other findings associated with myocardial ischaemia and infarction

In addition to RWMAs, other cardiac abnormalities are associated with myocardial ischaemia or infarction.

Myocardial rupture

Rupture of the ventricular septum (ischaemic VSD) causes left-to-right shunting, which is seen as a turbulent jet on colour Doppler and/or a visible defect on 2D imaging (Figure 6.17; see Online appendices 5.4.8–5.4.13). Rupture of the free wall of the LV results in acute pericardial tamponade and is often fatal.

Aneurysms and false aneurysms

About 80% of LV aneurysms occur in the territory of the left anterior descending (LAD) coronary artery; 10–15% are inferior, and the rest are lateral (see Online appendix 5.4.6). A **true aneurysm** is *lined by myocardium* that thins during systole, making the aneurysm appear slightly larger during systole (Figure 6.18). There is usually a smooth transition between normal myocardium and aneurysmal myocardium, and the neck of the aneurysm is typically as wide as the aneurysm is deep. Thrombus is commonly present within an aneurysm.

A **false aneurysm** represents a subacute or chronic rupture of the ventricular wall that has been contained by the pericardium (Figure 6.19). A false aneurysm has a well-defined, narrow neck, giving a 'walled-off' appearance. False aneurysms may also increase in size during systole due to the transmitted LV pressure, and may contain spontaneous echo contrast and/or thrombus. Colour Doppler typically demonstrates turbulent blood flow across the

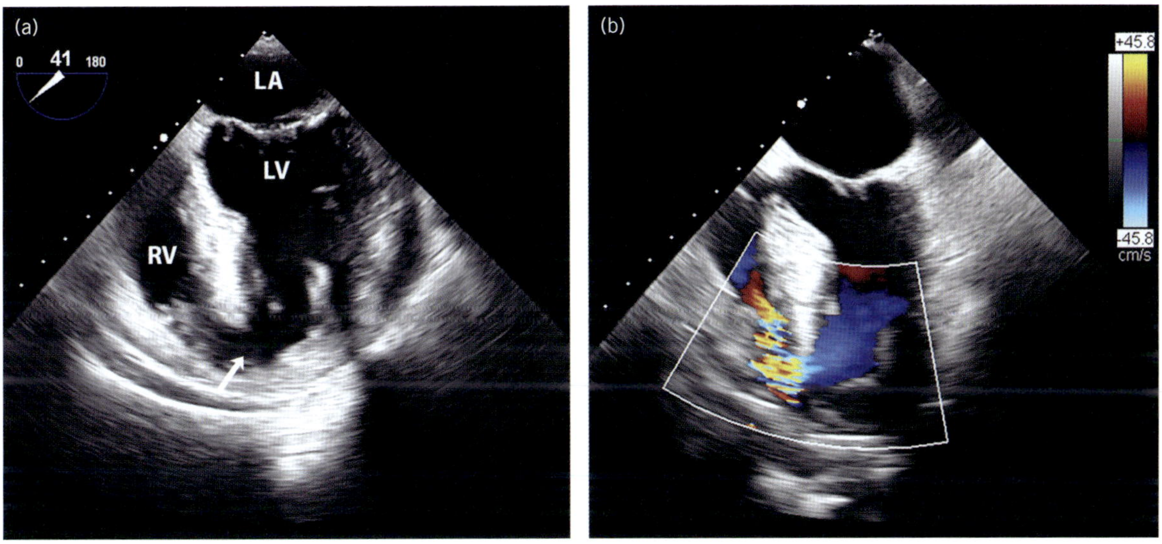

Figure 6.17 Post-myocardial infarction ventricular septal defect. Mid-oesophageal four-chamber view in (a) 2D and (b) with colour Doppler. (a) shows a large post-infarction apical VSD (arrow), and (b) shows a large colour jet representing a left-to-right shunt through the defect.

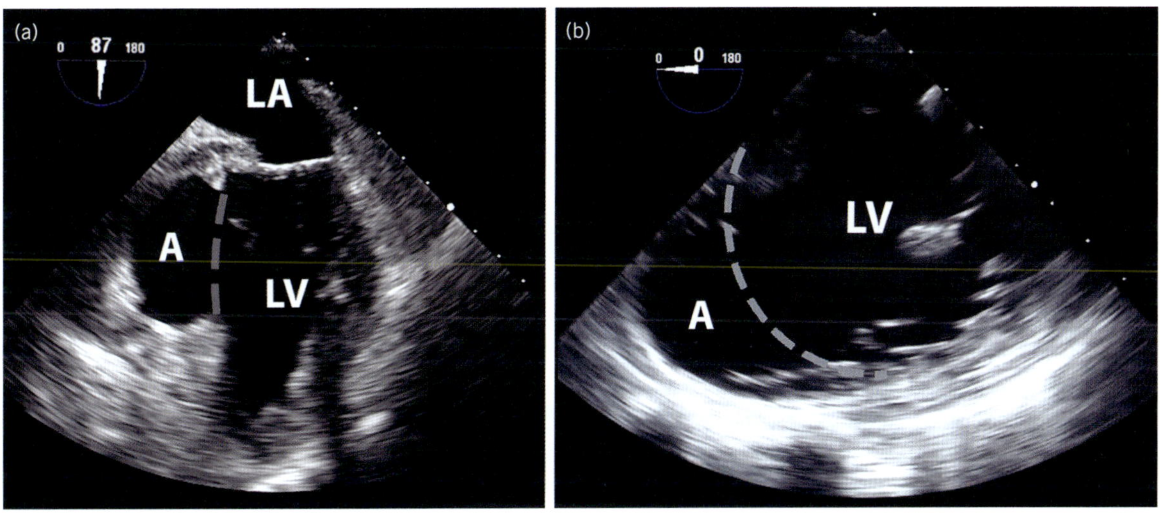

Figure 6.18 LV true aneurysms. Frame (a) is a mid-oesophageal two-chamber view, showing a large basal–inferior aneurysm. Frame (b) is a transgastric mid-papillary view, showing a large anterior/anteroseptal aneurysm (A). In both images, the dotted line represents approximately where the normal myocardial wall should be if there were no aneurysm. Note the wide neck of these true aneurysms.

neck of the aneurysm. False aneurysms have a high incidence of rupture and should be repaired surgically.

Cardiomyopathies

The term cardiomyopathy encompasses a heterogeneous group of heart muscle diseases that have proven difficult to classify. The traditional classification into dilated, hypertrophic, and restrictive has several limitations. For instance, DCM and HCM are anatomic definitions, whereas RCM is a functional classification. Some RCMs demonstrate hypertrophy, and some HCMs have restrictive filling. The system proposed by the European Society of Cardiology in 2008 is the simplest and remains the most widely used classification.[24] It groups the cardiomyopathies into

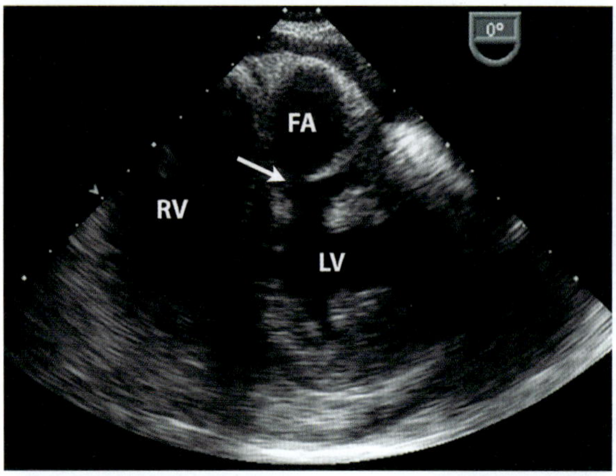

Figure 6.19 LV false aneurysm. In this transgastric mid-papillary view, one can see a rupture in the inferior LV wall into a false aneurysm cavity (FA). Note the narrow neck of this false aneurysm (arrow).

morphologic and functional phenotypes (dilated, hypertrophic, arrhythmogenic, hypertrophic, and unclassified), and separates each group into familial and non-familial subgroups. Recent developments in genomics have better defined the phenotypes of each cardiomyopathy, without major changes in these categories. Impaired LV function due to end-stage ischaemic or valvular heart disease is not considered a cardiomyopathy despite having similar echocardiographic appearances to DCM.

Dilated cardiomyopathy

DCM is defined as a dilated LV with impaired systolic function in the absence of loading conditions or coronary artery disease of sufficient severity to cause the findings. DCM accounts for 60% of all cardiomyopathies. The most common cause is familial/genetic or idiopathic in the absence of a known mutation. Other causes include infections, autoimmune disorders (e.g. scleroderma, systemic lupus erythematosus), endocrine, toxins (e.g. ethanol, doxorubicin), nutritional (e.g. thiamine), Kawasaki disease, radiation therapy, and pregnancy (peripartum cardiomyopathy).

Echocardiographic findings

The hallmarks of DCM are spherical LV dilation, LA dilation, and globally impaired LV systolic function. LV dimensions are frequently dramatically increased, and LVEF may be very low (<20%). LV wall thickness is usually normal or reduced, and the RV is usually also involved. Some degree of MR and TR is usually present. The TR jet velocity is usually elevated (>2.5 m/s), consistent with pulmonary hypertension. Thrombus may be present in the LA appendage or LV. The trans-mitral PW Doppler waveform usually demonstrates a restrictive filling pattern. LV strain is globally and symmetrically reduced.

Hypertrophic cardiomyopathy

HCM encompasses a heterogeneous group of genetic conditions characterized by autosomal dominant inheritance, myocardial disarray, and asymmetric LVH. Patients with HCM have a hypertrophied, non-dilated LV, with a maximum end-diastolic LV wall thickness of at least 15 mm in any wall segment (13 mm in patients with a family history of HCM or positive genetic testing). Hypertrophy of the ventricular septum is a common feature across phenotypes, present in >90% of patients.[25] Five variants are most common: sigmoid septum; reversed septal curvature; concentric; mid wall; and apical (Figure 6.20). LVOT obstruction (peak LVOT gradient ≥30 mmHg) can occur with all subtypes but is uncommon with the apical subtype. Patients with mid-wall HCM can demonstrate mid-cavity obstruction, and those with apical HCM are at increased risk of apical aneurysm formation. The mechanism of LVOT obstruction was previously thought to be solely due to the Venturi effect but is now known to be mostly from drag forces acting on an abnormal MV, causing displacement of the anterior (or, less frequently, posterior) mitral leaflet into the LVOT.[25]

Echocardiographic findings

The cardinal echocardiographic features of HCM are LVH, normal or reduced chamber size, diastolic dysfunction, abnormalities of the MV and subvalvular apparatus, and LVOT obstruction (see Online appendices 5.3.4 and 5.5).[26] The mid-oesophageal four-chamber view is the best image plane for visualizing the entire ventricular septum, but mid-septal measurements are best made in the transgastric mid-papillary short-axis view. End-diastolic septal thickness may be dramatically increased (≥15 mm). Hypertrophy may involve the other LV walls, but the inferolateral wall is usually spared. The septal-to-inferolateral wall thickness ratio is typically increased (>1.3). 3D echocardiographic measurements are superior to 2D measurements and closely correlate with MRI results. The MV leaflets are typically elongated, and the papillary muscles can be hypertrophied and displaced anteriorly and/or apically.

LVOT obstruction can be classified as: (1) non-obstructive; (2) obstructive at rest (peak gradient ≥30 mmHg); or (3) latent or inducible obstruction (peak gradient ≥30 mmHg only with provocation), with approximately

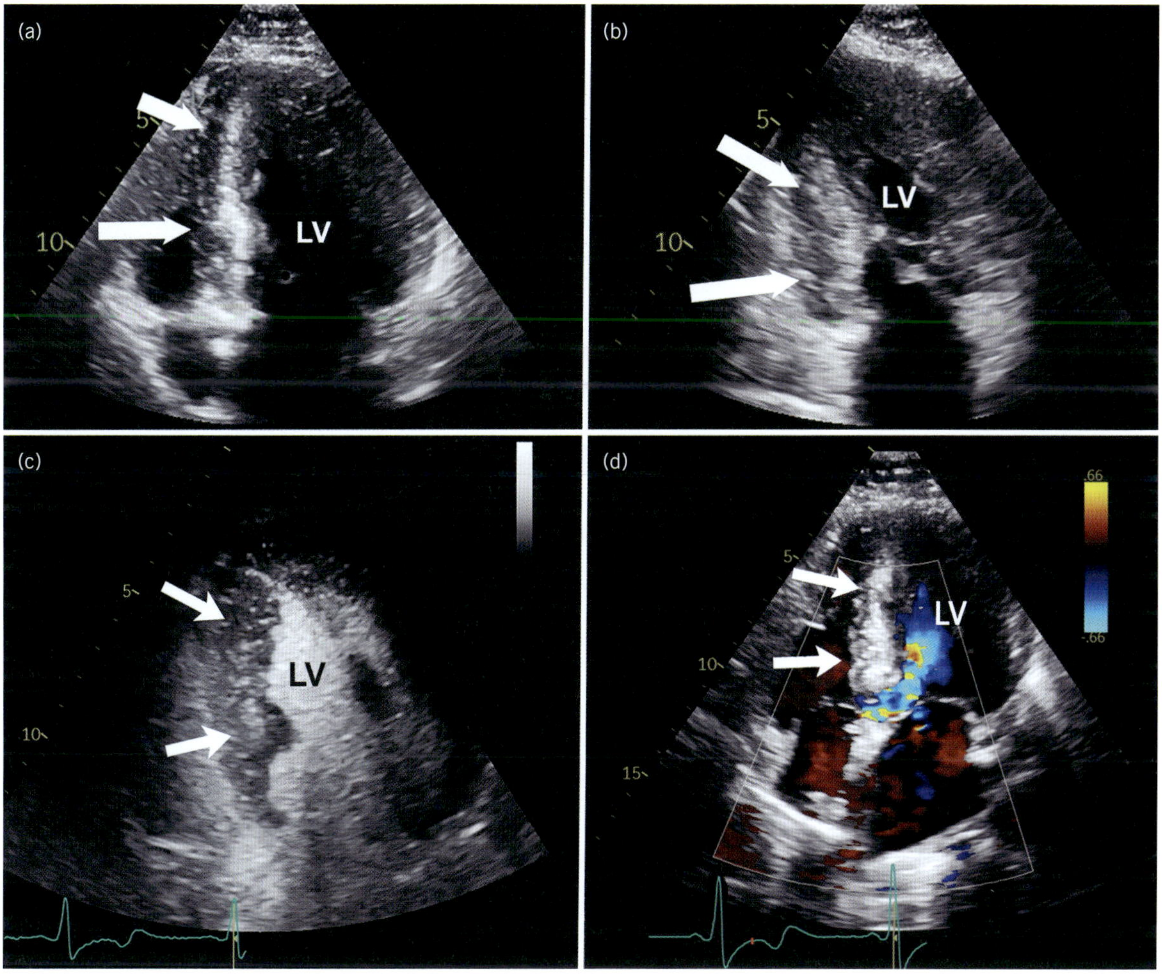

Figure 6.20 Hypertrophic cardiomyopathy. TTE apical four-chamber views, demonstrating examples of HCM. Note the severe thickening of the interventricular septum (arrows in frames (a) to (d)). Frame (c) uses intravenous echo contrast to improve the endocardial border resolution, which makes the LV cavity appear white. Frames (a) and (c) are examples of apical HCM.

equal numbers in each category.[25] LVOT obstruction is best appreciated in the mid-oesophageal long-axis view. With 2D imaging, the anterior mitral leaflet may be seen displaced into the LVOT in systole—a phenomenon called **systolic anterior motion** (SAM) (Figure 6.21a). With colour Doppler imaging, there is marked colour aliasing in the LVOT and usually a posteriorly directed jet of MR, which may be severe (Figure 6.21b). In addition to SAM, 10–20% of patients with HCM have MR secondary to intrinsic disease of the MV.[25]

The peak systolic velocity in the LVOT can be assessed with CW Doppler from a transgastric view. Because LVOT obstruction is maximal in *late systole*, the CW Doppler waveform is typically late-peaking and 'dagger-shaped' (Figure 6.21c), in contrast to the symmetrical waveform seen with valvular AS (see Figure 10.13). With marked obstruction, the LV is typically small, underfilled, and hyperdynamic. LVOT obstruction is exacerbated by hypovolaemia, arteriolar vasodilation, and increased myocardial contractility. In addition to LVOT obstruction, patients with HCM may also have outflow obstruction at the level of the mid LV, with corresponding marked colour aliasing.

Global LV systolic function is typically normal in both obstructive and non-obstructive HCM until late in the disease process. Strain can be reduced or normal in patients with HCM, even with normal ejection fraction. Reduced strain patterns frequently follow hypertrophied segments with reduced septal strain in the common sigmoid variant and reduced apical strain in the apical variant. Reduced strain has been shown to be an independent predictor of poor outcomes, including new-onset ventricular arrhythmias, heart failure, transplantation, and death. Doppler

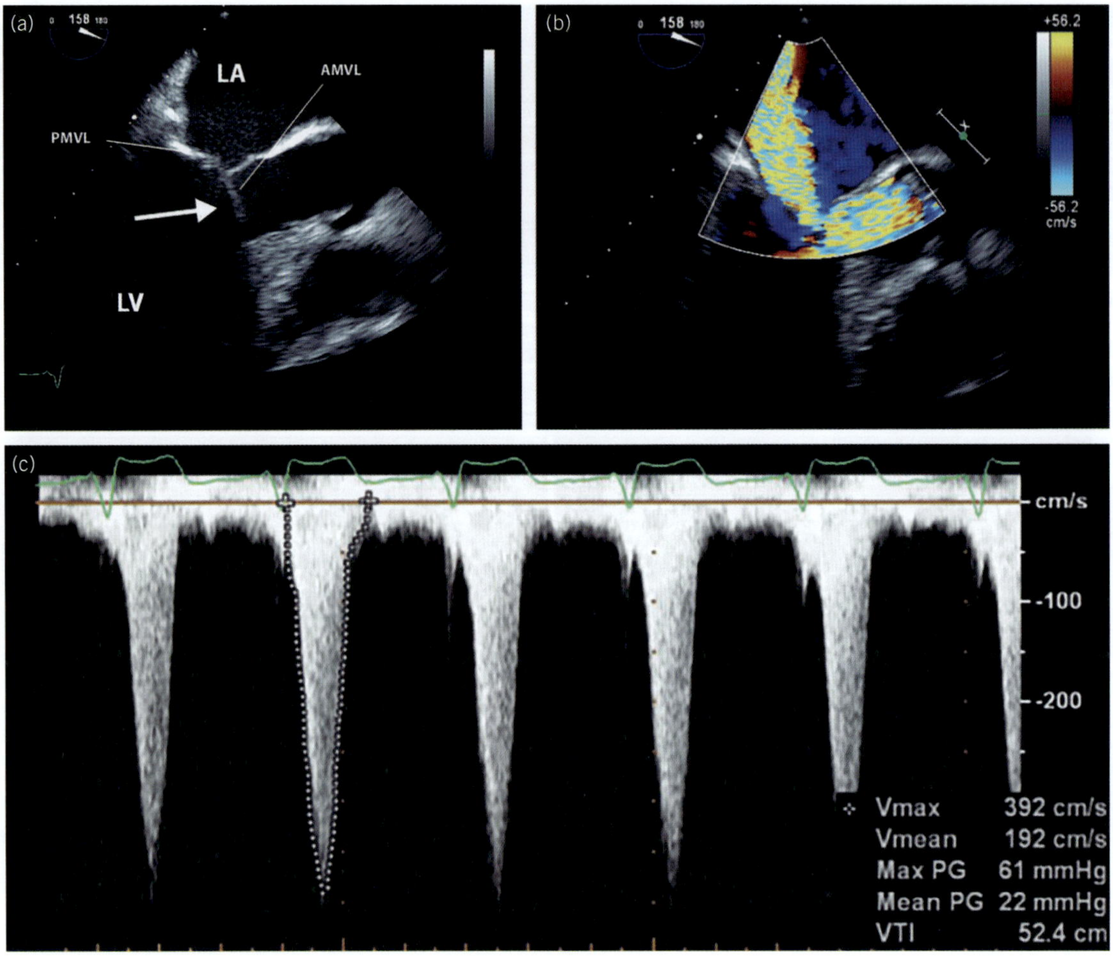

Figure 6.21 LVOT obstruction due to hypertrophic cardiomyopathy. (a) and (b) are mid-oesophageal long-axis views, showing simultaneous (a) 2D and (b) colour Doppler images of SAM with dynamic LVOT obstruction. On the 2D image, the anterior MV leaflet is seen obstructing the LVOT (arrow). The colour Doppler image shows accelerated (aliasing) flow in the LVOT, resulting in severe posteriorly directed MR. (c) shows a spectral display of the CW Doppler through that patient's LVOT (obtained in the transgastric view). Note the late-peaking LVOT velocity, producing the typical 'dagger shape' appearance. See also Online appendix 5.5.

assessment of diastolic function usually demonstrates a pattern of impaired relaxation, but patients with end-stage disease may have restrictive diastolic filling. LA enlargement is common.

Surgery for hypertrophic cardiomyopathy

Alcohol ablation or surgical myectomy is recommended for patients with HCM who have refractory symptoms and labile LVOT obstruction, defined as a resting peak gradient ≥30 mmHg and a peak gradient ≥50 mmHg with exercise.[25] Resection is typically performed with a myocardial incision between the nadir of the right coronary sinus and the anterior MV leaflet. This incision is extended beyond the mitral leaflet–septal contact point. After this initial resection, additional myocardium may be resected by extending the incision towards the apex. Abnormal MV leaflet lengths may require plication, and the papillary muscles may require reorienting. Useful measurements to guide resection include end-diastolic maximal septal thickness, distance of maximum thickness from the aortic annulus, location of the endocardial fibrous plaque, and apical extent of the septal bulge.

Careful post-procedure TOE assessment with 2D, colour Doppler, and CW Doppler should look for iatrogenic VSD, SAM, residual LVOT obstruction, and MR.

A provocative manoeuvre to simulate exercise should be performed by using rapid pacing or isoproterenol/dobutamine to achieve a heart rate >120 bpm. A provoked LVOT gradient ≥20 mmHg, significant residual SAM, severe MR (≥3+without SAM or LVOT obstruction), or a new VSD are indications for immediate surgical revision.[25] Apart from VSD, complications of septal myectomy include AR and damage to a septal perforator coronary artery. Uncorrected LVOT obstruction, VSD, AR, and a severed septal perforator artery *all* cause abnormal colour jets in the LVOT.

Expert tip: The origin, direction, and timing of the colour jet help to determine its aetiology—AR and LVOT obstruction are usually obvious. A severed perforator artery typically creates a diastolic jet, whereas a VSD typically creates a systolic jet.

Restrictive cardiomyopathy

RCM can be defined as the presence of restrictive diastolic filling (see Chapter 7) in association with normal or near-normal ventricular volume, systolic function, and wall thickness.[24] RCM may be idiopathic or familial, or occur as part of a systemic process (most commonly amyloidoisis in Western countries).

In most circumstances, the ventricles appear relatively normal; however, with amyloidosis, the myocardium may have a speckled or granular appearance. Chronically raised LA pressure results in LA enlargement and pulmonary hypertension. Amyloidosis may lead to paradoxically normal LA size in the presence of significant restrictive filling. Intracardiac thrombus is a frequent finding. Restrictive filling is diagnosed by a transmitral E/A ratio >2, E-wave deceleration time <140 ms, and a reduced mitral annular e'-wave or grade 3 criteria in ASE guidelines. Strain can be used to help differentiate pathology in patients with suspected RCM. Strain in patients with RCM secondary to amyloidosis reveals a unique pattern of *relative apical sparing* with a 'cherry-on-top' strain pattern consisting of normal strain in the apex and reduced strain elsewhere (Figure 6.22a). Patients with constrictive pericarditis demonstrate 'strain reversus' where the tethered lateral wall has reduced strain compared with other segments (Figure 6.22b). In contrast, patients with RCM typically have globally reduced strain.

Fulminant myocarditis

Viral myocarditis is one of the causes of DCM. However, the fulminant form of viral myocarditis does not present with DCM. Rather, patients rapidly develop severe acute heart failure *without* marked LV dilatation. Echocardiographic findings are of severe biventricular dysfunction, with relatively normal ventricular volumes (see Online appendix 5.3.7).[27] LV wall thickness is often increased due to myocardial oedema, and multiple RWMAs across coronary territories are common. Pericardial effusion, intracardiac thrombus, and secondary MR are also frequent findings.

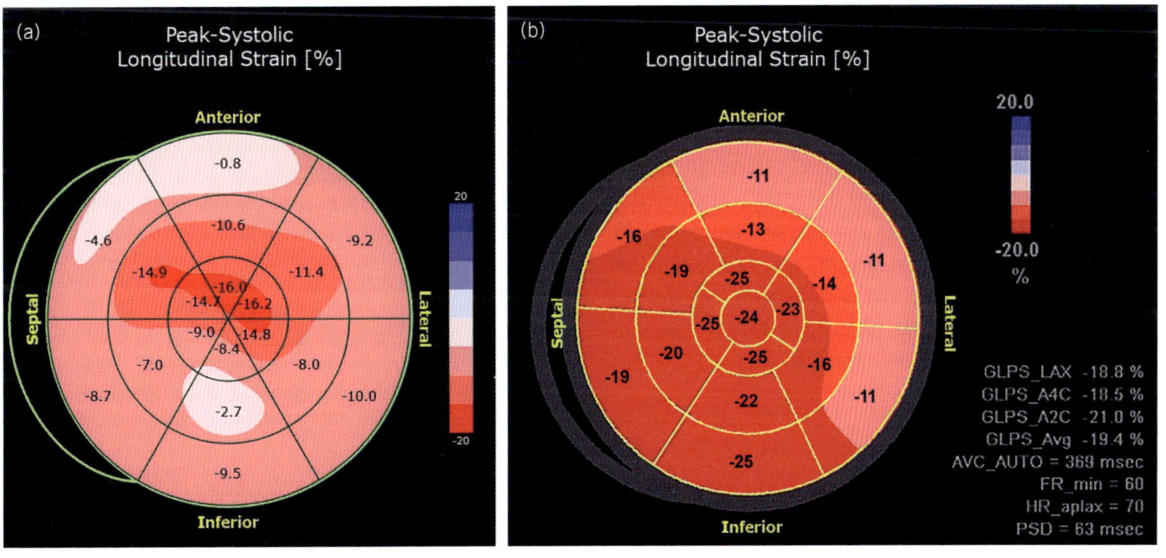

Figure 6.22 Strain pattern in amyloidosis and constrictive pericarditis. (a) Peak systolic longitudinal strain in a patient with amyloidosis, showing reduced longitudinal strain in all segments, except the apex ('cherry-on-top' pattern). (b) Peak systolic longitudinal strain in a patient with constrictive pericarditis. Note here the reduced lateral wall strain and preserved septal strain ('annulus strain reversus' pattern).

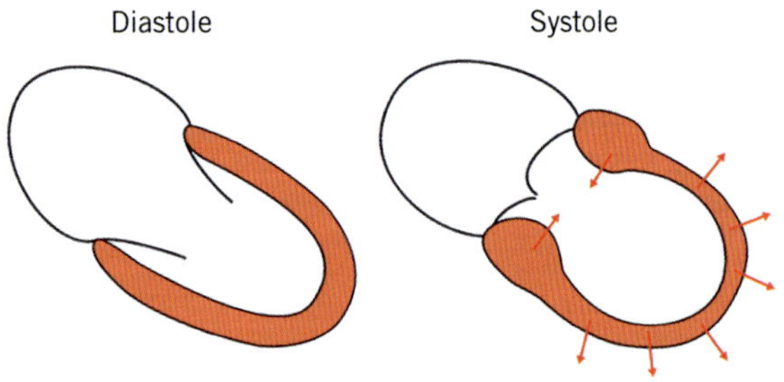

Figure 6.23 Schematic demonstrating Takotsubo cardiomyopathy. The characteristic feature is hypercontractility of the basal segments and systolic thinning and expansion of the mid and apical segments.

Left ventricular non-compaction

LV non-compaction is a congenital cardiomyopathy that may present in childhood or adulthood. The condition is characterized by prominent muscular trabeculations and deep inter-trabecular recesses within the LV chamber (see Online appendix 5.3.8). The LV wall itself is thinned, and ventricular size is typically increased. Global systolic function is severely impaired.

Takotsubo cardiomyopathy

Takotsubo cardiomyopathy (apical ballooning syndrome, stress-induced cardiomyopathy) is a sudden, usually transient cardiomyopathy associated with emotional stress. Echocardiographic findings are characteristic, with a circumferential pattern of myocardial dysfunction involving the apical and mid-LV segments (Figure 6.23).[28] Typically, there is akinesis or dyskinesis of the mid- and apical segments (hence the term 'apical ballooning'), with hypercontractility of the basal segments. Strain analysis demonstrates reduced strain in the apical regions. Other variants—such as mid-ventricular or inverted Takotsubo—have been described. The inverted form is associated with apical sparing, with either hypokinesis/akinesis of the basal segments only or hypokinesis/akinesis of the basal and mid walls. The mechanism of Takotsubo cardiomyopathy is thought to be catecholamine surges, and it typically spontaneously resolves over days to weeks.

Multiple choice questions

Discover interactive multiple choice questions to test your knowledge on this chapter by searching for this book's title or ISBN (9780198873686) at **https://academic.oup.com/** and going to the online appendix at the end of the book. Use your scratch-off code on the inside cover to access the material.

References

1. O'Brien SM, Shahian DM, Filardo G, *et al.* The Society of Thoracic Surgeons 2008 cardiac surgery risk models: part 2—isolated valve surgery. *Ann Thorac Surg.* 2009;**88**(1 Suppl):S23–42.
2. Rong LQ. An update on intraoperative three-dimensional transesophageal echocardiography. *J Thorac Dis.* 2017;**9**(Suppl 4):S271–82.
3. Lang RM, Badano LP, Mor-Avi V, *et al.* Recommendations for cardiac chamber quantification by echocardiography in adults: an update from the American Society of Echocardiography and the European Association of Cardiovascular Imaging. *Eur Heart J Cardiovasc Imaging.* 2015;**16**(3):233–71.
4. Hahn RT, Abraham T, Adams MS, *et al.* Guidelines for performing a comprehensive transesophageal echocardiographic examination: recommendations from the American Society of Echocardiography and the Society of Cardiovascular Anesthesiologists. *J Am Soc Echocardiogr.* 2013;**26**(9):921–64.
5. Wood PW, Choy JB, Nanda NC, Becher H. Left ventricular ejection fraction and volumes: it depends on the imaging method. *Echocardiography.* 2014;**31**(1):87–100.
6. Lee L, Cotella JI, Miyoshi T, *et al.* Normal values of left ventricular mass by two-dimensional and three-dimensional echocardiography: results from the World Alliance Societies of Echocardiography Normal Values Study. *J Am Soc Echocardiogr.* 2023;**36**(5):533–42.
7. Galderisi M, Henein MY, D'hooge J, *et al.* Recommendations of the European Association of Echocardiography: how to use echo-Doppler in clinical trials: different modalities for different purposes. *Eur J Echocardiogr.* 2011;**12**(5):339–53.
8. Manganaro R, Marchetta S, Dulgheru R, *et al.* Echocardiographic reference ranges for normal non-invasive myocardial work indices: results from the EACVI NORRE study. *Eur Heart J Cardiovasc Imaging.* 2019;**20**(5):582–90.
9. Abazid RM, Abohamr SI, Smettei OA, *et al.* Visual versus fully automated assessment of left ventricular ejection fraction. *Avicenna J Med.* 2018;**8**(2):41–5.
10. Thavendiranathan P, Popović ZB, Flamm SD, Dahiya A, Grimm RA, Marwick TH. Improved interobserver variability and accuracy of echocardiographic visual left ventricular ejection fraction assessment through a self-directed learning program using cardiac magnetic resonance images. *J Am Soc Echocardiogr.* 2013;**26**(11):1267–73.
11. Matos J, Kronzon I, Panagopoulos G, Perk G. Mitral annular plane systolic excursion as a surrogate for left ventricular ejection fraction. *J Am Soc Echocardiogr.* 2012;**25**(9):969–74.
12. Ichikawa N, Shiina Y, Kijima Y, Komiyama N, Niwa K. Severity classification of fractional area change (FAC) in the left ventricle. *Journal of Adult Congenital Heart Disease.* 2022;**11**(2):8–14. Available from: https://doi.org/10.34376/jsachd.O-2021-0005
13. Meris A, Santambrogio L, Casso G, Mauri R, Engeler A, Cassina T. Intraoperative three-dimensional versus

two-dimensional echocardiography for left ventricular assessment. *Anesth Analg.* 2014;**118**(4):711–20.
14. Mor-Avi V, Lang RM, Badano LP, *et al.* Current and evolving echocardiographic techniques for the quantitative evaluation of cardiac mechanics: ASE/EAE consensus statement on methodology and indications endorsed by the Japanese Society of Echocardiography. *J Am Soc Echocardiogr.* 2011;**24**(3):277–313.
15. Badran HM, Ahmed MK, Beshay MM, Zein FEA. A comparative study between transthoracic and transesophageal echo modalities in evaluation of left ventricular deformation. *Egypt Heart J.* 2019;**71**(1):4.
16. Brady B, King G, Murphy RT, Walsh D. Myocardial strain: a clinical review. *Ir J Med Sci.* 2023;**192**(4):1649–56.
17. Benson MJ, Silverton N, Morrissey C, Zimmerman J. Strain imaging: an everyday tool for the perioperative echocardiographer. *J Cardiothorac Vasc Anesth.* 2020;**34**(10):2707–17.
18. Kosaraju A, Muppidi V, Makaryus AN. *Stress Echocardiography.* Treasure Island, FL: StatPearls Publishing; 2023. Available from: http://www.ncbi.nlm.nih.gov/books/NBK448062
19. Youssef G, Saad Z, Ammar W, Sharaf Y. Assessment of left ventricular regional wall motion abnormalities using regional time-volume curves obtained by real time three-dimensional echocardiography. *Egypt Heart J.* 2018;**70**(3):189–94.
20. Abusaid GH, Ahmad M. Real time three-dimensional stress echocardiography advantages and limitations. *Echocardiography.* 2012;**29**(2):200–6.
21. Van Mourik MJW, Zaar DVJ, Smulders MW, *et al.* Adding speckle-tracking echocardiography to visual assessment of systolic wall motion abnormalities improves the detection of myocardial infarction. *J Am Soc Echocardiogr.* 2019;**32**(1):65–73.
22. Wang J, Zhang Y, Zhang L, *et al.* Assessment of myocardial fibrosis using two-dimensional and three-dimensional speckle tracking echocardiography in dilated cardiomyopathy with advanced heart failure. *J Card Fail.* 2021;**27**(6):651–61.
23. Altiok E, Tiemann S, Becker M, *et al.* Myocardial deformation imaging by two-dimensional speckle-tracking echocardiography for prediction of global and segmental functional changes after acute myocardial infarction: a comparison with late gadolinium enhancement cardiac magnetic resonance. *J Am Soc Echocardiogr.* 2014;**27**(3):249–57.
24. Elliott P, Andersson B, Arbustini E, *et al.* Classification of the cardiomyopathies: a position statement from the European Society of Cardiology Working Group on Myocardial and Pericardial Diseases. *Eur Heart J.* 2008;**29**(2):270–6.
25. Gersh BJ, Maron BJ, Bonow RO, *et al.* 2011 ACCF/AHA Guideline for the diagnosis and treatment of hypertrophic cardiomyopathy: a report of the American College of Cardiology Foundation/American Heart Association Task Force on Practice Guidelines. Developed in collaboration with the American Association for Thoracic Surgery, American Society of Echocardiography, American Society of Nuclear Cardiology, Heart Failure Society of America, Heart Rhythm Society, Society for Cardiovascular Angiography and Interventions, and Society of Thoracic Surgeons. *J Am Coll Cardiol.* 2011;**58**(25):e212–60.
26. Nagueh SF, Phelan D, Abraham T, *et al.* Recommendations for multimodality cardiovascular imaging of patients with hypertrophic cardiomyopathy: an update from the American Society of Echocardiography, in Collaboration with the American Society of Nuclear Cardiology, the Society for Cardiovascular Magnetic Resonance, and the Society of Cardiovascular Computed Tomography. *J Am Soc Echocardiogr.* 2022;**35**(6):533–69.
27. Shillcutt SK, Thomas WR, Sullivan JN, Duhachek-Stapelman A. Fulminant myocarditis: the role of perioperative echocardiography. *Anesth Analg.* 2015;**120**(2):296–9.
28. Citro R, Lyon AR, Meimoun P, *et al.* Standard and advanced echocardiography in takotsubo (stress) cardiomyopathy: clinical and prognostic implications. *J Am Soc Echocardiogr.* 2015;**28**(1):57–74.

7 Left ventricular diastolic dysfunction

Diastole is an active cardiac process that impacts overall cardiac performance. Diastolic dysfunction may occur independently of the clinical syndrome of congestive heart failure. It is important to distinguish between heart failure with preserved ejection fraction (HFpEF) and diastolic dysfunction; these terms are often used interchangeably, but they are not synonymous. Diastolic dysfunction can be present without symptoms of heart failure, whereas patients with HFpEF almost always have diastolic dysfunction. HFpEF is present in over 30% of patients aged 50 years and older and in >50% of people aged 70 years and older.[1] Conversely, not all patients with heart failure with *reduced* ejection fraction (HFrEF) have diastolic dysfunction. Diastolic dysfunction is independently associated with adverse cardiovascular outcomes and poor prognosis in patients with congestive heart failure.[2,3]

Diastolic dysfunction is characterized by impaired LV relaxation and/or increased LV stiffness. In 2016, the ASE and EACVI published updated guidelines for the assessment of LV diastolic dysfunction, with the objective of simplifying the approach for the grading of LV diastolic dysfunction.[4] In the perioperative setting, strict application of these guidelines may not be practical or accurate. Challenges, such as time constraints, limited TOE views of the LA, and variability in loading conditions, limit the acquisition of some recommended variables. However, the assessment of diastolic dysfunction remains important to guide diagnosis, prognosticate, and assist in clinical decision-making.

Physiology of diastole

LV diastole starts with closure of the AV and lasts until closure of the MV, and is divided into four phases (Figure 7.1):

1. ***Isovolumetric relaxation time (IVRT)***. Begins with closure of the AV, when aortic pressure exceeds pressure in the LV, and ends when LV pressure decreases below pressure in the LA, and the MV opens. Active myocardial relaxation causes a rapid drop in LV pressure, while LV volume remains unchanged (assuming no AR). IVRT is prolonged (>100 ms) by any condition that impairs active relaxation (e.g. myocardial ischaemia) and shortened (<60 ms) by any condition that raises LA pressure (e.g. MR). An abnormally early rise in LA pressure leads to premature opening of the MV, thereby shortening IVRT.
2. ***Early filling (E-wave)***. Starts with opening of the MV and ends with equalization of LA and LV pressures. After MV opening, the LV continues to relax, creating a suction effect, which leads to rapid transmitral flow. Under normal conditions, the largest diastolic pressure gradient between the LA and the LV occurs during early diastolic filling (E-wave). As much as 80% of ventricular filling may occur during this period. Early diastolic filling is decreased in impaired active relaxation of the LV and decreased elastic recoil of the myocardium, and increased with elevated LA pressure.
3. ***Diastasis*** *(mid diastole)*. Active LV relaxation ends, and LA to LV pressures begin to equalize. With a negligible gradient between the two chambers, diastasis is responsible for a small fraction of passive ventricular filling. The main contributor to ventricular filling during this phase is LV compliance. LV compliance is affected by intrinsic myocardial stiffness, RV size, pericardial restriction, ventricular mass, and LV chamber size. Occasionally, mitral inflow is triphasic with an **L-wave** (Figure 7.2) during diastasis. An L-wave can be a normal finding in bradycardic patients with normal hearts. Here, it is secondary to ongoing blood flow into the LA from the pulmonary veins. An L-wave may also be indicative of pathologic conditions that increase LV filling pressures or delay active relaxation (LV hypertrophy, LV systolic dysfunction, heart failure).[5]

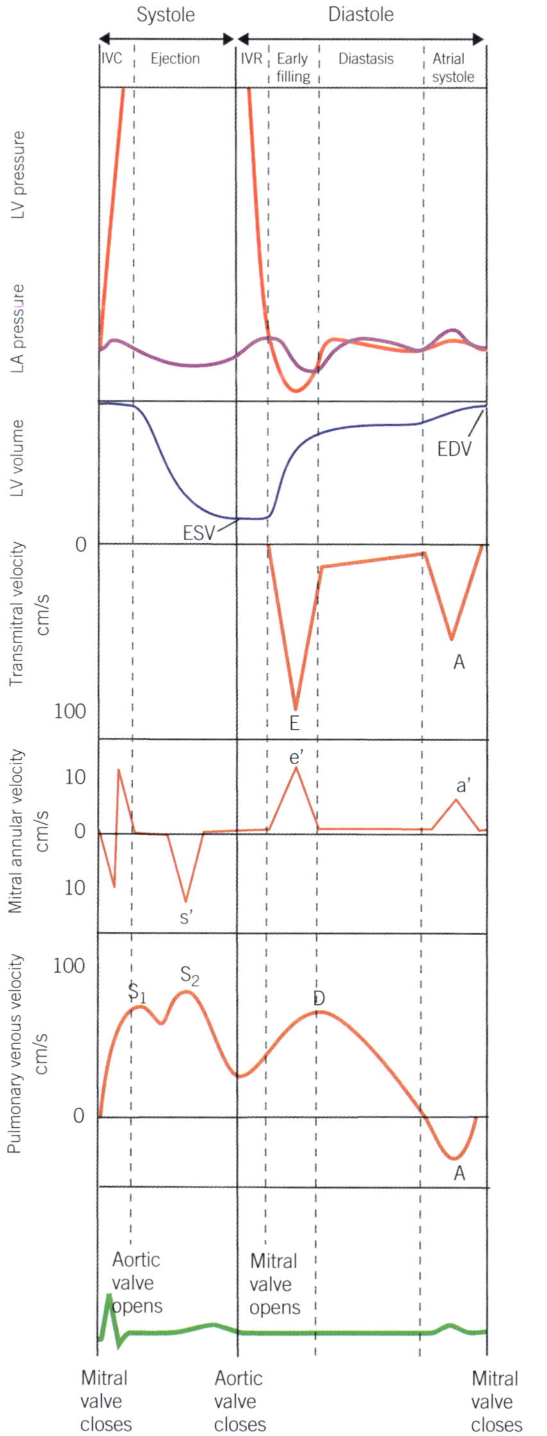

Figure 7.1 Changes in pressure and volume in the left heart during the cardiac cycle. The two phases of systole and the four phases of diastole are shown: isovolumetric contraction (IVC), ejection, isovolumetric relaxation (IVR), early filling, diastasis, and atrial systole. The normal transmitral, pulmonary venous, and tissue Doppler waveforms are shown. See text for details. EDV, end-diastolic volume; ESV, end-systolic volume.

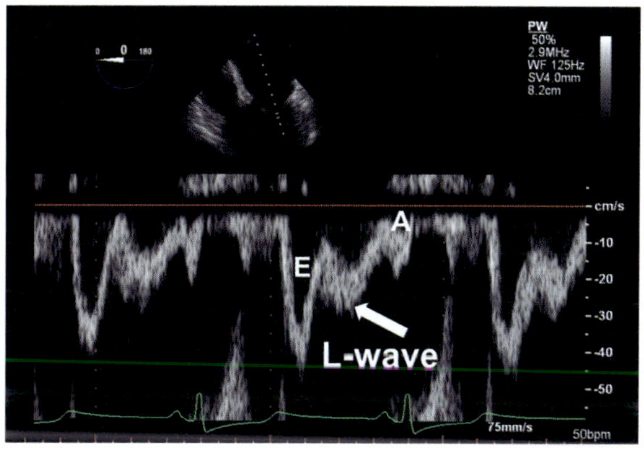

Figure 7.2 Transmitral pulsed-wave Doppler trace. E-wave, A-wave, and L-wave are demonstrated. See text for details.

4. ***Atrial contraction*** *(A-wave).* Late diastole begins with contraction of the LA (A-wave on transmitral PW Doppler) and ends with closure of the MV (onset of LV systole). Atrial systole increases the gradient between the LA and the LV, generating additional flow into the LV and retrograde flow into the pulmonary veins (AR wave on PW Doppler). Normally, atrial contraction is responsible for 20–25% of ventricular filling. In conditions that impair active relaxation (e.g. myocardial ischaemia, LV hypertrophy), the contribution of atrial systole to ventricular filling increases substantially. This phase is dependent on atrioventricular synchrony and is absent in atrial fibrillation.

Early LV filling is dependent on active relaxation of the LV, caused by reuptake of calcium ions into the myocyte sarcoplasmic reticulum, precipitating unlinking of actin–myosin cross-bridges in an adenosine triphosphate (ATP)-consuming process. Diastolic dysfunction initially manifests as reduction of the rate of active relaxation of the LV, leading to a decrease in early diastolic filling (**grade 1, impaired relaxation pattern**). Worsened dysfunction can lead to a decline in LV compliance and a compensatory rise in LA pressure (**grade 2, pseudonormal pattern**). Chronic and progressive decline in LV compliance causes LA pressure to rise further to maintain the LA-to-LV gradient (**grade 3, restrictive pattern**) (Figure 7.3).

Conditions that impair oxygen delivery (e.g. coronary artery disease) or increase oxygen demand (e.g. hypertrophic cardiomyopathy, hypertension, AS) predispose to diastolic dysfunction. Infiltrative processes affecting the LV (e.g. sarcoidosis, amyloidosis) and myocardial fibrosis act via a different mechanism, directly reducing compliance.

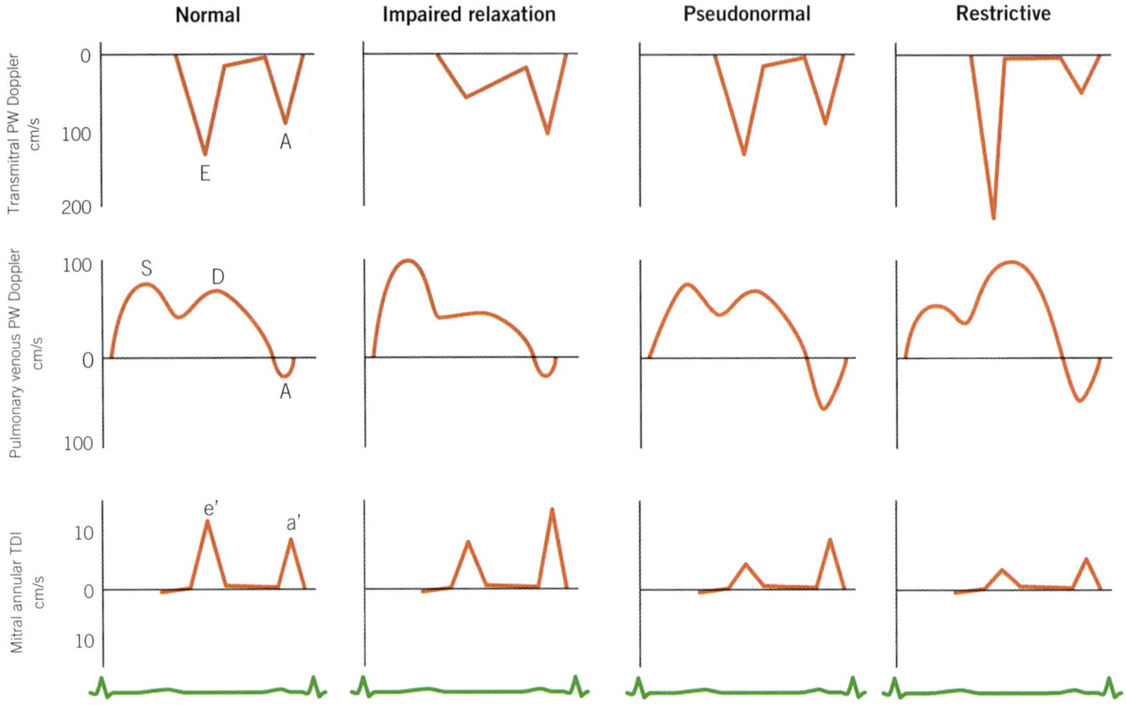

Figure 7.3 Normal and abnormal transmitral, pulmonary venous, and mitral annular tissue Doppler imaging waveforms. For simplicity, the systolic component of the mitral annular tissue Doppler imaging waveform is not shown. Stages of diastolic dysfunction and concomitant changes in pulmonary venous waveforms and mitral annular tissue Doppler imaging are shown.

Expert tip: Understanding the phases of diastole will aid in understanding of the clinical conditions that can affect diastolic performance.

Echocardiographic assessment of diastolic dysfunction

Echocardiographic assessment of LV diastolic dysfunction is based on the assessment of transmitral, pulmonary venous, and mitral annular Doppler waveforms. Doppler assessment is integrated with systolic function and volume status assessment from 2D imaging, including LVEF and subtle myocardial dysfunction detectable by global longitudinal strain (GLS), LA size and function, and valvular abnormalities. Clinical parameters and age are also integrated with echocardiographic information.

Transmitral PW Doppler imaging

The 2016 ASE/EACVI guidelines recommend that evaluation of diastolic dysfunction begin with assessment of LVEF.[4] In the guideline algorithm, an LVEF of 50% serves as a threshold to split assessment pathways.

Where LVEF is reduced (< 50%), the guidelines recommend proceeding to estimation of LV filling pressure with PW Doppler assessment of mitral inflow. A mitral E/A ratio >2 is likely due to elevated LA pressure and grade 3 diastolic dysfunction. Where the mitral E/A ratio is <2, further interrogation is recommended to determine the presence and grade of diastolic dysfunction. Assessment of three additional variables is recommended: average E/e' ratio; LA volume index; and peak TR jet velocity. If two or more of these variables are abnormal, LV diastolic dysfunction is present.

In patients with normal LVEF (≥50%), evidence of myocardial disease such as LV hypertrophy or coronary artery disease with regional wall motion abnormalities (RWMAs) is sought. In the presence of myocardial disease, examination of the following is recommended: mitral inflow E/A ratio; tissue Doppler velocities (septal and lateral mitral annulus e' and average E/e' ratio); peak TR jet velocity; and LA volume index. In the absence of myocardial disease, the guidelines recommend omitting the mitral inflow E/A ratio, and determining the presence of diastolic dysfunction by using tissue Doppler parameters, TR jet peak velocity, and LA volume index. This comprehensive algorithm has limited practical value in the operating room;

hence, a simpler algorithm better suited to the perioperative setting was developed in 2011.[3]

If diastolic dysfunction is present, LV filling pressures can be normal (grade 1 diastolic dysfunction) or elevated (grade 2 or 3 diastolic dysfunction).

Mitral inflow velocities

Ventricular filling depends on the LA-to-LV pressure gradient, which also determines the diastolic velocity profile across the MV. Mitral inflow patterns are therefore useful in the evaluation of diastolic dysfunction. Measurement of mitral inflow using PW Doppler is described in Chapter 4. The transmitral velocity waveform shows an early (E) wave reflecting early diastolic filling, and a second (A) wave due to atrial contraction. As noted, there may be a third wave (L-wave), discussed later. Mitral E velocity reflects the pressure gradient between the LA and LV during early diastole, and is affected by the rate of LV relaxation and LA pressure. E- and A-wave peak velocities and deceleration time (DT) of the E-wave are measured. **Deceleration time** is the time from the E-wave peak to baseline, and is influenced by LV relaxation, LV diastolic pressures following MV opening, and LV stiffness. A short DT with reduced LVEF indicates an elevated left ventricular end-diastolic pressure (LVEDP).

The **E/A ratio** is used to interpret LV filling pressures in patients with LVEF <50% (Figure 7.4):

- If E/A ratio is ≤0.8 and peak E velocity is ≤50 cm/s, then LA pressure (LAP) is low and grade 1 diastolic dysfunction is present (Figure 7.4a).
- If E/A ratio is >0.8 but <2, and peak E velocity is >50 cm/s, then LAP is elevated and grade 2 diastolic dysfunction is present (Figure 7.4b).
- If E/A ratio is ≥2 and peak E velocity is >120 cm/s, then LAP is elevated and grade 3 diastolic dysfunction is present (Figure 7.4c).

Note that an E/A ratio >2 may be a normal finding in individuals who are <40 years of age and is also seen in patients after recent cardioversion.

> ***Expert tip: When measuring mitral inflow with PW Doppler, care should be taken to align the ultrasound beam with the direction of blood flow across the MV.***

Mitral inflow filling patterns

Impaired relaxation: grade 1 diastolic dysfunction

Delayed LV relaxation in early diastole in the setting of normal LA pressure results in a reduced LA-to-LV gradient, since LV pressures show an abnormally slow decline. E-wave velocity is reduced, and DT is prolonged. A greater-than-normal proportion of diastolic filling occurs with atrial contraction, resulting in an increased A-wave velocity, with the E/A ratio decreasing to <0.8. Note that an impaired relaxation pattern is normal in individuals older than 50 years.

Pseudonormal: grade 2 diastolic dysfunction

Diastolic dysfunction progresses with a compensatory increase in LA pressure, resulting in 'normalization' of the LA-to-LV gradient. Consequently, the E-wave velocity appears normal, although the DT may be shortened. The E/A ratio is typically >0.8. A pseudonormal pattern can be distinguished from normal through the use of a Valsalva manoeuvre in awake patients, held for 10 seconds while recording mitral inflow. With Valsalva, mitral inflow filling

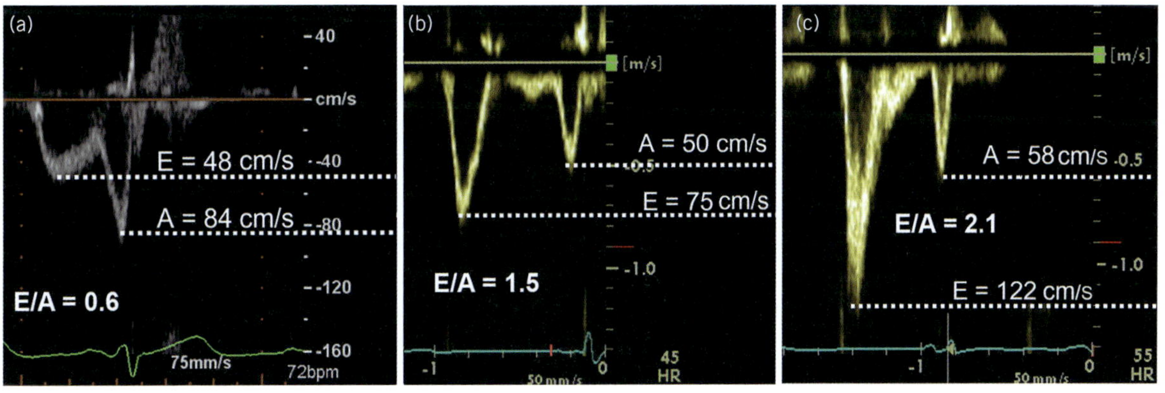

Figure 7.4 Transmitral PW Doppler patterns. Panel (a) shows mitral velocities and ratio consistent with grade 1 diastolic dysfunction (impaired relaxation). Panel (b) shows a pattern consistent with grade 2 diastolic dysfunction (pseudonormal pattern). Panel (c) shows a pattern consistent with grade 3 diastolic dysfunction (restrictive pattern).

pattern changes to an E/A ratio of <0.8, an impaired relaxation pattern. In the anaesthetized patient, LA pressure may be reduced by using the reverse Trendelenberg position or venodilators to reduce preload.

Restrictive filling: grade 3 diastolic dysfunction

Reduced LV compliance, increased LV stiffness, and elevated LA pressure result in a restrictive filling pattern. A wide LA-to-LV pressure gradient results in rapid early ventricular filling and greatly increased E-wave velocity. Decreased LV compliance results in a sharp deceleration of flow in mid diastole, leading to a short DT, and also results in a reduced A-wave velocity. The E/A ratio is typically >2. Restrictive filling is seen in patients with both normal (e.g. restrictive cardiomyopathy) and depressed (e.g. dilated cardiomyopathy) LVEF, and confers a poor prognosis, irrespective of the clinical scenario.

When the E/A ratio and peak E velocity are incongruent, other signals (e.g. TR jet velocity, tissue Doppler velocities) are necessary for estimation of LV filling pressure. A TR jet peak velocity >2.8 m/s and an E/e' ratio >14 support the presence of elevated filling pressures. Tissue Doppler velocities at the mitral annulus are represented by e' (described later). Mitral inflow velocities are unreliable in the presence of atrial fibrillation, moderate or severe MR or MS, mitral annular calcification, MV repair or replacement, LV assist devices, left bundle branch block, or ventricular pacing.

Mitral annular tissue Doppler imaging

Longitudinal shortening of the LV during systole causes descent of the mitral annulus towards the LV apex; longitudinal relaxation during diastole returns the annulus to its original position. TDI of the mitral annulus displays the velocity during the cardiac cycle, and provides information on systolic (see Chapter 6) and diastolic LV function. The diastolic component of mitral annular motion is biphasic, with early (e') and atrial (a') waves, analogous to mitral inflow velocity (Figure 7.3), but in the opposite direction—annular motion during diastole is towards the oesophageal transducer and therefore is displayed *above* the baseline. Important parameters for assessment are maximum e'-wave velocity and E/e' ratio. The normal septal e' velocity cut-off is >7 cm/s, whereas normal lateral e' velocity is >10 cm/s. The mitral annular e'-wave demonstrates progressive reduction in velocity, with worsening diastolic dysfunction, and so provides a useful method to distinguish normal (e'-wave >8 cm/s) from pseudonormal (e'-wave <8 cm/s). The Doppler settings and placement

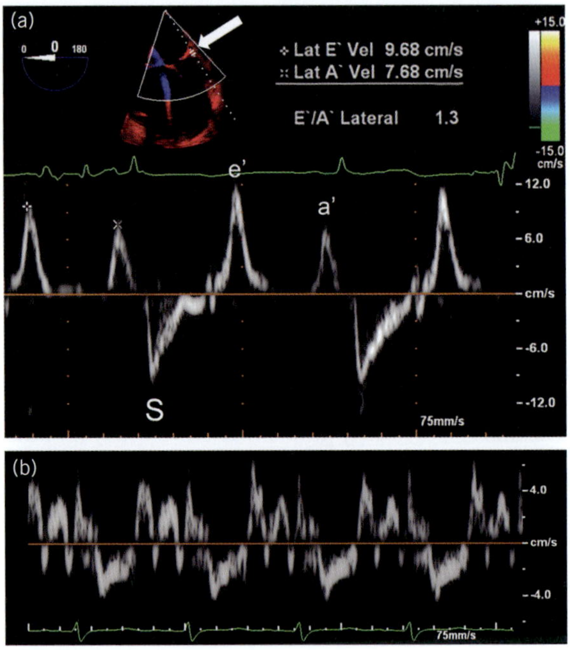

Figure 7.5 PW tissue Doppler imaging of the lateral mitral annulus. (a) demonstrates a PW tissue Doppler waveform from the lateral mitral annulus. The white arrow demonstrates the correct position of the sample volume on the 2D pilot image. The early (e') and atrial (a') waves are demonstrated, along with the systolic (s) wave. Note the clean signal, which is ideal. (b) is an example of a more erratic pattern, with spikes and feathering.

of sample volume must be precise—the sample volume (5–10 mm) must be non-angulated and placed at the annulus, avoiding myocardial wall tissue and LA and LV cavities. Ideally the spectral envelope should not display spikes or feathering (Figure 7.5). Early (e'-wave) velocity has limited accuracy in patients with regional dysfunction in the sample segments, significant mitral annular calcification, MS, MV prostheses, and pericardial disease.

> ***Expert tip: Carefully assess the underlying rhythm so as not to confuse early diastolic velocity with Isovolumetric relaxation velocity.***

Pulmonary vein PW Doppler imaging

Pulmonary vein systolic (S-wave) velocity is influenced by changes in LA pressure and compliance, and by LV and RV contractility.[6] Diastolic (D-wave) velocity is influenced by early diastolic LV filling and LV compliance. Abnormal relaxation is associated with increased S-wave and decreased D-wave, with an S/D ratio >1. Conversely, increased LA pressure is associated with decreased S velocity and increased D velocity, and an S/D velocity ratio <1. Pulmonary vein atrial reversal (AR) velocity duration is measured at zero baseline. The difference between AR duration and mitral A-wave duration (AR-to-A duration) correlates with LVEDP. The longer the time difference, the higher the LVEDP. Factors influencing pulmonary vein flow patterns are shown in Figure 7.6.

Expert tip: A 1- to 2-mm sample volume should be placed in the pulmonary vein at 1–2 cm from its entrance into the LA. Avoid mistaking intra-atrial flow for pulmonary vein flow by checking for the presence of an AR wave in patients in sinus rhythm.

Tricuspid regurgitation peak velocity

Peak TR velocity >2.8 m/s is used as a cut-off value for elevated pulmonary artery systolic pressure (PASP). Previous guidelines recommended calculating PASP by using indirect estimates of RA pressure (measurement of the IVC diameter and collapse with forced inspiration). In cardiac surgical cases where direct measurement of PA pressure is possible, indirect estimation becomes unnecessary. Elevation of PASP >35 mmHg is an indication of elevated LA filling pressure.

Left atrial volume index

Chronic elevation in LA filling pressure results in progressive LA dilation. Maximum LA volume index is measured by using Simpson's biplane method of discs with TTE. In the absence of congenital abnormalities, chronic MV disease, or atrial fibrillation, a maximum LA volume index >34 ml/m^2 is used as a cut-off and provides evidence to support diastolic dysfunction. Although TOE does not allow visualization of the entire LA, inferences can be made about LA volume based on the LA diameter. A diameter >5 cm in any view is considered enlarged.[7]

Colour M-mode flow propagation velocity

M-mode imaging displays the position of structures along a vertical scan line over time. Colour M-mode superimposes colour-encoded blood velocity data onto the same scan line. The information displayed on a colour M-mode recording of LV inflow can be used to assess diastolic

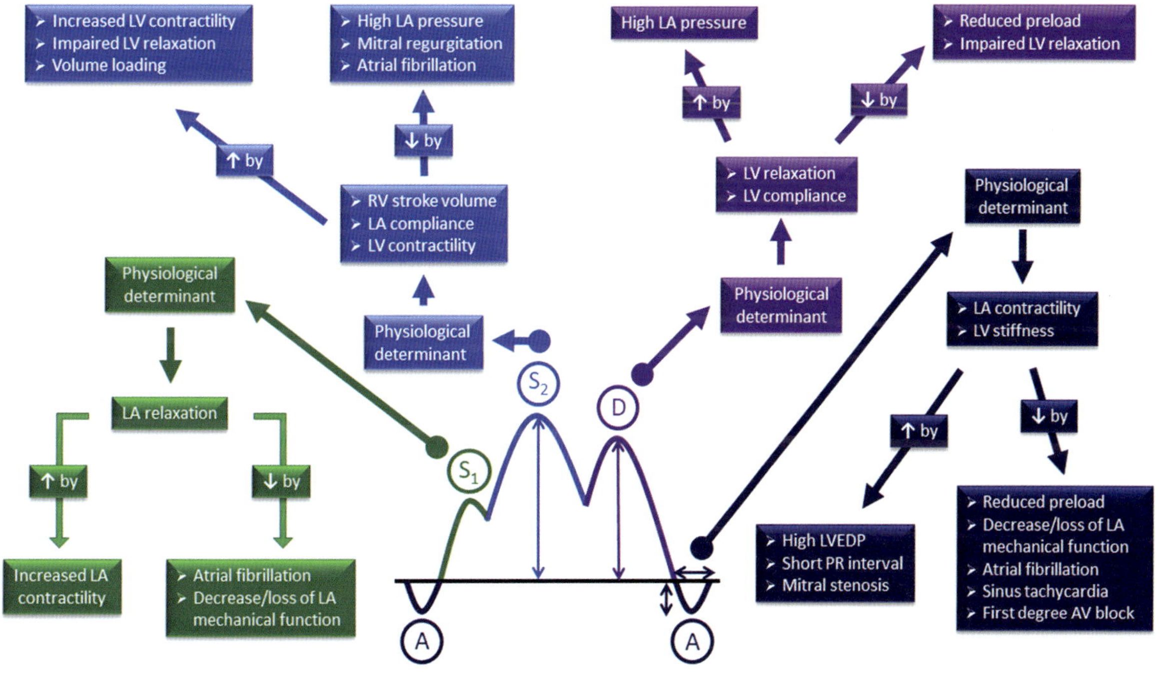

Figure 7.6 Influence of various physiological factors on individual pulmonary venous waveforms. AV, atrioventricular; ↑, increased; ↓, decreased.

Adapted with permission from *Journal of the American Society of Echocardiography*, **34**, 3, Fadel BM, Pibarot P, Kazzi BE, *et al.*, 'Spectral Doppler Interrogation of the Pulmonary Veins for the Diagnosis of Cardiac Disorders: A Comprehensive Review', pp. 223–236, Copyright 2021, with permission from Elsevier and the American Society of Echocardiography.

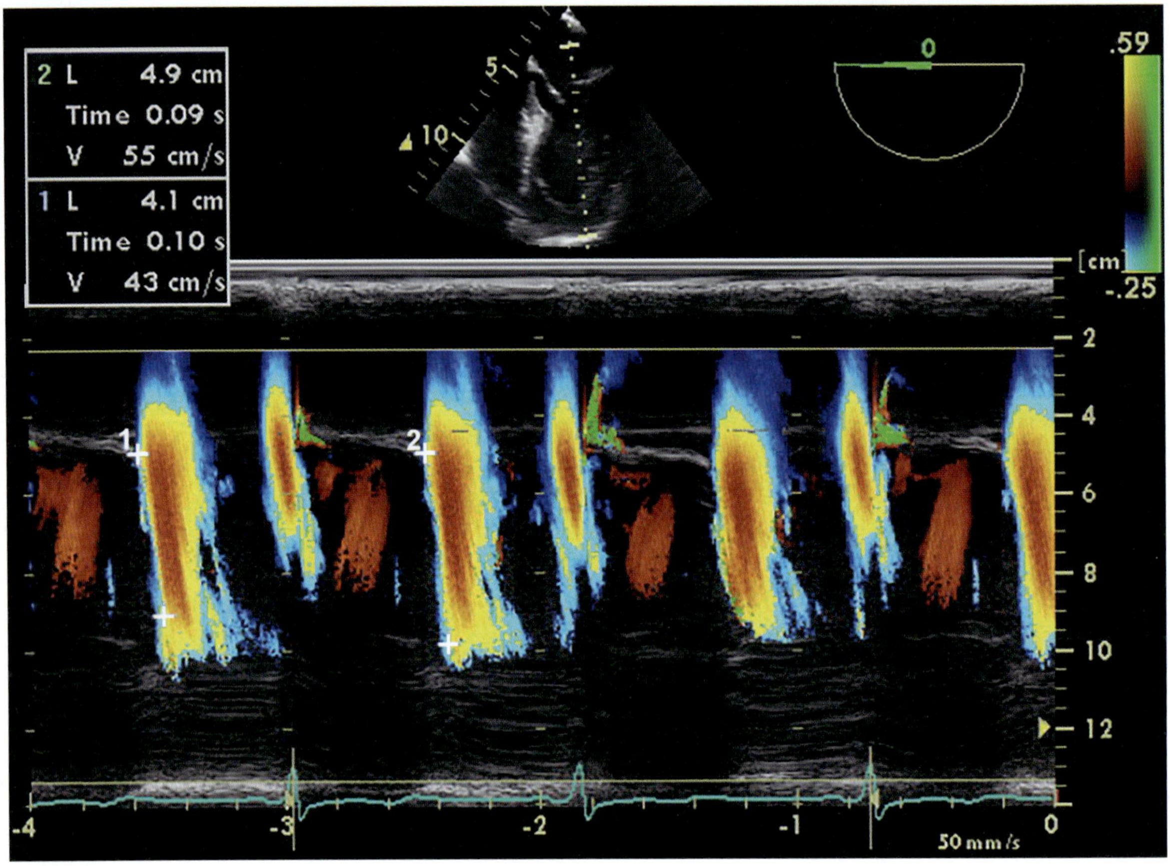

Figure 7.7 Color M-mode flow propagation velocity. See text for details.

function. The **propagation velocity** (Vp) of blood within the LV is the slope of any isovelocity line connecting the mitral leaflets to some point at least 4 cm within the ventricle (Figure 7.7) and is normally >50 cm/s. Diastolic dysfunction is associated with a low Vp (<50 cm/s). Colour M-mode is not reliably assessed clinically and has high inter-observer variability. Small differences in the position of the cursor along the isovelocity line can lead to large changes in the Vp. Furthermore, this method is not widely validated. For these reasons, colour M-mode flow propagation velocity has limited utility in the perioperative setting.[8]

Gender and ethnicity differences have been reported in the normal values for diastolic parameters, with the upper limit of normal for mitral E, septal e', and E/e' ratio higher in women compared with men.[9]

Factors that influence Doppler waveforms

Transmitral, pulmonary venous, and mitral annular tissue Doppler waveforms are influenced by several technical, physiologic, and pathologic factors, aside from diastolic dysfunction.

Doppler beam and sample volume position

Accurate and reproducible measurements are dependent on parallel alignment of the Doppler beam and direction of blood flow, or annular motion for tissue Doppler. As the angle between the Doppler beam and the path of blood flow increases, the error in the measured velocity of flow becomes greater. At angles >20°, an unacceptable level of error is introduced.[10] Optimal sample gate positioning will vary, based on the measurement being performed. For transmitral inflow PW Doppler, the sample volume should be placed *at the level of the leaflet tips in diastole* (the smallest opening). If the sample volume is placed proximal or distal to this point, lower velocities will be recorded. Mitral inflow is normally directed approximately 20° towards the lateral wall from the apex in the mid-oesophageal four-chamber view. The angle will increase further with progressive ventricular dilation and can become challenging to delineate in asymmetrically hypertrophied ventricles.

The left and right upper pulmonary veins are typically best suited for pulmonary venous PW Doppler measurement, as they have a more anterior–posterior alignment. The sample volume should be positioned *1–2 cm into the pulmonary vein* of interest. For mitral annulus TDI, the sample volume should be placed *2–3 mm into the lateral or septal annulus* to allow for intramyocardial velocities to be measured, as the annulus descends during systole. The lateral annulus is usually best aligned with the beam in the mid-oesophageal four-chamber view.

Age

Age is associated with an increase in LV stiffness and a decreased rate of myocardial relaxation.[11] In patients >60 years old, a mitral inflow pattern consistent with impaired relaxation (grade 1 diastolic dysfunction) is typical (Figure 7.8). Variables that are less age-dependent include mitral E/e' velocity, AR–A duration, and Valsalva-induced changes in mitral inflow velocities.[4] Mitral E/e' velocity is not entirely age-independent; however, the e' velocity can be used as a correction for the effects of decreased LV relaxation and values >14 have high specificity for increased LV filling pressures.

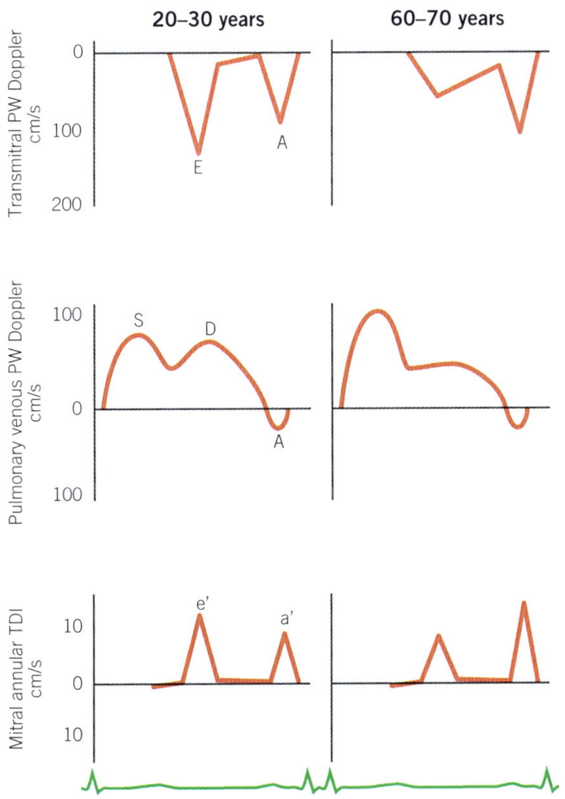

Figure 7.8 The effect of age on the transmitral, pulmonary venous, and mitral annular Doppler waveforms.

Expert tip: Many variables are influenced by age-related changes to the myocardium. Using multiple variables for assessment of diastolic dysfunction is recommended.

Loading conditions

Transmitral flow and Doppler variables such as peak E-wave velocity, E/A ratio, and pulmonary venous S- and D-waves vary with preload (Figure 7.9). In diastolic dysfunction, the pressure–volume curve is shifted to the left and upwards. A small change in preload corresponds to a larger-than-normal change in diastolic pressure in the ventricle. With increased preload, there is a concurrent increase in LA pressure, E- and A-wave velocities, and a shortened E-wave DT. The resulting pattern is similar to a restrictive filling pattern. Increased preload will also result in increased pulmonary vein S-, D-, and retrograde A-wave velocities, and an increased A-wave duration. In contrast, hypovolaemia is associated with a reduced transmitral E-wave, decreased A-wave, and reduced E/A ratio, similar to impaired relaxation. The pulmonary venous waveform in hypovolaemia demonstrates decreased pulmonary venous velocities and a shortened A-wave duration.

A Valsalva manoeuvre can be performed to temporarily reduce preload during the inspiratory hold (strain phase) and differentiate normal from pseudonormal filling. In normal patients, a reduction in E-wave velocity and, to a lesser extent, in A-wave velocity is observed, resulting in a relatively unchanged E/A ratio that remains >1. In patients with grade 2 diastolic dysfunction (pseudonormal pattern), a Valsalva manoeuvre leads to an impaired relaxation filling pattern, with an E/A ratio <1. If a Valsalva manoeuvre is performed in patients with grade 3 diastolic dysfunction (restrictive pattern), they would revert to grade 1 or 2 filling patterns. If patients with grade 3 diastolic dysfunction exhibit no change with Valsalva, they have irreversible or fixed diastolic dysfunction.[12]

Changing preload has less of an effect on mitral annular tissue Doppler e' velocity when compared with transmitral or pulmonary venous velocities. In patients with normal diastolic function, increases and decreases in preload have corresponding modest increases and decreases in e' velocity. However, in patients with abnormal diastolic function, e' velocity is less load-dependent, displaying minimal changes with preload variation.

Increasing LV afterload is associated with reduced E-wave velocity, prolonged E-wave DT, and decreased pulmonary venous S- and D-wave velocities.

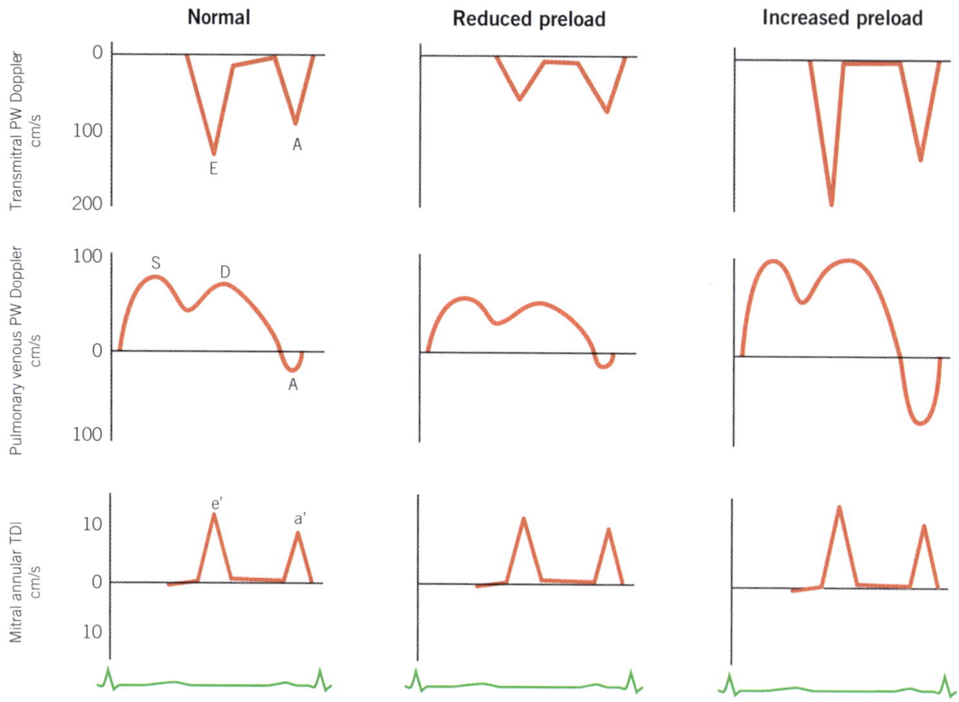

Figure 7.9 **The effect of preload changes on the transmitral, pulmonary venous, and mitral annular Doppler waveforms.**

Heart rate and rhythm

Sinus tachycardia is associated with reduced transmitral E-wave, increased A-wave, and reduced E/A ratio. At heart rates >100/min, or in the presence of first-degree atrioventricular block, E–A fusion occurs (Figure 7.10), making measurement of the E-wave DT impossible. In cases of marked fusion, diastolic MR may also be seen. An increase in the S-wave and a decrease in the D-wave are observed in the pulmonary venous waveform.

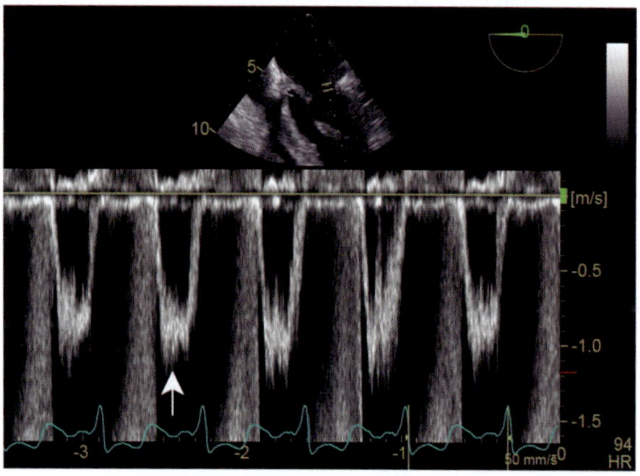

Figure 7.10 **Transmitral pulsed-wave Doppler tracing demonstrating fusion of E- and A-waves (arrow).** See text for details.

With atrial fibrillation, both transmitral and pulmonary venous A-waves are absent. Transmitral E-wave velocity and E-wave DT are highly variable, dependent on the overall cardiac cycle length. Isolated ventricular pacing and atrioventricular dissociation produce dissociated transmitral E- and A-waves. RV epicardial pacing causes asynchronous and prolonged LV myocardial relaxation, resulting in a decreased transmitral E-wave velocity.

Aortic and mitral valve disease

In general, LV diastolic dysfunction cannot be accurately assessed in the presence of significant MV disease. In patients with moderate or severe mitral annular calcification, transmitral velocities are increased, due to decreased mitral effective orifice area. Additionally, calcification of the mitral annulus limits excursion and the e' velocity is relatively low. The E/e' ratio is therefore not reliable in this setting. Transmitral flow velocities should be measured in patients who are in sinus rhythm to obtain the E/A ratio. IVRT should also be measured in the same cardiac cycle. IVRT is the time interval between the end of systolic flow through the LV outflow tract and the onset of mitral inflow. To precisely identify IVRT, the sweep speed should be set at 100 mm/s, and the velocity scale and filter settings should be adjusted appropriately. A short IVRT (<80 ms) suggests elevated filling pressure.

In MS, transmitral flow velocities and mitral annular dynamics are determined primarily by the degree of valvular disease rather than by LV disease. Increased transmitral E- and A-wave velocities and a prolonged E-wave DT are observed. Semiquantitative estimate of LAP can be provided by Doppler variables. The shorter the IVRT, the higher the LAP. The IVRT/$T_{E-e'}$ ratio ($T_{E-e'}$ is the time interval between the 'R'-wave on the ECG and E- and e'-waves) correlates well with mean pulmonary capillary wedge pressure (PCWP) and LA pressure in patients with MS. However, E/e' is not useful.[4] MR is associated with LV volume overload and increased LA pressure. The transmitral E-wave is increased, and the E-wave DT is decreased. The pulmonary venous waveform demonstrates decreased S-wave ('systolic blunting') and increased D-wave velocity (S/D <1). If regurgitation is severe, S-wave reversal may be seen and the effects on the pulmonary venous flow patterns may be uneven between the left and right pulmonary veins, depending on the MR jet direction. Pulmonary vein flow patterns do not accurately reflect diastolic function. The IVRT/$T_{E-e'}$ ratio again correlates well with PCWP here, with a ratio <3 predicting PCWP >15 mmHg.

In patients with severe AR, careful positioning of the sample volume is needed to avoid contamination of mitral inflow velocities measurement with the AR jet. In severe acute AR, LV diastolic filling time is shortened and the MV closes prematurely. In severe chronic AR, the mitral inflow pattern may show predominant early diastolic filling with short DT of the mitral E- velocity. An E/e' ratio >14, TR peak jet velocity >2.8 m/s, and LA enlargement support the presence of elevated LV filling pressures.

Ventilation

Changes in intrathoracic pressure during the respiratory cycle will alter LV loading conditions. During spontaneous ventilation, inspiration results in a fall in intrathoracic pressure, augmenting systemic venous return. An increase in tricuspid E-wave and A-wave velocities is seen, with a small decrease in transmitral E- and A-wave velocities, due to blood pooling in the pulmonary circulation (Figure 7.11). These changes are reversed during expiration. Certain conditions are associated with exaggerations of these normal respiratory variations, including pericardial tamponade, constrictive pericarditis (see Chapter 16), tension pneumothorax, and acute severe asthma. With mechanical ventilation, inspiration causes an increase in intrathoracic pressure, with resultant increases in transmitral flow and E- and A-wave velocities. However,

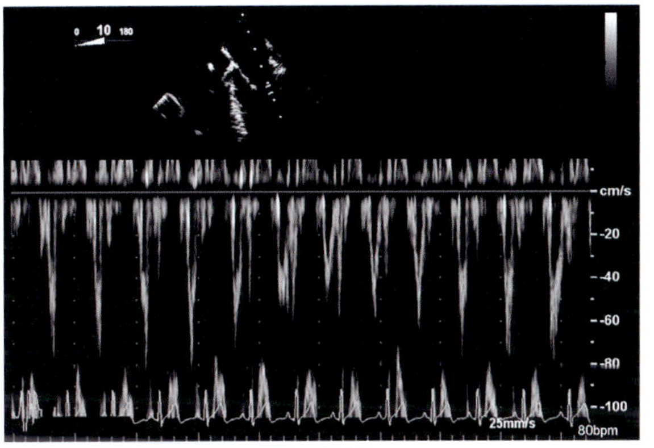

Figure 7.11 Transmitral pulsed-wave Doppler tracing demonstrating variable peak velocity of the transmitral E- and A-waves. See text for details.

this relationship is complex and incompletely defined. Additionally, positive pressure ventilation has the opposite effect on cardiac tamponade, reducing overall respiratory variation.[13] The effects of positive end-expiratory pressure (PEEP) have been more fully investigated, with increasing PEEP leading to a progressive fall in transmitral E- and A-waves and mitral annular e'- and a'-waves, with unchanged E/A and E/e' ratios.[14]

Heart transplantation

Heart transplantation presents different challenges when assessing diastolic function. The donor heart has an altered anatomy secondary to atrial anastomoses, which impairs atrial function, and is denervated, which is associated with resting sinus tachycardia and decreased heart rate variability. A restrictive filling pattern (grade 3 diastolic dysfunction) is common, even in hearts with normal diastolic function. These changes make diastolic parameters difficult to interpret and the usual cut-off values are not validated.[15] A trend of diastolic parameters may be more beneficial over time to assess progressive diastolic function.

Evaluating diastolic dysfunction in the perioperative period

The complexity of the ASE algorithm makes it less practical in the perioperative arena. A simplified algorithm that allows for rapid assessment during cardiac surgery was proposed by Swaminathan *et al.*[3] Using lateral mitral e' velocity, they stratified patients with values ≥10 cm/s as having normal diastolic function. Patients with lateral mitral annulus e' <10 cm/s were further stratified

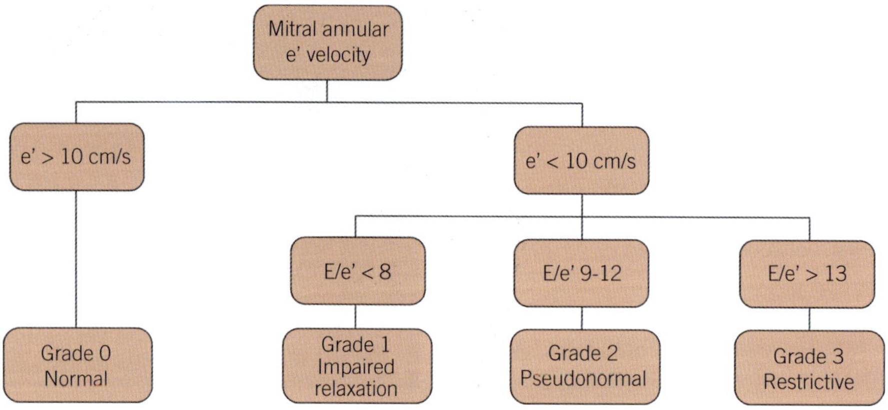

Figure 7.12 Simplified algorithm to grade severity of diastolic dysfunction.

Adapted with permission from *The Annuals of Thoracic Surgery*, **91**, 6, Swaminathan M, Nicoara A, Phillips-Bute BG, *et al.*, Utility of a simple algorithm to grade diastolic function and predict outcome after coronary artery bypass graft surgery, pp. 1844–1850, Figure 1, Copyright 2011, with permission from Society of Thoracic Surgeons and the Southern Thoracic Surgical Association.

based on their E/e' ratio (Figure 7.12). They found that this simple algorithm permitted characterization of LV diastolic dysfunction with TOE in the majority of patients undergoing coronary artery bypass grafting. Patients with normal diastolic function or impaired relaxation are preload-tolerant (i.e. cardiac output will increase with preload augmentation). Conversely, patients with restrictive filling are preload-intolerant (i.e. stroke volume is relatively fixed and preload augmentation may precipitate pulmonary oedema). Importantly, this algorithm was able to identify patients at risk of adverse post-operative outcomes, with the risk increasing with higher-grade diastolic dysfunction.

Multiple choice questions

Discover interactive multiple choice questions to test your knowledge on this chapter by searching for this book's title or ISBN (9780198873686) at **https://academic.oup.com/** and going to the online appendix at the end of the book. Use your scratch-off code on the inside cover to access the material.

References

1. Zile MR, Baicu CF, Gaasch WH. Diastolic heart failure—abnormalities in active relaxation and passive stiffness of the left ventricle. *N Engl J Med.* 2004;**350**(19):1953–9.
2. Bernard F, Denault A, Babin D, *et al.* Diastolic dysfunction is predictive of difficult weaning from cardiopulmonary bypass. *Anesth Analg.* 2001;**92**(2):291–8.
3. Swaminathan M, Nicoara A, Phillips-Bute BG, *et al.* Utility of a simple algorithm to grade diastolic dysfunction and predict outcome after coronary artery bypass graft surgery. *Ann Thorac Surg.* 2011;**91**(6):1844–50.
4. Nagueh SF, Smiseth OA, Appleton CP, *et al.* Recommendations for the evaluation of left ventricular diastolic function by echocardiography: an update from the American Society of Echocardiography and the European Association of Cardiovascular Imaging. *J Am Soc Echocardiogr.* 2016;**29**(4):277–314.
5. Ha JW, Oh JK, Redfield MM, Ujino K, Seward JB, Tajik AJ. Triphasic mitral inflow velocity with middiastolic filling: clinical implications and associated echocardiographic findings. *J Am Soc Echocardiogr.* 2004;**17**(5):428–31.
6. Fadel BM, Pibarot P, Kazzi BE, *et al.* Spectral Doppler interrogation of the pulmonary veins for the diagnosis of cardiac disorders: a comprehensive review. *J Am Soc Echocardiogr.* 2021;**34**(3):223–36.
7. Nicoara A, Skubas N, Ad N, *et al.* Guidelines for the use of transesophageal echocardiography to assist with surgical decision-making in the operating room: a surgery-based approach: from the American Society of Echocardiography in Collaboration with the Society of Cardiovascular Anesthesiologists and the Society of Thoracic Surgeons. *J Am Soc Echocardiogr.* 2020;**33**(6):692–734.
8. Djaiani GN, McCreath BJ, Ti LK, *et al.* Mitral flow propagation velocity identifies patients with abnormal diastolic function during coronary artery bypass graft surgery. *Anesth Analg.* 2002;**95**(3):524–30.
9. Miyoshi T, Addetia K, Citro R, *et al.* Left ventricular diastolic function in healthy adult individuals: results of the World Alliance Societies of Echocardiography Normal Values Study. *J Am Soc Echocardiogr.* 2020;**33**(10):1223–33.
10. Harris P, Kuppurao L. Quantitative Doppler echocardiography. *BJA Educ.* 2016;**16**(2):46–52.
11. Borlaug BA, Redfield MM, Melenovsky V, *et al.* Longitudinal changes in left ventricular stiffness: a community-based study. *Circ Heart Fail.* 2013;**6**(5):944–52.
12. Ghazal SN. Valsalva maneuver in echocardiography. *J Echocardiogr.* 2017;**15**(1):1–5.
13. Faehnrich JA, Noone RB Jr, White WD, *et al.* Effects of positive-pressure ventilation, pericardial effusion, and cardiac tamponade on respiratory variation in

transmitral flow velocities. *J Cardiothorac Vasc Anesth*. 2003;**17**(1):45–50.
14. Chin JH, Lee EH, Kim WJ, *et al*. Positive end-expiratory pressure aggravates left ventricular diastolic relaxation further in patients with pre-existing relaxation abnormality. *Br J Anaesth*. 2013;**111**(3):368–73.
15. Sciaccaluga C, Fusi C, Landra F, *et al*. Diastolic function in heart transplant: from physiology to echocardiographic assessment and prognosis. *Front Cardiovasc Med*. 2022;**9**:969270.

8
The mitral valve

The MV is ideally suited to examination with TOE because it lies in close proximity to the oesophagus and is separated from the transducer by the blood-filled LA, which acts as a superb acoustic window. In systole, the leaflets lie perpendicular to the ultrasound beam, enhancing the quality of the 2D image. Flow through the valve is nearly parallel to the ultrasound beam, creating excellent conditions for Doppler analysis. 3D is superior to 2D for predicting concordance with intraoperative findings during MV surgery,[1,2] and for this reason, 3D imaging should be performed routinely in patients undergoing MV surgery.

Anatomy

The MV should be thought of as a 'valve complex', or apparatus, consisting of the annulus, leaflets, chordae tendineae, papillary muscles, and the LV muscle that supports the papillary muscles. The relationship of the MV to surrounding cardiac structures is shown in Figure 8.1.

Annulus

The mitral annulus is a fibrofatty ring that approximates a hyperbolic paraboloid, a 3D shape that resembles a riding saddle (Figure 8.2). The annulus has two axes: a shorter and 'higher' (more basal) anteroposterior (AP) axis, and a longer and 'lower' (more apical) commissural axis (Figure 8.2). The AP axis is displayed in the mid-oesophageal long-axis view, while the commissural axis is visible in the mid-oesophageal mitral commissural view. The anterior pole of the AP axis can be thought of as the 'riding horn' of the saddle, and the commissural axis as the 'seat' of the saddle. The saddle shape of the annulus helps to reduce leaflet tension. During systole, radial shortening of the basal myocardial fibres causes sphincteric contraction of the posterior annulus, reducing the annular area by approximately 25%. Additionally, systolic folding takes place along the commissural axis, deepening the saddle. Sphincteric contraction and annular folding help to appose the mitral leaflets, particularly in early systole when ventricular pressure is low. Note that dilatation is associated with loss of the saddle shape of the MV, which contributes to annular dysfunction.

Anteriorly, the annulus is thickened and in direct continuity with the aortic root. This fibrous thickening is termed the intervalvular fibrosa or aorto-mitral curtain (Figure 8.1).

Leaflets

The MV has an anterior and a posterior leaflet. The leaflets do not lie in a true AP orientation; the anterior leaflet lies somewhat antero-medially, and the posterior leaflet somewhat postero-laterally, but for descriptive purposes, the terminology anterior and posterior is still used (Figure 8.3). The posterior leaflet has twice the annular attachment, but only half the base-to-tip length of the anterior leaflet.

The leaflets join at two **commissures**, based on their anatomic location: anterolateral and posteromedial. During systole, when the leaflet tips are apposed, a curved coaptation line forms between the two commissures. Under normal circumstances, the plane of coaptation is at, or slightly below, the level of the annulus, and there is normally 8–10 mm of leaflet overlap (called '*coaptation length*') at end-systole. The anterior MV leaflet is in fibrous continuity with the non-coronary and left coronary leaflets of the aortic valve.

In most people, the posterior MV leaflet comprises three distinct **scallops**, separated by more or less well-defined recessed areas called **indentations**. Pleating of the scallops at the site of these indentations aids in closure of the C-shaped posterior leaflet. By contrast, the anterior leaflet does not have distinct scallops per se, but it is divided into three segments for descriptive purposes. The anterior leaflet does not alter its circumferential length during systole, and no pleating mechanism is required. The leaflet segments are named using the Carpentier system (after Prof. Alain Carpentier, a French surgeon)—the anterolateral, middle, and posteromedial scallops of the posterior leaflet are named P1, P2, and P3, respectively, and the

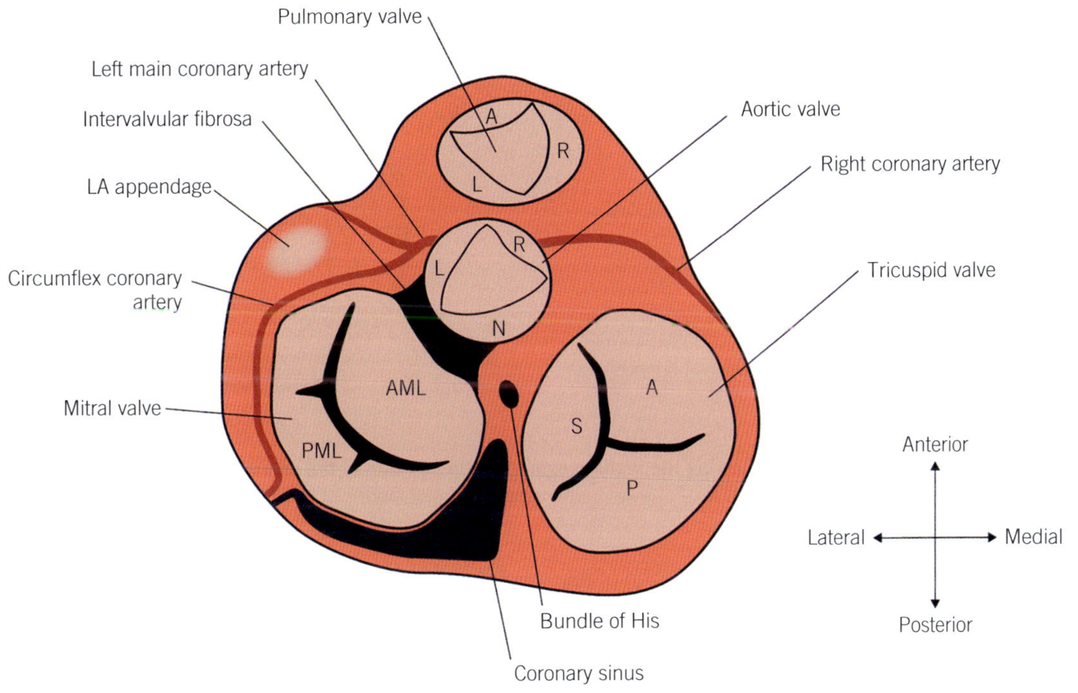

Figure 8.1 View of the four heart valves and surrounding structures. The base of the heart is shown in an anatomical orientation from the LA aspect. The relationships of the MV to the AV, LA appendage, circumflex coronary artery, coronary sinus, and bundle of His are demonstrated. Valve leaflets are labelled: AML, anterior mitral leaflet; PML, posterior mitral leaflet; A, anterior leaflet of the pulmonary and tricuspid valves; L, left leaflet of the pulmonary and aortic valves; R, right leaflet of the pulmonary and aortic valves; N, non-coronary leaflet of the aortic valve; S, septal leaflet of the tricuspid valve; P, posterior leaflet of the tricuspid valve.

opposing segments of the anterior leaflet are termed A1, A2, and A3, respectively (Figure 8.3). Other nomenclatures of the MV have been published but have not gained widespread acceptance.

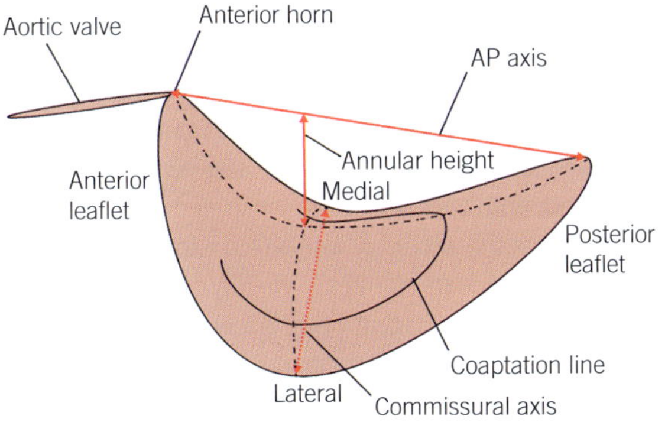

Figure 8.2 The mitral annulus. The 3D shape of the mitral annulus approximates a riding saddle. There are two axes: the anteroposterior (AP) axis, which is higher (more basal) and shorter, and the commissural axis, which is lower (more apical) and longer. The shorter AP axis is imaged in the mid-oesophageal long-axis view, while the longer commissural axis is imaged in the mid-oesophageal commissural view.

Papillary muscles, left ventricle, and chordae tendineae

Two papillary muscles—the anterolateral and posteromedial—support the mitral leaflets. Their orientation is similar to that of the commissures of the same names (Figure 8.3). The anterolateral muscle supports the anterolateral segments of both leaflets (A1/P1 and part of A2/P2), and the posteromedial muscle supports the posteromedial segments of both leaflets (A3/P3 and part of A2/P2). This allows for the A2/P2 segment (highest stress area) to have ample support; however, despite this, P2 prolapse/flail remain a common cause of MR. The anterolateral muscle has dual blood supply from branches of the left anterior descending and circumflex coronary arteries, whereas the posteromedial muscle (in most patients) is supplied entirely by the right coronary artery. This explains why ischaemic rupture of the posteromedial muscle is more common than the anterolateral muscle. In most patients, the anterolateral papillary muscle inserts into the mid-anterolateral region of the LV wall, and the posteromedial papillary muscle inserts into the mid-inferior or inferolateral segments. Adequate

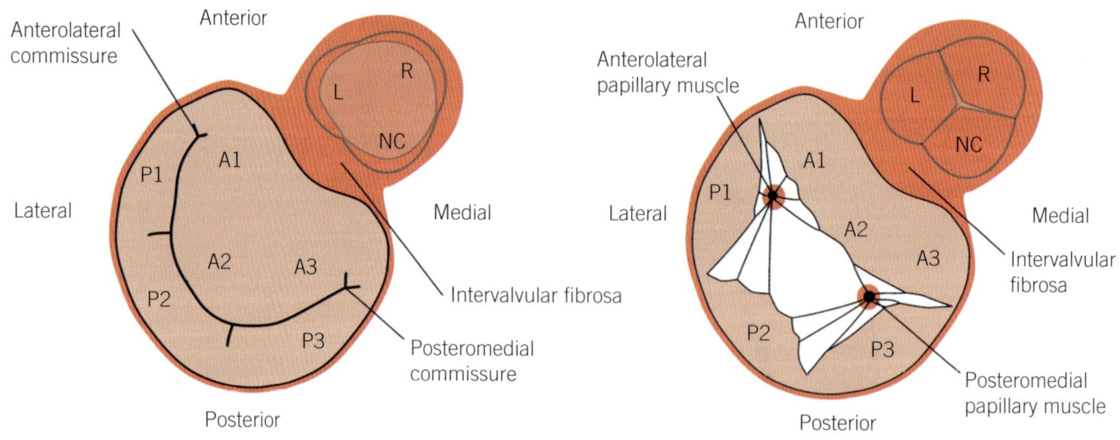

Figure 8.3 MV in systole and diastole showing the leaflet segments, the position of the commissures and papillary muscles, and the relationship to the AV leaflets. The MV is shown in the anatomic orientation.

LV function is important to maintain the orientation of the papillary muscles and prevent MR.

The papillary muscles attach to the valve leaflets via fibrous strands called **chordae tendineae**. Primary chordae attach to the free edges of the leaflets, and secondary chordae attach to the ventricular surface of the body of the leaflets. Primary chordae support the free edges of the leaflets, and their rupture usually causes acute MR. Secondary chordae help to maintain LV geometry, particularly the thicker strut chords that attach to the ventricular surface of the anterior leaflet. When they are shortened, or when the underlying LV wall is dilated, these chords also contribute to mitral leaflet *tethering*, which is a cause of MR (discussed later in this chapter and in Chapter 9). A substantial volume of blood passes through the interchordal space during diastole, and chordal thickening or fusion can contribute to mitral stenosis by causing subvalvular obstruction.

Systematic examination of the MV

Orientation of the MV can be confusing. The three main orientations used in this book are described in Figure 8.4. In the **anatomic view**, an *en face* view from the LA perspective, the valve is oriented in such a way that the left and right of the image correspond to the patient's left and right. The **surgeon's view** is rotated slightly to the left from the anatomic view. It is most commonly used with 3D echo, and it greatly facilitates communication with the surgical team. The **TOE view** corresponds to the 2D transgastric short-axis view of the MV, with the patient's left on the right of the image and the patient's right on the left of the image.

Echocardiographic–anatomic relationships

Identification of the various leaflet segments in the standard 2D TOE views of the MV are shown in Figure 8.5 and Online appendix 1.4. Using 2D imaging only, it can sometimes be difficult to be sure of which leaflet segments are visualized in each view. Some anatomical reference points in the heart can provide a general idea of which mitral segments are visualized; for example, the LVOT is an anterior cardiac structure, and when it is visible in a four-chamber view of the MV, one can reasonably assume that one is looking at the anterior segments of the MV (A1–2/P1–2). Likewise, if the LVOT is not present in a four-chamber view, one can generally assume that one is looking at the more posterior aspects of the MV (A2–3/P2–3). The LA appendage is another recognizable landmark usually adjacent to the anterolateral commissure (A1/P1). However, because of anatomical variants and distortion of the cardiac structures with long-standing valve disease, these reference points are not always reliable. Moreover, even small movements of the probe can also significantly alter the leaflet segments visualized. Mahmood and colleagues demonstrated that fact and reported that the accuracy with which experienced echocardiographers can correctly identify mitral segments from the mid-oesophageal views is low, particularly in the long-axis and four-chamber views.[3] Drake *et al.* described a technique of axial imaging of the MV, which relies on specific landmarks in the long-axis and commissural planes to confirm correct image orientation. Using this technique, they reported concordance with intraoperative findings of 94% for 2D imaging and of 100% for 3D imaging (Figures 8.6 and 8.7; see Online appendix 6.1).[2] Ultimately, the use of multi-plane 3D imaging software,

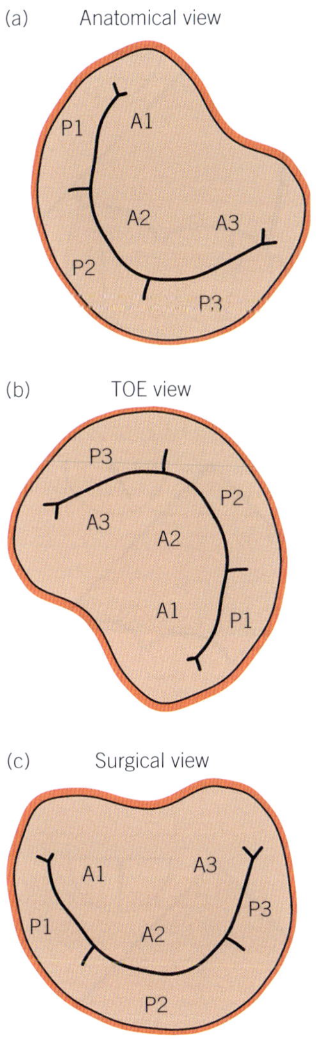

Figure 8.4 Orientation of the MV. In the anatomic view (a), the MV is viewed from the base of the heart (the LA side), with the atrium cut away. In this view, the valve is oriented such that the left and right of the image correspond to the patient's left and right, and the anterior and posterior leaflets appear in their correct anatomic positions. The lateral aspect of the valve is on the left, and the medial (or septal) aspect on the right. The anatomic view is used in line drawings throughout this chapter. Rotation of the anatomic view through 180° produces the TOE view (b), in which the observer's left and right are reversed, relative to the patient. This view corresponds to the orientation of the MV as it appears in the transgastric basal short-axis view. The surgical view (c) is the view the surgeon has, standing on the patient's right, looking through an LA incision. The AV is in the 12 o'clock position, and the LA appendage is in the 9 o'clock position. The surgeon's view is the standard view for displaying 3D data sets of the MV, which facilitates communication with the surgical team.

described later in this chapter, has made the precise identification of mitral segments much more reliable.

Mid-oesophageal views

Correct identification of the mid-oesophageal long-axis and commissural views is central to accurate 2D TOE imaging of the MV, as these views are aligned with the two main axes of the valve. Furthermore, in the long-axis view, the image plane passes perpendicularly to the coaptation line, allowing accurate measurements of leaflet height (the length from the annulus to the tip) to be obtained.

2D axial imaging uses the concept of the mitral–LV apex axis, an imaginary line running from the centre of the MV through the LV apex, along the intersection of the mid-oesophageal long-axis and commissural views. Using the landmarks described in Figure 8.6 and Online appendix 6.1.1, one confirms that both views are parallel to the mitral–LV apex axis and perpendicular to each other, ensuring that measurements are not distorted by oblique imaging. An essential component of 2D axial imaging is identifying the LV apex. However, optimal imaging of the mitral apparatus is best performed using a zoomed view of the valve. Therefore, the landmarks for axial imaging should be obtained, with the depth adjusted to include the LV apex; then, without moving the probe, the zoom function should be used to display the mitral apparatus in detail.

> ***Expert tip: A quick way to confirm that the long-axis view passes through the centre of the valve is to briefly turn on the 3D 'live' multi-plane mode and assess the alignment in the orthogonal plane (*Figure 8.7*).***

Live simultaneous multi-plane imaging is also helpful in obtaining accurate commissural and long-axis views. Because the landmarks for the commissural view are more readily apparent, this view should be obtained first. Then, by activating the multi-plane mode, an orthogonal long-axis view is displayed in the right-hand panel. By moving the cursor from left to right on the screen (from posteromedial to anterolateral on the valve), it is possible to accurately assess the entire MV anatomy.

When correctly obtained, the long-axis view is aligned with the AP ('higher', 'shorter') axis of the annulus. The

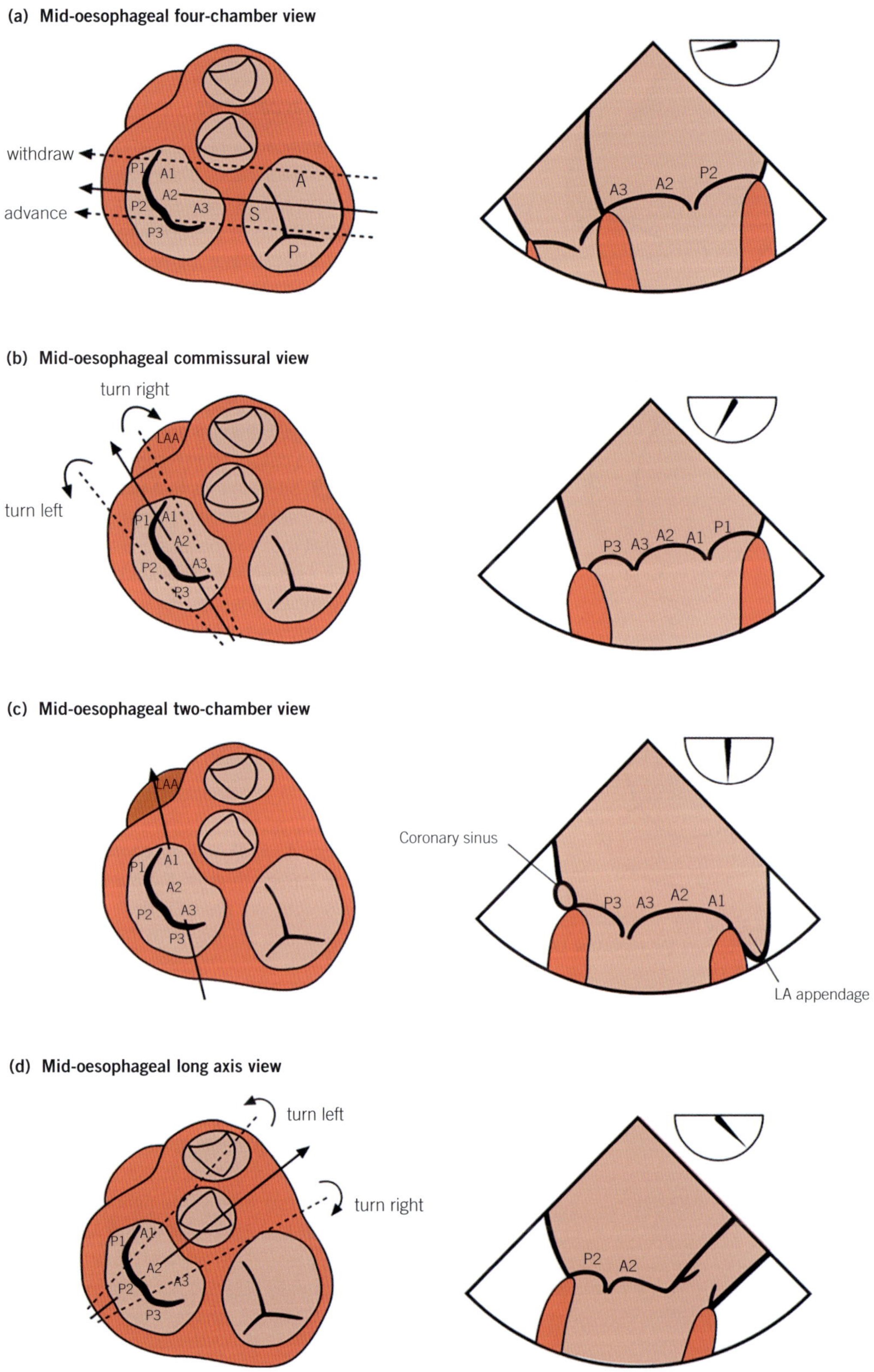

Figure 8.5 Standard image planes for assessing the MV. (a) Mid-oesophageal four-chamber view; (b) mid-oesophageal commissural view; (c) mid-oesophageal two-chamber view; (d) mid-oesophageal long axis view; (e) transgastric basal short axis view; (f) transgastric two-chamber view. See also Online appendix 1.4.

Reproduced with kind permission from David Sidebotham.

(e) Transgastric basal short axis view

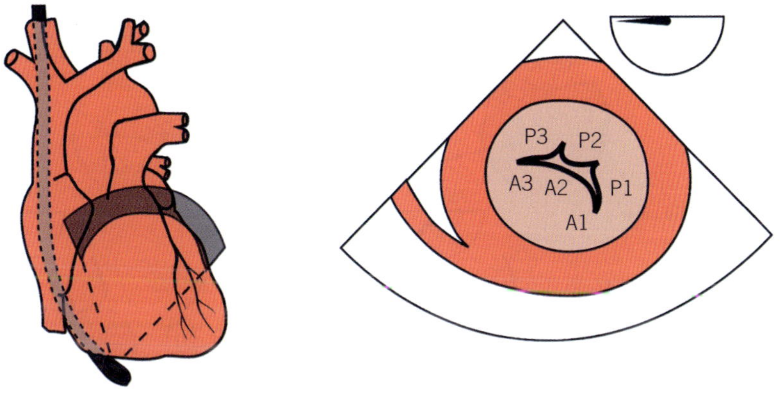

(f) Transgastric two-chamber view

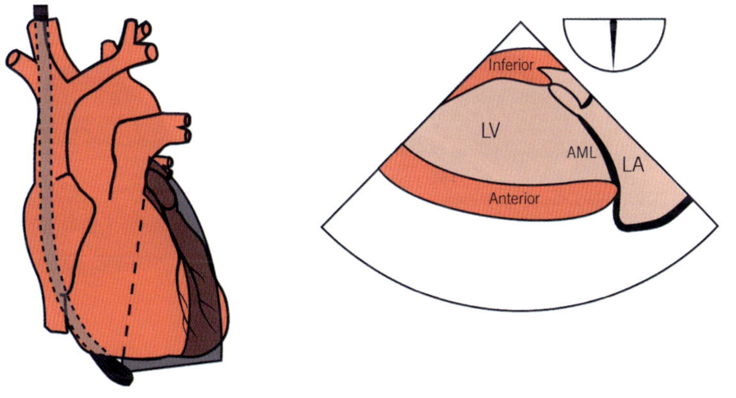

Figure 8.5 *Continued*

image plane runs perpendicular to the coaptation line and displays P2 on the left and A2 on the right (Figures 8.5 and 8.7). The mitral and aortic valves are both visible, but neither papillary muscle is seen. Turning the probe to the left (anticlockwise) sweeps the scan plane towards the anterolateral commissure, passing through P1/A1. Eventually the LA appendage comes into view. From the midline position, turning the probe to the right (clockwise) sweeps the scan plane towards the posteromedial commissure, passing through P3/A3 (note that these physical movements of the probe produce the same images as moving the multi-plane cursor on a commisural view described in the last paragraph). The long-axis view should be used for measuring the AP annular diameter and for assessing the P2/A2 coaptation surface. When colour Doppler is added, it is also the appropriate view for measuring the width of the vena contracta in 2D (described later).

If 3D imaging/live orthogonal imaging is not available, the method described by Drake *et al.* has been shown to reproducibly identify the MV segments and anatomy (Figures 8.6 and 8.7; see Online appendix 6.1).

When correctly obtained, the commissural view is aligned with the commissural axis of the annulus. Because of the semilunar shape of the coaptation, three mitral segments and two coaptation points are visible in this cross-section, with the P3 segment visible on the left, the A2 segment in the centre, and the P1 segment on the right. In diastole, the A2 segment appears to float freely in the centre of the annular plane and may disappear altogether. The leaflet segments visualized in the commissural view depend on the exact probe position. If the scan plane passes exactly through the centre of the valve, the P3/A3 coaptation is visualized on the left and the A1/P1 coaptation is visualized on the right (Figure 8.5). From the central position, turning the probe slightly to the right (clockwise) sweeps over the anterior leaflet and turning the probe slightly to the left sweeps over the posterior leaflet. The commissural view passes through the 'lower', 'longer' axis of the valve; therefore, in the normal MV, higher values

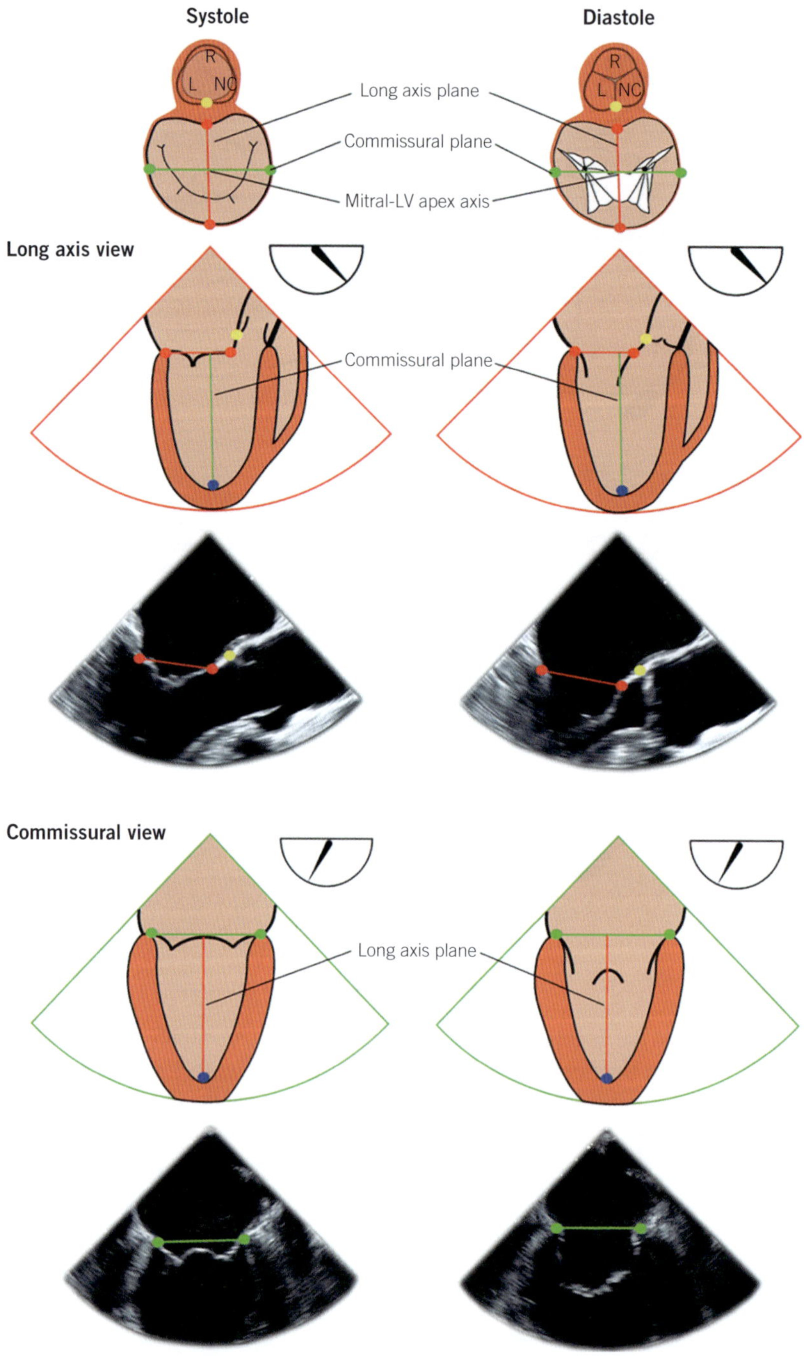

Figure 8.6 Landmarks for 2D axial imaging of the MV (see also Online appendix 6.1.1). The mitral–LV apex axis is an imaginary line running from the centre of the MV through the LV apex at the intersection of the mid-oesophageal long-axis and commissural views. The long-axis and commissural views are imaged in systole and diastole, with sufficient depth to incorporate the LV apex. The long-axis diastolic landmarks should include: (1) the commissure between the left and non-coronary leaflets of the AV (yellow dot); (2) the maximum anteroposterior annular width (red dots); and the LV apex (blue dot). The commissural diastolic landmarks should include: (1) the maximum annular width (green dots); (2) the free-floating A2 segment in the centre of the valve; and (3) the LV apex (blue dot). Subsequently, without moving the probe, the zoom function is used to focus on the MV. Zoomed views of the long-axis and commissural views in systole and diastole are shown. Measurements (e.g. annular dimensions, tenting height, etc.) are made on the zoomed images. In this diagram, the colour red denotes the long-axis plane, and the colour green denotes the commissural plane. This is the same colour scheme as used in Figure 8.11.

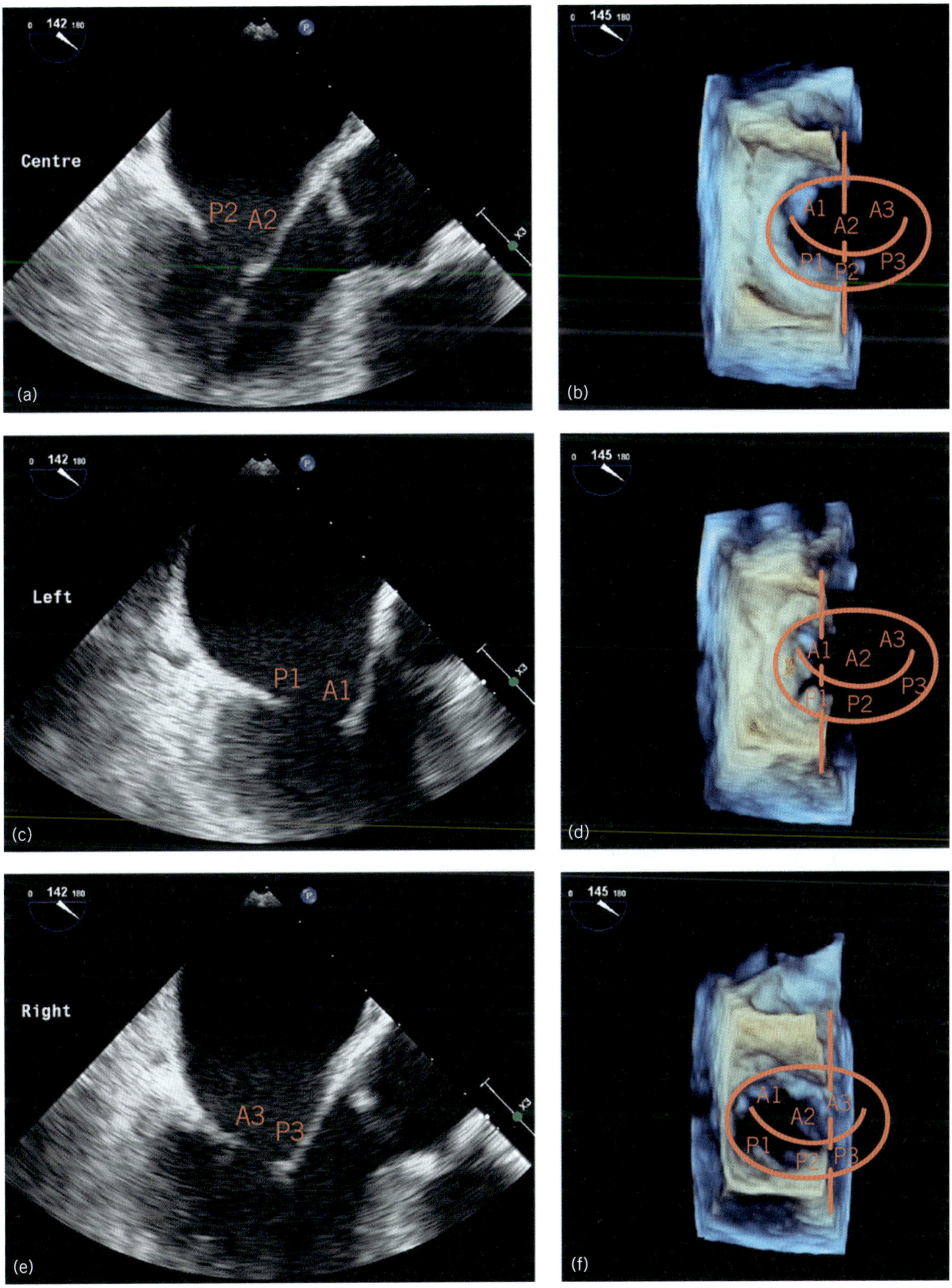

Figure 8.7 The use of 3D 'live' mode to help confirm correct positioning of the mid-oesophageal long axis view. The midoesophageal long-axis views are shown in (a), (c), and (e), and the resultant 3D 'live' views are demonstrated in (b), (d), and (f). In (b), 3D imaging demonstrates that the long-axis view passes through the centre of the valve (i.e. A2/P2). In (c) and (d), the probe has been turned to the left (anticlockwise) from the centre position, moving the sector scan towards the anterolateral commissure. 3D imaging shows the resultant long-axis view now passes through A1/P1. In (e) and (f), the probe has been turned to the right (clockwise) from the centre position, moving the sector scan towards the posteromedial commissure. 3D imaging indicates that the resultant long-axis view now passes through A3/P3.

for annular dimension are usually obtained in this view than in the long-axis view. This is not necessarily true in pathologic states where the poorly supported posterior wall may dilate and the anterior–posterior diameter can enlarge more than the commissural diameter.

Because the commissural view scans along the mitral coaptation line, if an MR jet is elliptical or long and thin (as opposed to circular), it may appear much broader than it actually is, or it may appear as a double jet or even multiple jets (Figure 8.8). For that reason, this view should not be used to measure the vena contracta (the long-axis view, which cuts perpendicular to the coaptation line, is preferred).[4]

Whether 2D imaging or 3D multi-plane is used, it is important to obtain long-axis and commissural views that pass through the *centre* of the valve. First, this ensures that all three coaptation surfaces (A1/P1, P2/A2, A3/P3) are visualized. Second, reproducible measurements of the minor (long-axis view) and major (commissural view) axes of the annulus can be obtained.

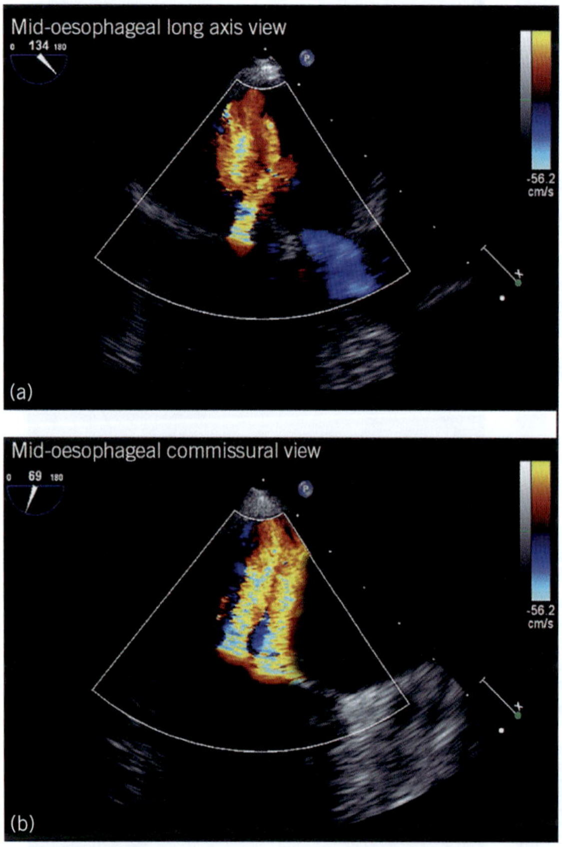

Figure 8.8 Mitral regurgitation demonstrated in the (a) mid-oesophageal long-axis and (b) commissural views in the same patient. This patient has a long, irregularly shaped jet of MR. (a) In the long-axis view, the image plane is perpendicular to the coaptation line, and a single jet of regurgitation is seen. (b) In the commissural view, the image plane is parallel to the coaptation line, showing a long, apparently double jet of MR.

In the standard four-chamber view, the anterior leaflet (usually A2) is on the left, and the posterior leaflet (usually P2) is on the right of the screen. Typically, the scan plane cuts the coaptation line slightly obliquely, and it can be difficult to be sure exactly which leaflet segments are visualized. Gently withdrawing or anteflexing the probe sweeps the image plane towards the anterolateral commissure (A1/P1) and displays the LVOT. Gently advancing or retroflexing the probe sweeps the image plane towards the posteromedial commissure (A3/P3).

In the standard two-chamber view at 90° of transducer rotation, P3 is to the left of the image and the three segments of the anterior leaflet (A3/A2/A1) are to the right. The P3/A3 coaptation surface is visualized.

Because the four-chamber and two-chamber views cut through the valve obliquely, these views should not be used for making annular measurements, measuring leaflet lengths, or evaluating the vena contracta.

Transgastric views

The basal short-axis view provides an *en face* view of the MV. With colour Doppler imaging in that view, it is possible to identify the location of a regurgitant jet, but not necessarily the pathological process *per se* (prolapse, restriction, etc.) (Figure 8.9). To visualize a regurgitant jet, the image plane must be sufficiently basal (at or above the annular plane in systole), which is sometimes not possible. The advent of 3D imaging has made the transgastric basal short-axis view less important in localizing segmental pathology, but it may still have some utility in the evaluation of transcutaneous edge-to-edge repair procedure. The transgastric two-chamber view is useful for visualizing the mitral subvalvular apparatus.

3D imaging

3D data sets of the MV are most commonly acquired using the 'zoom' mode. Apart from the annulus and leaflets, the AV and LA appendage should be included in the data set to help with image orientation. Single-beat acquisition is usually adequate for standard 3D imaging; however, for colour 3D imaging, multi-beat acquisition is necessary to ensure an adequate frame rate (ideally >15 Hz). The most intuitive format to display the MV is the 'volume' mode, in which the entire annulus and leaflets can be visualized simultaneously. The data sets should be displayed in

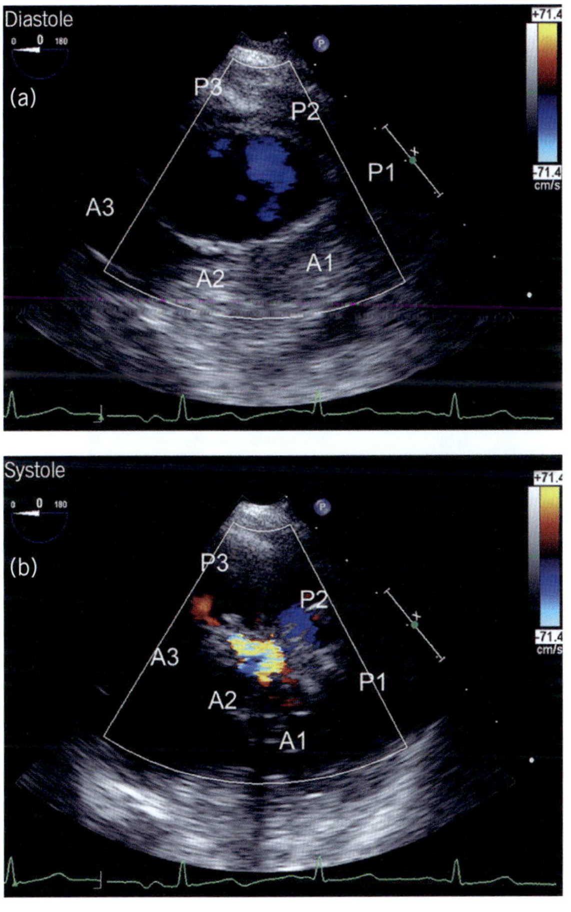

Figure 8.9 Mitral regurgitation in the (a) transgastric basal short-axis view. In (b) (systolic), a jet of MR can be seen in the central region of the valve (A2/P2). However, it is not obvious from these images what the mechanism of MR is or which leaflet is responsible for the regurgitation.

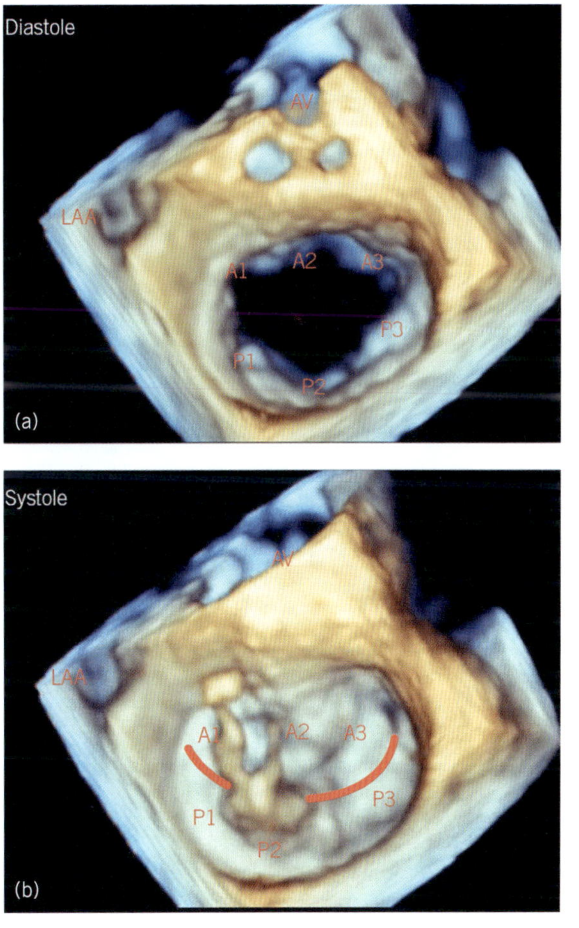

Figure 8.10 3D imaging of the MV, displayed in 'volume'-rendered mode. The images were acquired using 3D zoom. The data set is rotated to demonstrate the valve in the 'surgeon's view' (i.e. from the LA aspect, with the AV in the 12 o'clock position and the LA appendage (LAA) at 9 to 10 o'clock). The valve is shown in (a) diastole and (b) systole. The position of the six mitral segments is demonstrated. In the systolic frame, the approximate position of the coaptation line is also indicated. Note that this patient has a flail segment arising in the P1/P2 region of the valve. In systole, the flail segment and associated chordae can be seen extending over the A1/A2 region.

the surgical orientation from the LA aspect, as shown in Figure 8.10 and Online appendices 1.4.11 and 6.1.2.

Quantitative analysis is performed using multi-planar reconstruction (MPR), in which the 3D data set is displayed as three adjustable orthogonal two-dimensional slices (see Online appendix 6.1.3). Using the technique described in Figure 8.11, the AP and commissural image planes can be precisely located within the 3D structure. Once located, these 2D images display all surfaces of the valve, and reproducible measurements of the minor and major axes of the valve can be made. Furthermore, indices of leaflet dysfunction (prolapse height, coaptation height, tenting height and area) can be made at each coaptation surface. Indeed, the measurements obtained from these precisely located 2D images from within the 3D data set are perhaps of greater benefit to surgical decision-making than the elegant volume-rendered images, shown in Figure 8.10.

A key component in correctly identifying the long-axis and commissural image planes from within the 3D data set is the elimination of parallax. **Parallax** exists when one or both of the long-axis and commissural imaging planes are not exactly perpendicular, but rather oblique to the plane of the mitral annulus. This results in ambiguity about which surfaces are being examined in 2D MPR. To understand this ambiguity, it is useful in MPR to have one of the three planes reconstructing a short-axis view. This will allow the user to recognize when the long-axis and commissural views are not perpendicular to each other,

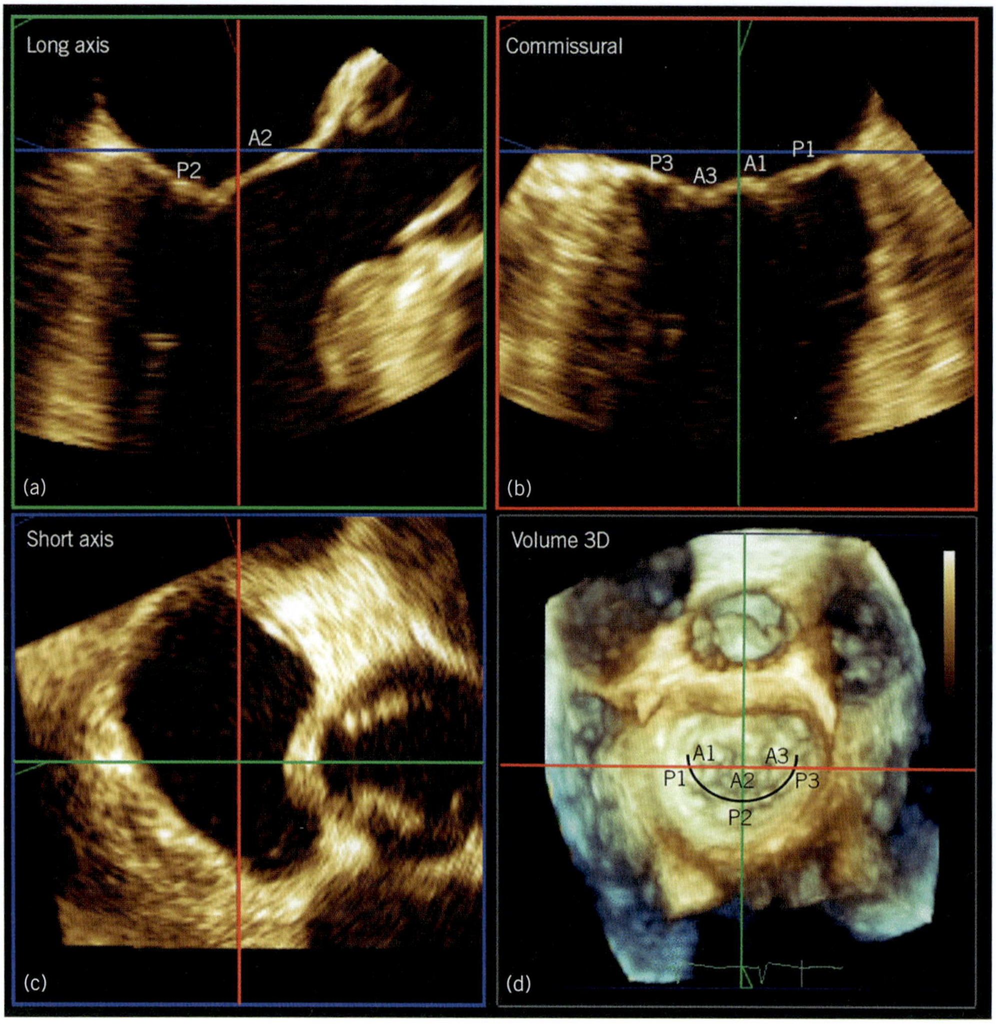

Figure 8.11 Method of 3D axial imaging using multi-planar reconstruction (MPR): a step-by-step guide. This figure should be viewed in conjunction with Online appendix 6.1. The (a) long-axis and (b) commissural landmarks (as shown in Figure 8.6) can be used as reference images for 3D acquisition. In the zoomed 3D data set, three orthogonal 2D slices are demonstrated—the long-axis plane is shown in (a) (green box); the commissural plane is shown in (b) (red box), and the short-axis view is shown in (c) (blue box). A volume-rendered view is shown in (d). Late systolic frames are chosen for analysis. The following steps provide a detailed practical guide to precisely identify the long-axis and commissural 2D slices from within the 3D data set:

1. The images should be magnified and, at least initially, the plane lock is set to keep the (b) red, (a) green, and (c) blue planes perpendicular to each other.
2. In (d), the volume-rendered image is adjusted to display the MV in the surgical orientation. Then, using the technique described in Figure 8.12, the image is toggled from volume mode to slice mode to check for parallax. The panel is then switched back to volume mode.
3. In the (a) long-axis and (b) commissural quadrants, the blue line is moved so it lies parallel to, and just above (i.e. on the LA side of), the annulus. In the long-axis quadrant (a), the blue line is further adjusted, so that the commissure between the left and non-coronary cusps of the AV is identified in the short-axis quadrant (c).
4. In the short-axis quadrant (c), the green line is adjusted so that it traverses the left/non-coronary commissure of the AV and, in the volume-rendered quadrant (d), traverses the MV centrally at the maximum anteroposterior width. The red line is adjusted, so it is perpendicular to the green line and, in the volume-rendered quadrant (d), traverses the MV centrally at the maximum commissural width.
5. Because plane lock ensures perpendicularity of the reconstructed views, and anatomic landmarks have been identified, parallax and leaflet ambiguity should no longer be present.

When the coloured lines are correctly positioned, the long-axis (green) slice a) crosses the A2/P2 coaptive surface and the commissural (red) slice b) traverses the A1/P1 and A3/P3 coaptive surfaces.

Reproduced with kind permission from Daniel Drake.

meaning that the visible reconstructions may be inaccurate. *It is extremely important to identify and eliminate parallax, as it can lead to significant diagnostic error.* The technique for identifying and eliminating parallax is outlined in Figure 8.12 and Online appendix 6.1.3.1.

Mitral regurgitation

Aetiology

Degenerative disease and secondary (functional) MR are the two most common causes of severe native MR in developed countries, accounting for 70% and 20% of surgical cases, respectively.[5] Rheumatic disease is the most common cause in developing nations. Other causes of native MR include endocarditis, congenital clefts, and papillary muscle rupture (most often ischaemic). Inflammatory diseases, post-radiotherapy fibrosis, and carcinoid disease are other rare causes of MR.

Degenerative

Degenerative MV disease (see Online appendix 6.2) is characterized by the proliferation of connective tissue and cellular elements within the leaflets and chordae, a process termed **myxomatous degeneration**. Degenerative change results in thickening and elongation of the leaflets and chordae, annular dilatation, chordal rupture, and sometimes calcification within the mitral apparatus. MR occurs due to leaflet prolapse or flail. Prolapse arises from thickening and elongation of the leaflets and chordae, while flail results from rupture of primary chords.

Two forms of degenerative MV disease are recognized: **fibroelastic deficiency** and **Barlow disease**. With fibroelastic deficiency, there is typically chordal rupture involving an isolated leaflet segment, most commonly P2. The leaflet segment itself may be morphologically normal or demonstrate myxomatous degeneration. The annulus is typically mildly dilated. Patients with fibroelastic deficiency are typically older (>60 years) than those with Barlow disease and have a shorter clinical history consistent with the abrupt onset of MR due to chordal rupture. Patients with Barlow disease tend to be younger (<60 years) and have a long clinical history consistent with slowly progressive disease. Barlow disease is characterized by widespread degenerative change involving multiple leaflet segments and the subvalvular apparatus. Annular dilatation is usually severe, particularly along the commissural axis.

Mitral annular disjunction (also termed mitral–annular disassociation or decoupling) is a common association with Barlow disease and involves migration of the posterior annulus off the LV shoulder into the LA (see Figure 9.7 and Online appendix 6.2.8). The posterior annulus appears hypermobile and displays highly abnormal annular dynamics, with paradoxical systolic expansion and flattening.[6] On TOE imaging, the mitral annulus ‘splays’ or ‘rolls’ outwards in late systole. This late-systolic splaying directly contributes to MR in a proportion of patients with Barlow disease.

Fibroelastic deficiency and Barlow disease are separate clinical entities but represent two ends of the same disease spectrum. Degenerative MV disease usually occurs in isolation but is also associated with systemic connective tissues disorders such as Marfan and Ehlers–Danlos syndromes.

Mild leaflet prolapse in the presence of normal leaflet morphology is a variation of normal and is usually associated with trivial regurgitation.

Secondary

Secondary (functional) MR (see Online appendix 6.5) refers to MR that occurs in the presence of *structurally normal* mitral leaflets. It may be ventricular in origin (termed ventricular functional MR (VFMR)) or atrial in origin (AFMR).

The most common mechanism of VFMR is LV dysfunction/dilatation, which causes lateral and/or apical displacement of the papillary muscles, decreased interpapillary shortening, and leaflet tethering in systole. VFMR can be ischaemic or non-ischaemic. Non-ischaemic VFMR is primarily due to dilated cardiomyopathy or is a consequence of chronic aortic valve disease. In ischaemic cardiomyopathy, secondary MR is more common following inferior or posterior myocardial infarction than following anterior infarction, despite greater ventricular dilatation with the latter. The reason for this lies in the fact that inferior/posterior infarction causes more displacement of the posteromedial papillary muscle than occurs to the anterolateral papillary muscle following anterior infarction (Figure 8.13).[7]

Annular dilatation and LV systolic dysfunction contribute to VFMR, but they are usually not the primary mechanisms. While systolic dysfunction is common in patients with secondary MR, there is an inconsistent relationship between LVEF and regurgitation severity. However, in the context of severe MR, LVEF should be supranormal and a declining ejection fraction should trigger a comprehensive assessment about suitability for intervention. Dilatation is common with secondary MR but tends to be less severe than with degenerative disease.

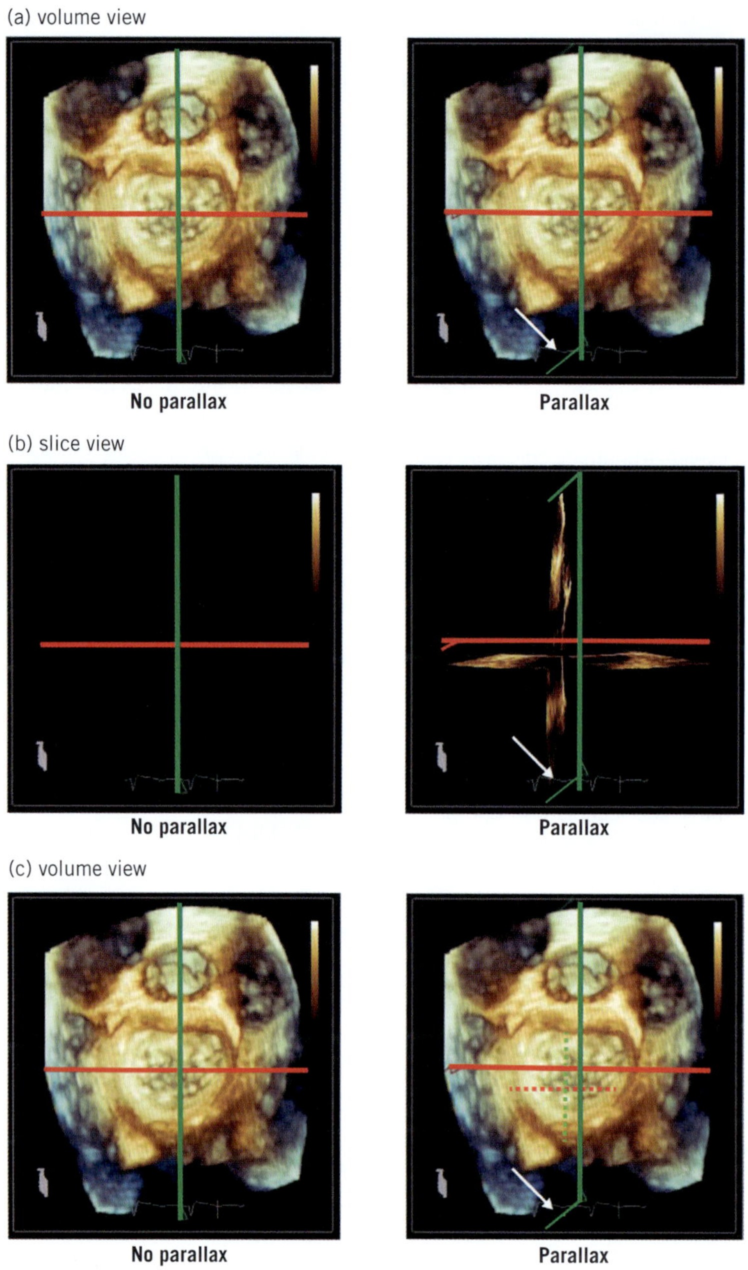

Figure 8.12 Technique for identifying and eliminating parallax with 3D imaging. Panel (a) shows a volume-rendered 3D data set of the MV in the surgical orientation. The pairs of coloured reference lines suggest that the long axis (green) and commissural planes (red) cross the centre of the MV in the correct position; however, note the slight perception of depth on the red and green lines in the right-hand image (identified by the white arrows), indicating that parallax is present (i.e. the planes are not orthogonal to the annular plane). Panel (b) shows the MV in slice mode. The left-hand image is perfectly perpendicular to the observer's line of sight and no parallax is present, therefore the 2D planes appear as coloured lines, with no echo data or depth perception evident. The right-hand image is not perpendicular to the observer's line of sight, meaning that parallax is present. In this circumstance, the 2D planes do show echo data and a perception of depth. When parallax is present, it is impossible to know for sure where the oblique 2D planes cross the 3D image. Panel (c) again shows the MV in volume-rendered mode. The dashed red and green lines in the right-hand image indicate the actual position where the 2D image planes intersect the MV, which is different from where the coloured reference lines indicate. To eliminate parallax, the position of the long-axis and commissural image planes are adjusted in slice mode, so that the echo data disappear and only the red and green lines remain. See also Online appendix 6.1.3.1.

Reproduced with permission from Daniel Drake.

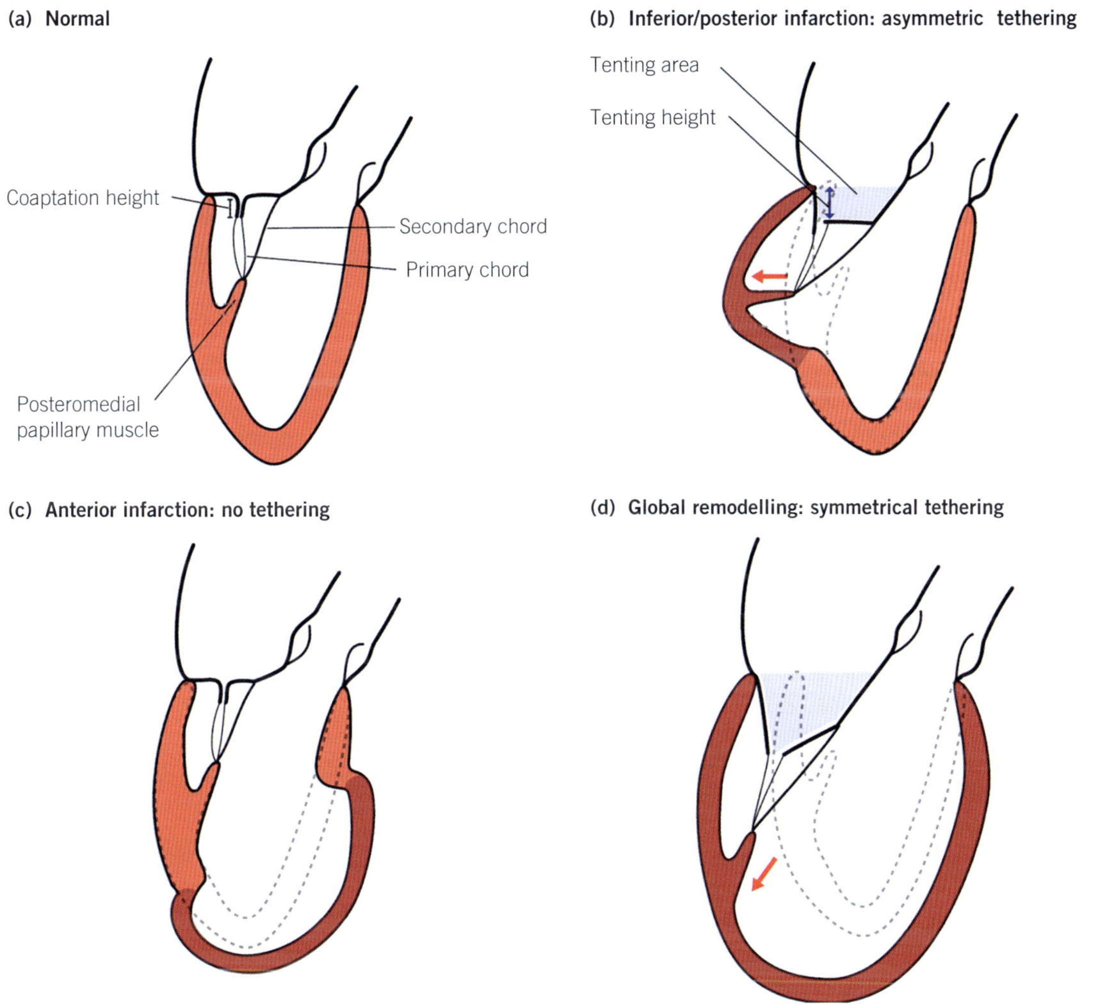

Figure 8.13 Leaflet tethering patterns and secondary MR. Panel (a) shows the normal appearances of the mitral leaflets in late systole. The plane of coaptation is at, or just below, the annular plane, and there is ample leaflet overlap (coaptation length). Panel (b) shows asymmetric leaflet tethering following inferior or posterior myocardial infarction. Localized remodelling causes lateral displacement of the posteromedial papillary muscle, leading to bileaflet tethering (but particularly of the posterior leaflet) and override of the anterior leaflet. Tension on the anterior leaflet from secondary chordae may cause bending of the mid portion of the leaflet ('seagull' sign). The MR jet is posteriorly directed. The severity of leaflet tethering can be quantified by measuring the tenting height and area. Tenting height is the distance from the coaptation point to the annular plane, and tenting area is the area bounded by the leaflets and annular plane. Note that tenting height and area are prognostic factors in ischaemic MR for difficulty of repair. Panel (c) shows the effect of anterior myocardial infarction. Remodelling following anterior infarction typically involves more myocardium than inferior infarction but causes less leaflet tethering. Panel (d) shows symmetrical leaflet tethering due to global LV remodelling. There is apical and lateral displacement of both papillary muscles, with bileaflet tethering. If present, MR tends to be central. Symmetrical tethering is associated with dilated cardiomyopathy and global remodelling following anterior myocardial infarction. See also Online appendices 6.5.2.1.

In recent years, AFMR has been increasingly recognized as an important and previously under-recognized cause of MR. A recent review proposed that the criteria for AFMR include MR with structurally normal leaflets, increased left atrial size (>34 mL/m^2), normal LV end-diastolic size, and an LVEF >60%. The pathophysiology remains incompletely understood but likely involves atriogenic leaflet tethering, in particular of the posterior leaflet. This tends to be seen primarily in patients with atrial fibrillation and heart failure with preserved ejection fraction (HFpEF). At the time of writing these lines, the treatment and implications of AFMR are an area of ongoing investigation.[8]

The various mechanisms involved in functional MR emphasize the fact that the MV is a complex 'apparatus' that begins with the atrial walls and ends with the ventricular walls that support the papillary muscles.

Rheumatic

Rheumatic heart disease (see Online appendix 6.3) is primarily a disease of the MV. Isolated involvement of the MV is common, but isolated involvement of other valves is relatively rare. Approximately 50% of rheumatic MV disease is mixed, with significant elements of both stenosis and regurgitation. For 'pure' lesions, regurgitation is more common in children and stenosis is more common in adults. Regurgitation occurs due to leaflet retraction and tethering, leading to reduced or absent leaflet coaptation.

Endocarditis

Endocarditis (see Online appendix 6.4) can occur on normal valves but is more common on diseased valves. Regurgitation can occur due to leaflet perforation, destruction, or deformity. Endocarditis may also cause aneurysm or abscess formation in the valve or surrounding tissues, which may perforate, causing MR. Streptococcal species and *Staphylococcus aureus* are the most common causative organisms in native endocarditis, although other organisms can be seen, especially in immunocompromised patients. Vegetations tend to be larger and tissue destruction greater with *S. aureus* infections.

Congenital clefts

Mitral clefts mostly involve the anterior leaflet and occur in association with endocardial cushion defects such as inlet VSD, primum ASD, and dysplastic atrioventricular valves (see Online appendix 6.2). Less commonly, anterior leaflet clefts occur as isolated findings. Clefts associated with endocardial cushion defects are usually diagnosed and treated in childhood. Posterior leaflet clefts are rare, with one large study reporting an incidence of 0.1%,[9] and they tend not to be associated with other congenital abnormalities. While there is no absolute consensus on what should be called a posterior cleft versus an indentation, most sources seem to agree that the two main characteristics of a cleft are: (1) the separation between two segments of the posterior leaflet extends *more than half of the distance* between the leaflet edge and the annulus; and (2) there is *some associated MR*. Thus, mitral clefts presenting in adulthood typically present as an isolated finding or in association with a minor endocardial cushion defect (e.g. a small ASD). Regurgitation through clefts can lead to mechanical injury and degenerative change in adjacent tissue, such that clefts presenting in adulthood commonly occur in association with degenerative disease.

Papillary muscle rupture

Papillary muscle rupture (see Online appendix 5.4) is most commonly due to myocardial infarction but occasionally arises as a consequence of chest trauma. Ischaemic rupture typically occurs a few days following a myocardial infarct, which itself may be relatively minor. Rupture of the posteromedial papillary muscle is associated with inferior myocardial infarction and occurs approximately 10 times more frequently than rupture of the anterolateral papillary muscle, reflecting the single-vessel blood supply to the former. In most cases, complete rupture occurs, although rarely partial rupture can happen. In cases of papillary rupture, the MR tends to be severe, both clinically and echocardiographically.

Systolic anterior motion

Systolic anterior motion (SAM) (see Online appendix 5.5) refers to displacement of the anterior mitral leaflet into the LVOT during systole, sometimes resulting in LVOT obstruction. The anterior motion of the anterior leaflet leads to failure of coaptation and MR. SAM tends to happen when the distance between the mitral coaptation point and the ventricular septum is very short. This typically occurs in the following clinical scenarios: (1) hypertrophic cardiomyopathy; (2) following AV replacement for aortic stenosis; and (3) following MV repair. However, SAM can occur in any patient with hypertrophy of the basal ventricular septum and can be precipitated or exacerbated by hyperdynamic states, inotropic support, and/or hypovolaemia.

Assessing valvular morphology and associated pathology

The goal when assessing MV morphology is to identify the pathologic mechanism (Figures 8.14 and 8.15) and the anatomical location of MR.

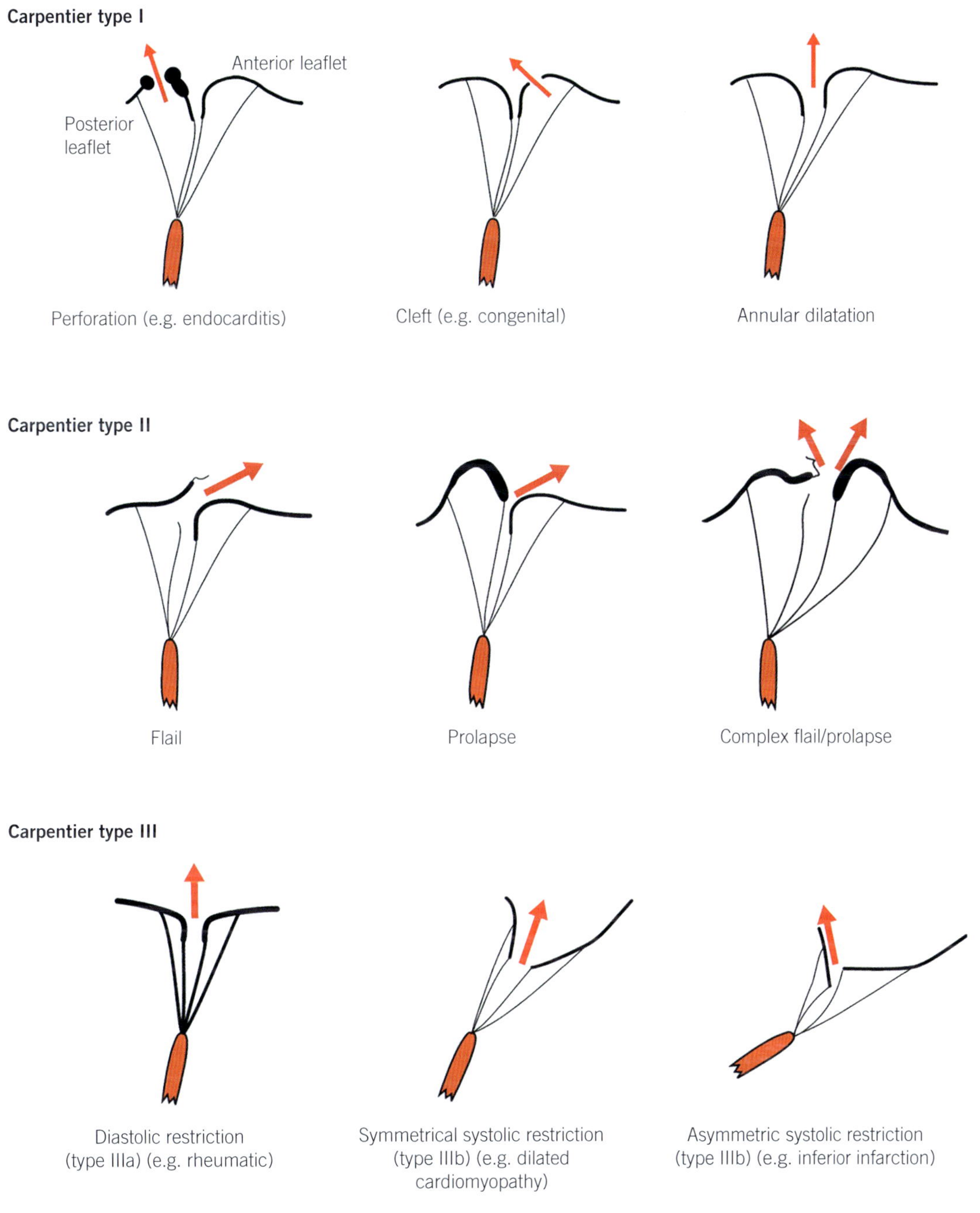

Figure 8.14 Carpentier classification of MV dysfunction based on leaflet motion. Arrows indicate the direction of the regurgitant jet. Type I lesions are associated with normal leaflet motion. Examples include leaflet perforation, leaflet cleft, and annular dilatation. Type II lesions are associated with excessive leaflet motion. Examples include leaflet flail, leaflet prolapse, and complex flail/prolapse. Type III lesions are associated with restrictive leaflet motion. Type IIIa refers to leaflet restriction that occurs predominantly in diastole. Examples include rheumatic disease and radiation-induced valvulopathy. Type IIIb refers to leaflet restriction that occurs predominantly in systole. Examples include dilated cardiomyopathy (symmetrical restriction), inferior myocardial infarction (asymmetric restriction), and systolic anterior motion (not shown). See also Online appendix 6.6.1.

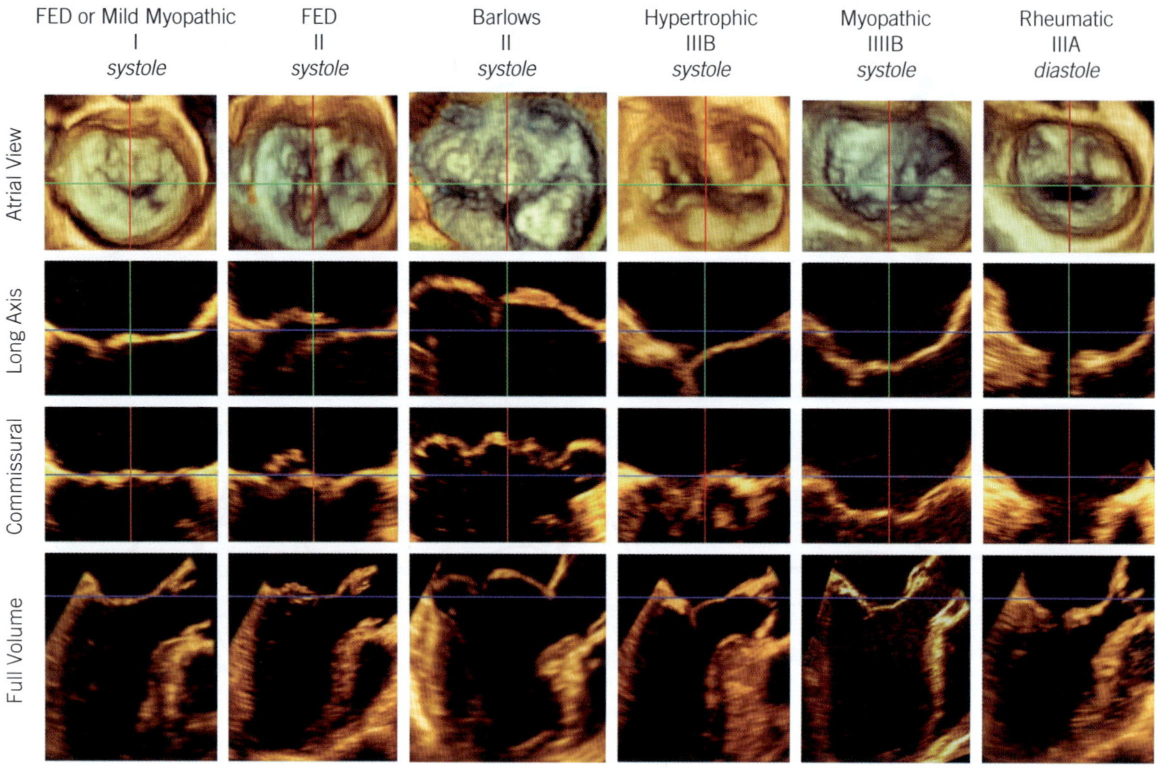

Figure 8.15 Differentiation of common MV diseases using 3D axial imaging. Images have been acquired using the techniques described in Figures 8.11 and 8.12 and demonstrated in Online appendix 6.1. Leaflet motion is classified using the Carpentier nomenclature (see Figure 8.14). Mild secondary MR and fibroelastic deficiency (FED) may result in mild annular dilatation and normal leaflet motion (type I). Advanced FED and Barlow disease are associated with excessive leaflet motion (type II). Note the dramatically enlarged commissural dimension with Barlow disease. Hypertrophic cardiomyopathy (with systolic anterior motion) and advanced myopathic disease are associated with leaflet restriction in systole (type IIIb). Rheumatic disease and radiation-induced valvulopathy are associated with leaflet restriction in diastole (type IIIa).

Annulus

The annulus should be measured in late systole in both the long-axis and commissural views, using 2D or 3D imaging. The callipers should be placed at the insertion point of the leaflet into the annulus. However, in the long-axis view, anteriorly, the calliper may be placed either at the hinge point of the anterior mitral leaflet (see red and yellow dots in Figure 8.6 and Online appendix 6.1.1) or at the base of the AV. Using the base of the AV includes the intervalvular fibrosa and therefore overestimates the true MV annular dimension by approximately 0.5 cm. Reported values vary, but for the AP axis, measured in late systole, the upper limit of normal is 3.5 cm (measured to the base of the AV) or 3.0 cm (measured to the anterior hinge point), and for the commissural axis, the upper limit of normal is 3.7 cm.[2,10]

Annular dilatation occurs with both degenerative and secondary disease. Marked dilatation along the commissural axis is a feature of Barlow disease. Mitral annular disjunction and late systolic splaying (described previously) should be specifically looked for in patients with Barlow disease (see Figure 9.7 and Online appendix 6.2.8).

Mitral annular calcification (see Online appendix 2.14) should also be noted and reported to the surgeon, as it can create difficulties when resecting valve segments or placing annuloplasty sutures. Annular calcification rarely causes functional abnormalities, although, if severe, it can extend into the leaflets themselves and cause stenosis.

Leaflets and chordae

MV dysfunction is commonly classified using the system proposed by Carpentier (Figure 8.14; see Online appendix 6.6.1). Normal leaflet motion (**type I**) is typically associated with clefts or perforations but may also be seen in AFMR. Clefts can be associated with degenerative disease or congenital anomalies of the MV, and perforations are common in patients with endocarditis. Both may be visualized directly, particularly with 3D imaging (Figures 8.16 and 8.17). The presence of a colour jet that originates away from the coaptation line, or appears to go *through* a leaflet, strongly suggests a cleft or perforation. Note that oblique imaging can cut the curved mitral coaptation line twice, giving the false impression of a cleft. Additionally, with severe degenerative disease, infolding of bulky leaflet tissue can result in jets that originate away from the coaptation line, also giving the false impression of a cleft. 3D imaging often helps to resolve these diagnostic challenges.

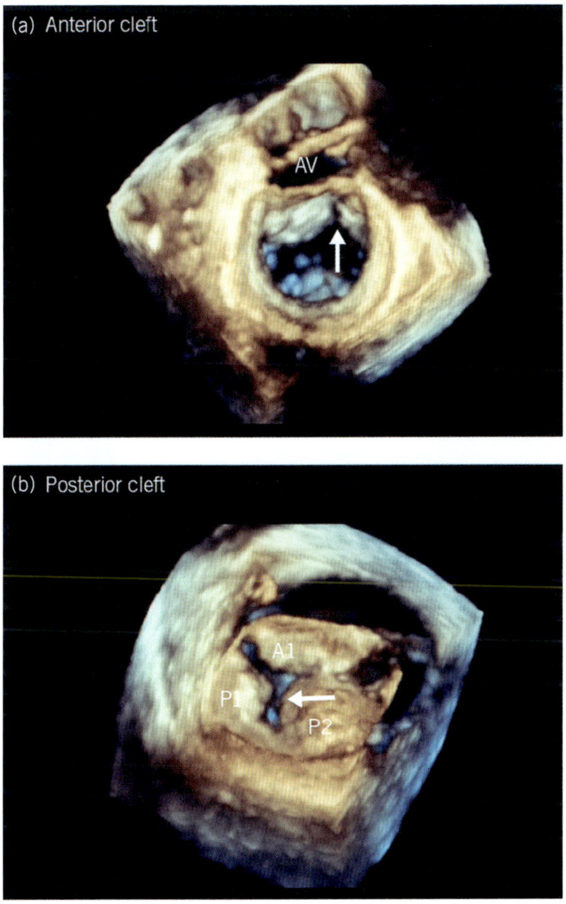

Figure 8.16 Mitral clefts. The MV is displayed in the 'surgical' orientation. An anterior leaflet cleft (arrow) involving A2/A3 is shown in (a), and a posterior cleft (arrow) involving P1/P2 is shown in (b). The posterior cleft is in the region of the indentation that normally separates P1 and P2 and may be considered a 'deep indentation'. Most sources use the term posterior cleft when the separation between mitral segments extends more than half of the distance between the leaflet edge and the annulus, and when there is associated MR. See also Online appendices 6.2.3 and 6.2.7.

Reprinted from *Journal of the American Society of Echocardiography*, **27**, 4, Sidebotham DA, Allen SJ, Gerber IL, Fayers T, Intraoperative transesophageal echocardiography for surgical repair of mitral regurgitation, Figure 12, pp. 345–366, Copyright 2014, with permission from American Society of Echocardiography.

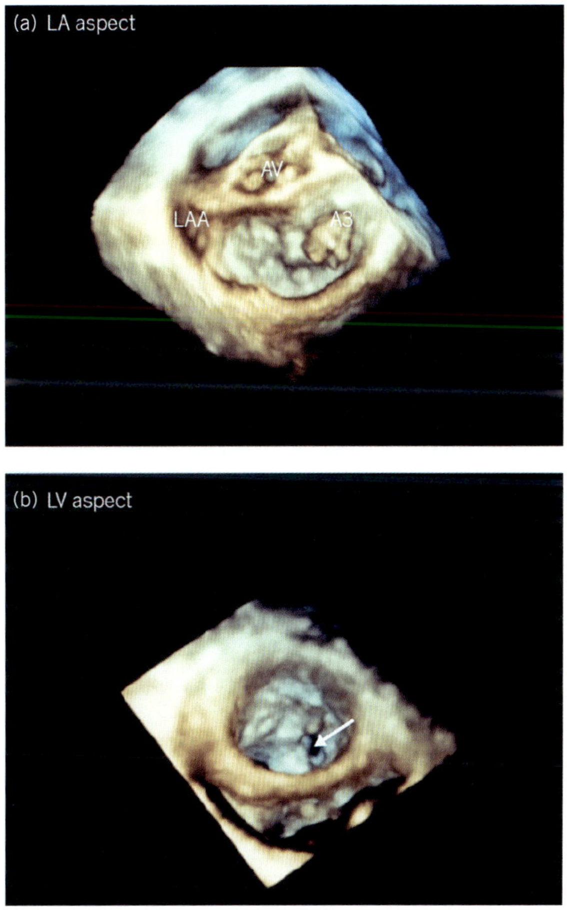

Figure 8.17 Mitral endocarditis. In panel (a), the MV is shown in 3D in the surgical orientation from the LA aspect. A large vegetation can be seen in the region of A3. In panel (b), the MV is shown in 3D from the LV aspect. A perforation (arrow) can be seen in the A3 segment, which was hidden by the vegetation in (a). See also Online appendix 6.4.

Reprinted from *Journal of the American Society of Echocardiography*, **27**, 4, Sidebotham DA, Allen SJ, Gerber IL, Fayers T, Intraoperative transesophageal echocardiography for surgical repair of mitral regurgitation, Figure 13, pp. 345–366, Copyright 2014, with permission from American Society of Echocardiography.

Vegetations from endocarditis typically occur on the LA (upstream) surface of the valve (Figure 8.17; see Online appendix 6.4), and leaflet perforation commonly occurs at the site of attachment of vegetations. With 3D imaging, visualizing the valve from the LV aspect may demonstrate perforations that are hidden by vegetations when the valve is viewed from the LA aspect. Again, 3D imaging with colour flow Doppler may point to the origin of the jet away from the coaptation line.

Excessive leaflet motion (**type II**) is associated with degenerative disease or papillary muscle rupture and results in prolapse or flail of one or more leaflet segments (see Online appendix 6.2). With prolapse (Figure 8.18), the body and tip of the leaflet lie above the annular plane at end-systole and the leaflet tip is directed towards the LV. With flail (Figures 8.10 and 8.19), the body and tip of the leaflet lie above the annular plane at end-systole and the tip of the leaflet is directed into the LA (the leaflet appears to be free-flowing in the LA during systole). One or more ruptured chordae may be visible in the LA during systole. With prolapse/flail, the regurgitant jet is directed *away* from the affected leaflet segment(s). Such jets are usually highly eccentric and may track along the wall of the LA for some distance (Figure 8.20). Myxomatous leaflet segments may appear thickened and elongated. Severely degenerative leaflet segments can be difficult to distinguish from vegetations.

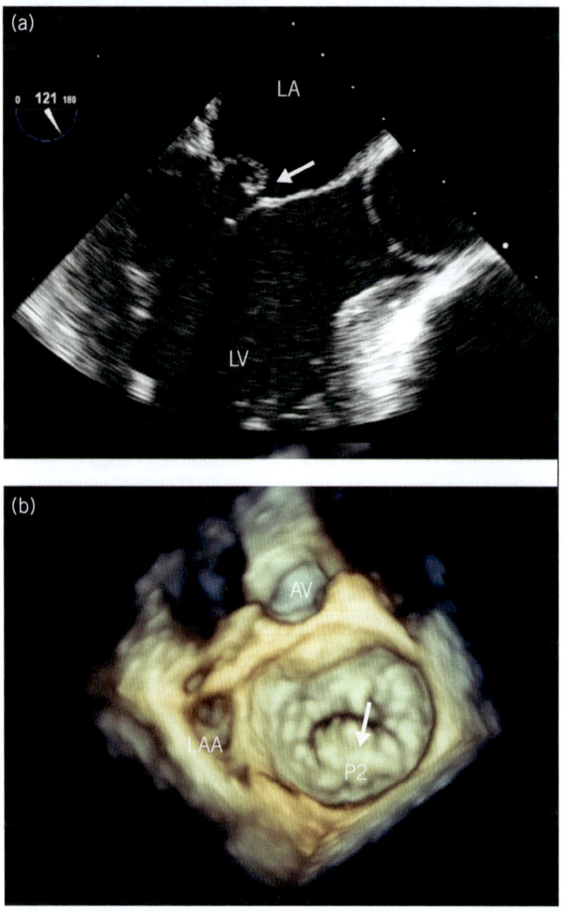

Figure 8.18 Leaflet prolapse. Panel (a) shows prolapse of P2 (arrow) in the mid-oesophageal long-axis view in late systole. Panel (b) shows the same lesion, also identified by an arrow, with 3D imaging from the atrial aspect in late systole. Examples are found in Online appendix 6.2.

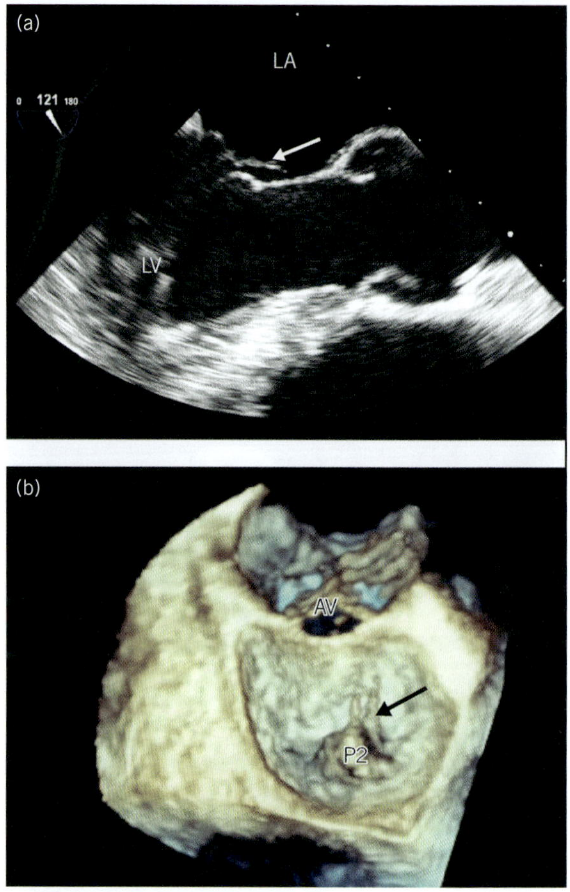

Figure 8.19 Leaflet flail. Panel (a) shows a flail P2 segment (arrow) in the mid-oesophageal long-axis view in late systole. Panel (b) shows the same lesion, also identified by an arrow, with 3D imaging from the atrial aspect in late systole. Note that in the 3D image, ruptured chordae can be seen passing over the A2 region of the valve. See multiple examples in Online appendix 6.2.

Leaflet prolapse and flail are readily localized with 3D imaging (see Online appendices 6.2.1.5 and 6.2.4.8). It is useful to confirm the origin of the jet(s) with 3D colour imaging, particularly in patients with Barlow disease, as not all myxomatous segments necessarily contribute to regurgitation (Figure 8.21). In most cases, a flail segment passes over the corresponding segment of the opposite leaflet; for instance, a flail P2 passes over A2 in late systole. This common scenario is demonstrated in Figures 8.10 and 8.19. Occasionally, confusion may arise when the flail segment passes obliquely across the opposite leaflet in late systole. An example of this phenomenon is shown in Figure 8.22 and Online appendix 6.2.6, where a flail involving A2 passes obliquely over P1, rather than over P2. While the precise origin of a flail segment may sometimes be difficult to pinpoint with 2D imaging

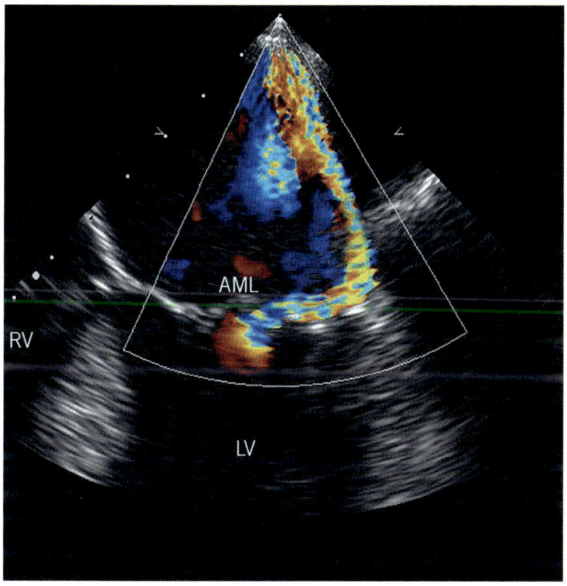

Figure 8.20 Wall-hugging jet. In this mid-oesophageal four-chamber view, there is a flail anterior mitral leaflet (AML), resulting in a posteriorly directed, wall-hugging jet of mitral regurgitation.

alone, 3D usually makes it easy to distinguish between these various scenarios.

Papillary muscle rupture typically results in torrential MR due to bileaflet regurgitation (see Figure 6.13 and Online appendix 5.4). The head of the papillary muscle may be seen floating in the LA during systole. Imaging in the transgastric two-chamber view helps to identify which muscle is ruptured.

Leaflet motion that is restricted in systole and diastole (**type IIIa**) is typically due to rheumatic or radiation-induced MV disease (see Online appendix 6.3). The leaflets are thickened and retracted, and often have a rolled-edge appearance with a visible coaptation defect in late systole. The regurgitant jet is often central; however, if one leaflet is more severely affected than the other, the jet may be eccentric and directed *towards* the affected side.

Leaflet restriction in systole (**type IIIb**) is typically due to secondary MR (see Online appendices 6.5 and 6.6 S) but may also be caused by SAM (see Online appendix 5.5). Two patterns of secondary MR are recognized: symmetric and asymmetric (Figure 8.13). Symmetric restriction occurs due to global LV remodelling (e.g. from dilated cardiomyopathy or large anterior infarction). There is bileaflet tethering due to apical and lateral displacement of both papillary muscles and decreased interpapillary shortening. The regurgitant jet tends to be mostly central. Asymmetric restriction refers to disproportionate tethering of the posterior leaflet, particularly the P2–P3 junction,

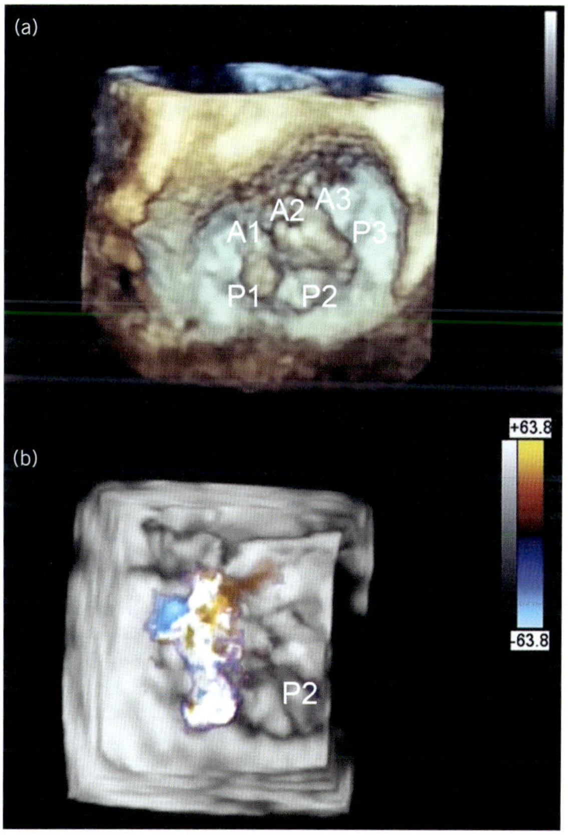

Figure 8.21 3D imaging in a patient with complex degenerative MV disease. (a) With standard 3D imaging, the P1 and P2 segments demonstrate prolapse/flail. Torn chordae can be seen extending over the body of the anterior mitral leaflet. (b) With colour 3D imaging, mitral regurgitation is most marked in the region of P1/A1. The clips related to this image are demonstrated in Online appendix 6.2.4 . Another example of complex degenerative disease is demonstrated in Online appendix 6.2.8 .

Reprinted from *Journal of the American Society of Echocardiography*, **27**, 4, Sidebotham DA, Allen SJ, Gerber IL, Fayers T, Intraoperative transesophageal echocardiography for surgical repair of mitral regurgitation, Figure 11, pp. 345–366, Copyright 2014, with permission from American Society of Echocardiography.

due to lateral displacement of the posteromedial papillary muscle. The anterior leaflet may override the posterior leaflet, and the regurgitant jet is typically posteriorly directed (i.e. towards the affected side). Asymmetric restriction occurs following inferior/posterior infarction due to localized remodelling of the basal inferior and/or inferolateral walls. Tethering of P3 and basal inferior SWMAs are best seen in the mid-oesophageal two-chamber view.

With both forms of leaflet tethering, the plane of coaptation lies below the annular plane and coaptation is reduced or non-existent. A coaptation length of <0.5 cm indicates that coaptation is significantly reduced. The severity of leaflet tethering may be quantified by measuring the

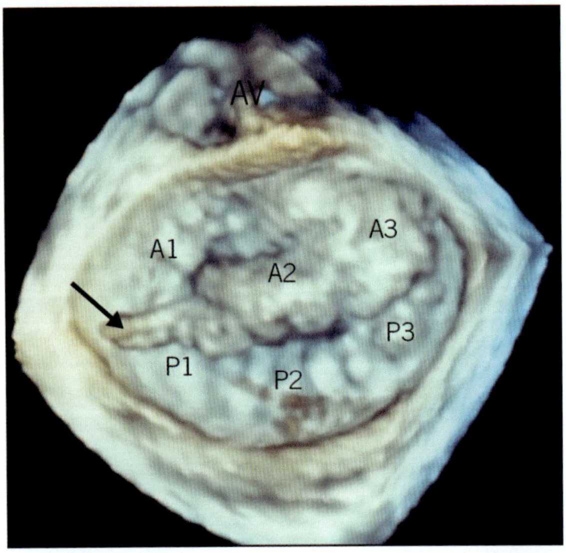

Figure 8.22 Flail segment involving A2 with oblique extension of the chordae. A 3D view of the MV from the LA aspect in late systole is demonstrated. A flail segment originating from A2 is evident. A ruptured chord (arrow) can be seen over P1 and extending towards the anterolateral commissure. Contrast this finding with the more usual appearances of ruptured chordae demonstrated in Figures 8.10 and 8.19 where the chordae extend over the same segments on the opposite leaflet. Oblique extension of the chordae is easily identified with 3D imaging but can cause confusion as to the origin of the flail segment with conventional 2D imaging. Note the A3 segment also appears to prolapse slightly.

tenting height and area (Figures 8.13; see Figure 9.4 and Online appendices 6.5 and 6.6). A **tenting height** >1.0 cm and a **tenting area** >1.60 cm^2 indicate severe leaflet tethering. Measurements should be made in the mid-oesophageal long-axis view in late systole.

Multiple abnormalities of leaflet function may coexist. Clefts can occur in patients with degenerative disease (see Online appendices 6.2.3 and 6.2.7). Endocarditis often occurs on abnormal valves and is therefore associated with degenerative and rheumatic disease. Degenerative disease can also be associated with leaflet tethering. Advanced degenerative disease causes LV dilatation, which may cause prolapsing segments to return towards the annular plane or lead to tethering of non-affected segments. With degenerative disease, the presence of complex or multiple jets suggests either multi-segment involvement (most likely) or the presence of additional pathology such as cleft or leaflet tethering. The *timing* of jets is also important when considering concomitant tethering. Jets due to leaflet prolapse or flail tend to be maximal in late systole, whereas regurgitation due to tethering is often maximal in early systole (see later).

Associated features

Haemodynamically significant MR, especially when chronic, tends to be associated with LA and LV dilatation, LV systolic dysfunction, and/or pulmonary hypertension. Severe pulmonary hypertension can lead to secondary right heart dysfunction. LV enlargement that occurs as a *consequence* of MR tends to be global and spherical, whereas ventricular dilatation that *causes* MR may be regional (i.e. asymmetric tethering).

MR imposes a volume load on the LV but also provides a low-resistance pathway for systolic ejection into the low-pressure LA. These combined effects lead to an increased end-diastolic dimension and, at least initially, a reduced end-systolic dimension, resulting in an apparent supranormal LVEF. The first sign of systolic impairment is an increased end-systolic dimension, which initially occurs despite an apparent 'normal' LVEF. Therefore, when reporting the LVEF as measured by TOE, one should consider adding the caveat '*in the presence of severe MR*', in order to alert the reader to the possibility of a worse LV contractile function than actually measured.

Grading severity

Several methods of grading MR may be used in the operating room. Because different methods may provide somewhat different, and sometimes conflicting, information, it is important to use multiple methods, and to consider these methods collectively and in context.

The impact of general anaesthesia (GA) on the appearance of MR is important and should not be overlooked. It is a well-known fact that GA can decrease the apparent severity of MR by as much as a full grade.[11] For that reason, in a procedural setting, the severity of MR should ideally be graded by a pre-procedure study. When this is not possible, haemodynamic manipulations should be undertaken in the operating room to counteract the effect of GA on LV preload and afterload, in an attempt to simulate the 'awake state'.

MR is graded as trivial, mild, moderate, and severe. Depending on the measuring technique, it may be appropriate to subcategorize moderate regurgitation into mild-to-moderate or moderate-to-severe. It can also be useful to consider the different components of regurgitant flow, namely flow convergence (PISA), flow acceleration (VC), turbulence (jet size and area), and downstream effects (pulmonary venous flow). Guidelines for assessing severity have been published by various international organizations.[12]

Jet area

Colour flow Doppler is the simplest and most obvious way to screen for MR, and it also provides a qualitative assessment of the severity of MR. Jet area (and jet length) have been used to quantify MR, but they are imprecise and should be confirmed by other methods. In general, small jets (<20% of LA area) are consistent with mild regurgitation and large jets (>40% of LA area) are associated with severe regurgitation. However, absolute jet area measurements are affected by Doppler gain settings, loading conditions, ventricular function, and atrial size and compliance, among other factors. Jet area is also affected by the acuity of the MR, and the resulting LA remodelling and dilation in chronic MR. Moreover, jet area greatly underestimates the severity of eccentric, wall-hugging jets due to the Coanda effect (see Chapter 3). For all those reasons, jet area should be used as a preliminary assessment and it should be confirmed by other methods.

Special mention must be made of **wall-hugging jets**—these eccentric high-energy MR jets follow the atrial wall for some distance and they often point to a significant structural issue with a mitral leaflet.

> ***Expert tip: As a general rule, all wall-hugging MR jets should be considered severe until proven otherwise, and they warrant careful evaluation.***

Vena contracta width

Vena contracta width (Figure 8.23; see Online appendices 6.3.4.3 and 6.5.1.2) is the most widely used validated technique for quantifying MR severity. The **vena contracta** (VC) is the narrowest part of a jet as it passes through an orifice, and should be measured *perpendicular* to the coaptation line in the mid-oesophageal long-axis view. If multiple jets are present, the largest jet should be measured. The zoom or depth controls should be adjusted to focus on the mitral leaflets, and the Nyquist limit set to 40–70 cm/s. The colour box should be centred on the origin of the jet. The probe should be slightly turned from left to right, scanning along the coaptation line in order to identify the widest jet; then the image is frozen, and the narrowest part of that jet is measured. The average of at least three measurements is reported. A VC width <0.3 cm is associated with mild regurgitation, and a value ≥0.7 cm usually indicates severe regurgitation.[12]

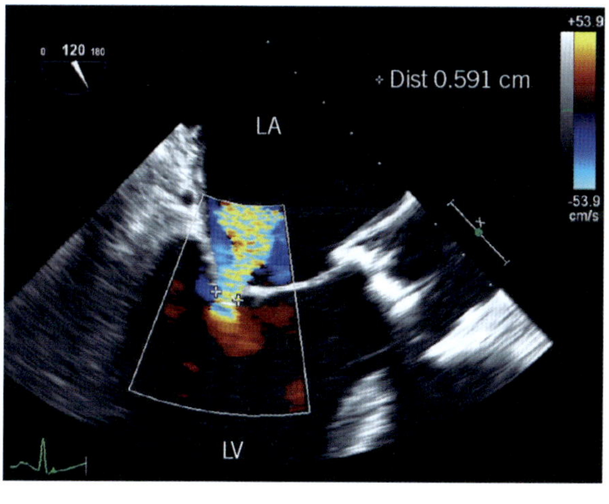

Figure. 8.23 Vena contracta width. In this mid-oesophageal long-axis view, the vena contracta is identified. The value of 0.591 cm suggests mitral regurgitation is moderate. See also examples in Online appendices 6.5.1.2 and 6.3.4.3.

VC width is reliable for evaluating both central and eccentric jets, and is less influenced by loading conditions than jet area and jet length. The main limitation of the technique is the assumption that the regurgitant orifice is relatively circular, and that the AP diameter of the VC is actually representative of the total size of the orifice, which may not be the case (see later). In some patients, it may not be possible to obtain a VC that is suitable for measurement. VC width is also not valid when there are multiple jets.

Vena contracta area

A more robust technique for quantifying severity of MR is the measurement of **vena contracta surface area** (VCA) (Figure 8.24) using multi-plane analysis of a 3D data set with colour Doppler. Like the flow convergence technique, described later, the VCA provides a measure of the **effective regurgitant orifice area** (EROA), although it is slightly smaller than the EROA. VCA has the advantage over other techniques that no assumption needs to be made regarding the shape of the regurgitant orifice. It is simply measured by planimetry. Also, a total VCA can be measured when there are multiple jets. The main difficulty with this technique is obtaining a suitable 3D data set and measuring the VCA at the proper level. It is also more time-consuming in the busy environment of the operating theatre. It is essential that the VC be well visualized with standard colour Doppler imaging before acquiring a 3D data set. If the frame rate is too low, it is possible that a frame demonstrating the real VC will not be captured. The frame rate is improved by using a narrower sector width and multi-beat acquisition.

Flow convergence

The flow convergence method (Figure 8.25; see Online appendices 6.2.2.2 and 6.5.1.3) is a quantitative

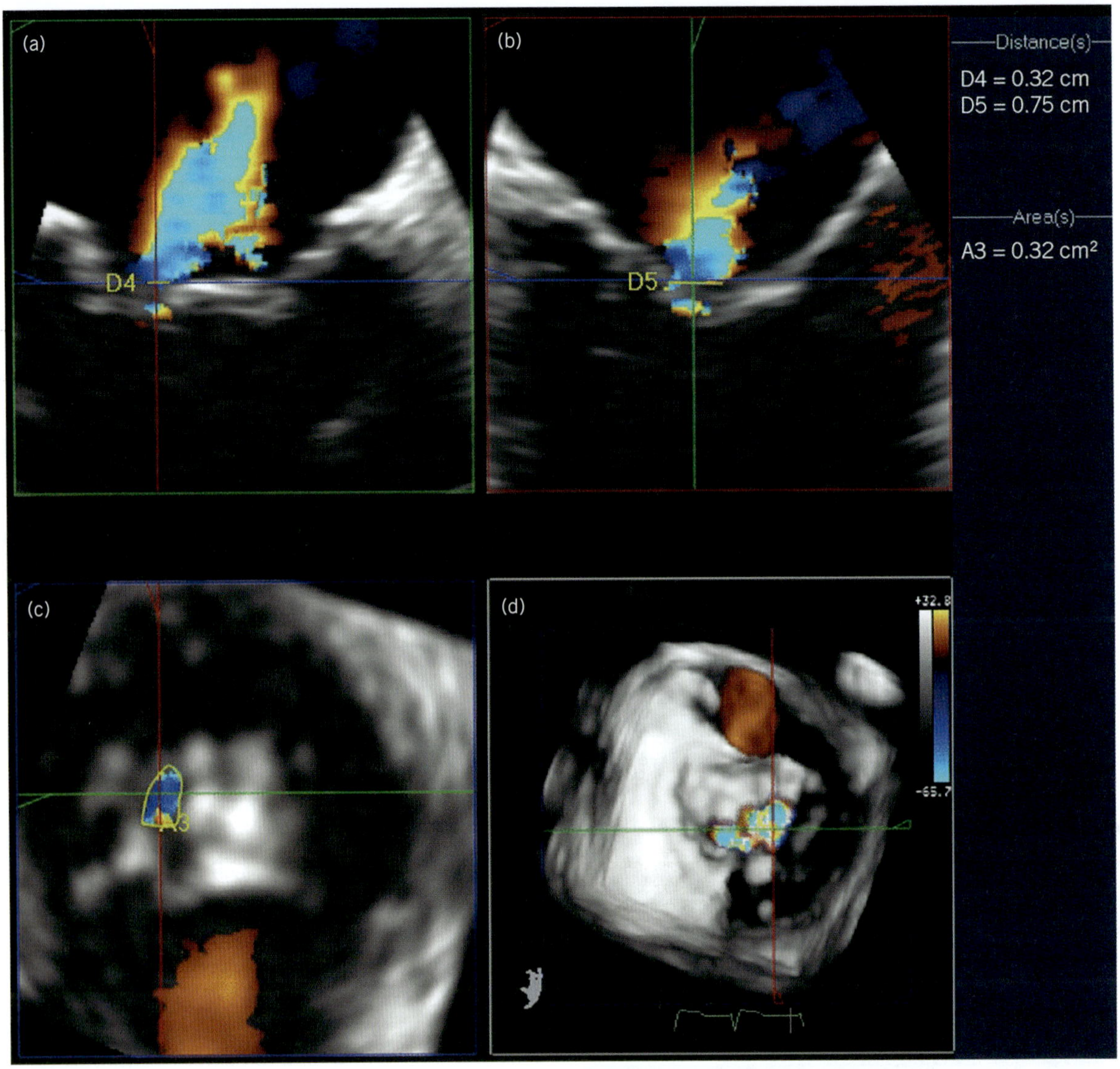

Figure 8.24 Measurement of vena contracta area by multi-planar reconstruction. Axial 3D images of the MV with colour Doppler imaging are shown. A late systolic frame has been chosen for analysis. Panel (a) shows a commissural 2D slice. Panel (b) shows a long-axis 2D slice. Panel (c) shows a short-axis slice at the level of the vena contracta. Panel (d) shows a volume-rendered colour 3D image in the surgical orientation from the LA aspect. In the (a) commissural and (b) long-axis quadrants, the red and green lines have been adjusted so they are positioned through the centre of the jet, and the blue lines have been adjusted so they pass through the narrowest part of the jet (i.e. the vena contracta). (c) The vena contracta area has then been measured with planimetry. The value of 0.32 cm^2 indicates moderate regurgitation. See text for details.

technique for estimating EROA that can be performed rapidly in the operating room. The technique is based on the continuity principle, which states that flow along the length of a regurgitant jet is constant. Since flow is the product of area and velocity, if the flow can be measured at one point along the regurgitant jet, and if the velocity at the site of the regurgitant orifice is known, then the regurgitant orifice area can easily be calculated.

Fluid dynamics dictate that when blood is forced from the large LV into the much smaller regurgitant mitral orifice during systole, blood cells accelerate along a continuum of concentric hemispheric shells, which show on colour Doppler as a zone of colour aliasing proximal to the valve. This is called the **flow convergence area**. In that area, colour will appear as shades of red/orange/yellow (towards the transducer) until the velocity of blood reaches the Nyquist limit, at which point the colour will abruptly shift to a shade of blue (Figure 8.25). The distance between this point and the regurgitant orifice represents the radius (r) of the *hemispheric shell* defined by the colour change. This radius is used to calculate the surface area of the hemisphere termed the **proximal isovelocity surface area** (PISA). The velocity of blood at that particular point in space equals the Nyquist limit (NL). The velocity of the MR jet at the regurgitant orifice is then measured with CW Doppler, aligned with the regurgitant jet (V_{MR}).[13]

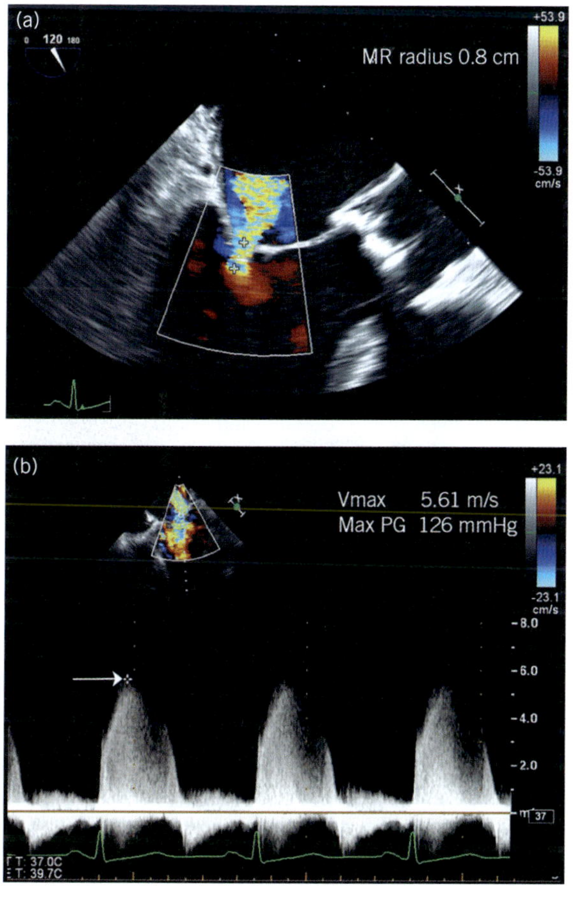

Figure 8.25 Measurement of effective regurgitant orifice area by the flow convergence method. See text for details. In (a), the Nyquist limit is 53.9 cm/s; the radius of the proximal isovelocity surface area is 0.8 cm, and in (b), the peak regurgitant velocity is 5.61 m/s. From Equation 8.2, the effective regurgitant orifice area is 0.39 cm^2, which is just below the threshold for severe MR. Note the regurgitant CW Doppler waveform in (b) is incomplete, which may indicate the peak regurgitant velocity is under-recorded. Under-recording the peak regurgitant velocity overestimates the regurgitant orifice area and regurgitation severity. See examples in Online appendices 6.2.2.2 and 6.5.1.3.

Since flow equals velocity times area, and since flow at the PISA equals flow at the regurgitant orifice, we have the following equation (Equation 8.1):

$$V_{PISA} \times CSA_{PISA} = V_{orifice} \times EROA \qquad \text{Equation 8.1}$$

The surface area of the PISA hemisphere is $2\pi r^2$ where r is the PISA radius. Blood flow at the PISA is equal to the NL$\times 2\pi r^2$. Regurgitant flow through the orifice is the product of peak jet velocity (V_{MR}) and EROA, the unknown quantity. Therefore (Equation 8.2):

$$EROA = \frac{2\pi r^2 \times NL}{V_{MR}} \qquad \text{Equation 8.2}$$

PISA radius should be measured in the mid-oesophageal long-axis view. Adjusting the Nyquist limit to approximately 40 cm/s helps to display a well-defined PISA hemisphere. Careful measurement of the PISA radius is essential, as this value is squared in the calculation. Underestimating the PISA radius underestimates EROA, and vice versa. Peak regurgitant velocity is measured using CW Doppler through the mitral leaflets. The CW Doppler signal must be well aligned with the regurgitant jet (may be challenging with eccentric jets) to minimize underestimating the peak velocity. Underestimating peak regurgitant velocity overestimates EROA.

Once EROA is known, measuring the velocity–time integral of the regurgitant jet in systole (VTI_{MR}) allows the regurgitant volume (RV) to be calculated (Equation 8.3):

$$RV = EROA_{MR} \times VTI_{MR} \qquad \text{Equation 8.3}$$

An EROA <0.2 cm^2 defines mild MR, and an EROA >0.4 cm^2 (and a regurgitant volume ≥60 mL) defines severe regurgitation. The flow convergence technique can be used to distinguish mild-to-moderate (EROA 0.2–0.3 cm^2) and moderate-to-severe regurgitation (EROA 0.3–0.4 cm^2). Note that previous guidelines had considered an EROA of 0.2 cm^2 to be severe in *secondary* MR, but the 2017 guidelines on native valvular regurgitation no longer have separate EROA criteria for secondary MR.[12]

The flow convergence technique has many limitations: (1) it is more accurate for central jets than for eccentric jets; (2) like VC width, it assumes a circular regurgitant orifice (if the orifice is not circular, the hemishell is not a true hemisphere and $2\pi r^2$ does not define its surface area); (3) changing the colour map (Nyquist limit) changes the shape of the measured hemishell (again, if the hemishell is not a true hemisphere, $2\pi r^2$ may not apply); (4) it does not work with multiple orifices; and (5) any small error in measuring the radius of the hemishell is squared (remember that spatial resolution of colour Doppler is lower than 2D, because of the reduced number of scan lines—see Chapter 1). Consequently, making conclusions about MR severity based on PISA alone should be approached with caution.

> ***Expert tip: Despite all the quantitative limitations discussed, the qualitative presence of a zone of flow convergence ('PISA shell') should always raise suspicion that MR is haemodynamically significant and warrants a careful examination of the valve. The same rule of thumb can be applied to any PISA shell across any valve in any direction.***

Setting the Nyquist limit to 40 cm/s and assuming that the LV-to-LA pressure difference is 100 mmHg (i.e. $V_{MR} = 5$ m/s), Equation 8.2 can be reduced to **EROA = $r^2/2$**. Using this super-simplified form, a PISA radius of 1.0 cm indicates an EROA of 0.5 cm^2. Thus, a PISA radius ≥1.0 cm suggests that regurgitation is severe. This simplification is not valid when LV function is severely impaired, as the LV-to-LA pressure difference may be <100 mmHg. For a detailed discussion of PISA, the reader is referred to this review.[13]

> ***Expert tip: A PISA radius >1 cm at a Nyquist limit of 40 cm/s or less suggests severe MR.***

Semiquantitative spectral Doppler methods

Moderate and severe MR alters the pulmonary venous PW Doppler waveform. Moderate regurgitation is associated with *blunting* of the S-wave, and severe regurgitation with systolic flow *reversal* from the atria into the pulmonary vein (see Online appendix 6.2.3.7). Elevated LA pressure (e.g. due to MS or LV diastolic dysfunction) can also cause S-wave blunting. Systolic blunting or reversal may affect the pulmonary veins unequally, particularly with eccentric MR jets. Therefore, both left- and right-sided pulmonary veins should be interrogated, with the finding of systolic flow reversal being specific for severe MR if found in two or more pulmonary veins.

The severity of MR also influences the *density* of the signal obtained with CW Doppler along the MR jet. Comparing the signal density in systole and diastole provides a qualitative guide to regurgitation severity that is independent of Doppler gain setting. A systolic CW waveform with a complete envelope of bright white density, similar to the diastolic waveform, suggests that regurgitation is significant.

MR imparts an additional volume load on the LA, resulting in increased diastolic flow across the MV and an increased peak velocity of early diastolic filling. A peak E-wave velocity >1.2 m/s is associated with severe regurgitation. This sign is unreliable in the presence of hyperdynamic circulation or even minor degrees of MS (e.g. following MV repair). By contrast, an inflow velocity that is A-wave dominant (i.e. A > E) is highly suggestive of non-severe (at worst moderate) MR.

Additional considerations when assessing severity

Several factors must be considered when assessing the severity of MR. First, the haemodynamic state can significantly affect severity, particularly for secondary MR. The apparent severity is minimized when arterial blood pressure, preload, afterload, and contractility are low. As discussed earlier, reduced preload and afterload associated with GA lead to a significant reduction in regurgitation severity.[14]

Second, many measurements described previously involve the analysis of a single frame. However, MR severity varies throughout systole. With degenerative disease, severity typically increases throughout systole, peaking just prior to the end of systole. By contrast, for secondary MR, regurgitation is typically greatest in early systole, diminishes and may cease in mid-systole (as LV closing forces overcome the leaflet tethering), and then has a smaller peak in late systole.[15] Most clinicians choose the frame showing the worst regurgitation for analysis. However, this approach can overestimate severity when regurgitation is highly dynamic. In patients with atrial fibrillation, in whom stroke volume (and regurgitant volume) varies from beat to beat, several measurements should be performed and the average reported.

Third, VC width and the flow convergence method assume a circular shape to the regurgitant orifice, which is a reasonable assumption for isolated segmental prolapse or flail. However, with secondary MR—and, to a lesser extent, with rheumatic disease—the regurgitant orifice is typically elliptical or slit-like; thus, VC width and flow convergence tend to underestimate severity. VCA is not affected by the shape of the MR jet, and the technique is particularly useful for assessing secondary MR.

While each of the above methods has its own limitations and pitfalls, the use of *multiple redundant methods* helps to avoid inaccurate diagnosis.

Considerations for secondary mitral regurgitation

Assessing secondary MR in the operating room is particularly difficult, as it is highly influenced by loading conditions and tends to be underestimated by the two most commonly used quantification techniques: VC width and flow convergence. Furthermore, there is evidence that for patients with secondary regurgitation, an EROA ≥0.2 cm², obtained by the flow convergence technique, is an independent predictor of cardiac death.[16] For these reasons, the 2014 American Heart Association (AHA)/American College of Cardiology (ACC) guidelines on the management of patients with valvular heart disease recommended using an EROA ≥0.2 cm² for defining severe secondary MR. However, in the 2017 focused update on these guidelines, the recommendation was reversed and a value >0.4 cm² was reinstituted. Nevertheless, the guideline authors acknowledged the difficulty in defining severe secondary MR and commented that *'an EROA cut-off of >0.2cm² is more sensitive and >0.4cm² is more specific for severe secondary MR'*.[12] One should also consider the potential to incite early intervention by calling lesions severe that are, in fact, moderate, and there is evidence that surgery on patients with moderate functional MR is associated with worse outcomes.

> ***Expert tip: The best time to evaluate secondary (functional) MR is preoperatively, when the patient is awake, with normal loading conditions.***

Notwithstanding these issues, accurate intraoperative quantification of secondary regurgitation may still be necessary, as it may have been insufficiently assessed preoperatively, it may have changed since an earlier evaluation, or urgent surgery may not have allowed time for preoperative workup. In such circumstances, it is essential that the patient's haemodynamics be adjusted to mimic the awake state. Information from multiple sources should be obtained when quantifying severity, including, where possible, VCA.

Mitral stenosis

Aetiology

In the vast majority of cases, haemodynamically significant native mitral stenosis (MS) is due to rheumatic heart disease, although calcific disease is happening with increasing frequency. Less common causes include congenital abnormalities (e.g. parachute MV deformity, cor triatriatum) and inflammatory diseases (rheumatoid arthritis, systemic lupus erythematosus). Physical obstructions, like a large atrial myxoma or an atrial thrombus, may mimic the clinical presentation of MS, but they are not diseases of the MV per se. MS can also occur in prosthetic valves (see Chapter 13) and as a complication of valve repair (see Chapter 9).

Assessing valvular morphology and associated pathology

2D and 3D appearances

(See Online appendix 6.3.) The echocardiographic features of rheumatic MS include commissural fusion (an important distinguishing feature from calcific MS), thickening and reduced mobility of the leaflets, chordal thickening and shortening, and calcification of the annulus, leaflets, and chordae. Thickening is most pronounced at the free edges of the leaflets. Commissural fusion and chordal shortening impart a funnel shape to the valve. While the free edge of the anterior leaflet is usually restricted, the body often moves freely, resulting in diastolic *doming* ('hockey stick' sign).

Leaflet morphology and diastolic doming are best appreciated in the mid-oesophageal long-axis view (Figure 8.26). Subvalvular involvement is best visualized in the transgastric two-chamber view. With 3D imaging, commissural fusion is easily identified from the LA aspect, while displaying the valve from the LV aspect demonstrates the funnel shape to the mitral orifice (Figure 8.27).

Colour Doppler

Colour aliasing and a zone of flow convergence can usually be identified on the LA side of the valve during diastole (Figure 8.26).

Associated features

Significant MS is virtually always associated with LA dilatation, sometimes severe, which often leads to atrial fibrillation. Blood velocity within the LA is reduced, with slow-swirling flow visible as spontaneous echo contrast (SEC). LA thrombus formation, particularly in the LA appendage (see Figure 5.15 and Online appendix 3.1), is not uncommon, due to the combined effects of blood stasis and/or atrial fibrillation. The risk of thrombus formation is highest in patients with marked SEC and when peak blood velocity in the LA appendage is <20 cm/s (normal >40 cm/s). LV function is often abnormal in patients with MS, with RV dilatation and paradoxical motion of the interventricular septum adversely

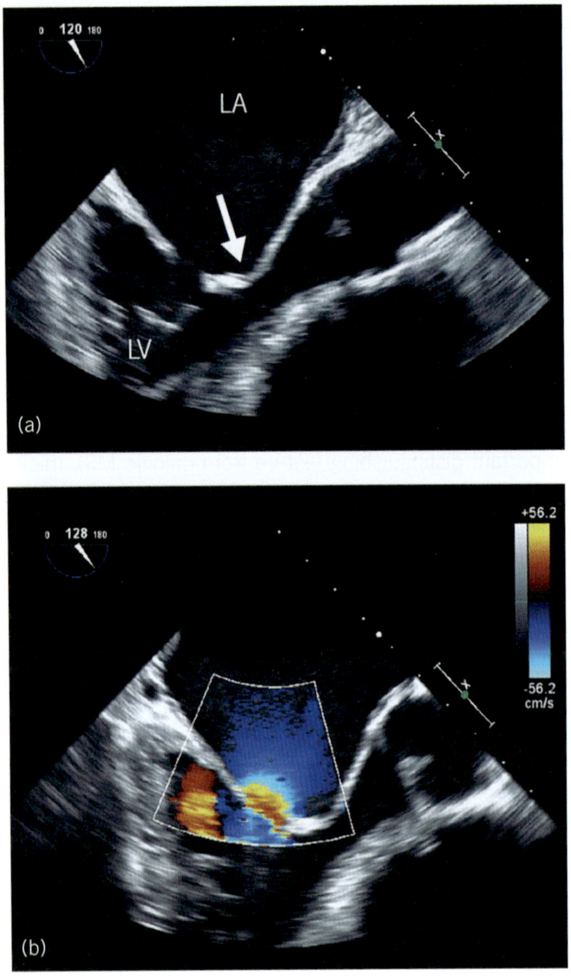

Figure 8.26 Rheumatic mitral stenosis. (a) With 2D imaging (mid-oesophageal long-axis view, late diastole), there is diastolic doming of the anterior mitral leaflet (arrow). Both leaflets are thickened and demonstrate reduced diastolic excursion. (b) With colour Doppler, a proximal flow convergence zone (PISA shell) can be seen on the LA side of the valve, consistent with severe stenosis. See more examples in Online appendix 6.3.

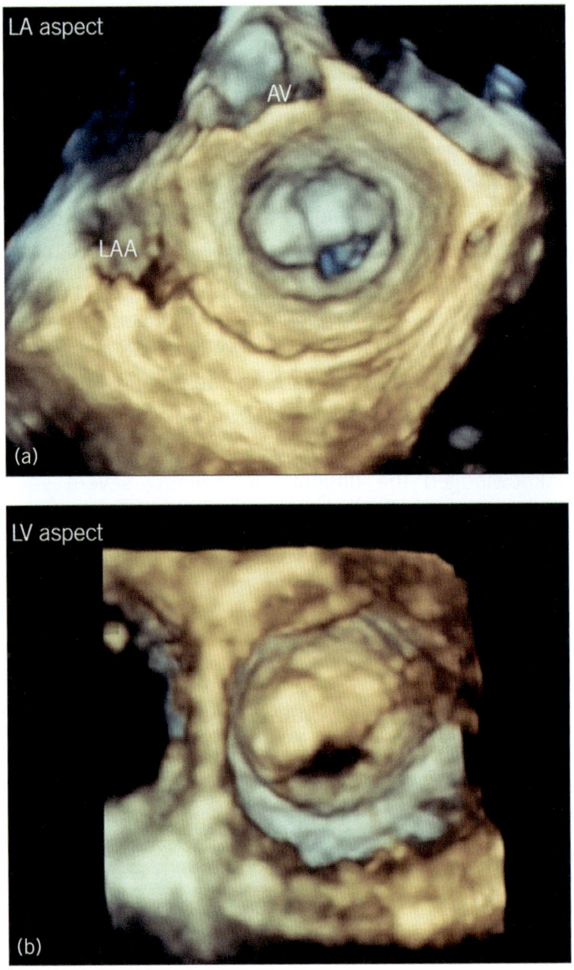

Figure 8.27 Rheumatic mitral stenosis with 3D imaging. In panel (a), the 3D data set has been orientated to display the MV from the LA aspect, and a late diastolic frame has been chosen for analysis. Marked commissural fusion can be seen, resulting in a narrowed mitral orifice. In panel (b), the data set has been orientated to display the valve from the LV aspect. Doming of the leaflets with commissural fusion can be clearly identified. The valve has a funnel-like appearance and the leaflets appear thickened. See more examples in Online appendix 6.3.

affecting LV filling and contractility. Calcification of the mitral annulus may also impair contractility of the basal segments. Typical echocardiographic features of RV pressure overload and pulmonary hypertension may also be present (see Chapter 14).

Assessing severity

The severity of MS is graded on the basis of diastolic pressure gradients and MV area (MVA), recalling that normal MVA is 4–5 cm^2 (Table 8.1). Recent guidelines have indicated MVA <1.5 cm^2 should be considered severe MS.[17]

The 2020 ACC guidelines moved to a staging of MS from A to D, based on features including anatomy, symptoms, and Doppler findings. Stage A (at risk of MS) refers to early in the disease process, prior to elevated gradients or symptoms, but with diastolic doming of the mitral leaflets being present on echocardiography. Trans-mitral flow is normal. When this progresses to stage B (progressive MS), symptoms are not yet present, pressure half-time (PHT) remains <150 ms, and MVA remains >1.5 cm^2; however, commissural fusion is present, along with elevated trans-mitral velocities. Stages C and D correspond to severe MS, with stage C being asymptomatic and stage

Table 8.1 Grading severity in mitral stenosis

	Mean diastolic pressure gradient (mmHg)	Mitral valve area (cm^2)
Mild	<5	>2.5
Moderate	5–9	1.6–2.5
Severe	>10	<1.5

Data from Pandian NG, Kim JK, Arias-Godinez JA, Marx GR, Michelena HI, Chander Mohan J, *et al.* Recommendations for the Use of Echocardiography in the Evaluation of Rheumatic Heart Disease: A Report from the American Society of Echocardiography. *J Am Soc Echocardiogr.* 2023;**36**(1):3–28.

D being symptomatic. At these stages, PHT >150 ms, MVA <1.5 cm^2, in addition to the previous anatomical features being present.[18]

Trans-mitral pressure gradient

Pressure gradients across the MV are estimated from the transmitral CW Doppler diastolic waveform. Once a representative Doppler envelope has been saved, peak and mean transmitral pressure gradients can be estimated using the trace function. Only the *mean* gradient should be used for quantifying and reporting the severity of MS, as it is less influenced by atrial compliance and LV diastolic function than by peak gradient. However, even the mean gradient is influenced by the haemodynamic state, being increased by elevated cardiac output, tachycardia, restrictive diastolic function, and MR. Given its heart rate dependence, the mitral gradient should always be reported with the heart rate. For patients in atrial fibrillation, where the diastolic time changes from beat to beat, an average of five measurements should be reported.

Pressure half-time

Calculation of the PHT is the preferred technique for rapidly estimating the MVA (see Figure 3.6 and Online appendix 6.3.1.4). On CW Doppler, the transmitral E-wave normally undergoes rapid deceleration due to the abrupt fall in pressure gradient as the LV fills during early diastole. The rate of diastolic pressure equalization (and therefore flow) between the LA and LV across a structurally normal MV is largely determined by LV compliance and LA pressure. Thus, in the absence of significant flow limitation (i.e. stenosis), the PHT is not a useful method of measuring the MVA. With MS, however, the pressure gradient is maintained much later in diastole, resulting in a greatly prolonged E-wave and slower deceleration of flow across the valve. The PHT is the time in milliseconds (ms) for the diastolic pressure (not velocity) to fall by 50% from the peak of the E-wave. More severe MS results in a flatter deceleration curve and a longer PHT, which, in turn, translates into a smaller calculated MVA. The empiric relationship between MVA and PHT is (Equation 8.4):

$$MVA = \frac{220}{PHT} \qquad \text{Equation 8.4}$$

Thus, a PHT of 220 ms equates to an MVA of 1 cm^2. Once a representative CW Doppler profile has been obtained, the E-wave descent is evaluated at two points. The machine software then automatically calculates the PHT and MVA (see Figure 3.6 and Online appendix 6.3.1.4). Because even small variations in the measurement can result in significant differences in the calculated MVA, an average of at least three recordings should be reported. Sometimes the E-wave deceleration slope is bimodal, being steeper in early diastole and tapering down later on. In this circumstance, the slope in *mid diastole* should be used for assessment of PHT. Occasionally, the slope is concave, in which case determining the PHT is not possible. Again, atrial fibrillation causes significant beat-to-beat variation in E-wave descents. PHT measurements from heartbeats with short diastoles should not be used, and an average of five long cycles reported.

While the effects are less pronounced than for pressure gradient, the haemodynamic state and other valve lesions also influence PHT measurements. Factors that increase LV end-diastolic pressure (tachycardia, restrictive diastolic filling, severe mitral and aortic regurgitation, high preload, and poor LA compliance) all reduce the PHT and *overestimate* the MVA. Bradycardia and impaired LV relaxation (as opposed to restrictive filling) prolong the PHT and *underestimate* the MVA. PHT is generally felt to be unreliable when the haemodynamic state changes rapidly such as in the early post-procedure period following MV repair or balloon mitral valvotomy.

Mitral planimetry

Planimetry of the mitral orifice is not recommended for 2D TOE imaging, because it is hard to be sure that the scan cuts the valve at right angles to the leaflets (an oblique cut overestimates the MVA) or that the measurement is made at the narrowest point of the valve (usually the leaflet tips) to avoid overestimating the MVA. Planimetry from a 3D MPR avoids these pitfalls and provides more reliable measurements of the MVA[19] (Figure 8.28; see Online appendix 6.3.1.8). Planimetry is a direct measurement, independent of loading conditions, chamber

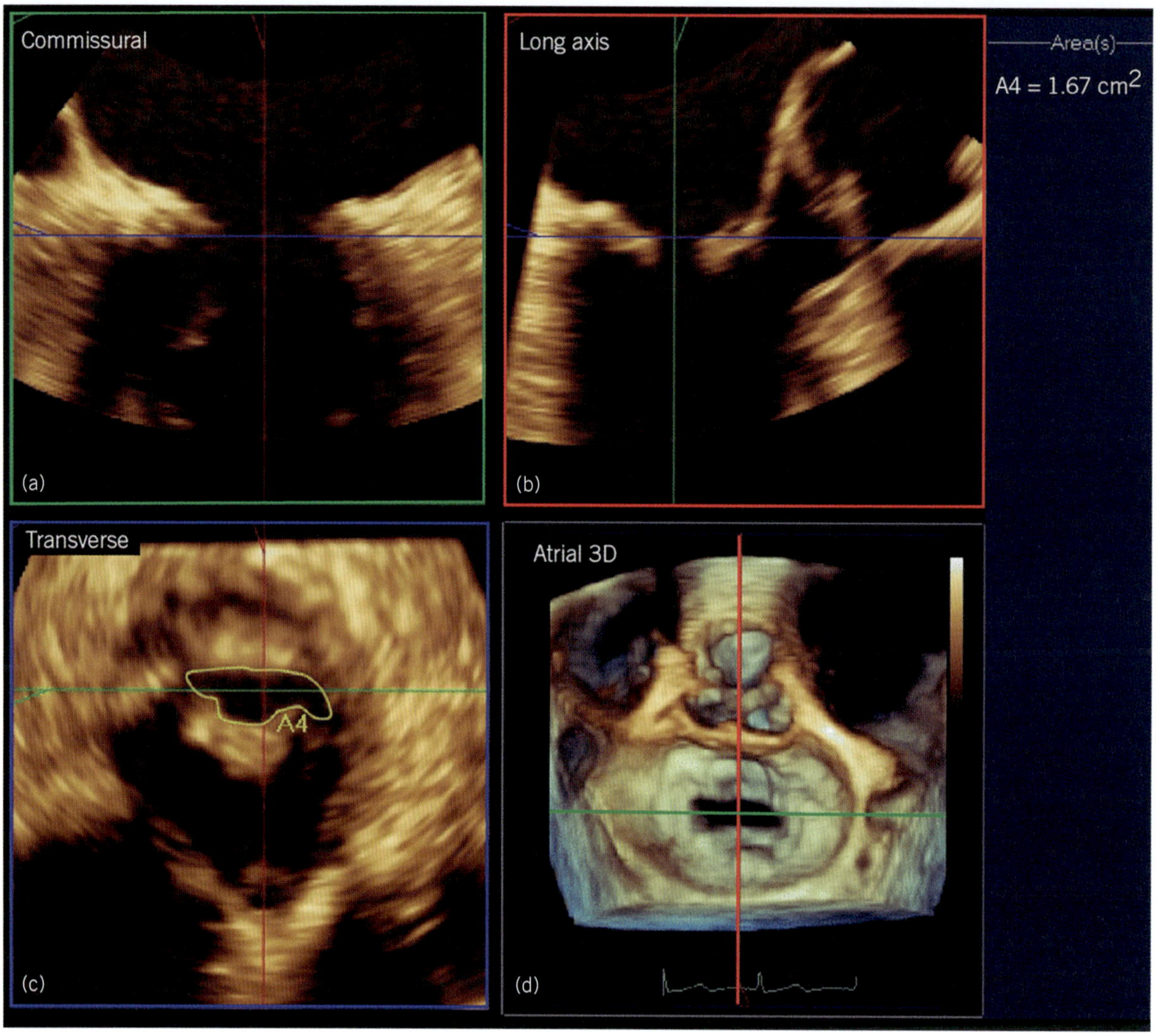

Figure 8.28 Measurement of mitral valve area (MVA) using multi-planar reconstruction. Axial 3D images of the MV are shown. The frame with the largest diastolic opening of the MV has been chosen for analysis. Panel (a) shows a commissural 2D slice. Panel (b) shows a long-axis 2D slice. Panel (c) shows a short-axis slice at the level of the leaflet tips. Panel (d) shows a volume-rendered 3D image in the surgical orientation from the LA aspect. In the (a) commissural and (b) long-axis quadrants, the red and green lines have been adjusted so they are positioned through the centre of the mitral orifice, and the blue lines have been adjusted so they pass through the narrowest part of the mitral orifice. (c) The MVA has then been measured with planimetry. The area measurement of 1.67 cm^2 indicates mild mitral stenosis. See example in Online appendix 6.3.1.

stiffness, and concomitant AV disease. If properly aligned using 3D MPR, it reliably correlates with the size of the anatomic orifice, and it is the preferred method of evaluation of the MVA.[17]

Flow convergence

MVA can also be estimated from analysis of the PISA that forms on the LA side of the valve during diastole. This is the same principle described previously for quantifying MR, except that a correction factor must be used when calculating the surface area of the PISA to account for the funnel shape of the mitral orifice in diastole. Thus, Equation 8.2 becomes Equation 8.5:

$$MVR = \frac{2\pi r^2 \times (\alpha / 180) \times NL}{V_E} \qquad \text{Equation 8.5}$$

where α is the angle between the mitral leaflets in diastole and V_E is the peak velocity across the MV in diastole (i.e. E_{max}).

The Nyquist limit should be adjusted to obtain a clear PISA shell, which usually involves reducing the aliasing velocity to about 40 cm/s. In contrast to MR, the PISA hemishell in MS is not a complete hemishell because it is restricted on either side by the mitral leaflets. Given that 180° defines a complete hemisphere, $\alpha/180$ represents the fraction of a hemisphere defined by the mitral leaflets.

Because the technique is limited by the same factors as for MR (shape of the orifice, small error being squared in the equation), *plus* the fact that the α angle is difficult to measure accurately and is a source of significant error, and the fact that the technique is not valid in patients with atrial fibrillation or concurrent MR, the PISA technique is rarely used for assessing MS.

Continuity equation

The continuity principle can theoretically be used with MVA as with any other valvular calculation. The formula here is (Equation 8.6):

$$MVA = \frac{\pi r^2 \times \mathrm{VTI}_{Ao}}{\mathrm{VTI}_{mitral}} \quad \text{Equation 8.6}$$

There are, however, significant limitations to using the continuity equation in MS, including the number of measurements decreasing accuracy and the presence of concurrent MR, AR, or atrial fibrillation. Due to these limitations, its routine use is not recommended by guidelines.[20]

Multiple choice questions

Discover interactive multiple choice questions to test your knowledge on this chapter by searching for this book's title or ISBN (9780198873686) at **https://academic.oup.com/** and going to the online appendix at the end of the book. Use your scratch-off code on the inside cover to access the material.

References

1. Chandra S, Salgo IS, Sugeng L, *et al.* Characterization of degenerative mitral valve disease using morphologic analysis of real-time three-dimensional echocardiographic images: objective insight into complexity and planning of mitral valve repair. *Circ Cardiovasc Imaging.* 2011;**4**(1):24–32.
2. Drake DH, Zimmerman KG, Hepner AM, Nichols CD. Echo-guided mitral repair. *Circ Cardiovasc Imaging.* 2014;**7**(1):132–41.
3. Mahmood F, Hess PE, Matyal R, *et al.* Echocardiographic anatomy of the mitral valve: a critical appraisal of 2-dimensional imaging protocols with a 3-dimensional perspective. *J Cardiothorac Vasc Anesth.* 2012;**26**(5):777–84.
4. Sidebotham DA, Allen SJ, Gerber IL, Fayer T. Intraoperative transesophageal echocardiography for surgical repair of mitral regurgitation. *J Am Soc Echocardiogr.* 2014;27(4):345–66.
5. Enriquez-Sarano M, Akins CW, Vahanian A. Mitral regurgitation. *Lancet.* 2009;**373**(9672):1382–94.
6. Lee APW, Jin CN, Fan Y, Wong RHL, Underwood MJ, Wan S. Functional implication of mitral annular disjunction in mitral valve prolapse: a quantitative dynamic 3D echocardiographic study. *JACC Cardiovasc Imaging.* 2017;**10**(12):1424–33.
7. Kumanohoso T, Otsuji Y, Yoshifuku S, *et al.* Mechanism of higher incidence of ischemic mitral regurgitation in patients with inferior myocardial infarction: quantitative analysis of left ventricular and mitral valve geometry in 103 patients with prior myocardial infarction. *J Thorac Cardiovasc Surg.* 2003;**125**(1):135–43.
8. Farhan S, Silbiger JJ, Halperin JL, *et al.* Pathophysiology, echocardiographic diagnosis, and treatment of atrial functional mitral regurgitation. *J Am Coll Cardiol.* 2022;**80**(24):2314–30.
9. Wyss CA, Enseleit F, van der Loo B, Grünenfelder J, Oechslin EN, Jenni R. Isolated cleft in the posterior mitral valve leaflet: a congenital form of mitral regurgitation. *Clin Cardiol.* 2009;**32**(10):553–60.
10. Caldarera I, Van Herwerden LA, Taams MA, Bos E, Roelandt JR . Multiplane transoesophageal echocardiography and morphology of regurgitant mitral valves in surgical repair. *Eur Heart J.* 1995;**16**(7):999–1006.
11. Sidebotham DA, Allen SJ, Gerber IL, Fayers T. Intraoperative transesophageal echocardiography for surgical repair of mitral regurgitation. *J Am Soc Echocardiogr.* 2014;**27**(4):345–66.
12. Zoghbi WA, Adams D, Bonow RO, *et al.* Recommendations for noninvasive evaluation of native valvular regurgitation. *J Am Soc Echocardiogr.* 2017;**30**(4):303–71.
13. Lambert AS. Proximal isovelocity surface area should be routinely measured in evaluating mitral regurgitation: a core review. *Anesth Analg.* 2007;**105**(4):940.
14. Chin JH, Lee EH, Choi DK, Choi IC. The effect of depth of anesthesia on the severity of mitral regurgitation as measured by transesophageal echocardiography. *J Cardiothorac Vasc Anesth.* 2012;**26**(6):994–8.
15. Grayburn PA, Chandrashekhar YS. Functional mitral regurgitation: more questions than answers. *JACC Cardiovasc Imaging.* 2021;**14**(4):711–14.
16. Lancellotti P, Troisfontaines P, Toussaint AC, Pierard LA. Prognostic importance of exercise-induced changes in mitral regurgitation in patients with chronic ischemic left ventricular dysfunction. *Circulation.* 2003;**108**(14):1713–17.
17. Pandian NG, Kim JK, Arias-Godinez JA, *et al.* Recommendations for the use of echocardiography in the evaluation of rheumatic heart disease: a report from the American Society of Echocardiography. *J Am Soc Echocardiogr.* 2023;**36**(1):3–28.
18. Otto CM, Nishimura RA, Bonow RO, *et al.* 2020 ACC/AHA Guideline for the management of patients with valvular heart disease: a report of the American College of Cardiology/

American Heart Association Joint Committee on Clinical Practice Guidelines. *Circulation.* 2020;**143**(5):72–227.

19. Sugeng L, Weinert L, Lammertin G, *et al.* Accuracy of mitral valve area measurements using transthoracic rapid freehand 3-dimensional scanning: comparison with noninvasive and invasive methods. *J Am Soc Echocardiogr.* 2003;**16**(12):1292–300.
20. Baumgartner H, Hung J, Bermejo J, *et al.* Echocardiographic assessment of valve stenosis: EAE/ASE recommendations for clinical practice. *J Am Soc Echocardiogr.* 2009;**22**(1):1–23.

9

Surgical repair of the mitral valve

Mitral valve (MV) repair is an important—if not the most important—indication for intraoperative TOE. Examination prior to repair influences the surgical technique, while the post-repair assessment may identify problems necessitating further surgery or medical intervention. 3D imaging allows the location and mechanism of regurgitant lesions to be more accurately determined than with 2D imaging, and therefore should be performed routinely on patients undergoing MV repair.

The majority of adults undergoing MV repair do so for degenerative disease and secondary (functional) MR. Mitral repair is also performed for endocarditis, congenital lesions, and, in certain circumstances, rheumatic heart disease.

A major review of TOE for patients undergoing MV repair, co-written by one of the authors of this chapter, was published in 2014.[1] Readers may find this article a useful reference source.

Indications for repair

For patients with degenerative MV disease and severe MR, surgery is indicated for symptoms or impaired LV systolic function (LVEF ≤60%, end-systolic diameter >4.0–4.5 cm).[2,3] Surgery should be considered in asymptomatic patients with preserved LV function who develop atrial fibrillation or have a systolic pulmonary artery pressure >50 mmHg. The management of patients with asymptomatic severe regurgitation and preserved LV function is controversial. A critical factor is the likelihood of successful repair. Current recommendations are that surgery is reasonable in this circumstance if the likelihood of successful repair is >95%.[2,3]

Treatment of secondary MR is somewhat controversial due to reduced durability of valve repair, compared to degenerative disease, and high perioperative mortality in patients with severe LV dysfunction (LVEF <30%). For patients undergoing coronary artery bypass grafting (CABG), MV surgery is indicated for severe secondary MR and should be considered when regurgitation is moderate.[2,3,4] Recent publications have provided conflicting data on intervening for secondary MR. A small randomized trial involving 300 patients with moderate secondary regurgitation found the addition of an annuloplasty ring at the time of CABG surgery was associated with increased post-operative morbidity.[5] Counted against this is a recent publication of patients enrolled in the STICH trial, in which patients with low LVEF were randomized to medical therapy alone, CABG surgery, or CABG plus ventricular reconstruction. Among the 1460 CABG patients, 234 also underwent MV surgery for moderate or severe MR, which involved valve repair in 94% of cases. MV surgery at the time of CABG was associated with significantly improved 30-day survival.[6]

When CABG surgery is not indicated, MV surgery should be considered in patients with severe secondary MR who have symptomatic heart failure despite optimal medical therapy.[2,3]

For native valve endocarditis, in addition to regurgitation severity, factors such as heart failure, recurrent embolism, persisting sepsis, resistant microorganisms, vegetation size, and extravascular involvement (e.g. heart block or abscess) must be considered.

Axial imaging

Preintervention imaging is mandatory for all MV repairs. This is especially important for secondary disease because the surgeon cannot accurately assess the severity of tethering once the heart is arrested. Axial imaging uses the long-axis and commissural views to symmetrically traverse the centre of the MV and ventricular apex (Figure 9.1).[7,8] These orthogonal views have been successfully applied for guiding surgical MV repair and are also used for guiding transcatheter repair (see Chapter 17).[7,9] 3D post-acquisition multi-planar reconstruction (MPR) allows for highly reproducible valve analysis and facilitates

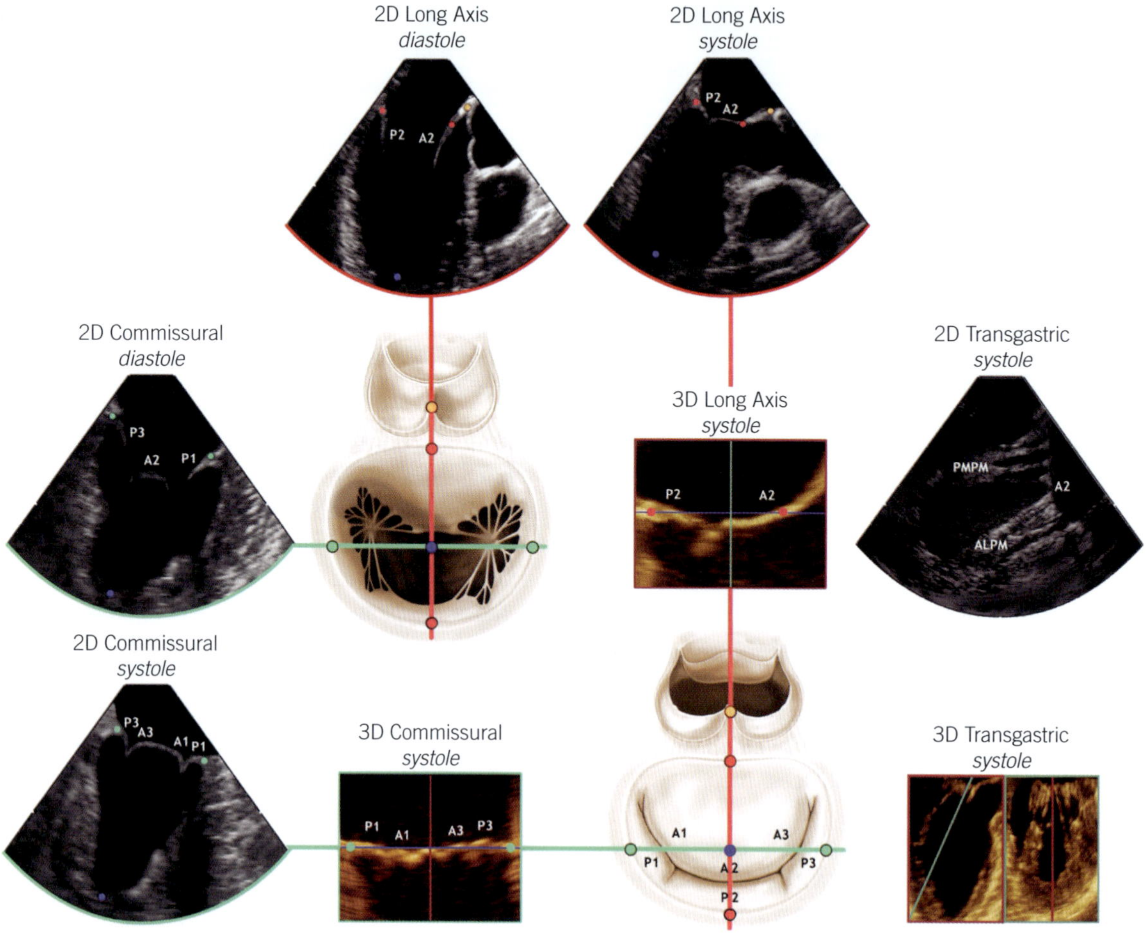

Figure 9.1 Image acquisition for axial imaging of the MV and examples of common mitral pathologies. Image acquisition for 2D and 3D axial imaging. The 2D images are shown as grey-scale pyramidal sectors. Landmarks for axial imaging are obtained from diastolic frames. The diastolic landmarks ensure the long-axis and commissural views are perpendicular to each other in systole, which is when measurements are made. Diastolic landmarks for the long-axis view are: (1) the commissure between the left and non-coronary leaflets of the aortic valve (yellow dot); (2) the maximum anteroposterior annular width (red dots); and (3) the apex of the LV (blue dot). Diastolic landmarks for the commissural view are: (1) the free-floating central A2 segment; (2) the maximum annular width (green dots); and (3) the apex of the LV (blue dot). Measurements of annular dimensions and leaflet distortion are then made from systolic frames. In systole, the long-axis view demonstrates the anteroposterior axis, the A2 and P2 segments, and the A2/P2 coaptive surface. In systole, the commissural view demonstrates the commissural axis, the A1, P1, A3, and P3 segments, and the A1/P1 and A3/P3 coaptive surfaces. It is important that all landmarks remain within view throughout the cardiac cycle. Each grey-scale acquisition is followed by an acquisition using colour flow Doppler of approximately the same cycle length. Then, without moving the probe, the zoom function is used to acquire axial 2D and colour images focusing on the mitral apparatus. The landmarks for 3D acquisition are the same as for standard multi-plane imaging. The initial 3D data sets are acquired using full-volume mode with and without colour Doppler imaging. Without moving the probe, additional 3D data sets are acquired using the zoom mode, again with and without colour Doppler imaging. 3D data sets are then analysed using multi-planar reconstruction (MPR) to obtain 2D axial long-axis and commissural images. Systolic frames obtained using MPR from 3D data sets are shown as rectangular boxes in the figure.

procedural planning (see Figure 8.11).[8] Parallax must be eliminated prior to MPR interpretation (see Figure 8.12). A video outlining an approach to echo-guided mitral repair is demonstrated in the online material (see Online appendix 6.6.2).

It is helpful to have a sonographer skilled in 3D acquisition and rapid post-acquisition analysis present at the time of MV repair. The presence of a skilled sonographer is particularly helpful for patients undergoing repair of secondary MV disease, for transcatheter intervention, and for minimally invasive procedures, including robotic MV repair.

Surgical technique and outcome

The primary goal for any repair technique is to restore an adequate systolic coaptation surface. An annuloplasty ring should be placed in all patients to increase the coaptation height, to correct annular dilatation, and to prevent further annular dilatation.

Degenerative disease

The classical approach to MV repair for degenerative disease is to resect prolapsing or flail segments and their associated chordae (Figure 9.2)—the 'French correction' popularized by Carpentier. The extent of resection parallels the spectrum of disease from fibroelastic deficiency (FED) to Barlow disease. Localized posterior leaflet prolapse/flail typical of FED requires nothing more than narrow triangular resection. More extensive posterior leaflet prolapse/flail characteristic of Barlow disease may be corrected with segmental resection and sliding posteroplasty, which, in addition to segment resection, requires that the annulus at the base of the remaining segments is compressed to allow approximation of the remaining leaflet tissue without reducing the posterior leaflet tissue available for coaptation. Very advanced Barlow disease, with bileaflet prolapse, may be treated with limited anterior triangular resection, posterior segmentectomy, sliding posteroplasty, and/or papillary muscle shortening. Potential problems with leaflet resection, particularly when there is minimal excess tissue, are reduced coaptation and increased leaflet tension, which may reduce the durability of the repair. Despite these concerns, excellent long-term outcomes have been observed with leaflet resection and papillary shortening.[7,10]

Replacing ruptured or elongated chordae with polytetrafluoroethylene neochordae has become a popular alternative to leaflet resection. Potential advantages of chordal replacement over leaflet resection are the creation of a greater coaptation surface, preserved leaflet mobility, reduced leaflet tension, and use of a larger

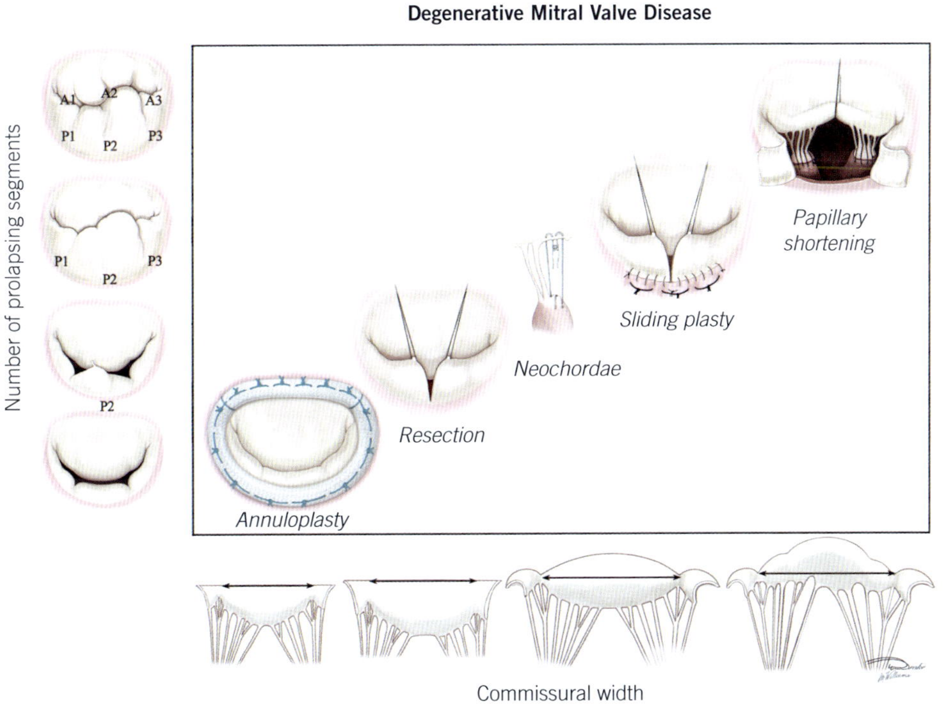

Figure 9.2 Surgical techniques for repair of degenerative MV disease. Annular dilation from mild fibroelastic deficiency requires nothing more than a simple ring. Resection with or without sliding posteroplasty or neochordae are the most common procedures for isolated posterior leaflet prolapse. Advanced Barlow disease with bileaflet prolapse frequently requires papillary muscle shortening or multiple neochordae and oversized ring annuloplasty.

From *New England Journal of Medicine*, Drake DH, Zimmerman KG, Sidebotham DA, Surgical treatment for moderate ischemic mitral regurgitation, **372**, 18, Figure 1, pp. 1771–1773. Copyright © 2015 Massachusetts Medical Society. Reprinted with permission from Massachusetts Medical Society.

annuloplasty ring. Conversely, neochordal length, even if pre-measured, introduces an additional variable that is a risk for repair failure. Similar results have been obtained with both techniques.[11,12]

Successful repair of degenerative MR is possible in most patients, particularly when disease is limited to the posterior leaflet. Anterior leaflet and bileaflet repairs are more challenging, and are associated with a lower rate of initial success and a higher need for reoperation.[2,13,14] However, success rates for all types of repair are increasing, and approach 100% for isolated posterior leaflet repairs.[15] For complex anterior and bileaflet repairs, success rates >90% have been reported from high-volume centres.[7,14]

Modifications to surgical technique for patients at increased risk of systolic anterior motion

Systolic anterior motion (SAM) is an important potential complication of MV repair for degenerative disease, particularly Barlow disease. SAM refers to movement of the anterior mitral leaflet into the LVOT during systole, resulting in outflow tract obstruction and MR. The primary mechanisms for post-repair SAM are excess leaflet tissue relative to annular size and an anterior (i.e. close to the LVOT) coaptation point. An *excess of either anterior or posterior leaflet tissue* predisposes to SAM (Figure 9.3a, b); however, the risk is greatest with an excess of posterior leaflet tissue, as this displaces the coaptation point anteriorly, towards the LVOT.[16] Other anatomic risk factors for SAM are a *pre-repair non-enlarged annulus*, a small LV, hypertrophy of the basal anterior septum, and a *narrow aorto-mitral angle* (Figure 9.3c).[17]

Modifications to standard surgical techniques may be employed for patients at risk of SAM. Avoiding undersizing the annuloplasty ring is important, as a small annuloplasty ring moves the coaptation point closer to the LVOT. When there is excess posterior leaflet tissue, resection of posterior leaflet tissue may be undertaken. If posterior chordal replacement is performed, displacing bulky posterior leaflet tissue into the LV with shortened neochordae moves the coaptation point posteriorly, away from the LVOT. Ideally, the atrial surface of the posterior leaflet should be ≤1.5 cm and should never exceed 2.0 cm. For excess anterior leaflet tissue, an annuloplasty ring with a larger AP diameter may be chosen. If neochordae are used to correct anterior leaflet prolapse, it is important that the neochordae are not too short, as this displaces the anterior leaflet into the LV, thereby bringing the coaptation point closer to the LVOT.

Secondary mitral disease

Common causes of secondary MR are annular dilation from atrial enlargement, ischaemic disease resulting in regional

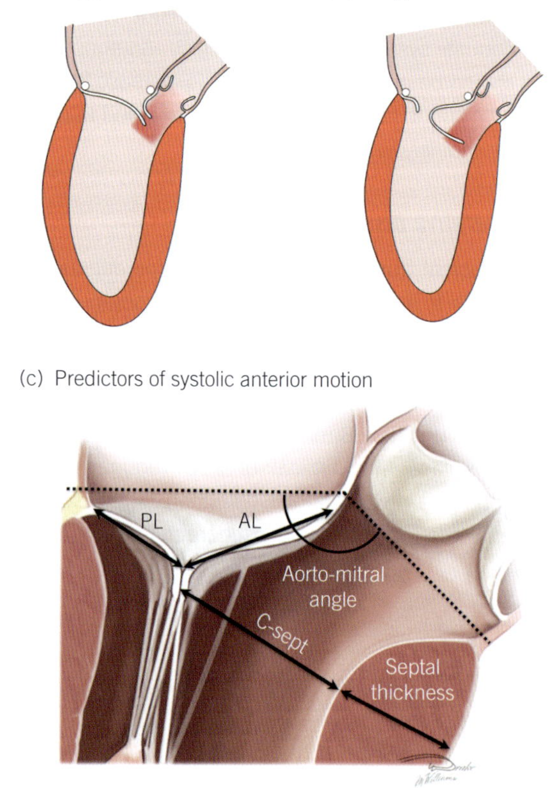

Figure 9.3 Mechanisms of systolic anterior motion (SAM) demonstrated in the long-axis view. (a) Effect of a long posterior leaflet. A long posterior leaflet, in combination with an undersized annuloplasty ring, moves the coaptation line anteriorly, displacing the anterior mitral leaflet into the LVOT. This is the classical mechanism for post-repair SAM. The shaded pink area represents systolic blood flow in the LVOT. (b) Effect of a long anterior leaflet. A long anterior leaflet, in combination with an undersized annuloplasty ring, can also result in the anterior leaflet being exposed to the LVOT, with resultant SAM. (c) Echocardiographic predictors of systolic anterior motion (SAM) in the long-axis view. An increased risk of post-operative SAM is indicated by: (1) posterior leaflet length >1.5 cm; (2) anterior leaflet length >2.0 cm; (3) posterior leaflet (PL) relative to anterior leaflet (AL) length (AL/PL) <1.3; (4) C-sept <2.5 cm; (5) an aorto-mitral angle <120°; (6) septal thickness >1.5 cm; and (7) LV end-diastolic diameter (LVEDD) <45 mm. C-sept is the shortest distance between the coaptation point and the anterior septal wall. Other than LVEDD, all measurements should be obtained in late systole in the mid-oesophageal long-axis view.

b) Adapted with permission from Kahn RA, Mittnacht AJ, and Anyanwu AC, Systolic anterior motion as a result of relative 'undersizing' of the mitral valve annulus in a patient with Barlow's disease, *Anesthesia and Analgesia*, **108**, 4, pp. 1102–1104, Figure 3, Copyright 2009, International Anesthesia Research Society. http://journals.lww.com/anesthesia-analgesia/pages/default.aspx)

ventricular wall motion abnormalities, global cardiomyopathy associated with decreased ventricular function, and hypertrophic cardiomyopathy. A large observational study involving >14000 patients undergoing surgical MV repair for both primary and secondary disease demonstrated that 10-year survival was equivalent to that of the age- and sex-matched population in the United States and concluded that MV repair was durable and restored long-term survival to normal.[18] Countered against this is the high rate of recurrence when a restrictive annuloplasty is used in isolation.[4] A recent meta-analysis demonstrated that durable MV repair can be obtained as long as the repair technique is tailored to the degree of anatomic valvular distortion.[19]

The simplest approach to valve repair for secondary MR is placement of an undersized annuloplasty ring. The risk of recurrence is increased when leaflet tethering is severe or there is marked annular dilation. This finding is explained by the fact that anterior displacement of the posterior annulus by a restrictive annuloplasty ring can worsen leaflet tethering (Figure 9.4).

A recent meta-analysis suggested that simple ring annuloplasty for secondary disease should be limited to patients with minimal tethering.[19] Various echocardiographic indices of leaflet tethering (Figure 9.5a) can help to identify patients at risk of recurrence when a restrictive annuloplasty is used in isolation. Risk factors that have been validated for TOE are a tenting height >1.0 cm, a tenting area ≥1.6 cm² (long-axis view), and an annular diameter ≥3.7 cm (four-chamber view). Parameters that have been validated with TTE are a tenting height >1.0 cm, a tenting area >2.5 cm², and a posterior leaflet closing angle ≥45° (apical four-chamber view).

Several surgical adjuvants have been developed in an attempt to overcome the high failure rate associated with

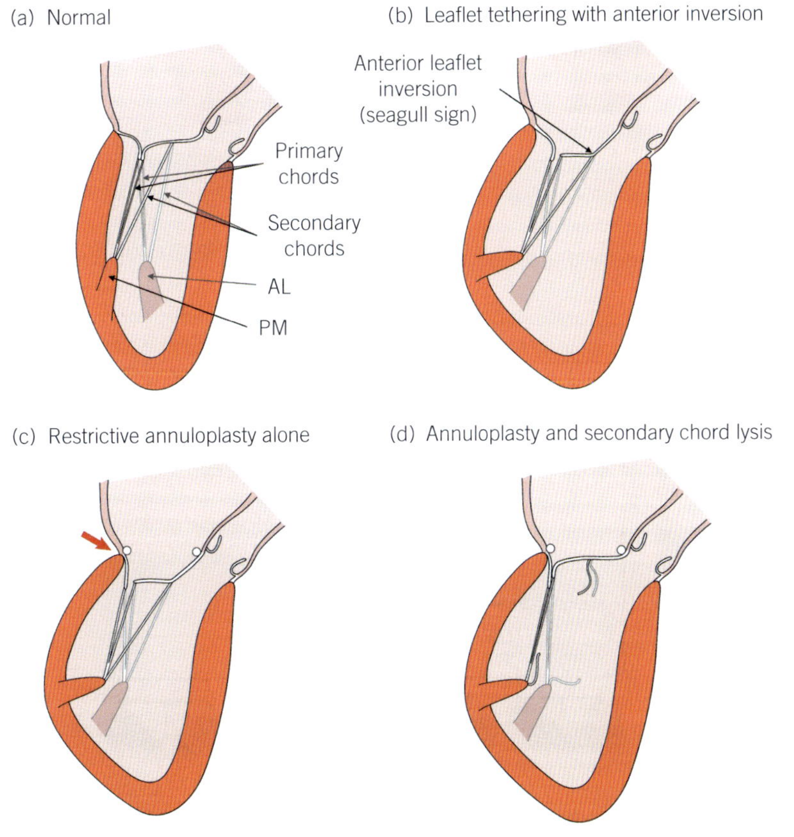

Figure 9.4 Effect of a restrictive annuloplasty and secondary chord lysis on leaflet tethering shown in the long-axis view. Note that the papillary muscles are normally symmetrically displaced posteromedially (PM) and anterolaterally (AL) from the midline of the mitral valve and are consequently not seen in the long-axis view. Both papillary muscles provide primary and secondary chords to the anterior and posterior leaflets. (a) Normal appearances of the mitral leaflets in late systole. (b) Severe leaflet tethering due to lateral displacement of the posteromedial papillary. Note inversion of the anterior leaflet (seagull sign) due to tension from secondary chordae. (c) Effect of a restrictive annuloplasty alone. The annuloplasty ring has displaced the posterior annulus anteriorly (red-direction arrow), reducing the annular dimension. However, the distance between the head of the posteromedial papillary muscle and the leaflet margins has increased, worsening leaflet tethering. (d) Effect of secondary chord lysis. Secondary chord lysis has reduced tension on the anterior leaflet, eliminated leaflet inversion, and improved leaflet coaptation.

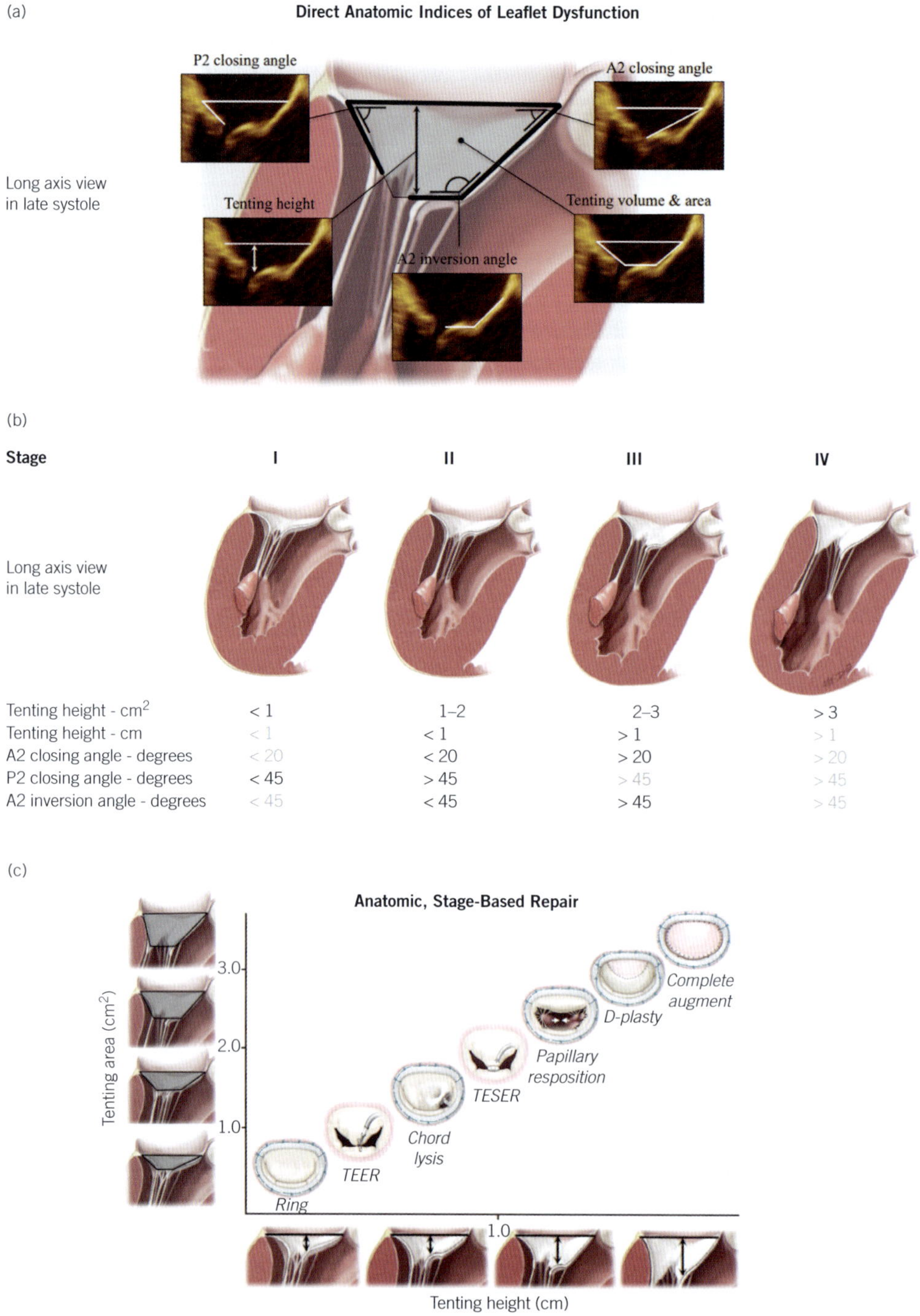

Figure 9.5 Index-based staging and stage-based recommendations for mitral repair. (a) The direct indices of mitral dysfunction from secondary disease are illustrated in the long-axis view during late systole. Echocardiographic images appear in the inserts. The direct indices include tenting area, tenting height, A2 closing angle, P2 closing angle, and A2 inversion angle. (b) A simple, evidence-based anatomic staging system is demonstrated. (c) Simple surgical ring annuloplasty should be limited to stage I disease. Transcatheter edge-to-edge is effective for stages I and II, but not for stages III and IV. Anterior leaflet augmentation, papillary approximation, surgical edge-to-edge repair, and other advanced surgical techniques combined with ring annuloplasty are effective for stage III. Carpentier nomenclature is used to identify leaflet segments.

a restrictive annuloplasty when leaflet tethering is severe. These include sectioning of secondary chordae, chordal translocation, reorientation of the papillary muscles, LV aneurysmectomy, patch extension of the anterior leaflet, and edge-to-edge repair. While secondary chordae are important in maintaining LV geometry, they can also contribute to anterior leaflet tethering. Following inferior/posterior infarction, lateral displacement of the posteromedial papillary muscle causes distortion (inversion) of the anterior leaflet (seagull sign; Figure 9.4). Selective sectioning of secondary chordae can reduce anterior leaflet distortion, thereby improving leaflet coaptation (Figure 9.4).[7,20] A recently reported meta-analysis supports a stage-based graduated protocol progressing from restrictive ring annuloplasty to sectioning of secondary chordae, and ultimately patch extension of the anterior leaflet, depending on the severity of leaflet tethering (Figure 9.5b, c).[7,19] Currently, these adjuvant techniques are not fully established, and many surgeons elect to perform MV replacement when leaflet tethering is severe.[2]

Endocarditis

Valve repair is possible in the majority of patients with MV endocarditis and is associated with low mortality and high freedom from reoperation.[21] Surgery involves excision of vegetations, leaflet debridement, suture or pericardial patch closure of perforations, and placement of an annuloplasty ring. Chordal replacement may be required if there is chordal involvement or significant leaflet destruction. Abscess formation or severe leaflet destruction may necessitate valve replacement.

Rheumatic disease

Patients with rheumatic MV disease may have predominantly stenosis, predominantly regurgitation, or mixed disease. The primary pathologic mechanism of rheumatic MS is commissural fusion. Nowadays, rheumatic MS is usually treated with balloon mitral valvotomy (BMV) (see Chapter 17). If the anatomy is unsuitable for BMV, surgical repair typically involves open commissurotomy, chord fenestration, leaflet augmentation, placement of an annuloplasty ring, and excision of LA thrombus (if present). However, more commonly, valve replacement is performed in patients unsuitable for BMV.

Valve repair for rheumatic MR is technically demanding and associated with lower durability, compared to repair of other mitral lesions.[22] However, in experienced hands and in appropriate clinical circumstances—notably women of childbearing age wishing to avoid warfarin anticoagulation, surgical repair can be a good option. The repair technique depends on the pathology. The leaflets and subvalvular apparatus may require debridement and decalcification. Patch augmentation may be required if there is marked leaflet retraction. An annuloplasty ring is indicated in all patients.

Considerations for minimally invasive and robotic mitral repair

TOE has a specific role for patients undergoing minimally invasive and robotic MV surgery in guiding and confirming correct placement of cannulae and wires (Figure 9.6). CPB is usually established via the femoral vessels. For venous drainage, a long cannula is advanced from the femoral vein over a guidewire and positioned so that the tip lies in the SVC, close to the SVC–RA junction. Before advancing the cannula over the wire, it is important to confirm the guidewire is positioned in the SVC and has not passed across the atrial septum (Figure 9.6a) or TV (Figure 9.6b). When correctly positioned, the cannula can be seen traversing the IVC, RA, and SVC in the mid-oesophageal bicaval view (Figure 9.6c). Sometimes a second venous drainage cannula is advanced from the right internal jugular vein, with the tip positioned at the SVC–RA junction. In this circumstance, the tip of the femoral cannula should be positioned in the RA, close to the RA–IVC junction (Figure 9.6d). For arterial return, a short cannula is typically placed in the femoral artery. Confirmation of the guidewire in the descending aorta is important to rule out a false passage or iatrogenic dissection.

Aortic cross-clamping may be performed externally, via a clamp inserted through a small chest wall incision, or internally, via an **endoclamp** inserted via the femoral artery. Endoclamping is technically demanding to use but has the advantage of facilitating redo surgery when adhesions may preclude placement of an external clamp. An endoclamp should be positioned in the proximal ascending aorta just distal to the sinotubular junction (Figure 9.6e). The position of the endoclamp should be assessed throughout the case to ensure it does not move, particularly during balloon inflation and during initiation of CPB.

The presence of more than trivial aortic regurgitation may preclude the use of antegrade cardioplegia and increase the risk of LV distension during CPB. Retrograde cardioplegia is delivered via a coronary sinus cannula inserted either through a chest wall incision or percutaneously via the right internal jugular vein. Correct positioning of a coronary sinus catheter can be confirmed in the deep mid-oesophageal four-chamber view (Figure 9.6f).

Cardiac exposure is severely reduced during minimally invasive robotic surgery. Thus, TOE is useful for assessing

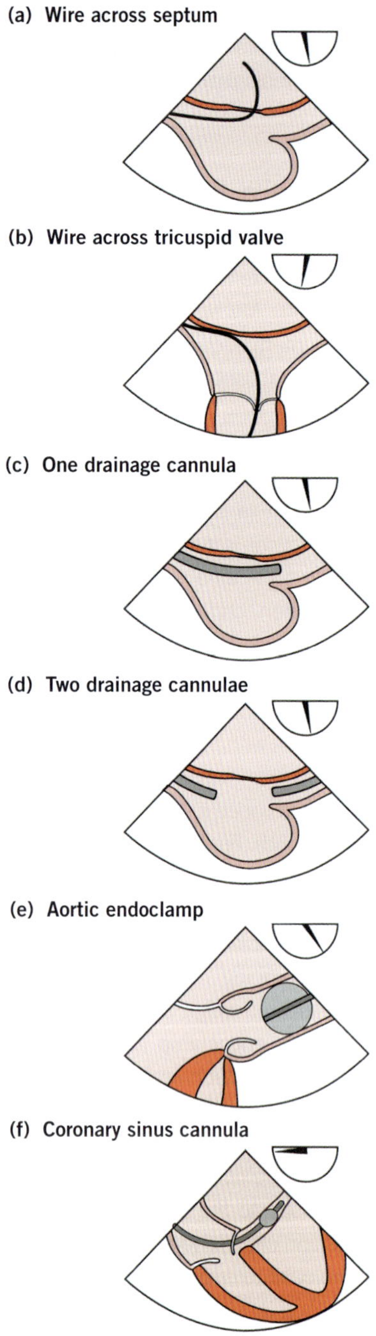

Figure 9.6 TOE imaging of wires and cannulae for minimally invasive MV repair. (a) Wire across septum; (b) wire across tricuspid valve; (c) one drainage cannula; (d) two drainage cannulae; (e) aortic endoclamp; (f) coronary sinus cannula. See text for details.

ventricular distension during CPB and for evaluating ventricular function following separation from CPB. TOE is also useful to assess the effectiveness of de-airing of the heart at completion of surgery.

Robotic MV repair is associated with excellent results that compare favourably to outcomes from other minimally invasive procedures and sternotomy.[23] However, the instrumentation is considerably more complex and, at least initially, requires additional personnel, training, and organization. During robotic surgery, exposure is even more severely limited than in other minimally invasive procedures, and the surgeon has no tactile feedback to prevent unintended tissue injury. There are numerous blind spots, in which robotic manoeuvres may result in occult injuries. And finally, the robot must be undocked and removed from the surgical field prior to performing an emergency thoracotomy or sternotomy. For these reasons, robotic surgery requires that a dedicated robotic team undergo comprehensive training, simulation, rehearsal, and operative proctoring for at least the first 5–6 cases.[24] Anaesthetic and haemodynamic management during robotic procedures often demands the full attention of the anaesthesia provider. A second echocardiographer who is skilled at rapid 3D axial acquisition and post-acquisition analysis is recommended.

Although frequently simplified, the techniques used for robotic MV repair are largely the same as for conventional repair, other than the instrumentation. A summary of the sequence of robotic MV repair is presented in Box 9.1.

Examination prior to repair

TOE views and axial imaging of the MV are reviewed in Chapter 8 and Online appendices 1.4 and 6.1. Several features on the pre-repair TOE examination influence surgical decision-making (Box 9.2).

To avoid misdiagnosis, it is essential that leaflet segments are correctly identified and leaflet pathology is accurately diagnosed. Measurement of the mitral annulus is important and is described in Chapter 8.

Degenerative disease

(See Online appendix 6.2.) The most common degenerative lesion requiring surgery is isolated flail of a single leaflet segment due to chordal rupture (see Figure 8.19). The posterior leaflet is more commonly affected than the anterior leaflet, and P2 is more commonly involved than P1 or P3. In patients with FED, there is typically minimal excess leaflet tissue and annular dilatation is usually mild. 3D imaging is extremely useful to delineate the extent of the lesion.

Patients with Barlow disease are easily identified because of increased annular dimensions and numerous prolapsing segments. The commissural diameter is typically dramatically enlarged. Axial imaging allows

Box 9.1 Robotic MV repair procedural summary

Anesthesia, echocardiography, positioning, and line/cannula placement

- Induce general anaesthesia and place a double-lumen endotracheal tube
- Insert a right internal jugular pulmonary artery catheter and superior vena cava cannula
- Introduce a TOE probe; complete 2D and 3D TOE examinations
- Position for right thoracotomy (right chest elevated by 30°)
- Introduce right femoral venous and arterial cannulae under TOE guidance
- Introduce coronary sinus catheter under TOE guidance
- Initiate one-lung anaesthesia (right lung deflated)

Port access and docking

- Port access or mini-thoracotomy in the right fifth intercostal space
- Insert trocars for the camera, instruments, and left atrial retractor
- Dock robotic instruments, and deploy the camera and instruments

Cardiopulmonary bypass and mitral repair

- Initiate cardiopulmonary bypass with systemic cooling
- Apply endovascular balloon or transthoracic aortic clamp, and infuse cardioplegia
- Open and suspend the pericardium by using transthoracic sutures
- Left atriotomy, and insert robotic retractor to expose the mitral valve
- Perform mitral valve repair
- Place pacing wire(s) on the right ventricle
- Close atriotomy, meticulously de-air, and release aortic clamp
- Wean patient from cardiopulmonary bypass (with both lungs inflated)

Echocardiography, decannulation, and endotracheal tube management

- Confirm satisfactory repair with complete echocardiographic study
- Remove the coronary sinus catheter
- Undock the robot
- Decannulate vessels and close incisions
- Extubate or exchange the double-lumen for a single-lumen endotracheal tube
- Transfer patient to intensive care unit

reproducible measurement of the severity of leaflet segment prolapse. Prolapse ≤0.5 cm typically does not require correction. It is important to identify which segment(s) is/are functionally regurgitant, as not all myxomatous segments are necessarily regurgitant. Colour 3D imaging is very useful to confirm the site(s) of regurgitation (see Figure 8.21). Once a 3D data set has been acquired, it is useful to crop down onto the valve from the LA surface to determine the origin of the jet(s).

Mitral clefts are associated with degenerative MV disease and are suggested by colour jets that are displaced from the coaptation line. However, caution is required when interpreting such jets, as infolding bulky leaflet tissue can create the false impression of a cleft. Again, 3D imaging is useful for identifying clefts (see Figure 8.16).

Severe degenerative disease is associated with **mitral annular disjunction**, in which there is a wide separation (0.5–1.5 cm) between the LV and the posterior mitral annulus (Figure 9.7; see Online appendix 6.2.8), resulting in hypermobility of the annulus.[25] If mitral annular disjunction is identified, it can be corrected during the repair procedure.

Several measurements on the pre-repair examination indicate an increased risk of developing SAM (Figure 9.3).[17] These are: (1) a posterior leaflet length >1.5 cm; (2) an anterior leaflet length >2.0 cm; (3) a long posterior leaflet (PL) relative to anterior leaflet (AL) length (AL/PL <1.3); (4) a C-sept <2.5 cm; (5) an aorto-mitral angle <120°; and (6) septal bulge >1.5 cm.[26] Measurements should be obtained in *late systole* in the mid-oesophageal long-axis view.

Secondary mitral regurgitation

(See Online appendix 6.5.) Patients with secondary MR are usually scheduled for CABG surgery, and

Box 9.2 Features on the pre-repair TOE examination that may influence surgical decision-making in patients undergoing MV repair

Degenerative mitral disease

- Severity of mitral regurgitation
- Annular dimensions (anteroposterior and commissural axes)
- Amount of redundant tissue (i.e. fibroelastic deficiency vs Barlow disease)
- Anatomical location of leaflet segment prolapse/flail
- Prolapse height in non-flail segments
- Anatomical location of regurgitation jet(s) (Barlow disease)
- Ventriculo-annular disjunction
- Unexpected cleft
- Leaflet tethering in non-prolapsing segments
- Presence of mitral annular calcification
- Presence of mitral annular disjunction
- Risk factors for systolic anterior motion
- Tricuspid regurgitation severity and tricuspid annular dimensions

Secondary mitral disease

- Severity of mitral regurgitation
- Annular dimensions (anteroposterior and commissural axes)
- Pattern of leaflet tethering (symmetric versus asymmetric)
- Severity of leaflet tethering (tenting height, tenting area, A2 closing angle, P2 closing angle, degree of anterior leaflet inversion)
- Interpapillary distance and shortening
- Ventricular dimension, area, and volume (end-systole, end-diastole)
- Left ventricular ejection fraction
- Pulmonary artery pressure
- Tricuspid regurgitation severity and tricuspid annular dimensions

Endocarditis

- Severity of mitral regurgitation
- Pre-existing mitral valve disease (was the valve normal prior to infection?)
- Annular dimensions (anteroposterior and commissural axes)
- Degree of tissue destruction
- Presence and location of leaflet perforations
- Presence and location of fistulae or abscesses

Rheumatic mitral disease

- Severity of mitral regurgitation and stenosis
- Annular dimensions (anteroposterior and commissural axes)
- Presence of annular, leaflet, and subvalvular calcification
- Leaflet mobility
- Leaflet retraction (regurgitation)
- Commissural fusion (stenosis)
- Involvement of other valves/structures

the severity of their MR may have been inadequately determined—or have changed—since the preoperative study. Thus, intraoperative assessment of both the mechanism and severity of the regurgitation may be critically important. Assessing the mechanism of secondary MR involves measuring annular dimensions, evaluating the pattern of leaflet tethering (symmetric or asymmetric), and measuring the tenting height, area, A2 closing angle, P2 closing angle, and degree of anterior leaflet inversion (quantitate 'seagull sign') (Figure 9.5; see Online appendix 6.6.3). Measurements should be made in late systole in the mid-oesophageal long-axis view or with 3D imaging by using MPR (see Figures 8.11 and 8.12). Assessment of regurgitant jet direction is also helpful—central jets suggest symmetric tethering with dilated cardiomyopathies, whereas posterior jets suggest asymmetric tethering commonly associated with posterior or inferior infarctions.

Endocarditis

(See Online appendix 6.4.) In patients with endocarditis, it is important to identify the presence and location of any leaflet perforations, as these must be closed as part of the repair procedure. 3D imaging from the LV aspect is useful for identifying perforations that are obscured by vegetations when imaging the valve from the atrial aspect (see Figure 8.17). Valve repair may not be feasible when there is extensive leaflet destruction or when an abscess or a fistulous connection has formed. These

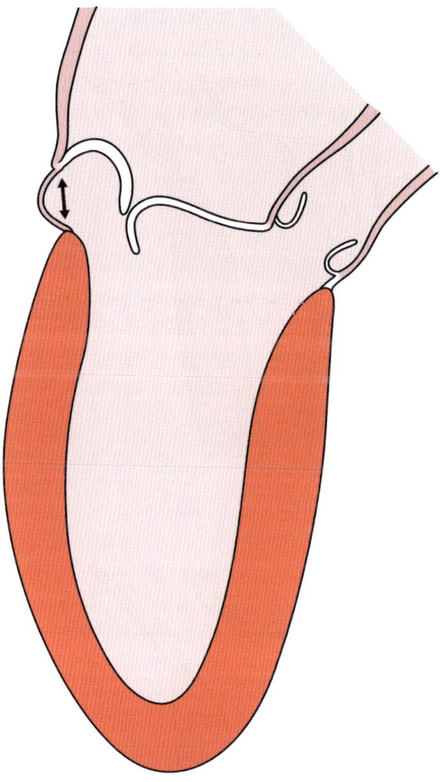

Figure 9.7 Schematic showing mitral annular disjunction. The arrow indicates the extent of separation between the posterior mitral annulus and the posterior mitral leaflet. See Online appendix 6.2.8.

complications should be excluded by careful inspection of the valve with colour Doppler imaging.

Rheumatic disease

(See Online appendix 6.3.) Patients presenting for surgical repair of rheumatic MV disease are a selected group, with surgical repair having been chosen over BMV (for stenosis) or valve replacement (for stenosis or regurgitation). Most of the features listed in Box 9.2 are visualized with 2D and colour Doppler imaging (see Figure 8.26). The exception is commissural fusion, which is best seen with 3D imaging (see Figure 8.27).

Examination following repair

The post-repair examination should focus on identifying any residual MR and ruling out complications such as MS, SAM, and ventricular dysfunction. Coaptation, leaflet motion, and the correct seating of the annuloplasty ring should be assessed in the mid-oesophageal long-axis view or with 3D imaging using MPR.

Normal appearances following mitral repair

It is useful to recognize the normal appearances of the MV following repair (Figures 9.8 and 9.9; see Online appendix 9.1.4). The annuloplasty ring is usually easily identified, particularly posteriorly. Annuloplasty rings may be flexible or rigid, and complete or incomplete (see Online appendices 9.1.4.5– 9.1.4.10). Incomplete rings are deficient anteriorly in the region of the intervalvular fibrosa. However, even complete rings are more easily visualized posteriorly where the annulus is thinner. With posterior leaflet resection, echo dropout from the annuloplasty ring creates difficulties in visualizing the residual posterior leaflet, making the valve appear unicuspid (Figures 9.2, 9.8a, and 9.9a; see Online appendix 9.1.4.1). There is generally a small coaptation surface (<0.5 cm) and the plane of coaptation is at, or just below, the annular plane. The surface of coaptation is more normal when posterior leaflet sliding plasty is performed (Figure 9.2).

Similar to sliding plasty, repair with neochordae tends to produce a more normal-looking valve (compare panels (A) and (B) in Figure 9.9; see Online appendix 9.1.4.3). However, subtle differences exist, depending on the leaflet pathology and neochord technique. For posterior leaflet repairs where there is significant leaflet redundancy, it is usual to displace the leaflet into the LV by using shortened neochordae (Figure 9.8b). The coaptation point is displaced posteriorly, away from the LVOT, and the plane of coaptation lies below the annular plane. There is usually a large coaptation surface (>1.0 cm). For posterior chordal replacement where there is minimal excess leaflet tissue (Figure 9.8c), the plane of coaptation is typically at, or just below, the annular plane and the coaptation point is generally more anterior than when the posterior leaflet has been displaced into the ventricle. A similar appearance is seen when chordal replacement is used for anterior leaflet prolapse/flail (Figure 9.8d). In both circumstances, coaptation >0.8 cm is ideal. Neochordae are more echogenic than normal chordae—a feature that is best appreciated when the ultrasound beam is perpendicular to the chordae, in the transgastric two-chamber view.

When patch augmentation of a leaflet has been performed (e.g. for rheumatic MR, endocarditis, or severe secondary MR), the patch may appear hypermobile and sometimes billow above the annular plane. Although not ideal, if there is no MR and satisfactory coaptation (>0.8 cm), the repair can be considered acceptable.

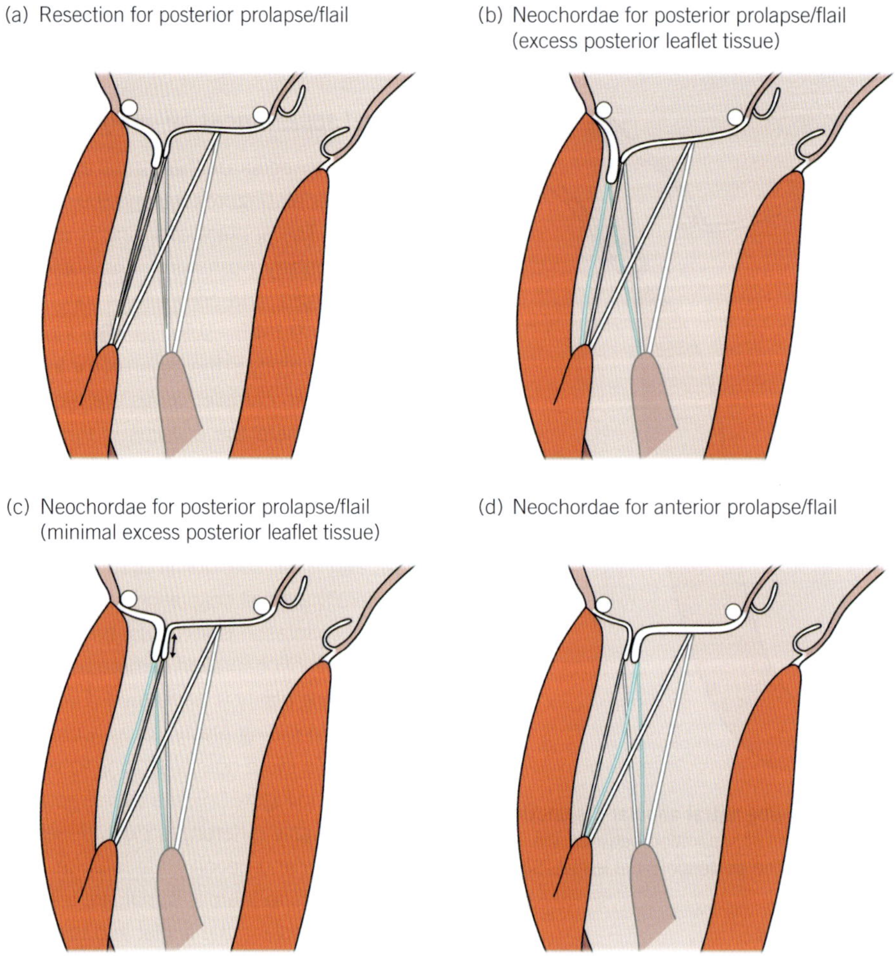

Figure 9.8 Schematic showing the normal appearances following different types of mitral repair. (a) Resection for posterior prolapse/flail; (b) neochordae for posterior prolapse/flail (excess posterior leaflet tissue); (c) neochordae for posterior prolapse/flail (minimal excess posterior leaflet tissue); (d) neochordae for anterior prolapse/flail. Neochords are represented in green.

Residual regurgitation

Residual regurgitation should be assessed once the heart has been fully de-aired, ventricular function recovered from the effects of CPB, and appropriate inotropic and fluid therapy administered. The haemodynamic state should try to match the 'awake' state.

The presence of residual regurgitation that is more than mild is an indication to revise the repair or replace the valve, as this finding is associated with an increased need for future reoperation.[27,28] However, there are little data to guide decision-making when residual regurgitation is mild. In general, the goal of MV repair surgery should be to achieve nil or trivial residual regurgitation, and the treatment decision for mild regurgitation must take into account the overall clinical picture. Factors to consider when deciding whether to reoperate are the likelihood of improving the repair, the risks of a second CPB run, and the risks associated with late reoperation.

Severity should be quantified by measuring the vena contracta (VC) width or the VC area. VC area is measured with 3D imaging using MPR, and it has the added advantage of demonstrating the anatomical location of the leak (Figure 9.10). The flow convergence method is not appropriate for assessing milder degrees of MR, as the flow convergence zone is too small to measure accurately. Unfortunately, distinguishing mild from more severe regurgitation can be difficult. The width of the VC can vary, depending on the imaging plane, haemodynamic state, and systolic frame chosen for analysis, straddling the cut-off (0.3 cm) for mild regurgitation. It is important to obtain a true long-axis view (see Chapter 8) and to turn the probe left and right to scan along the entire coaptation line. The narrowest part of the widest jet should be used

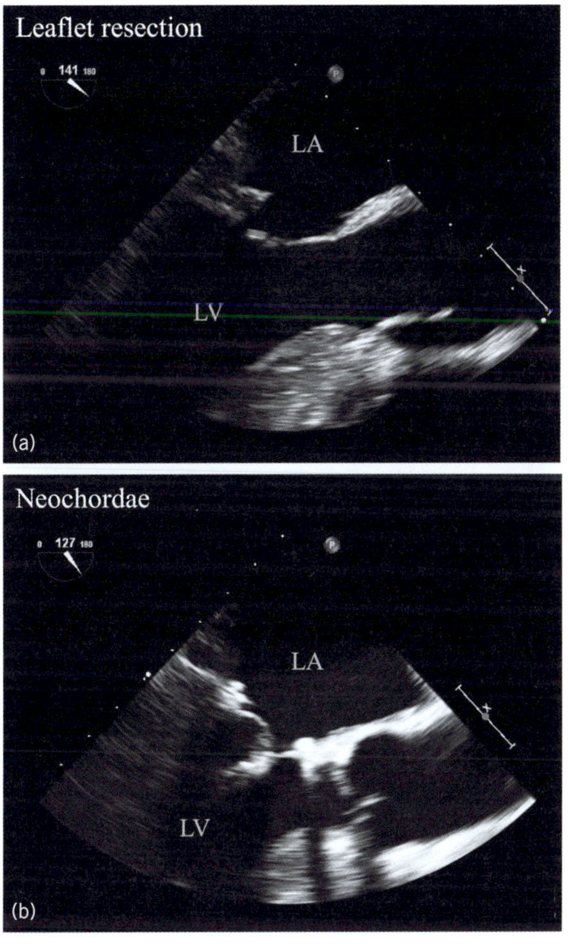

Figure 9.9 Normal 2D long-axis appearances following leaflet resection and neochordal replacement for P2 flail. Frames (a) and (b) were obtained from the mid-oesophageal long-axis view in late systole. (a) With leaflet resection, the posterior leaflet is not seen, giving the appearance of a unicuspid valve. The annuloplasty ring is also not well visualized but is responsible for the bulky echo-density in the region of the posterior leaflet. Poor visualization of the posterior leaflet is partly due to echo dropout from the annuloplasty ring and partly due to the reduced leaflet length following resection. (b) With neochordae, both leaflets and the annuloplasty ring are clearly seen, and there is significant leaflet overlap (coaptation). See Online appendix 9.1.4.

for measurement. It is common to see brief jets that are present for only one or two frames in early systole. Such jets usually diminish over time and can be ignored. In difficult cases, it is important to wait for up to 30 minutes following separation from CPB before making a final decision, as residual regurgitation may significantly improve with recovery of ventricular function.

If unacceptable residual regurgitation is present, it is important to identify the *mechanism* (Figure 9.11). Causes of residual regurgitation are persistent prolapse, inadequate coaptation, excessive leaflet tension causing separation of the posterior scallops, persistent tethering (secondary regurgitation), leaflet tethering due to excessively short neochordae, SAM, uncorrected clefts, and leaflet perforation from the annuloplasty ring. Uncorrected clefts and separation of the posterior scallops may be identified with colour 3D imaging. Jets due to perforation from the annuloplasty ring should be repaired, even if trivial.

In addition to the mechanism, it is important to identify the *anatomical location* of the residual regurgitation. 3D imaging with colour Doppler is extremely useful in this regard (see video case study in Online appendix 6.6.4). A closely cropped, magnified 3D data set displayed from the atrial aspect can direct the surgeon to the area of concern (Figure 9.11).

Mitral stenosis

New MS is rare following MV repair but can occur with the use of small annuloplasty rings and when there has been extensive commissural plication. Evaluation of post-repair stenosis is complicated by the fact that diastolic pressure gradients are typically elevated in the early period following separation from CPB due to a hyperdynamic circulation, tachycardia, and reduced LV compliance. Mean diastolic gradients of up to 5 mmHg are common in the early post-repair period. While data are limited, in one study of 557 patients undergoing MV repair, a mean diastolic pressure gradient of ≥7 mmHg and a peak gradient of ≥17 mmHg reliably identified the need for reoperation.[29]

Systolic anterior motion

SAM is a particular risk factor for patients with Barlow disease but is very uncommon in patients with FED. SAM is best appreciated in the mid-oesophageal long-axis view. With 2D imaging, the anterior mitral leaflet bends into the LVOT in systole and a mitral coaptation defect may be visible. 3D imaging in MPR mode is also useful to characterize SAM (Figure 9.12). With colour Doppler imaging, there is marked turbulence in the LVOT and (usually) a posteriorly directed jet of MR. With CW Doppler imaging in the deep transgastric or transgastric long-axis views, a high-velocity waveform may be identified across the LVOT/AV. Peak velocity is typically maximal in *late systole*, imparting a 'dagger' shape to the waveform. Velocities of up to 6 m/s may be seen.

Mild SAM, as evidenced by a peak LVOT velocity of <2 m/s and mild MR, can be safely ignored. More severe forms of SAM should be treated with fluid loading,

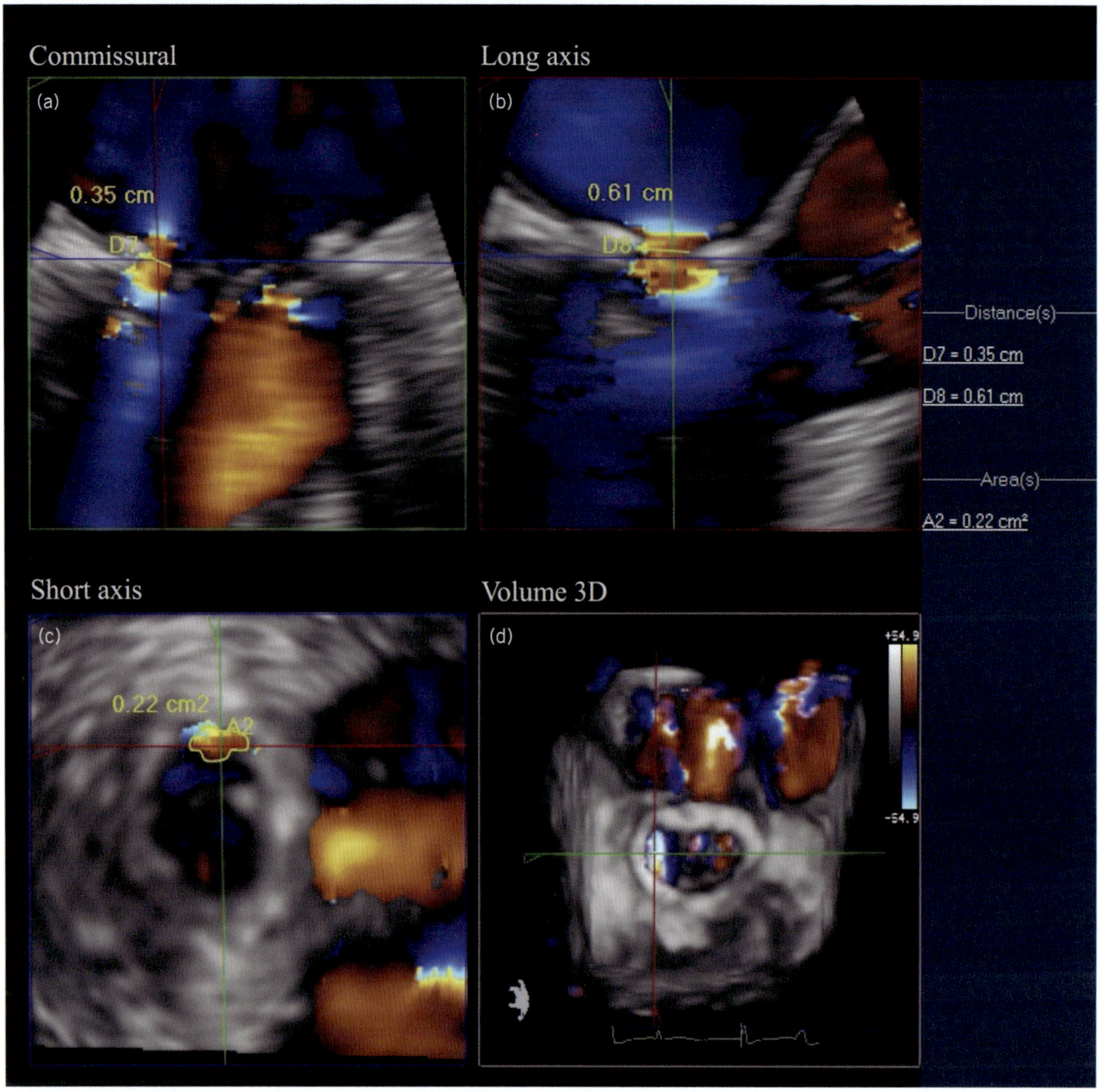

Figure 9.10 Localization and quantification of residual mitral regurgitation using colour 3D imaging in multi-planar reconstruction mode. Vena contracta (VC) width should be measured perpendicular to the surface of coaptation in the mid-oesophageal long-axis view (0.61 cm^2, (b). VC area is measured in the short-axis view (0.22 cm^2, (c). Measuring the jet width in the commissural view (0.35 cm^2, (a) helps to confirm that VC area and width are concordant (0.35×0.61=0.21). The area measurement is consistent with mild-to-moderate regurgitation, whereas the width measurement is consistent with moderate regurgitation (see Chapter 8). (d) In the volume-rendered 3D view, the data set has been orientated and cropped onto the valve to display the origin of the jet from the atrial aspect in the surgical orientation. The site of residual regurgitation is A1/P1. The position of the long-axis and commissural planes has been adjusted to obtain the largest VC area. While the commissural plane (green line) passes through the centre of the valve, the long-axis plane (red line) passes through A1/P1 (note the positions of the red and green lines in panel (d) and compare with Figure 8.24). Adjusting the long-axis and commissural planes to obtain the largest VC area is the 3D equivalent of turning the probe left and right with standard 2D imaging to obtain the largest VC width. See also Online appendix 6.6.4.

vasoconstrictors, and cessation of inotropic support. Medical therapy is usually effective, and only rarely is surgical revision necessary.[30] Indications for surgical revision are an LVOT velocity >3.5 m/s and MR that is more than mild despite optimal medical management.[31]

Ventricular dysfunction

Ventricular dysfunction is common following MV repair. Correction of mitral regurgitation increases LV afterload, which may unmask or exacerbate pre-existing LV systolic

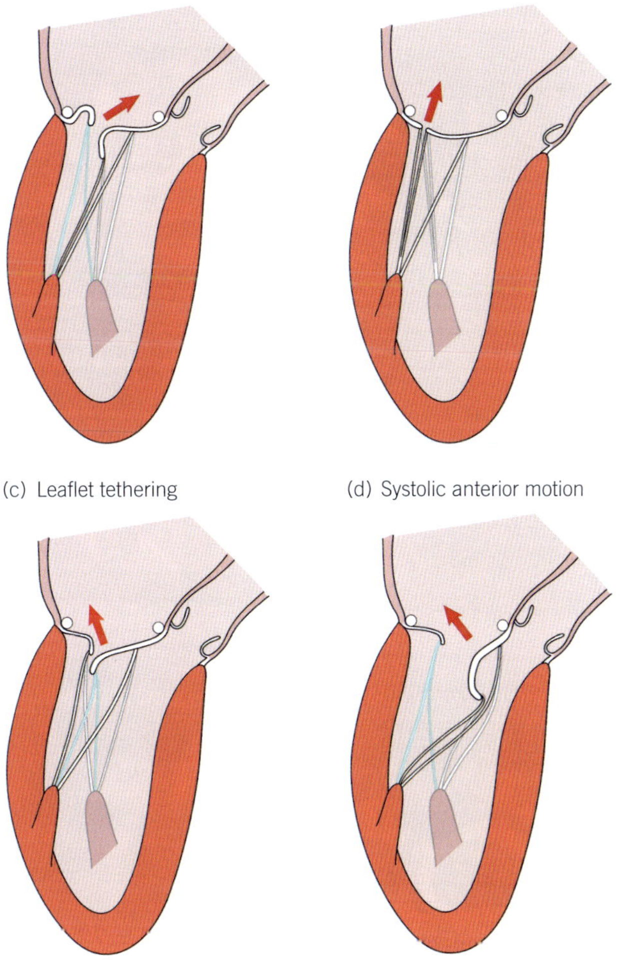

Figure 9.11 Mechanisms of residual mitral regurgitation. (a) Residual prolapse due to overly long neochordae. Note that with the leaflet resection technique, residual prolapse can also arise due to inadequate resection (not shown). (b) Inadequate coaptation following leaflet resection. This situation suggests either that leaflet resection has been excessive or that the annuloplasty ring is too large. Revision using a smaller annuloplasty ring may correct the problem. (c) Leaflet tethering due to overly short neochordae. (d) Systolic anterior motion.

dysfunction. Injury to the circumflex coronary artery (see Figure 8.1) is a rare cause of LV dysfunction but should be kept in mind, especially if a new RWMA is noted, with or without accompanying ST segment changes. RV dysfunction can arise from poor myocardial protection, gas embolus down the anteriorly positioned right coronary artery, and exacerbation of pre-existing pulmonary hypertension.

Other complications

Very occasionally, MV repair is associated with posterior atrioventricular rupture or LA dissection (see Online appendix 9.2.6).

Multiple choice questions

Discover interactive multiple choice questions to test your knowledge on this chapter by searching for this book's title or ISBN (9780198873686) at **https://academic.oup.com/** and going to the online appendix at the end of the book. Use your scratch-off code on the inside cover to access the material.

References

1. Sidebotham DA, Allen SJ, Gerber IL, Fayers T. Intraoperative transesophageal echocardiography for surgical repair of mitral regurgitation. *J Am Soc Echocardiogr.* 2014;**27**:345–66.

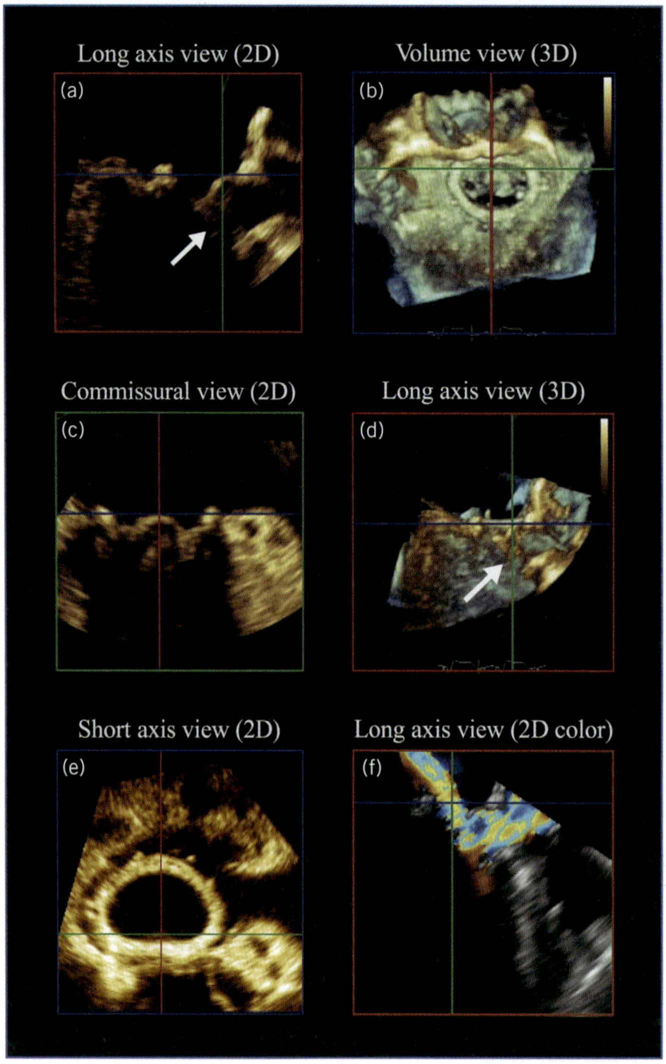

Figure 9.12 Systolic anterior motion (SAM) following MV repair. The images have been obtained from a 3D data set using multi-planar reconstruction (MPR). The left column contains the three orthogonal 2D images required for axial MPR: the long-axis view (a), commissural view (c), and short-axis view (e). (b) shows a 3D view of the mitral valve from the atrial perspective in the surgical orientation. The annuloplasty ring is clearly visible. Parallax has been eliminated, so the long axis (red line) and commissural (green line) views are perpendicular to the plane of the volume view image and traverse the mitral valve as shown. SAM is typically identified in the long-axis view and is clearly identified in the 2D, 3D, and colour Doppler long-axis views (a, d, f, respectively). The arrows indicate the anterior mitral leaflet bending into the LVOT. LVOT turbulence and a posterior jet of mitral regurgitation can be seen with colour Doppler imaging. (c) is a 2D commissural view close to the LVOT. SAM is not obvious in most commissural views, but has a very unique and characteristic appearance when the 2D commissural plane traverses both the anterior portion of the MV and the LVOT, as shown by the green line in the (a, d, f) long-axis, (e) short-axis, and (b) volume views. (e) is the short-axis view in the plane of the prosthetic annulus.

2. Otto CM, Nishimura RA, Bonow RO, *et al.* 2020 ACC/AHA guideline for the management of patients with valvular heart disease: executive summary: a report of the American College of Cardiology/American Heart Association joint committee on clinical practice guidelines. *J Am Coll Cardiol.* 2021;**77**:450–500.
3. Vahanian A, Beyersdorf F, Praz F, *et al.* 2021 ESC/EACTS Guidelines for the management of valvular heart disease. *Eur J Cardiothorac Surg.* 2021;**60**:727–800.
4. Acker MA, Parides MK, Perrault LP, *et al.* Mitral-valve repair versus replacement for severe ischemic mitral regurgitation. *N Engl J Med.* 2014;**370**:23–32.
5. Smith PK, Puskas JD, Ascheim DD, *et al.* Surgical treatment of moderate ischemic mitral regurgitation. *N Engl J Med.* 2014;**371**:2178–88.
6. Wrobel K, Stevens SR, Jones RH, *et al.* Influence of baseline characteristics, operative conduct, and postoperative course on 30-day outcomes of coronary artery bypass grafting

among patients with left ventricular dysfunction: results from the surgical treatment for ischemic heart failure (STICH) trial. *Circulation*. 2015;**132**:720–30.
7. Drake DH, Zimmerman KG, Hepner AM, Nichols CD. Echo-guided mitral repair. *Circ Cardiovasc Imaging*. 2014;**7**:132–41.
8. Drake DH, Zimmerman KG, Sidebotham DA. Transesophageal echocardiography for surgical repair of mitral regurgitation. In: Otto C, editor. *Practice of Clinical Echocardiography*, 6th edition. Philadelphia, PA: Elsevier; 2022, pp. 541–66.
9. Stone GW, Lindenfeld J, Abraham WT, *et al*. Transcatheter mitral-valve repair in patients with heart failure. *N Engl J Med*. 2018;**379**:2307–18.
10. Braunberger E, Deloche A, Berrebi A, *et al*. Very long-term results (more than 20 years) of valve repair with carpentier's techniques in nonrheumatic mitral valve insufficiency. *Circulation*. 2001;**104**:I8–11.
11. David TE, Armstrong S, McCrindle BW, Manlhiot C. Late outcomes of mitral valve repair for mitral regurgitation due to degenerative disease. *Circulation*. 2013;**127**:1485–92.
12. Seeburger J, Falk V, Borger MA, *et al*. Chordae replacement versus resection for repair of isolated posterior mitral leaflet prolapse: à égalité. *Ann Thorac Surg*. 2009;**87**:1715–20.
13. David TE, Ivanov J, Armstrong S, Christie D, Rakowski H. A comparison of outcomes of mitral valve repair for degenerative disease with posterior, anterior, and bileaflet prolapse. *J Thorac Cardiovasc Surg*. 2005;**130**:1242–9.
14. Castillo JG, Anyanwu AC, Fuster V, Adams DH. A near 100% repair rate for mitral valve prolapse is achievable in a reference center: implications for future guidelines. *J Thorac Cardiovasc Surg*. 2012;**144**:308–12.
15. Johnston DR, Gillinov AM, Blackstone EH, *et al*. Surgical repair of posterior mitral valve prolapse: implications for guidelines and percutaneous repair. *Ann Thorac Surg*. 2010;**89**:1385–94.
16. Kahn RA, Mittnacht AJ, Anyanwu AC. Systolic anterior motion as a result of relative 'undersizing' of a mitral valve annulus in a patient with Barlow's disease. *Anesth Analg*. 2009;**108**:1102–4.
17. Hymel BJ, Townsley MM. Echocardiographic assessment of systolic anterior motion of the mitral valve. *Anesth Analg*. 2014;**118**:1197–201.
18. Badhwar V, Peterson ED, Jacobs JP, *et al*. Longitudinal outcome of isolated mitral repair in older patients: results from 14,604 procedures performed from 1991 to 2007. *Ann Thorac Surg*. 2012;**94**:1870–7; discussion 1877–9.
19. Drake DH, Zhang P, Zimmerman KG, Morrow CD, Sidebotham DA. Anatomic, stage-based repair of secondary mitral valve disease, *J Thorac Cardiovasc Surg*. 2024;**167**:1733–44.
20. Magne J, Senechal M, Dumesnil JG, Pibarot P. Ischemic mitral regurgitation: a complex multifaceted disease. *Cardiology*. 2009;**112**:244–59.
21. Shimokawa T, Kasegawa H, Matsuyama S, *et al*. Long-term outcome of mitral valve repair for infective endocarditis. *Ann Thorac Surg*. 2009;**88**:733–9.
22. Chauvaud S, Fuzellier JF, Berrebi A, Deloche A, Fabiani JN, Carpentier A. Long term (29 years) results of reconstructive surgery in rheumatic mitral valve insufficiency. *Circulation*. 2001;**104**:I12–15.
23. Almeida A, Tutungi E, Moten S, Chen Y. Minimally invasive and robotic approaches to mitral valve: robotic is best. *JTCVS Tech*. 2021;**10**:75–9.
24. Chitwood WR Jr. Robotic mitral valve repair: how I teach it. *Ann Thorac Surg*. 2019;**107**:1297–301.
25. Eriksson MJ, Bitkover CY, Omran AS, *et al*. Mitral annular disjunction in advanced myxomatous mitral valve disease: echocardiographic detection and surgical correction. *J Am Soc Echocardiogr*. 2005;**18**:1014–22.
26. Said SM, Schaff HV, Suri RM, Greason KL, Dearani JA, Nishimura RA. Bulging subaortic septum: an important risk factor for systolic anterior motion after mitral valve repair. *Ann Thorac Surg*. 2011;**91**:1427–32.
27. Meyer MA, von Segesser LK, Hurni M, Stumpe F, Eisa K, Ruchat P. Long-term outcome after mitral valve repair: a risk factor analysis. *Eur J Cardiothorac Surg*. 2007;**32**:301–7.
28. Suri RM, Schaff HV, Dearani JA, *et al*. Survival advantage and improved durability of mitral repair for leaflet prolapse subsets in the current era. *Ann Thorac Surg*. 2006;**82**:819–26.
29. Riegel AK, Busch R, Segal S, Fox JA, Eltzschig HK, Shernan SK. Evaluation of transmitral pressure gradients in the intraoperative echocardiographic diagnosis of mitral stenosis after mitral valve repair. *PLoS One*. 2011;**6**:e26559.
30. Kuperstein R, Spiegelstein D, Rotem G, *et al*. Late clinical outcome of transient intraoperative systolic anterior motion post mitral valve repair. *J Thorac Cardiovasc Surg*. 2015;149:471–6.
31. Varghese R, Anyanwu AC, Itagaki S, Milla F, Castillo J, Adams DH. Management of systolic anterior motion after mitral valve repair: an algorithm. *J Thorac Cardiovasc Surg*. 2012;**143**:S2–7.

10 The aortic valve and left ventricular outflow tract

Positioned in the centre of the heart and separated from the midoesophagus by the LA, the AV lends itself to excellent TOE imaging. While 2D and Doppler imaging remain the most important imaging techniques, 3D imaging provides additional information not otherwise available, most notably when measuring the aortic root and LVOT.

The focus of this chapter is on native AV disease. AV repair is discussed in Chapter 11, diseases of the aorta in Chapter 12, prosthetic AV valves in Chapter 13, and percutaneous AV replacement in Chapter 17.

Anatomy and nomenclature of the AV and LVOT

The AV is a complex three-dimensional structure nestled in the aortic root. It has many components (Figures 10.1 and 10.2).

The **aortic root** is the most proximal part of the aorta, bound by the **ventriculo-aortic junction** (VAJ) and **sinotubular junction** (STJ), and it contains the aortic leaflets, interleaflet triangles, leaflet attachments, and **sinuses of Valsalva** (SoVs).[1]

The normal AV has three **leaflets** (left, right, and non-coronary), inserted proximally into the VAJ and distally into the STJ, and forming a *crown-shaped* attachment. Behind each leaflet is the respective SoV, a dilatation of the aortic root that functions as a reservoir for coronary blood flow in diastole and ensures separation of the leaflet from the coronary ostium in systole. Each sinus is named according to the adjacent AV leaflet (left, right, or non-coronary). The left and right SoVs give rise to the left and right coronary arteries, respectively. The non-coronary SoV, as its name implies, does not give rise to a coronary artery and is adjacent to the inter-atrial septum. Each leaflet joins the adjacent leaflets at a **commissure**, and in diastole, the free edge of each leaflet apposes to the two adjacent leaflets along a **coaptation line**. The central portion of the free edge of each leaflet has a localized thickening called the **nodule of Arantius**.

Note that the leaflets of the AV and pulmonic valves are often referred to as '**cusps**' (abbreviated LCC for left-coronary cusp, RCC for rightcoronary cusp, and NCC for non-coronary cusp), and the terms tend to be used interchangeably. Both are used in this book.

Some authors differentiate between the VAJ and the basal ring. The **basal ring** represents the basal attachment of the leaflets in the LV. It is not an anatomic structure, but a virtual plane connecting the nadirs of the cusp's insertion line; hence, it is sometimes called the *virtual* basal ring. By contrast, the VAJ is the true anatomic junction between the ventricular muscle and the aortic media, and it is *slightly above* the nadirs of the cusps. The distinction between the VAJ and the basal ring is important surgically, but in echocardiography, the term **aortic annulus** is often used as a surrogate to designate the VAJ or the basal ring. The entire crown-shaped structure, from the VAJ to the STJ, is sometimes referred to as the '**functional aortic annulus**', especially in the context of AV repair (see Chapter 11).[2]

The funnel-shaped region below the aortic annulus is termed the left ventricular outflow tract (LVOT). The walls of the LVOT comprise the intervalvular fibrosa/anterior mitral leaflet, the membranous ventricular septum, and the muscular ventricular septum (Figure 10.2). The left- and non-coronary leaflets are in continuity with the base of the anterior leaflet of the MV and the intervalvular fibrosa (see Figures 8.1 and 8.3).

The aortic root is at the centre of the heart, surrounded by several structures (Figure 10.2). Knowledge of the relationship between the aortic root and adjacent structures is important when evaluating root abscesses and fistulae, VSDs (see Chapter 18), and SoV aneurysms.

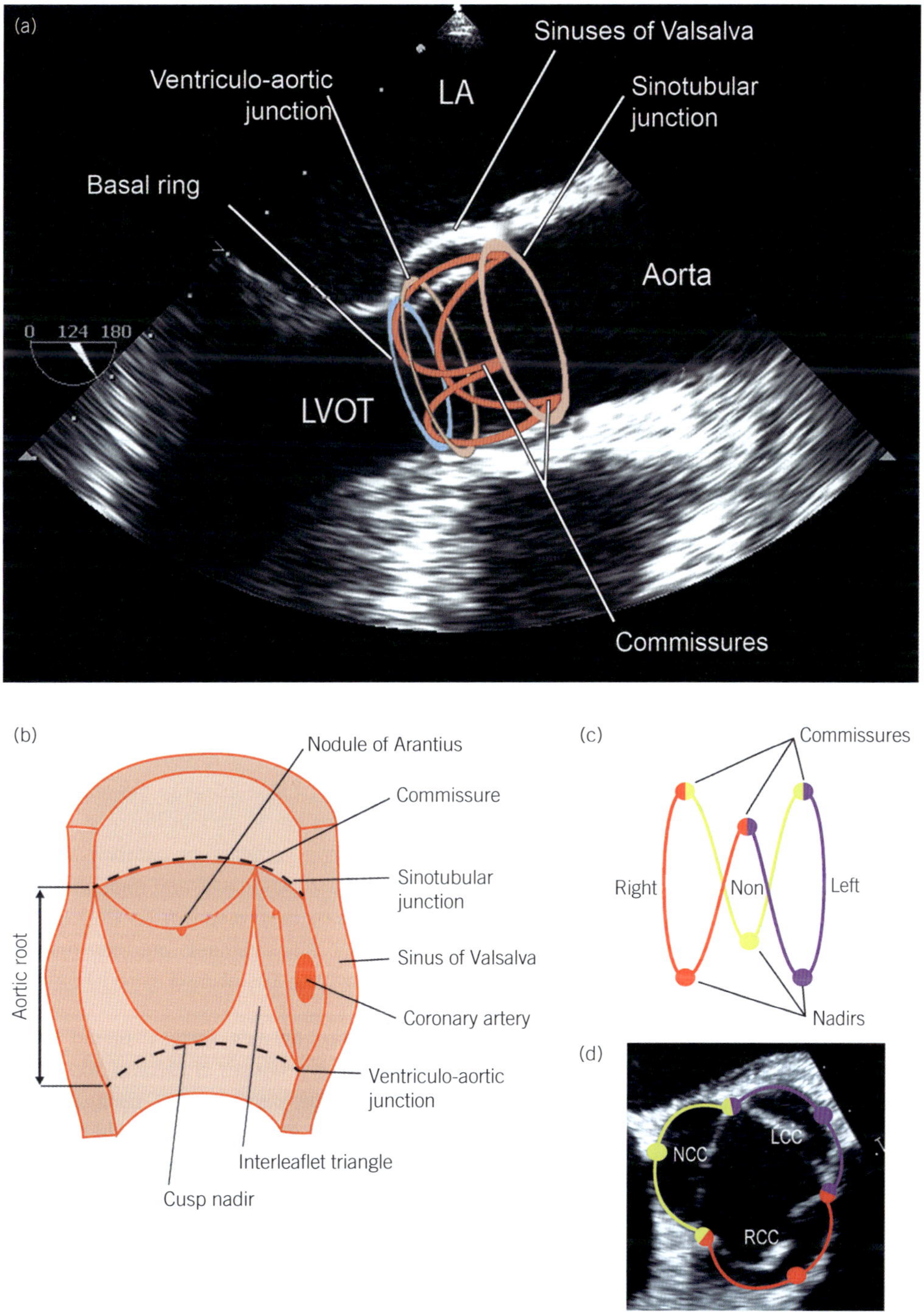

Figure 10.1 Anatomy of the aortic valve. (a) is a schematic view of the AV nestled in the aortic root, with its crown-shaped attachments to both at the ventriculo-aortic junction (VAJ) and at the sinotubular junction (STJ). (b) and (c) show the various components of the AV. The cusp nadirs are just below the actual VAJ (see text for details). Note the commissures between the three leaflets at the level of the STJ. (d) Note also that the crown-shaped attachment creates three interleaflet triangles, which project above the basal ring echocardiographically, but they are part of the LVOT.

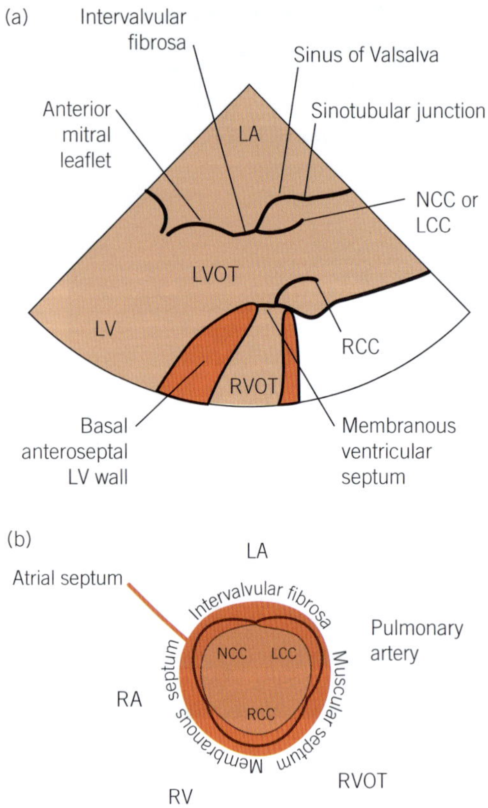

Figure 10.2 Anatomy of LV outflow and adjacent structures. (a) is a schematic representation of the mid-oesophageal AV long-axis view demonstrating the components of the aortic root and their relationship to surrounding structures. (b) is in the same orientation as in the mid-oesophageal AV short-axis view. The relationship of the aortic cusps to surrounding structures is shown. NCC, non-coronary cusp; LCC, left coronary cusp; RCC, right coronary cusp.

Echocardiographic examination

Four standard views are used for assessing the LVOT and aortic root: the mid-oesophageal AV short- and long-axis views; the deep transgastric five-chamber view; and the transgastric long-axis view (see Figures 4.4 and 4.6 and Online appendix 1.6).

The mid-oesophageal AV short-axis view is useful for defining the anatomical location of leaflet pathology. Off-axis imaging produces asymmetrical leaflets and can give the false impression of a coaptation defect or leaflet perforation. Slightly withdrawing or advancing the probe, or adjusting the angle of rotation might help with full visualization at the leaflet tips of the AV. Once the view is obtained at the tip of the leaflets, withdrawing the probe slightly will demonstrate the origin of the coronary arteries. The left coronary artery (Figure 10.3) is easier to visualize than the right in this view. The right coronary artery is better seen in the mid-oesophageal AV long-axis view (colour Doppler will facilitate the identification of both coronary arteries).

The mid-oesophageal AV long-axis view, with and without colour Doppler, is used to assess the mechanism and severity of AR, and to measure the dimensions of the aortic annulus and aortic root (see discussion that follows, and Figures 10.2 and 10.4). Simultaneous biplane imaging may also help to accurately localize the origin of a regurgitant jet with colour Doppler.

Measurement of the aortic annulus

Accurate measurement of the aortic annulus and root is an important part of the TOE examination, and one must ensure that the imaging plane passes through the *exact centre* of the root, so that the measurements reflect the true diameter. This can be achieved with 2D imaging but is greatly facilitated by using 3D biplane imaging or a reconstructed 3D dataset.

Using 2D imaging, the probe is gently turned left and right in the AV long-axis view to ensure that the maximum diameter is visualized. Note that being off-axis will result in underestimation of the maximum annular diameter (see Figure 12.2).

Using 3D biplane imaging, the cursor is adjusted on the short-axis plane, so that the measuring plane passes*through the commissure between the left and non-coronary cusp posteriorly, and through the centre of the right coronary cusp anteriorly* (in the case of a trileaflet valve).[3] The measurements are then made on the corresponding long-axis plane (Figure 10.5).

> ***Expert tip: Off-axis images should be suspected whenever two sinuses of Valsalva and two leaflets are visible in the long-axis view, because when properly centred, the long-axis view should pass between the LCC and NCC, so the posterior part of the aortic root should be relatively flat and no posterior leaflet (NCC or LCC) should be seen (*Figure 10.5*).***

The LVOT and aortic annulus should be measured in *mid-systole* at the hinge points where the leaflets insert into the annulus. All other measurements of the aortic root should be made at *end-diastole* (Figure 10.6; see Online appendix 7.3.13). The LVOT and aortic annulus should be measured by using the inner edge-to-inner edge convention, and the aortic root and aorta should be measured by using the leading edge-to-leading edge convention.[3] In valve-sparing aortic root procedures, 3D measurements must be made for each SoV separately (see Chapter 11).

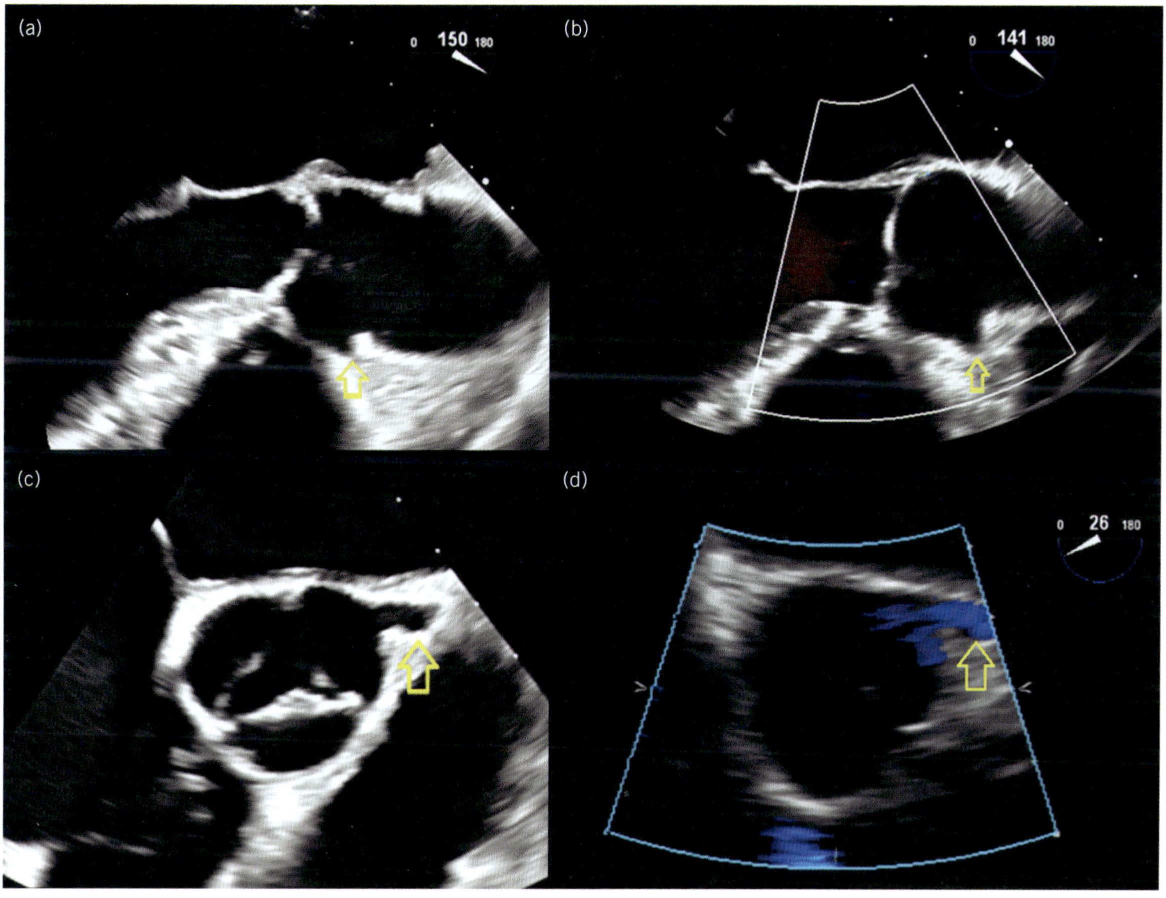

Figure 10.3 Imaging the coronary arteries. (a) and (b) are the mid-oesophageal long-axis views, and (c) and (d) are the mid-oesophageal short-axis views, with slight withdrawal of the probe above the leaflet tips. (a) and (c) are in 2D, and (b) and (d) are with colour Doppler. In (a) and (b), the arrows demonstrate the right coronary artery. In (c) and (d), the arrows demonstrate the left main coronary artery. See also Online appendix 1.6.2.

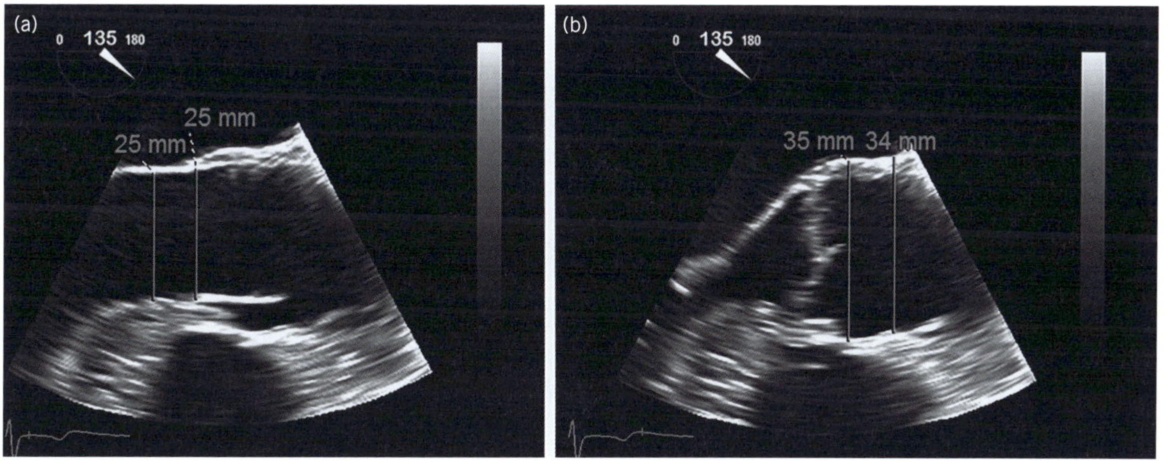

Figure 10.4 Aortic annulus and aortic root measurements with 2D imaging. In this mid-oesophageal AV long-axis view, (a) is frozen in systole and demonstrates the correct position to measure the LVOT and aortic annulus. (b) is frozen in diastole and demonstrates the measurement of the sinuses of Valsalva and the sinotubular junction. See also Online appendix 7.3.13.

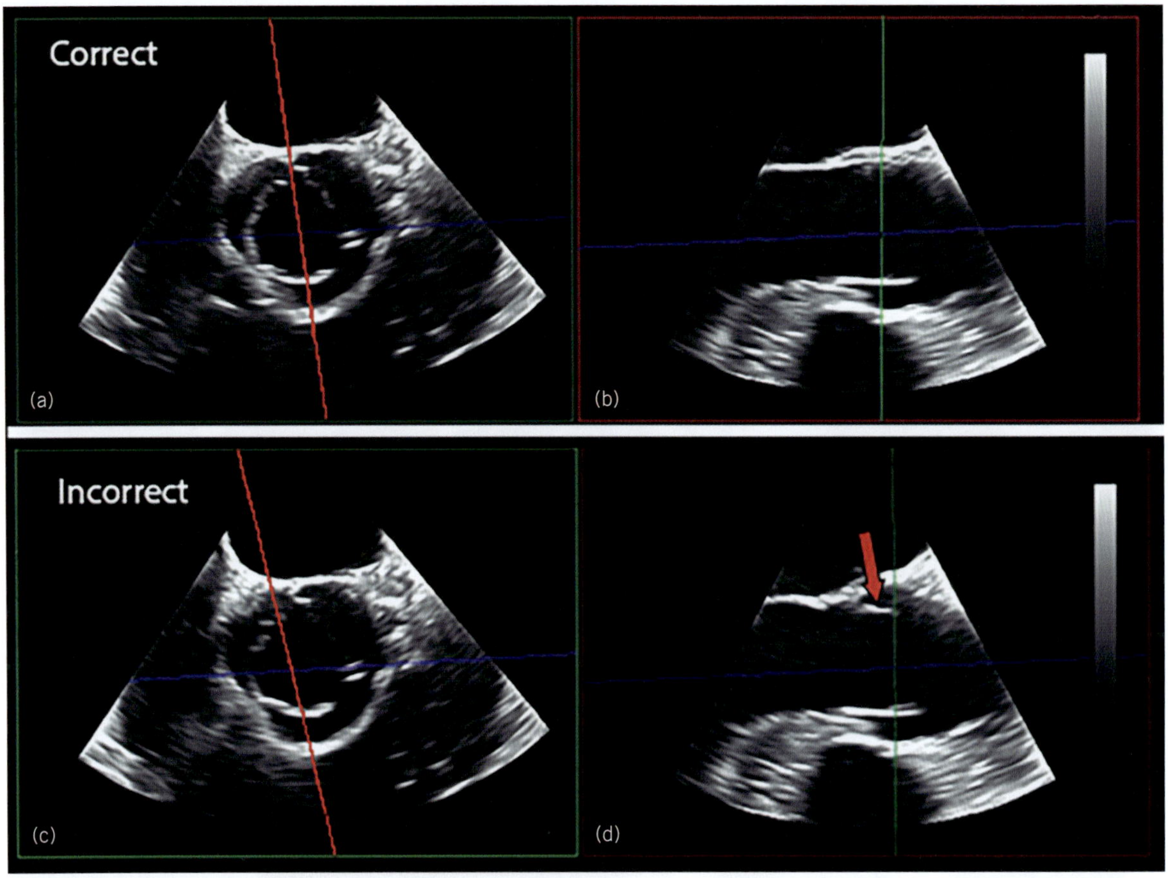

Figure 10.5 Measuring the aortic annulus. Whether one uses 3D biplane imaging or a full 3D data set, it is important to measure the correct plane. This composite image displays (a, c) short-axis views of the AV, and (b, d) the corresponding long-axis image in biplane mode. The image is frozen in mid systole, and the imaging plane (red line) is adjusted in short axis to produce a long-axis image. (a) and (b) demonstrate the CORRECT plane where the red line passes through the commissure between the LCC and NCC posteriorly, and through the centre of the RCC anteriorly. Note that in the corresponding long-axis image, no SoV and no leaflet are visible posteriorly, because the plane passes between the LCC and the NCC. (c) and (d) show the INCORRECT alignment where the plane passes through the NCC and the non-coronary SoV, resulting in a leaflet and the SoV being visible posteriorly (arrow).

An alternate way to measure the annulus using a standard 3D dataset is shown in Figure 10.7. This approach is more time-consuming, but it yields the most accurate results.

It is important to remember that the aortic annulus is *elliptical*, not circular, being smaller in the anteroposterior diameter than in the medial–lateral dimension, and measurements of the annulus obtained with 3D imaging yield larger values than those obtained with 2D imaging.[4] The difference between the major and minor axes can be as much as 6 mm.[3] To reconcile this difference, especially in cases where the aortic annular measurement is critical (e.g. Ross procedure), some experts recommend using the *mean* annular diameter in systole. This can be calculated from the surface area of the aortic annulus, measured on a 3D dataset by using the technique described in Figure 10.7. Then one usesEquation 10.1:

$$\text{Mean diameter} = \sqrt{\left(\frac{\text{area}}{\text{p}}\right)} \times 2 \qquad \text{Equation 10.1}$$

Using Figure 10.7 as an example, where the elliptical annulus has a short axis of 2.46 cm, a long axis of 2.71 cm, and a surface area of 5.01 cm^2:

$$\text{Mean diameter} = \sqrt{(5.01/\pi)} \times 2 = 2.5\,\text{cm}$$

Normal values for aortic root dimensions obtained from 2D TTE are shown in Table 12.1.

Transgastric views allow the AV to be displayed from the ventricular aspect, which is useful when acoustic shadowing and reverberations (e.g. from calcification or a prosthetic valve) prevent visualization of the valve or LVOT in the mid-oesophageal views. Transgastric views are also the only views from which a spectral Doppler signal can

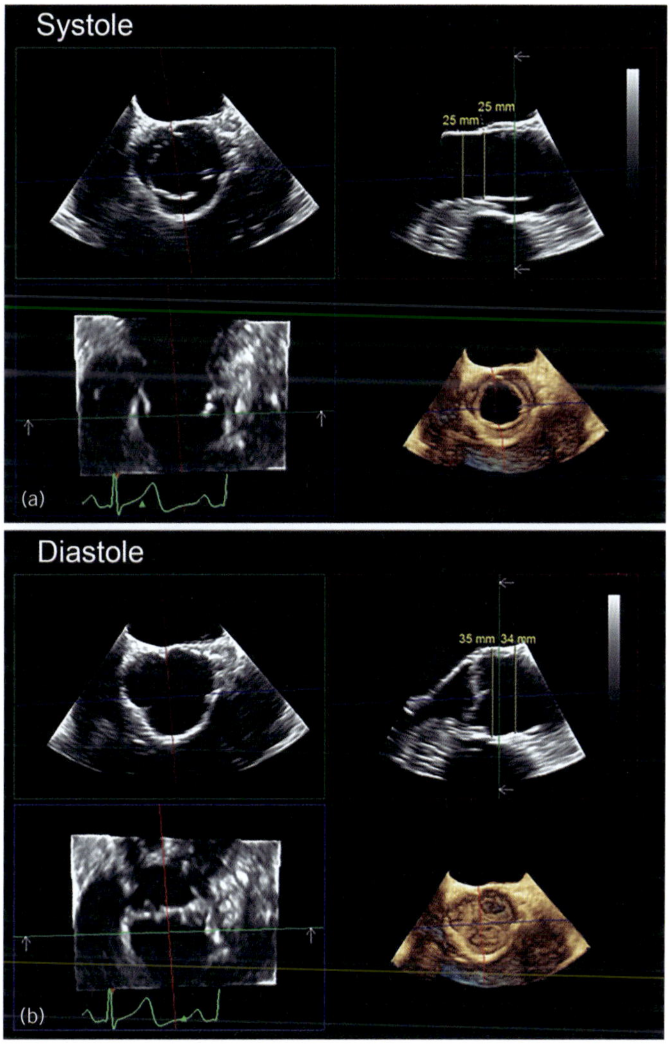

Figure 10.6 Measuring the annular diameter using a standard 3D data set. Using multi-planar reconstruction, the orthogonal planes are aligned with the centre of the aortic root, making sure that the red plane passes through the LCC/NCC commissure and through the centre of the RCC (see Figure 10.5). The LVOT and aortic annulus should be measured in systole (data set in panel (a)), while the SoV and STJ should be measured in diastole (data set in panel (b)).

be adequately aligned with blood flow across the LVOT/AV when assessing valve gradients and areas. Unfortunately, transgastric views may be difficult to obtain in some patients, and even if a view is obtained, precise alignment with the Doppler signal is not always possible.

3D imaging includes narrow sector ('live') and focused wide sector ('zoom') modes (see example in Online appendix 1.6.6). Because the AV leaflets are relatively thin, echo dropout may give a false impression of defects in the leaflets. The AV can be viewed in shortaxis (*en face*) or longaxis (from the side). The main advantage of 3D imaging over 2D imaging is in measuring aortic root and LVOT dimensions, and in the evaluation of anatomical or congenital defects.

Congenital abnormalities of the AV

Congenital abnormalities of the AV include unicuspid, bicuspid, and quadricuspid valves (Figure 10.8; see Online appendix 7.1). Bicuspid AV (BAV) is the most common form, occurring in 0.5–2% of the population, with a male-to-female ratio of 3:1.[5] The most common form of BAV involves fusion of the left and right leaflets. Fusion of the right and non-coronary cusps is less common, and rarely the left and non-coronary cusps are fused. A **raphe**, or fibrous ridge, is usually present between fused leaflets. Occasionally, the two leaflets are of equal size and no raphe is present. Sievers and colleagues classified bicuspid and unicuspid valve morphology based on

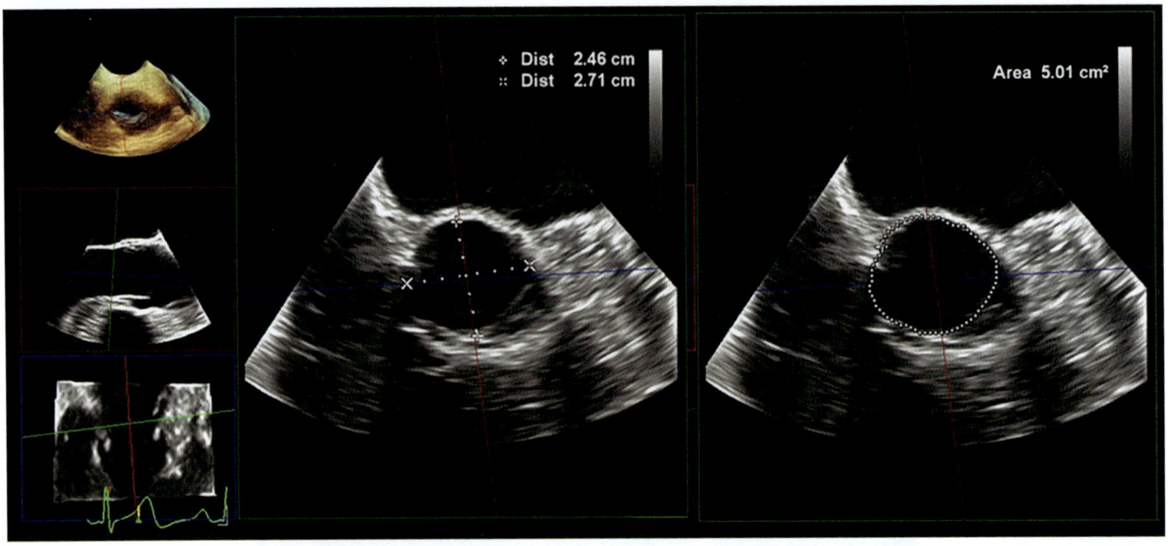

Figure 10.7 The aortic annulus is elliptical. In this 3D multi-planar reconstruction, the green box has been magnified to show the short-axis view of the annulus. After the long-axis planes (red and blue lines in this case) have been aligned with the centre of the AV, the short-axis plane (green cursor) is moved towards the LVOT until the AV leaflets are no longer visible. Note how the measurements of 2.46cm in the anteroposterior diameter and of 2.71cm in the medial–lateral diameter demonstrate that the annulus is not round. Once this view is acquired, the annulus can also be measured by planimetry and its surface area calculated, in (e). The LVOT diameter and surface area can be measured in the same manner, by moving the short-axis plane a further 0.5–1.0cm below the aortic annulus. When the LVOT is very short, the aortic annular diameter can be substituted for the LVOT measurement.

cusp fusion and the number of raphes (Figure 10.9).[6] This classification is simple and widely used, but other classifications of BAV exist in the literature, and to harmonize communication between clinicians and researchers, an international consensus was recently published, which offers a more detailed classification and associations of different forms of BAV with aortopathies and clinical states. A more detailed discussion of BAV morphology is beyond the scope of this chapter, but readers can refer to it if needed.[7] Ultimately, the use of common terminology facilitates communication between the echocardiographer and the surgeon.

Secondary calcification of the leaflets occurs in many cases of BAV, leading to the development of premature AS, AR, or mixed disease. Onset of clinically significant AV dysfunction usually occurs between the ages of 40 and 60 years. Patients with BAV are also at increased risk of endocarditis.

Finally, BAV is associated with pathology of the thoracic aorta, notably aneurysms of the aortic root and ascending aorta, coarctation, and, rarely, more complex forms of congenital heart disease. Specific cusp morphology may correlate with specific pathologic valvular complications and with various aortopathies.[7]

Bicuspid morphology can usually easily be confirmed with 2D (Figure 10.8) or 3D imaging (Figure 10.10). The characteristic echocardiographic sign is that of two usually unequal-sized (but sometimes equal) leaflets opening in systole, resulting in an elliptical, rather than a triangular-shaped, orifice. If a valve is calcified and stenosed, it may appear echocardiographically bicuspid, but one cannot tell if the fusion was congenital or acquired. Moreover, heavily calcified BAV may be impossible to distinguish from calcified unicuspid or trileaflet valves. When imaging the valve in longaxis, a doming appearance of one or both leaflets may be seen due to eccentric closure of the cusps. If BAV is identified, it is important to search for associated abnormalities of the aortic root and thoracic aorta.

Unicuspid or quadricuspid valves are much less common than bicuspid valves. Quadricuspid AVs frequently become regurgitant, and the diagnosis is usually made as an incidental finding in patients presenting for AV replacement in adulthood. Quadricuspid valves are associated with congenital anomalies of the coronary arteries.

Unicuspid valves typically present in childhood or early adulthood with either aortic stenosis or regurgitation. They may have one commissure only (*unicommissural*) or no commissure at all (*acommissural*), and two raphes may be seen. Unicuspid valves are also associated with aortopathies.

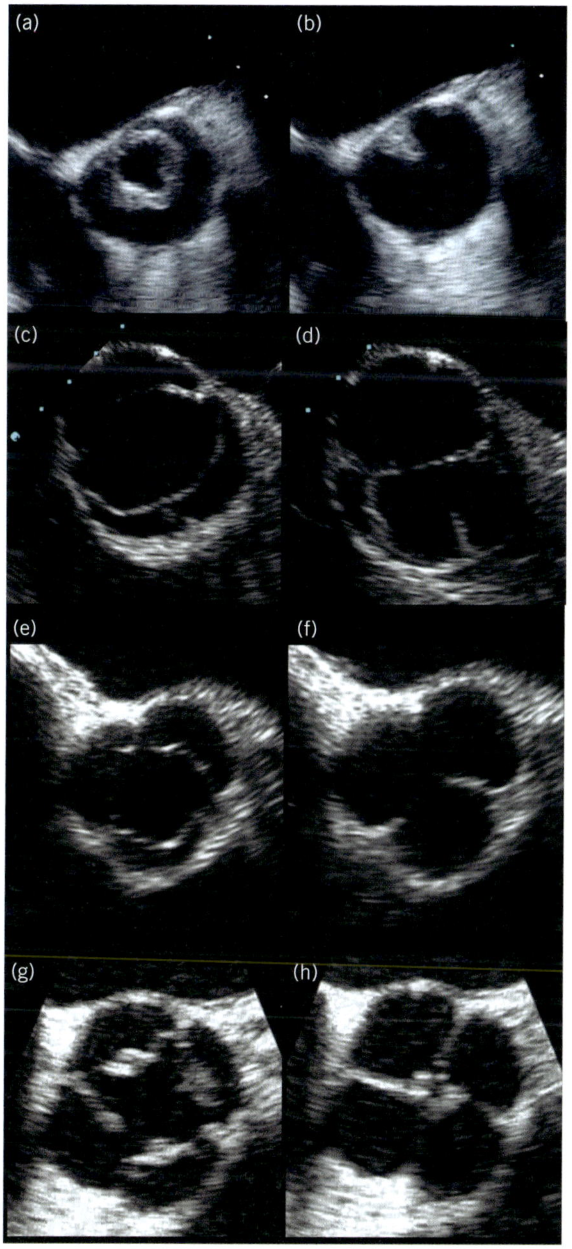

Figure 10.8 Congenital abnormalities of the AV. Three abnormalities (unicuspid, bicuspid, quadricuspid) are shown, with a normal tricuspid valve for comparison. Images (a), (c), (e), and (g) are in systole, and images (b), (d), (f), and (h) are in diastole. See also Online appendix 7.1.

Aortic stenosis

Aortic stenosis (AS) may occur as a consequence of calcific degeneration of a normal trileaflet valve, rheumatic AV disease, or calcific degeneration of a bicuspid (or unicuspid) valve (see Online appendix 7.2). Calcific degeneration of a trileaflet valve is the most common aetiology and tends to occur in patients over the age of 70 years, and it is often seen in patients with coronary artery disease. Some degree of AR is also common, but it is rarely severe. Rheumatic AS tends to occur in younger patients and is usually associated with MV disease; here, concomitant AR is common and may be severe.

Classification of aortic stenosis severity

In the 2020 American College of Cardiology (ACC)/American Heart Association (AHA) guidelines on the management of patients with valvular heart disease,[8] AS is classified into four stages:

- Stage A: at risk of AS
- Stage B: progressive AS
- Stage C: asymptomatic, severe AS
- Stage D: symptomatic, severe AS.

Stage A represents patients with AV disease (e.g. sclerosis, BAV) who are at risk of developing AS but who have not yet done so. **Stage B** represents patients with mild and moderate AS. Such patients are typically asymptomatic. **Stage C** is subdivided into C1 (asymptomatic, severe AS with *normal* LV systolic function) and C2 (asymptomatic, severe AS with *reduced* LV systolic function). **Stage D** includes all patients with *symptomatic*, severe AS and is subdivided into patients with high-gradient stenosis (D1), low-flow, low-gradient (LFLG) AS with reduced LVEF (D2), and low-gradient AS with normal LVEF (D3; so-called *paradoxical* low-flow severe AS). Stages D2 and D3 are discussed in more detail later. The echocardiographic findings associated with mild, moderate, and severe AS (including stages D2 and D3) are summarized in Table 10.1.

The best measures of severity are the peak transvalvular velocity, mean pressure gradient, and calculated valve area, with values >4 m/s, >40 mmHg, and $\leq 1\,cm^2$, respectively, defining severe stenosis. Calculation of the valve area is particularly useful if the transvalvular velocity and mean pressure gradient are lower than expected due to low LVEF or low stroke volume (SV) (see later). Indexing the AV area for patients with an unusually small or large body surface area has been suggested (cut-off of $0.6\,cm^2/m^2$ for severe AS), and this is especially important in children, adolescents, and very small adults.[9]

Indications for surgery

According to the same 2020 AHA/ACC guidelines,[8] AV replacement is *indicated* for patients with:

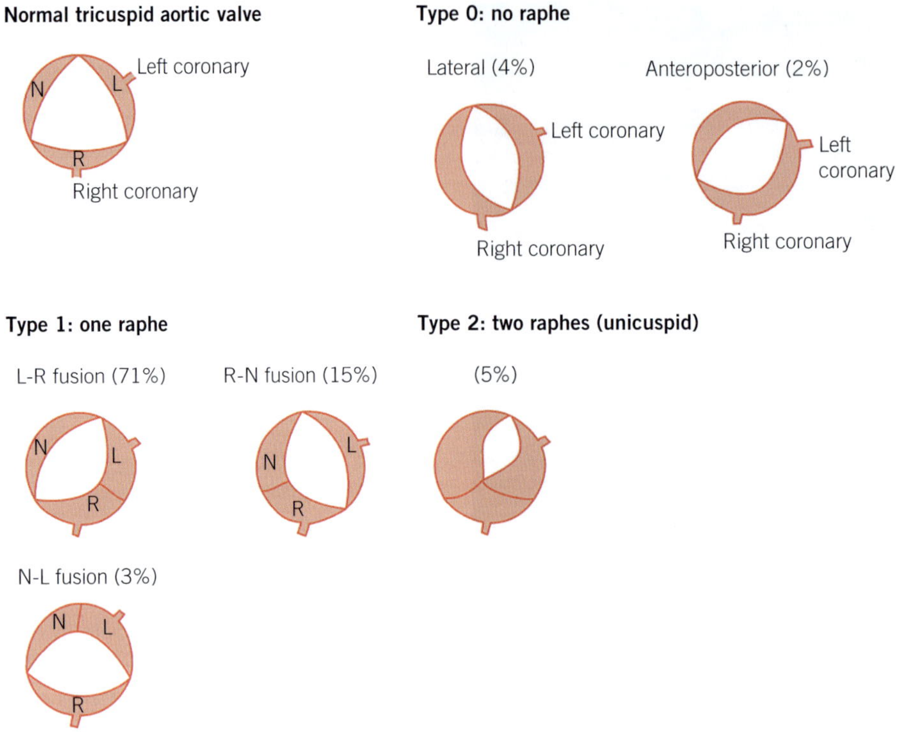

Figure 10.9 Classification of bicuspid AVs. Sievers and colleagues[5] classified bicuspid and unicuspid valves into three types. With type 0 (relatively uncommon), there are two equal-sized cusps and no raphe, and the leaflets may be arranged medial-to-lateral or anteroposteriorly. With type 1, there is one raphe and fusion of two leaflets, creating an asymmetric bicuspid valve with one large cusp and one small cusp. Type 1 defects constitute >90% of all bicuspid valves, with fusion of the left and right cusps being the most common. With type 2 defects, there are two raphes, creating a unicuspid valve. The incidences of the various morphologies in Sievers' series of 304 surgical specimens are shown. The AV is shown in the same orientation as in the mid-oesophageal AV short-axis view.

1. Symptomatic, severe high-gradient AS (stage D1)
2. Asymptomatic, severe AS with LVEF <50% (stage C2)
3. Asymptomatic, severe AS (stage C1) who are undergoing cardiac surgery for other indications
4. Symptomatic low-flow, low-gradient with LVEF <50% (stage D2)
5. Symptomatic low-flow, low-gradient with normal LVEF (paradoxical or stage D3) if AS is the most likely cause of symptoms.

Additionally, AV replacement is *reasonable* for patients with:

1. Asymptomatic AS (stage C1) and low surgical risk with:
   a. Decreased exercise tolerance (exercise test)
   b. Serum B-type natriuretic peptide (BNP) level >3 times normal
   c. Serial testing showing an increase in aortic velocity ≥0.3 m/s per year
2. Asymptomatic with very severe AS (stage C1) and low surgical risk.

In the past decade, rapid expansion of transcatheter aortic valve implantation (TAVI) has offered an alternative to surgical AV replacement, and the criteria for TAVI are discussed in Chapter 17.

Echocardiographic imaging for aortic stenosis

2D and 3D imaging

The hallmarks of AS are leaflet calcification and leaflet restriction. With degeneration of a trileaflet or bicuspid valve, there is typically extensive calcification involving the bodies and free edges of the leaflets (Figures 10.11a and 10.11c; see Online appendix 7.2). Calcification is frequently asymmetric and may extend over the intervalvular fibrosa to involve the anterior mitral leaflet. In short-axis view, the systolic orifice is typically star-shaped and irregular (Figure 10.11b). Commissural fusion is rare. By contrast, in rheumatic disease, calcification tends to be less

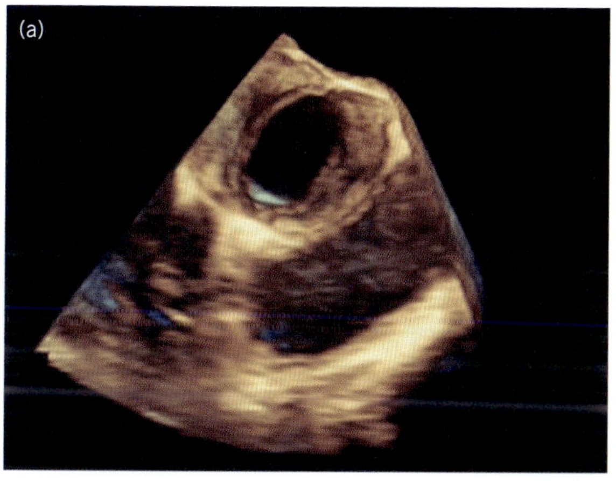

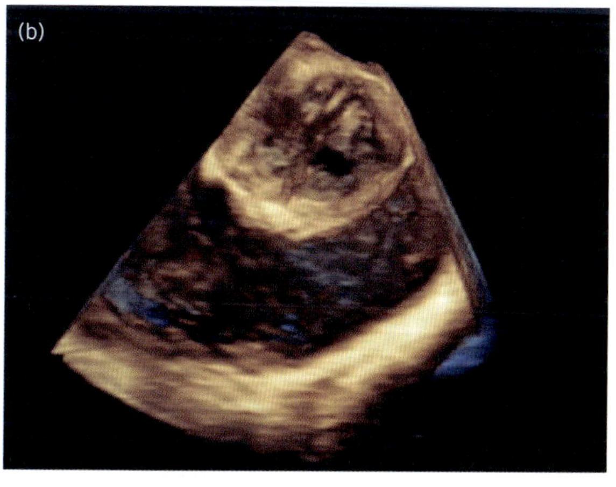

Figure 10.10 Bicuspid AV with 3D imaging. The images were obtained using the narrow sector (3D 'live') mode. The AV is shown from the aortic perspective in the same orientation as in the mid-oesophageal AV short-axis view. The morphology of the AV is type 0 (no raphe) with an anteroposterior orientation (see Figure 10.9). Note the elliptical shape of the opening in systole (a). The valve closure line in diastole is indicated. Note in diastole (b), apparent defects can be seen in the AV leaflets. This is due to echo dropout, rather than abnormalities with the leaflets themselves. See Online appendix 7.1.5 S.

marked, but commissural fusion is more pronounced. The systolic orifice is typically circular or triangular.

While marked leaflet calcification can occur without significant AS, the absence of valvular calcification makes significant stenosis very unlikely. An increased transvalvular velocity in the absence of significant valvular pathology on 2D imaging can be seen in very high-flow states, or it raises the possibility of obstruction at the level of the LVOT.

Direct planimetry of the AV orifice may be helpful if Doppler interrogation is suboptimal. However, with 2D imaging, it can be difficult to reliably obtain a true short-axis view of the valve at the level of the leaflet tips, particularly when calcification is marked, and oblique views may lead to erroneous measurements. Moreover, if the image plane is not at the narrowest point of the valve (usually the leaflet tips), the AV area may be overestimated. 3D imaging with multi-plane reconstruction allows the plane of the leaflet tips in systole to be more reliably determined than with 2D imaging (Figure 10.12). In a study by Machida and colleagues, AV planimetry with 3D TOE yielded excellent correlation and agreement with the AV area calculated by the continuity equation. By contrast, correlation was less for planimetry by 2D TOE, particularly for bicuspid valves.[10]

AS may be associated with dilatation of the aortic root and ascending aorta due to associated aortopathy or the effects of turbulent post-stenotic flow. Thus, careful measurement of aortic dimensions (SoV, STJ, proximal ascending aorta) is indicated. Mitral annular calcification and atheroma of the thoracic aorta are other findings commonly associated with AS.

Concentric LV remodelling and hypertrophy are common in AS. Hypertrophy of the basal anteroseptal wall ('septal knuckle') can occur, which predisposes to dynamic LVOT obstruction following AV replacement. In most patients, ventricular volume and LVEF are normal. Impaired LV systolic function implies advanced disease or another pathological process (e.g. concomitant severe AR or coronary artery disease). Assessment of diastolic function typically demonstrates impaired relaxation.

Colour Doppler imaging

Colour Doppler imaging cannot be used to quantify the severity of AS, but it is nevertheless a useful screening technique. Intense aliasing in the proximal aorta is typical with AS and occurs due to the turbulent, high-velocity post-stenotic flow pattern. Absence of such intense aliasing suggests AS is not severe. As previously noted, aliasing in the proximal aorta may occur in hyperdynamic, high-flow states and does not necessarily indicate AS. Post-stenotic aliasing is best seen in the mid-oesophageal AV long-axis view (Figure 10.11d; see Online appendix 7.2.4). If planimetry is performed, colour Doppler imaging in shortaxis often helps to define the shape of the valve orifice in systole (Figure 10.11b; see Online appendix 7.2.2). In diastole, colour Doppler is used to evaluate any associated AR (Figure 10.11e).

Spectral Doppler imaging: peak transvalvular velocity and mean pressure gradient

In most patients, peak transvalvular velocity and mean pressure gradient can be measured with CW Doppler from a transgastric view. Once an adequate CW Doppler

Table 10.1 Severity and type of aortic stenosis

Severity and type	Valve haemodynamics	Associated echo features	Symptoms
Mild AS	V_{max}: 2.0–2.9 m/s P_{mean}: <20 mmHg	• Early diastolic dysfunction • Normal LVEF • Mild/moderate leaflet calcification with some reduced leaflet motion	• Asymptomatic
Moderate AS	V_{max}: 3.0–3.9 m/s P_{mean}: 20–39 mmHg	• As per mild AS	• Asymptomatic
Severe, high-gradient AS	V_{max}: ≥4 m/s P_{mean}: ≥40 mmHg AVA: ≤1.0 cm^2(may be higher with mixed AS/AR)	• Diastolic dysfunction • LV hypertrophy • LVEF typically normal but may be <50% • May have pulmonary hypertension • Severe leaflet calcification with severely reduced leaflet motion	• May or may not be symptomatic • Symptoms: exertional dyspnoea, exertional angina, syncope
Very severe, high-gradient AS	V_{max}: ≥5 m/s P_{mean}: ≥60 mmHg AVA: ≤1.0 cm^2(may be higher with mixed AS/AR)	• As per severe high-gradient AS	• As per high-gradient AS
Severe low-flow, low-gradient, low-LVEF AS	V_{max}: <4 m/s (resting) P_{mean}: <40 mmHg (resting) AVA: ≤1 cm^2 (resting) With dobutamine stress: AVA <1.0 cm^2 with V_{max}>4 m/s (at any flow rate)	• LV diastolic dysfunction • LV hypertrophy • LVEF <50% • Severe leaflet calcification with severely reduced leaflet motion	• Heart failure, angina, syncope
Severe, low-gradient, normal-LVEF AS (paradoxical low-flow severe AS)	V_{max}: <4 m/s P_{mean}: <40 mmHg AVA: ≤1 cm^2 SVI: ≤35 mL/m^2(measured when normotensive, i.e. SBP <140 mmHg)	• Restrictive diastolic dysfunction • Small LV chamber size with reduced SV • Increased relative LV wall thickness • LVEF ≥50% • Severe leaflet calcification with severely reduced leaflet motion	• Heart failure, angina, syncope

AVA, aortic valve area; P_{mean}, mean transvalvular systolic pressure gradient; SBP, systolic blood pressure; SVI, stroke volume index; V_{max}, maximum transvalvular systolic pressure gradient.
Data from Otto *et al.*, 2020 ACC/AHA Guideline for the Management of Patients With Valvular Heart Disease: A Report of the American College of Cardiology/American Heart Association Joint Committee on Clinical Practice Guidelines, *Journal of the American College of Cardiology*, 2021;**77**:e25–197.

signal has been obtained, the velocity–time curve is traced and the machine automatically calculates the mean pressure gradient (Figure 10.11f; see Online appendix 7.2.7) by using the simplified Bernoulli equation (see Equation 3.29).

The main limitations of CW imaging across the AV are:(1) obtaining good *alignment* between the Doppler beam and blood flow through the AV; and (2) ensuring the Doppler beam interrogates the *central* flow pattern. Off-axis measurements lead to transvalvular velocity being underestimated. Because velocity is squared in the Bernoulli equation, pressure calculations are even more affected by poor alignment than velocity. As discussed in Chapter 1, if the intercept angle between the Doppler beam and the blood flow is <20°, underestimation of velocity is <6%. As it is not possible to overestimate velocity with Doppler, the *highest* value of several measurements should be used.

Failure to interrogate the central region of flow results in an incomplete waveform, which can also lead to velocity

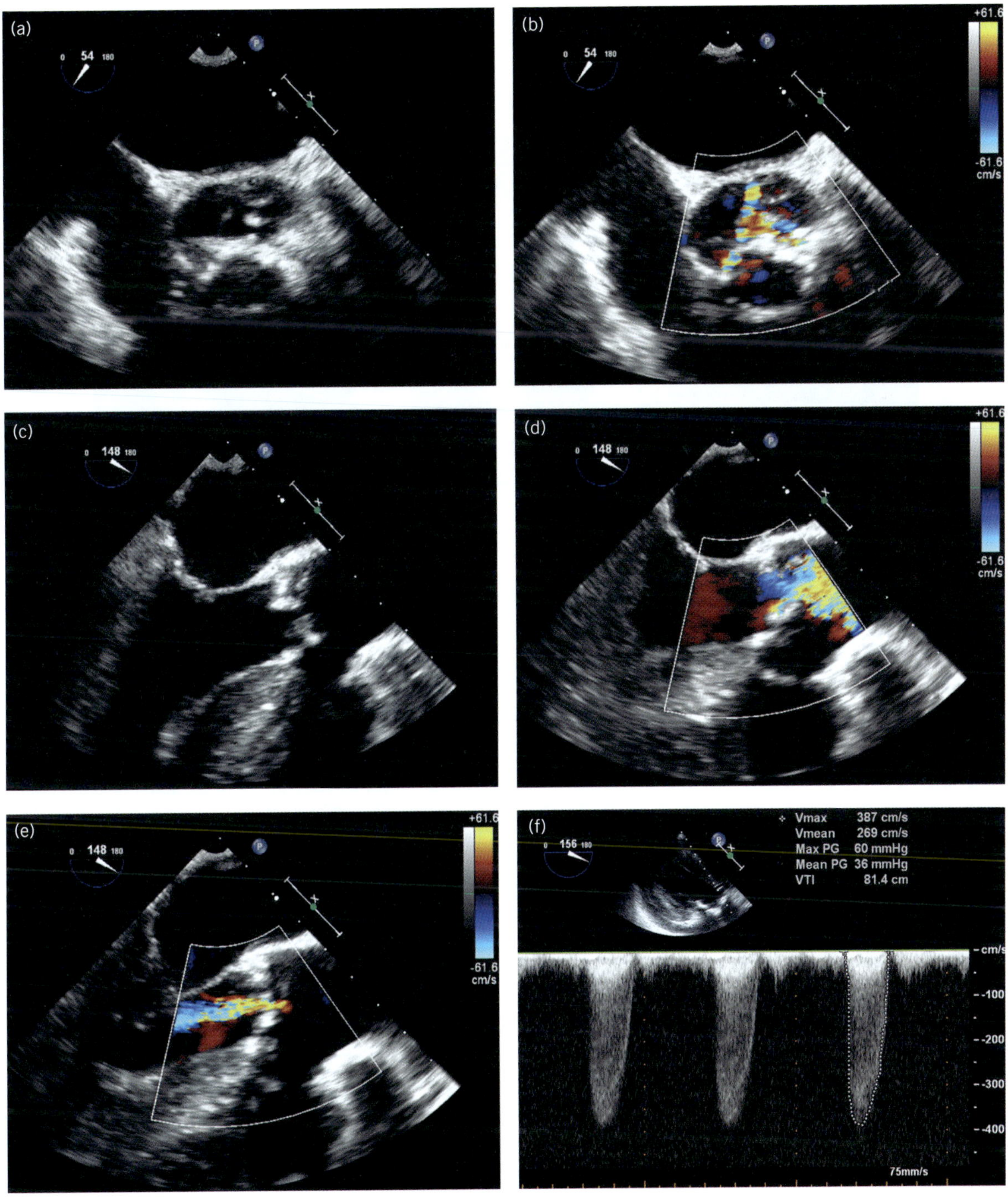

Figure 10.11 Calcific aortic stenosis. Frame (a) is a mid-oesophageal AV short-axis view in systole demonstrating asymmetric leaflet calcification, predominantly involving the right cusp. (b) With colour Doppler imaging in systole, an irregular-shaped orifice is seen, typical of calcific AS. (c) In the mid-oesophageal AV long-axis view in systole, heavy calcification of the leaflets can be seen, along with a narrowed orifice. (d) With colour Doppler imaging, marked turbulence can be seen in the proximal aorta in systole. (e) In diastole, there is mild central AR. Frame (f) is a CW Doppler waveform obtained from the transgastric long-axis view, showing a peak velocity of 3.87 m/s and a mean gradient pressure gradient of 36 mmHg, consistent with at least moderate AS. See also Online appendix 7.2.

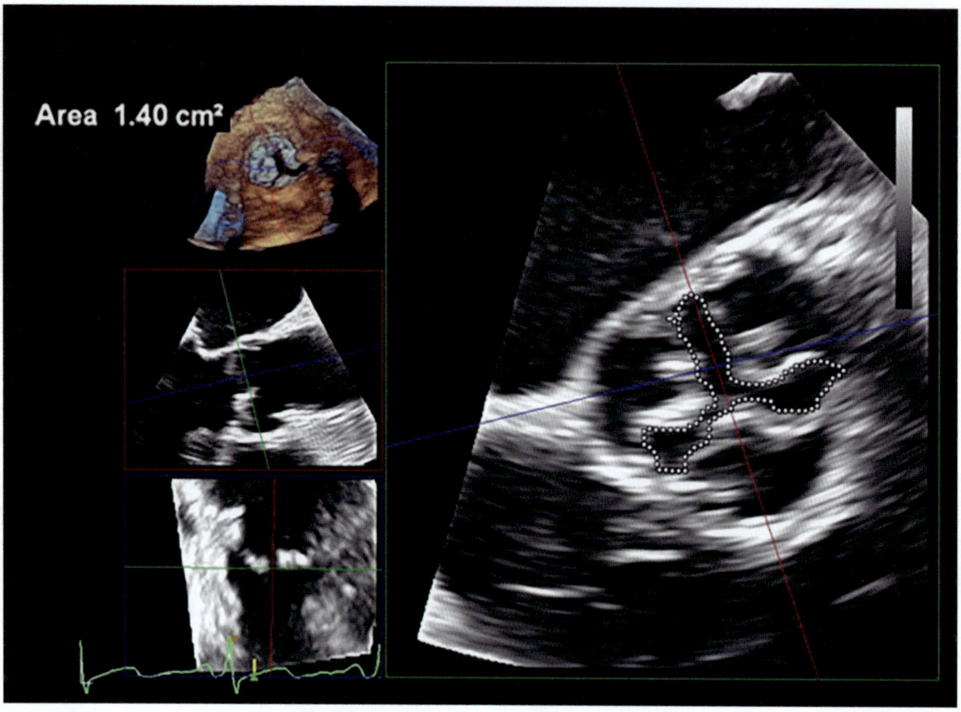

Figure 10.12 Planimetry of the AV using 3D MPR. In this multi-planar reconstruction, the two long-axis planes (blue and red in this example) are carefully aligned with the aortic valve, producing a perfect short-axis view of the valve in the remaining plane. The short-axis cursor (green in this example) is positioned at the very tip of the leaflets, where the valve area is smallest. The stenotic valve opening is then measured with the trace function, in this case $1.40\,cm^2$.

being underestimated. Moreover, if the velocity in the LVOT is elevated (>1.5 m/s—for instance, due to a subvalvular membrane or dynamic LVOT obstruction), the long form of the Bernoulli equation (see Equation 3.28) should be used (see Chapter 13 for details). Lastly, in the transgastric views, it is easy to mistake the signal of an MR jet for an AS waveform. Since MR jets are typically >5 m/s, there is the potential for confusion. The timing and shape of the velocity curves can help to differentiate them (Figure 10.13).[9]

Spectral Doppler: calculation of AV area by the continuity equation

The AV area is calculated by using the continuity principle (see Chapter 3), which states that, in the absence of an intracardiac shunt, the net forward SV through any part of the heart equals the net forward SV at any other part. For calculating the AV area by the continuity method, the SV is compared across the LVOT and AV. Thus (Equation 10.2):

$$SV_{LVOT} = SV_{AV} \qquad \text{Equation 10.2}$$

SV is the product of the cross-sectional area (CSA) and the velocity–time integral (VTI), which is the area bounded by the spectral Doppler velocity–time curve. Thus (Equation 10.3):

$$SV_{LVOT} = CSA_{LVOT} \times VTI_{LVOT} \qquad \text{Equation 10.3}$$

And (Equation 10.4):

$$SV_{AV} = CSA_{AV} \times VTI_{AV} \qquad \text{Equation 10.4}$$

Combining Equations 10.2, 10.3, and 10.4 (Equation 10.5):

$$CSA_{AV} = \frac{CSA_{LVOT} \times VTI_{LVOT}}{VTI_{AV}} \qquad \text{Equation 10.5}$$

The CSA_{LVOT} can be calculated from an LVOT diameter measured in 2D in the mid-oesophageal AV long-axis view in mid-systole at approximately the same distance from the aortic annulus as the VTI recording is made (about 0.5–1.0 cm from the valve). As the LVOT is somewhat elliptical and any errors in this measurement are squared when calculating the area, the mean LVOT diameter using 3D data set may be used to improve accuracy, as described earlier. The LVOT size is usually constant in the 1 cm proximal to the valve, so the aortic annular

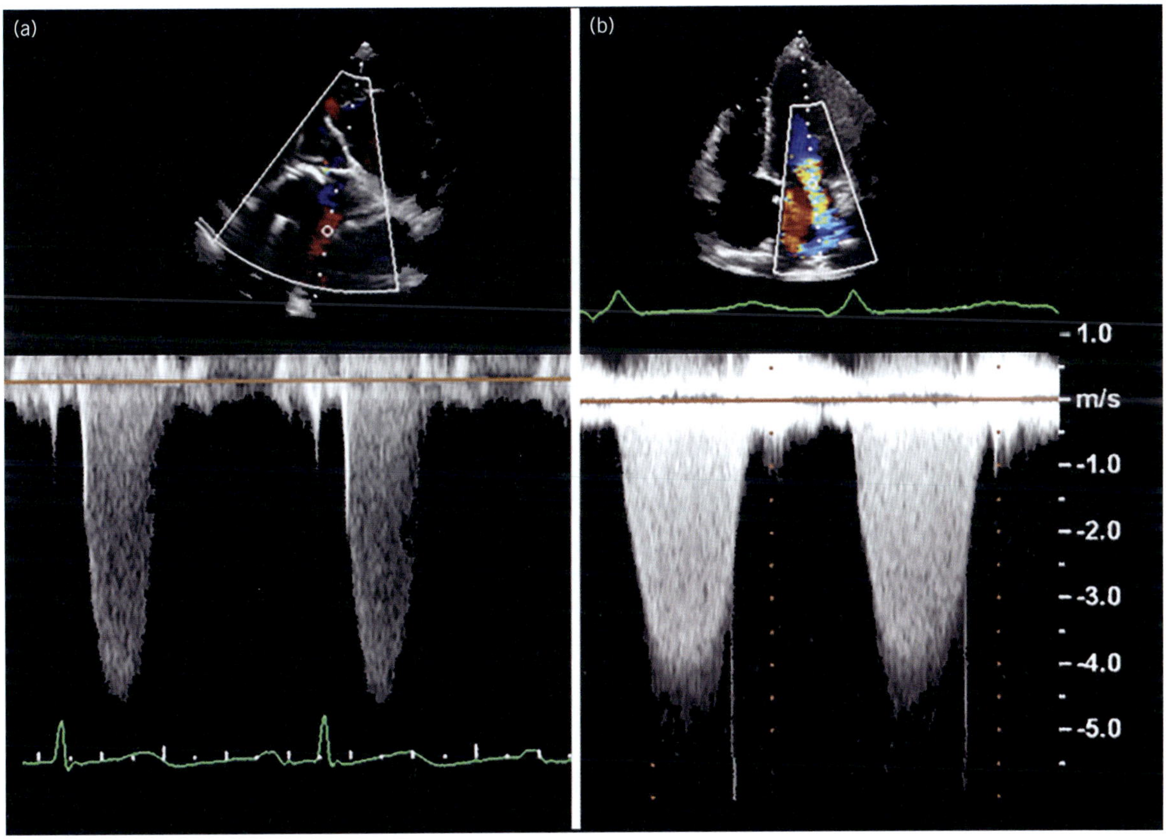

Figure 10.13 CW Doppler of AS versus MR. (a) shows a CW signal of AS. (b) shows a CW signal of MR. Note the holosystolic nature and the typically more rounded shape of the MR signal. See text for details.

diameter (Figure 10.7; see Online appendix 7.2.7) can be used as a surrogate for the LVOT diameter.

VTI measurements are obtained in thetransgastric view. The VTI_{AV} is measured with CW Doppler (see earlier), and the VTI_{LVOT} is measured with PW Doppler. Care must be taken when measuring the VTI_{LVOT} to avoid placing the sample volume within the flow convergence zone proximal to the valve.

> ***Expert tip: Colour Doppler is useful in the deep transgastric view or transgastric long-axis view to help align the CW and PW Dopplers. Aligning the cursor with the aliasing colour flow through the AV ensures that the highest velocity is sampled. Colour Doppler also helps in positioning the PW sample volume to avoid the flow convergence zone.***

One simple approach is to use the 'double envelope technique'. In Figure 10.8f and Online appendix 7.28, a bright, lower-velocity region can be seen within the CW Doppler waveform due to flow in the LVOT. If this region is clearly visible, it is possible to trace the VTI_{AV} and the VTI_{LVOT} from the same CW waveform, with the so-called 'double envelope'. As for any other PW measurement, for patients in sinus rhythm, the VTI_{AV} retained for the calculation should be the *highest* of three recorded beats, and for patients in atrial fibrillation, the *average* values from ≥5 beats should be taken.[9]

Because the ratio of the VTIs across the AV and LVOT is used in Equation 10.5, errors due to poor alignment between the Doppler beam and blood flow tend to cancel out. Thus, off-axis imaging is less important for valve area calculations than for simple pressure measurements.

When measuring the AV area by the continuity equation, maximum velocity (V_{max}) can be substituted for VTI. Since the LVOT area tends to remain relatively constant over time, Equation 10.5 can be simplified to the ratio of the VTI (or V_{max}) across the LVOT to the VTI (or V_{max}) across the AV. This ratio is known as the '**Doppler velocity index**' (DVI) or the '**dimensionless index**' (Equation 10.6):

$$DVI = \frac{VTI_{LVOT}}{VTI_{AV}} \text{ or } \frac{Vmax_{LVOT}}{Vmax_{AV}} \qquad \text{Equation 10.6}$$

A DVI <0.25 is consistent with severe AS. The DVI can be rapidly measured by using the 'double envelope' technique.

The valve area calculated by the continuity equation measures the *effective* orifice area, which is the area of the stream of blood as it passes across the valve. The effective orifice area is typically a little smaller than the anatomical orifice area, as measured by planimetry or angiography.

The effect of flow

It is essential to interpret Doppler velocity waveforms in light of the patient's LV function and stroke volume. Transvalvular velocity and pressure measurements are influenced by flow (see Chapter 3), whereas the valve area calculated by the continuity equation is relatively independent of flow. Thus, factors that increase systolic transaortic flow (high cardiac output, AR) lead to increased velocity and pressure measurements for any given valve area, whereas factors that decrease systolic transaortic flow (low cardiac output, MR) reduce velocity and pressure measurements.

Low-flow/low-gradient AS

Low-flow/low-gradient (LFLG) AS may be defined as:[8,9]

- AV area (calculated by continuity equation) ≤1 cm^2
- Measured peak velocity <4 m/s and mean gradient <40 mmHg
- LVEF <50% (or normal LVEF in cases of paradoxical LFLG AS).

There are two possible explanations for these findings: (1) low LVEF due to true severe AS; and (2) moderate AS with another cause of low LVEF (e.g. cardiomyopathy). In both scenarios, the transvalvular velocity and pressure gradient are low due to low cardiac output. In the first scenario, the LV is overwhelmed by a severely stenosed AV, resulting in low LVEF. In the second scenario, the AV is only moderately stenosed, but the calculated area is low because the LV does not generate enough flow to fully open the valve leaflets. AV replacement is beneficial in the first scenario, but not in the second.

The following approach was recommended by the EACVI and the ASE for the evaluation of LFLG AS.[9] Whenever a valve appears significantly stenosed on examination, the AV area should be calculated by the continuity equation. If the AV area is ≤1 cm^2, but the velocity/gradient across the valve are low (assuming that measurement errors are ruled out), the first step is to determine the flow across the valve by calculating the stroke volume index (SVI) (see Chapter 3). A low AV gradient with normal flow (SVI>35 mL/m^2) all but rules out severe AS. If flow is low (SVI<35 mL/m^2), the next step is to evaluate LV function. If depressed, flow reserve should be evaluated with a dobutamine stress echocardiography. By increasing the SV, dobutamine will help to distinguish between true severe AS and pseudo-severe AS. In the former, dobutamine results in an increased transvalvular velocity (>4 m/s) and the valve area remains low (≤1 cm^2) (=true severe AS). In the latter, transvalvular velocity remains low and the calculated valve area increases to >1 cm^2 (=pseudo-severe or moderate AS). Note that the absence of contractile reserve (i.e. the SV does not increase >20% from baseline with dobutamine) is a predictor of higher surgical mortality, although AVR might improve the LV function and outcome in these patients.[9]

Severe low-velocity AS can also occur in patients with normal LVEF, so-called 'paradoxical low-flow AS' (stage D3). Patients typically have a small, hypertrophied LV and increased systemic vascular resistance (i.e. hypertension). High LV afterload, in combination with low SV, results in a low transvalvular velocity (<4 m/s) despite severe AS. The diagnosis is confirmed by the finding of a low calculated AV area (≤1 cm^2 or ≤0.6 cm^2/m^2), in combination with a low SVI (<35 mL/m^2). Such patients do benefit from AV replacement.

Both patients with LFLG AS with no flow reserve and patients with paradoxical LFLG AS present a diagnostic challenge. The combination of clinical, radiological, and echocardiographic findings helps to grade the severity.

It must be noted that reduced pressure gradients are often seen on the pre-cardiopulmonary bypass TOE examination of patients with true severe AS. The effects of general anaesthesia (GA) on AV gradients and flows are not well defined, but one study showed that as much as 54% of patients with severe AS had a mean pressure gradient of <40 mmHg under GA.[11] So care must be taken when assessing AS severity in the operating room and one should rely on the preoperative echocardiography assessment if possible. Relying on multiple criteria is helpful in the operating room to confirm the diagnosis of severe stenosis, especially 3D AV planimetry and flow-independent indices such as the VTI ratio.

Aortic regurgitation

Aortic regurgitation (AR) results from congenital or acquired disease of either the AV leaflets and/or the aortic

Table 10.2 Aetiology and mechanism of AV regurgitation

Classification	Specific aetiology	Mechanism
Congenital leaflet abnormalities	Bicuspid, unicuspid, or quadricuspid aortic valve	Leaflet calcification and restriction or prolapse
	Ventricular septal defect	Leaflet prolapse
Acquired leaflet abnormalities	Senile calcification	Leaflet calcification and restriction
	Rheumatic disease	Leaflet thickening and restriction
	Radiation or toxin-induced valvulopathy	Leaflet calcification, retraction, and restriction
	Infective endocarditis	Leaflet perforation and prolapse
Congenital aortic root abnormalities	Connective tissue disease (e.g. Marfan syndrome, Loeys–Dietz, Ehlers–Danlos)	Aortic root dilatation
Acquiredaortic root abnormalities	Systemic hypertension	Aortic root dilatation
	Idiopathicaortic root dilatation	Aortic root dilatation
	Autoimmune disease (e.g. systemic lupus erythematosus, rheumatoid arthritis, Reiter's syndrome)	Leaflet thickening and restriction Aortic root dilatation
	Aortitis (e.g. Takayasu's arteritis, giant cell arteritis)	Aortic root dilatation
	Aortic dissection	Aortic root dilatation Leaflet prolapse or restriction

Adapted from *Journal of the American Society of Echocardiography*, 30, 4, Zoghbi WA, Adams D, Bonow RO, *et al.*, 'Recommendations for noninvasive evaluation of native valvular regurgitation. A report from the American Society of Echocardiography developed in collaboration with the Society for Cardiovascular Magnetic Resonance', pp. 303–371, Copyright 2017, with permission from American Society of Echocardiography.

root that results in valve malcoaptation (Table 10.2).[12] Acute AR can arise due to endocarditis or aortic dissection. However, in most cases, AR is chronic and slowly progressive. The mechanisms of AR are discussed in more detail in Chapter 11.

Classification of aortic regurgitation severity

As with AS, the AHA/ACC classifies AR into four stages (A–D).[8] Stage A represents patients at risk of developing AR (e.g. congenital valve anomaly, disease of the aortic root or ascending aorta, rheumatic heart disease, or infective endocarditis). Stage B encompasses mild and moderate AR. Stage C is asymptomatic, severe AR, and stage D is symptomatic, severe AR. The echocardiographic findings associated with mild, moderate, and severe AR are outlined in Table 10.3.

Indications for surgery

According to the same AHA/ACC guidelines,[8] AV replacement or repair is *indicated* for:

1. All symptomatic patients with severe AR (stage D)
2. Asymptomatic patients with chronic severe AR (stage C) and LV systolic dysfunction (LVEF ≤55%)
3. Patients with severe AR (stage C or D) undergoing cardiac surgery for other indications.

Additionally, surgery is *reasonable* for:

1. Asymptomatic patients with severe AR and normal LV systolic function, but severe LV dilatation (LV end-systolic diameter (LVESD)>50 mm or indexed LVESD >25 mm/m^2)
2. Patients with moderate AR (stage B) undergoing other cardiac surgery.

For many years, most patients requiring surgical intervention for AR received valve replacement with a mechanical or bioprosthetic valve.[8] However, advances in surgical AV repair and valve-sparing root replacement in the past decade are providing good long-term results in selected patients.[13] This is discussed in Chapter 11.

Table 10.3 Severity of aortic regurgitation

Severity	Valve haemodynamics	Associated echo features	Symptoms
Mild AR	Jet width <25% of LVOT Vena contracta<0.3 cm RV <30 mL/beat RF <30% ERO ≤0.10 cm^2 Angiography 1+	Normal LV systolic function Normal or mildly increased LV size and volume May have dilated aortic sinuses or other pathology (leaflet calcification, rheumatic changes, endocarditis, leaflet prolapse/ restriction)	Asymptomatic
Moderate AR	Jet width 25–64% of LVOT Vena contracta 0.3–0.6 cm RV 30–59 mL/beat RF 30–49% ERO 0.10–0.29 cm^2 Angiography 2+	As per mild AR	Asymptomatic
Severe AR	Jet width ≥65% of LVOT Vena contracta>0.6 cm RV ≥60 mL/beat RF ≥50% ERO ≥0.30 cm^2 Angiography 3+ or 4+ Holodiastolic flow reversal in proximal abdominal aorta	Moderate/severe LV dilatation LV systolic function may be normal or abnormal (mild, moderate, or severely depressed) May have dilated aortic sinuses or other pathology (leaflet calcification, rheumatic changes, endocarditis, leaflet prolapse/ restriction)	May or may not be symptomatic Symptoms include: exertional dyspnoea, exertional angina, and heart failure symptoms

ERO, effective regurgitant orifice; RF, regurgitant fraction; RV, regurgitant volume.

Data from Otto *et al.*, 2020 ACC/AHA Guideline for the Management of Patients With Valvular Heart Disease: A Report of the American College of Cardiology/American Heart Association Joint Committee on Clinical Practice Guidelines, *Journal of the American College of Cardiology*, 2021;**77**:e25–197.

Echocardiographic evaluation

2D and 3D echocardiography should be used in an integrated approach to identify both the aetiology and the mechanism of AR. The AV should be examined for specific pathology such as congenital abnormalities (e.g. BAV) and acquired defects (e.g. vegetations or abscesses). The leaflets should be inspected, looking for evidence of thickening, calcification, restriction, perforation, or prolapse. The dimensions of the aortic root and proximal aorta should be carefully measured. LV volume overload is a consistent finding in chronic severe AR, and a comprehensive assessment of LV size and function should be performed (see Chapter 6).

Colour Doppler imaging

Colour Doppler is useful to screen for AR, grade the severity, elucidate the mechanism, and identify the precise location of regurgitant jet(s). In the AV short- and long-axis views, turning the colour map on and off may help to define the anatomical location and mechanism of regurgitation. With symmetrical cusp restriction or commissural fusion, the AR jet is usually central (see Online appendices 7.4.2 and 7.4.6). Asymmetric cusp restriction typically results in an eccentric regurgitant jet that is directed *towards* the affected leaflet. With cusp prolapse,

Box 10.1 Central versus eccentric jet

The distinction between central and eccentric jet is important. The term 'eccentric' refers to anything that is not central. However, it may refer to the *origin* of the jet (i.e. central vs commissural) or to the *direction* of the jet (directed down the centre of the LVOT or off to one side), and these can have very different clinical implications. The reader is encouraged to be specific in their description of AR jets (e.g.*the jet originates centrally but is directed eccentrically in a posterior direction*, or *the origin of the jet is eccentric, at the LCC/NCC commissure*—see Chapter 11 for more details).

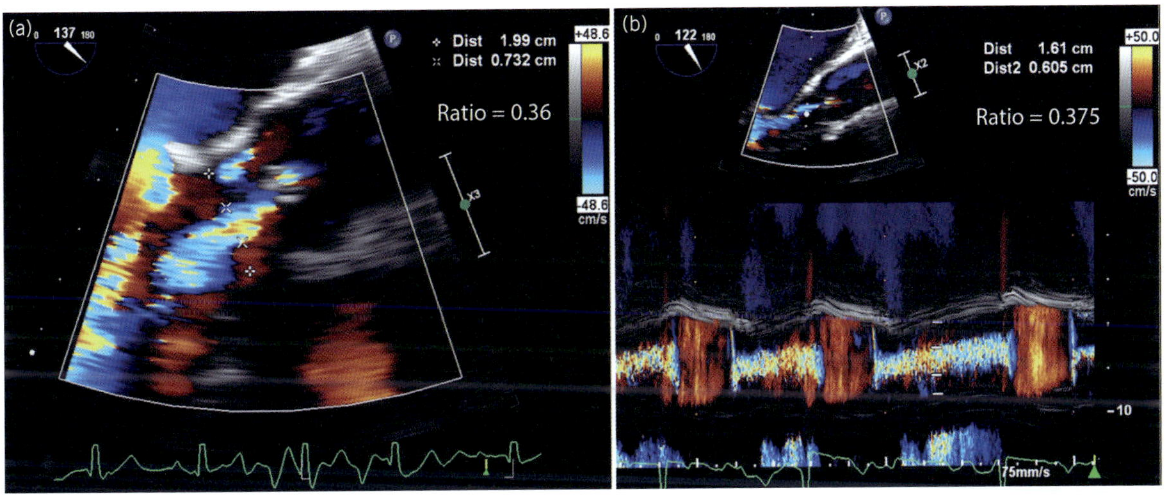

Figure 10.14 Jet width-to-LVOT width ratio. (a) is a zoomed mid-oesophageal AV long-axis view in mid diastole, showing an AR jet. The width of the jet (0.732 cm) was measured just below the AV, which is not well seen in this frame. The width of the LVOT (1.99 cm) was measured at the same level. The ratio of 0.36 suggests moderate AR. (b) The same measurement can be made on a colour M-mode scan. Here an M-mode cursor was placed across the LVOT just below the AV. Note the M-mode cursor is not exactly perpendicular to the LVOT, which is not ideal, but very common with TOE imaging. The width of the AR jet (0.605 cm) was measured in mid diastole. The width of the LVOT (1.61 cm) was measured at the same point in time. The ratio of 0.37 again suggests regurgitation is moderate.

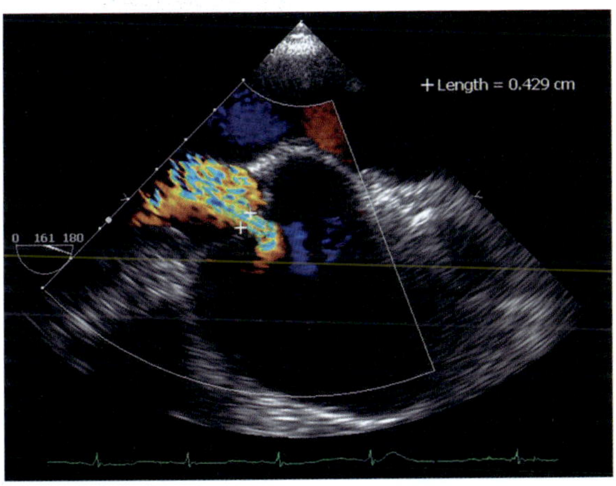

Figure 10.15 Vena contracta width. In this modified mid-oesophageal AV long-axis view in mid diastole, the width of the VC was measured at the narrowest part of the jet as it traverses the AV. The VC width of 0.429 cm suggests regurgitation is moderate.

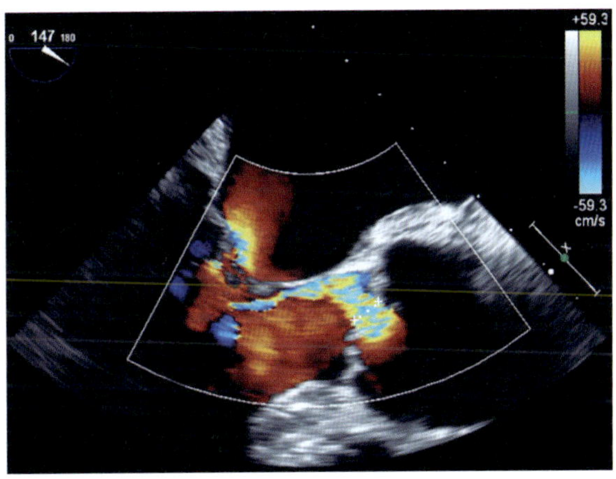

Figure 10.16 Eccentric aortic regurgitation. In this mid-oesophageal AV long-axis view in mid diastole, an eccentric AR jet can be seen passing under the anterior mitral leaflet. The appropriate site of measurement for VC is shown. However, using the jet width-to-LVOT width ratio in this patient would significantly underestimate AR severity, as the jet is confined by the LVOT (see Chapter 3).

the regurgitant jet is usually eccentric and directed *away* from the affected leaflet (see Online appendices 7.3.6 and 7.3.12). With symmetric dilatation of the aortic root and/or cusp perforation (see Online appendix 7.3.2), the regurgitant jet is usually central.

Several colour Doppler-based techniques can be used to quantify AR severity.[8,14] These techniques have been mainly validated for TTE but are widely used with TOE.

Jet width/LVOT ratio

In centrally directed jets, the width of the regurgitant jet can be estimated in the AV long-axis view and compared with the width of the LVOT. A ratio >65% is consistent with severe regurgitation, and a ratio <25% with mild regurgitation. The technique can be performed by using standard colour Doppler imaging or with colour M-mode

(Figure 10.14). Measurements should be made immediately below the AV.[14] Severity is overestimated if measurements are made more proximally in the LVOT, after the jet has splayed out. The technique assumes a circular shape to the jet and is therefore less reliable if the regurgitant orifice is elliptical (e.g. BAV) or irregular (e.g. calcific degeneration). The technique is also unreliable with eccentric jets directed towards the septum or anterior MV leaflet, or with multiple jets.

Vena contracta

The **vena contracta** (VC) is the narrowest part of the regurgitant jet as it traverses the aortic orifice and is normally numerically smaller than the jet width in the LVOT. The VC width is measured in a zoomed AV long-axis view (Figure 10.15) and is independent of flow rate and driving pressure. A value >6 mm is consistent with severe AR, and a value <3 mm with mild AR. Over- or underestimation of severity can occur if the regurgitant orifice is elliptical or irregular, depending on the orientation of the orifice and scan plane. The VC width is generally reliable for eccentric jets (Figure 10.16) but is unreliable when there are multiple jets.

Like for the MV, the 3D **vena contracta area** (VCA) measurement shows better correlation with regurgitant volume, angiographic grades, and effective regurgitant orifice area (EROA), compared to jet width/LVOT or VC width (Figure 10.17).[15] In most recent studies, the cut-off value of 3D VCA for severe AR has been established at >0.32 cm^2.[15,16] The VCA is proportional to the EROA, and in relevant clinical guidelines, severe AR is defined as EROA ≥0.30 cm^2.[12]

Flow convergence (PISA)

Similar to the method described for MR (see Chapter 8), quantification of the size of the proximal isovelocity surface

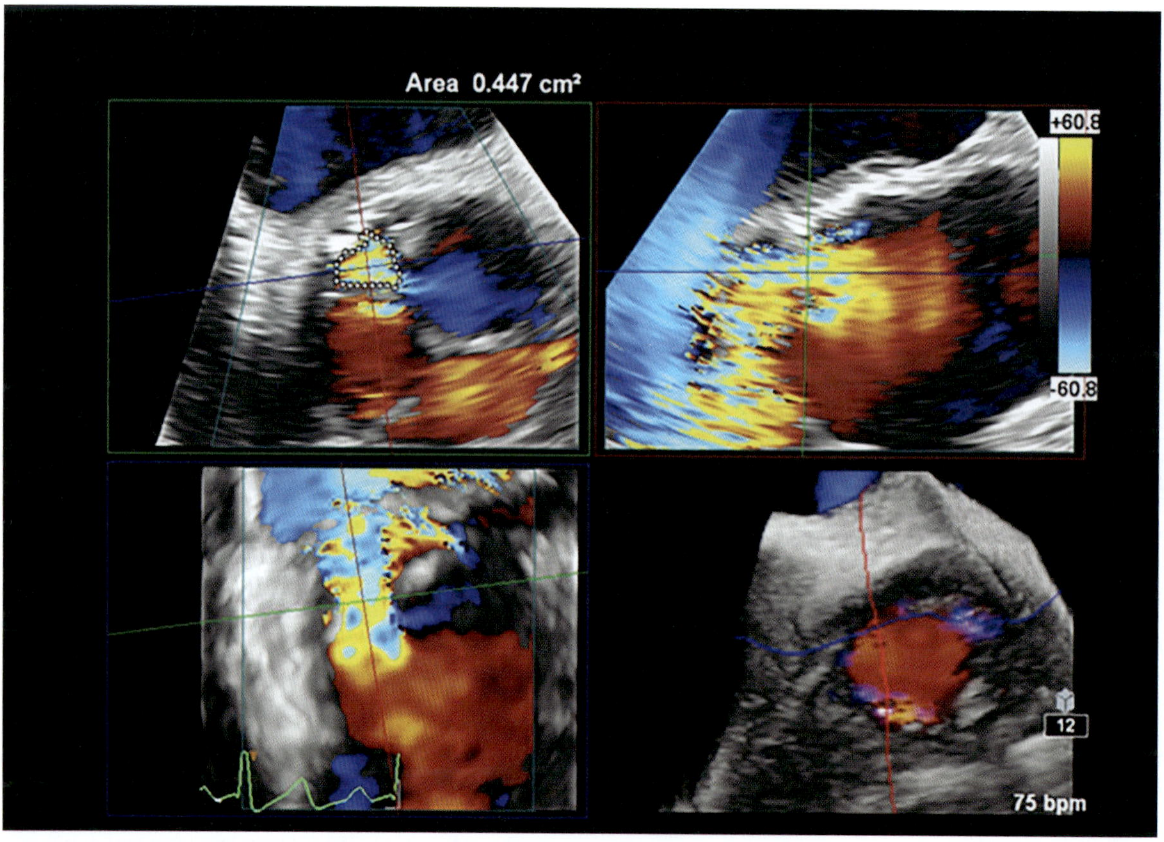

Figure 10.17 3D vena contracta area. This is a 3D MPR of the AV with colour Doppler. Here the structure of interest is the AR jet (not the AV itself or the LVOT). Therefore, the long-axis planes are aligned with the regurgitant jet, creating an orthogonal short-axis view of the jet in the short-axis plane. The level of the short-axis plane is then carefully moved to the narrowest point of the AR jet, and the VCA is measured in the short-axis plane. In this example, a value of 0.45 cm^2 is consistent with severe AR.

area (PISA) on the aortic side of the valve in diastole can be used to quantify the severity of AR. Practically, there are several problems with this method. First, acoustic shadowing from the diseased valve frequently obscures the flow convergence zone in the AV long-axis view, so a deep transgastric view must be used. Second, the technique requires measuring the peak regurgitant velocity with CW Doppler imaging, which is frequently difficult to properly align with TOE. Finally, non-planar or confined flow convergence zones (which invalidate the hemispheric assumptions of the technique) are common with AR and can lead to severity being over- or underestimated.[14] Nevertheless, if a suitable flow convergence zone can be identified, a simplified form of the technique may be applied. In one small study, a PISA radius ≥7 mm at an alias velocity of 33 cm/s was always associated with severe AR.[17]

> ***Expert tip: As previously noted for MR, the qualitative presence of a flow convergence zone is always significant and should prompt the operator to carefully investigate the AR.***

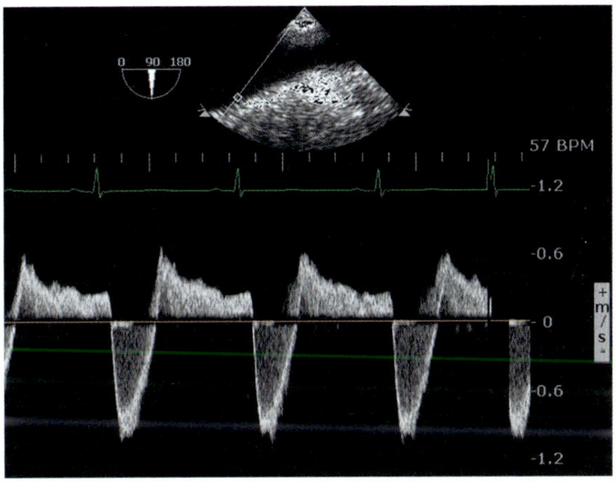

Figure 10.18 Holodiastolic flow reversal in the descending thoracic aorta. In this descending aorta long-axis view, a PW Doppler sample volume has been placed in the mid descending thoracic aorta. Flow in systole is directed away from the transducer and displayed below the baseline. Flow reversal (towards the transducer) throughout diastole is due to AR. The end-diastolic velocity of approximately 0.25 cm/s suggests regurgitation is severe.

Spectral Doppler imaging

Two spectral Doppler techniques may be used to help define the severity of AR:

1. Diastolic flow reversal in the descending thoracic aorta
2. Pressure half-time (PHT) of the regurgitant jet.

Aortic diastolic flow reversal

Early diastolic flow reversal within the descending thoracic aorta is a normal finding and can be readily evaluated with PW Doppler from the descending aorta long-axis view. Increasing severity of AR is associated with a more prolonged reversal of diastolic flow. Holodiastolic flow reversal in the proximal descending thoracic aorta, with an end-diastolic velocity of >20 cm/s, is a sensitive sign of severe AR (Figure 10.18; see Online appendix 7.5.6).[14] Care must be taken to ensure the angle of incidence between the Doppler beam and blood flow is <20°; otherwise end-diastolic velocity will be underestimated.

Pressure half-time of the regurgitant jet

Sampling of the regurgitant jet can be performed with CW Doppler from a transgastric view (see Figure 3.6). In that view, flow is directed towards the transducer and displayed above the baseline. Peak velocity is typically 3–5 m/s, reflecting the diastolic pressure gradient between the aorta and the LV in early diastole. Off-axis imaging is common with TOE, which underestimates the peak velocity, as in Figure 3.6.

The *slope* of the regurgitant waveform is indicative of the rate of pressure equalization between the aorta and the LV, and is dependent on the severity of the regurgitation. The rate of decline (i.e. deceleration) of the diastolic pressure gradient is quantified by the PHT, which is defined as the time, in milliseconds, for the peak transvalvular *pressure gradient* (not velocity) to decrease by half of its maximal value (see Chapter 3). PHT is inversely related to the size of the regurgitant orifice. Severe AR is associated with a rapid fall in the diastolic pressure gradient, and therefore a *short* PHT (typically <200 ms). With mild AR, PHT is typically much longer (>500 ms). No empiric relationship exists between PHT and severity of AR (like there is for MS).

In practice, this technique is limited by the fact that it is often difficult to obtain a clear spectral envelope with TOE, and the slope of the waveform is heavily influenced by LV compliance, vascular resistance, and loading conditions.

Endocarditis

TOE is the investigation of choice for evaluating suspected AV endocarditis (see Online appendix 7.5).

AV vegetations typically appear as echogenic masses of soft tissue density, usually attached to the LV side of the leaflet(s). Vegetations typically move back and forth between the LVOT and aortic root with the cardiac cycle and are usually more easily identified in the LVOT in diastole than in the aorta in systole (Figure 10.19). Their motion typically has a fluttering quality. There is often a pre-existing abnormality of the AV, and vegetations may be more difficult to detect on a calcified disorganized valve. Metastatic vegetations can occur in the LVOT or on the anterior leaflet of the MV, typically in the path of the AR jet.

AV endocarditis is associated with several important complications. There may be destruction of leaflet tissue, causing perforation or rupture of one or more cusps. AR is typically severe in these circumstances (Figure 10.19). An abscess may form, appearing as one or more echolucent cavities around the valve (Figure 10.20). Rupture of an abscess can create fistulae to adjacent structures, notably the LA, RA, RV (Figure 10.20), and pulmonary artery. Careful imaging with colour Doppler using non-standard views may be required to track the path of a fistula. Finally, vegetations on one valve should always prompt a careful evaluation of other valves.

LVOT obstruction

Subaortic stenosis (SAS) differs from valvular stenosis in that the site of the narrowing is in the outflow tract rather than the valve itself. It may be dynamic or fixed.

Dynamic LVOT obstruction is due to a systolic reduction in the distance between the anterior leaflet of the MV and the ventricular septum and may occur with hypertrophic cardiomyopathy, following MV repair, or following AV replacement for AS. With dynamic SAS, the obstruction develops predominantly in mid-to-late systole, resulting in a *late peaking* velocity curve on spectral Doppler. Dynamic obstruction also varies with loading conditions, with obstruction being worse with tachycardia and small ventricular volumes, and/or when ventricular contractility is increased. Hypertrophic cardiomyopathy and surgical myectomy are discussed in Chapter 6. Dynamic LVOT obstruction following MV repair is discussed in Chapter 9. Fixed SAS is usually the result of a thin, crescent-shaped membrane just below the AV in 75–85% of cases, or a thick fibromuscular ridge (Figure 10.21). On Doppler assessment, the haemodynamics are similar to an obstruction at the valvular level.[18] A fixed SAS should be

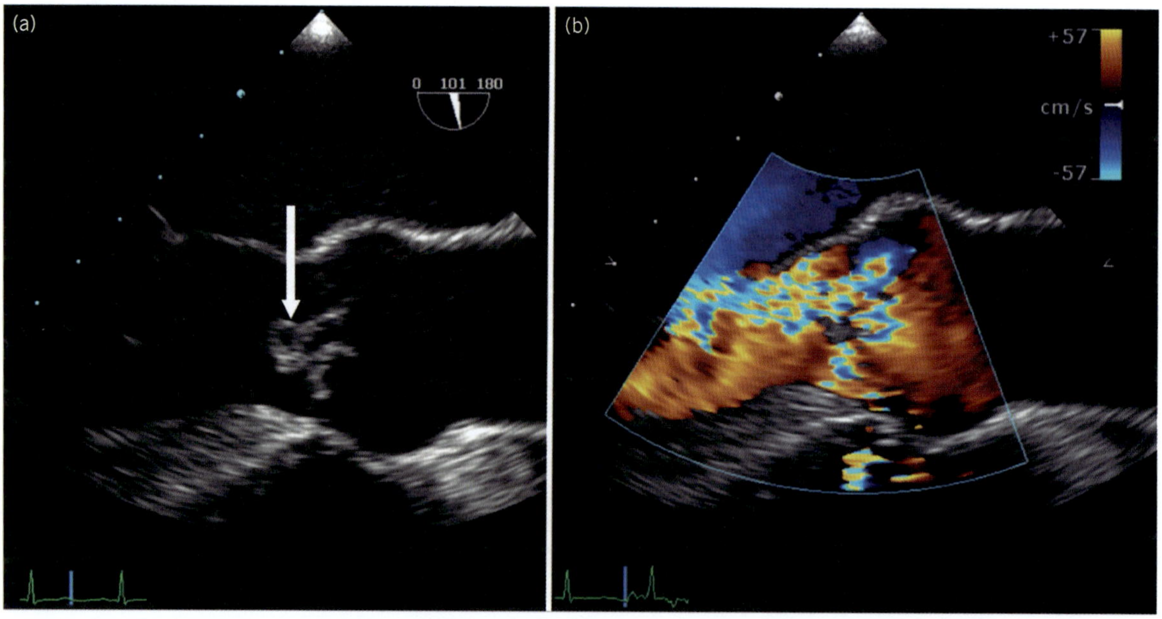

Figure 10.19 AV endocarditis. This is a mid-oesophageal long-axis view of the AV. In systole (not shown here), the AV opened normally and no abnormality was apparent. (a) In diastole, an echogenic mass (arrow) due to vegetations can be seen on the 2D image. It is not obvious in this view which leaflet(s) is/are involved. (b) A broad jet of aortic regurgitation can be seen with colour Doppler imaging. See Online appendix 7.5.

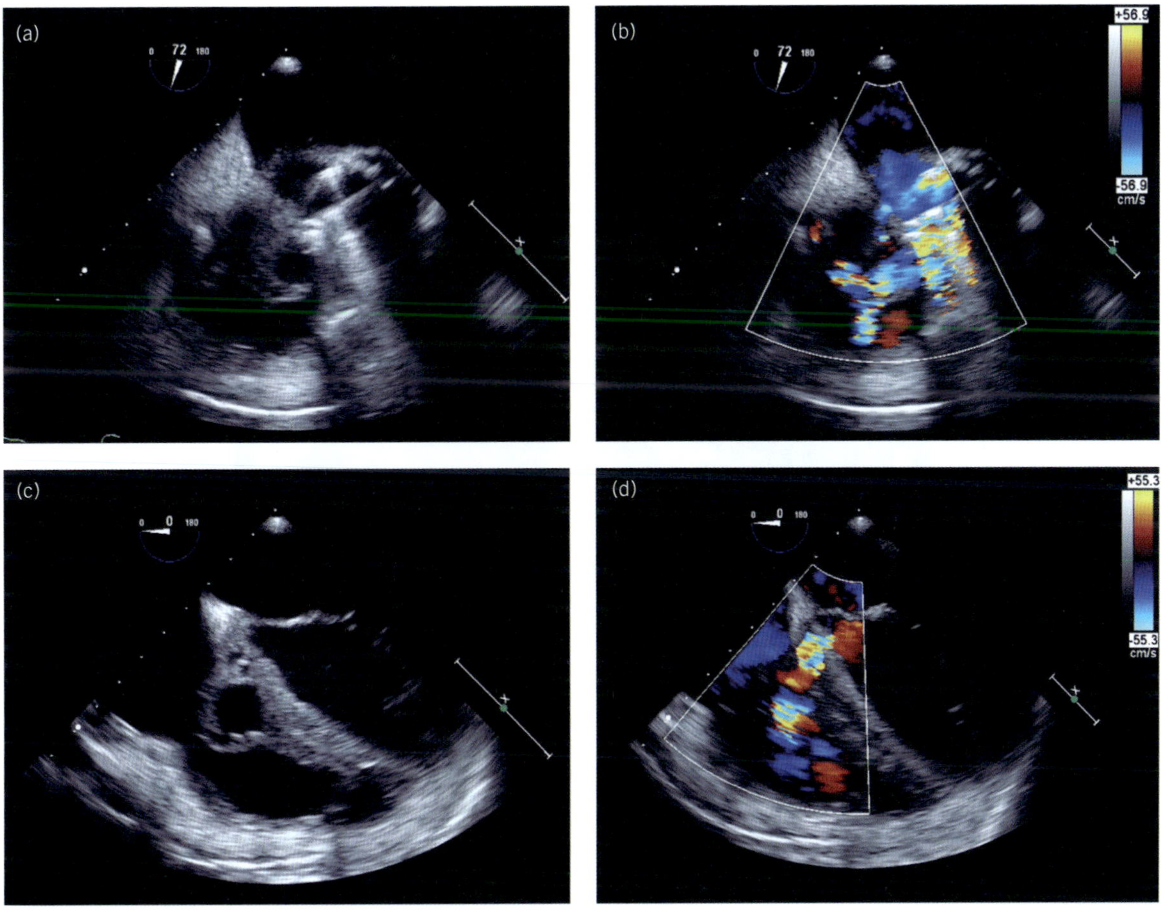

Figure 10.20 Aortic root abscess with a fistulous connection between the LVOT and the RV in a patient with a bileaflet mechanical AV replacement. Frame (a) shows a mid-oesophageal AV short-axis view in systole. The mechanical AV can be seen with associated reverberation artefact and acoustic shadowing in the far field. Abscess spaces can be seen around the valve, most notably bulging into the RV. Frame (b) shows the same view with colour Doppler imaging. A high-velocity jet can be seen passing from the abscess space into the RV. Frame (c) shows a mid-oesophageal four-chamber view. An abscess space in the region of the ventricular septum is clearly seen. (d) With colour Doppler imaging, flow can be seen between the LVOT and the RV. See also Online appendix 9.3.1.

suspected whenever there is an increased velocity within the LVOT (>1.5 m/s), peaking in *early to mid-systole*, with apparently unrestricted motion of the AV leaflets on 2D examination. Echocardiography is ideally suited to diagnose fixed SAS, to define the anatomy of the subaortic tissue, and to determine the haemodynamic impact of the lesion.

Colour Doppler showing aliasing in the LVOT in the absence of turbulence in the proximal aorta also suggests the diagnosis of SAS. The gradient across the subaortic obstruction may be measured with CW Doppler from a transgastric window. Unlike valvular AS, alignment of the beam may sometimes be challenging. Intraoperative TOE can guide the surgeon to the site of the stenosis, the degree of resection required, and the adequacy of repair. Following resection, it is important to rule out any residual obstruction, VSD, or valvular regurgitation.

Multiple choice questions

Discover interactive multiple choice questions to test your knowledge on this chapter by searching for this book's title or ISBN (9780198873686) at **https://academic.oup.com/** and going to the online appendix at the end of the book. Use your scratch-off code on the inside cover to access the material.

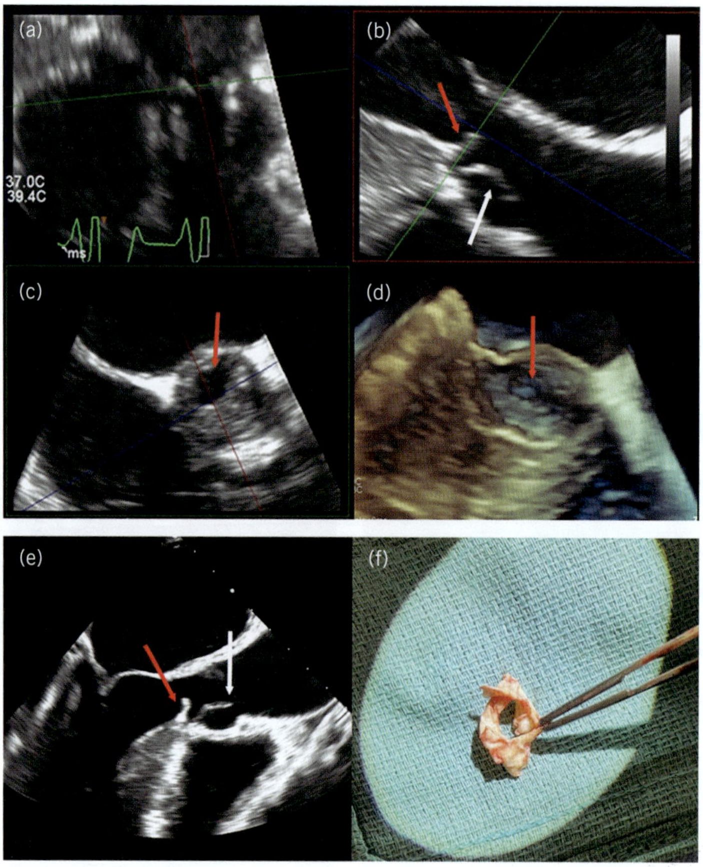

Figure 10.21 Subaortic membrane. This composite image shows a subaortic membrane. Frames (a), (b), and (c) show a 3D MPR of the AV. With the long-axis planes (frames (a) and (b)) aligned with the LVOT, the short-axis plane (frame (c)) shows a subaortic membrane with a narrow opening. Frame (d) is a volume-rendered image of the LVOT from the ventricular aspect, showing the same membrane with its opening. Frame (e) is a 2D mid-oesophageal long-axis view. In all frames, the red arrows point to the subaortic membrane, and the white arrows point to the RCC. Frame (f) shows the membrane after being surgically removed from the patient.

References

1. Charitos EI, Sievers HH. Anatomy of the aortic root: implications for valve-sparing surgery. *Ann Cardiothorac Surg*.2013;**2**:53–6.
2. El Khoury G, de Kerchove L. Principles of aortic valve repair. *J Thorac Cardiovasc Surg*.2013;**145**:S26–9.
3. Lang RM, Badano LP, Mor-Avi V, *et al.* Recommendations for cardiac chamber quantification by echocardiography in adults: an update from the American Society of Echocardiography and the European Association of Cardiovascular Imaging. *J Am Soc Echocardiogr*.2015;**28**:1–39 e14.
4 Hagendorff A, Evangelista A, Fehske W, Schafers H-J. Improvement in the assessment of aortic valve and aortic aneurysm repair by 3-dimensional echocardiography. *JACC CardiovascImaging*2019;**12**(11 Pt 1):2225–44.
5. Siu SC, Silversides CK. Bicuspid aortic valve disease. *J Am Coll Cardiol*.2010;**55**:2789–800.
6. Sievers HH, Schmidtke C. A classification system for the bicuspid aortic valve from 304 surgical specimens. *J Thorac Cardiovasc Surg*.2007;**133**:1226–33.
7. Michelena HI, Della Corte A, Evangelista A, *et al.* International consensus statement on nomenclature and classification of the congenital bicuspid aortic valve and its aortopathy, for clinical, surgical, interventional and research purposes. *Eur J Cardiothorac Surg*. 2021;**60**(3):448–76.
8. Otto CM, Nishimura RA, Bonow RO, *et al.* 2020 AHA/ACC Guideline for the management of patients with valvular heart disease: a report of the American College of Cardiology/ American Heart Association Joint Committee on Clinical Pratice Guidelines. *Circulation*.2021;**143**:72–227.
9. Baumgartner H, Hung J, Bermejo J, *et al.* Echocardiographic assessment of valve stenosis:afocus update from the EACVI and the ASE. *J Am Soc Echocardiogr*.2017;**30**:372–92.
10. Machida T, Izumo M, Suzuki K, *et al.* Value of anatomical aortic valve area using real-time three-dimensional transoesophageal echocardiography in patients with aortic stenosis: a comparison between tricuspid and bicuspid aortic valves. *Eur Heart J Cardiovasc Imaging*.2015;**16**:1120–8.
11. Whitener G, McKenzie J, Akushevicj I, *et al.* Discordance in grading methods of aortic stenosis by pre-cardiopulmonary bypass transesophageal echocardiography. *AnesthAnalg*2016;**122**:953–8.

12. Zoghbi WA, Adams D, Bonow RO, *et al.* Recommendations for noninvasive evaluation of native valvular regurgitation. A report from the American Society of Echocardiography developed in collaboration with the Society for Cardiovascular Magnetic Resonance. *J Am Soc Echocardiogr.* 2017;**30**:303–71.
13. Arnaoutakis GJ, Sultan I, Siki M, Bavaria JE. Bicuspid aortic valve repair: systematic review on long-term outcomes. *Ann Cardiothorac Surg.*2019;**8**:302–12.
14. Lancellott iP, Tribouilloy C, Hagendorff A, *et al.* Recommendations for the echocardiographic assessment of native valvular regurgitation: an executive summary from the European Association of Cardiovascular Imaging. *Eur Heart J Cardiovasc Imaging.*2013;**14**:611–44.
15. Yanagi Y, Kanzaki H, Yonezawa R, *et al.* Diagnostic value of vena contracta area measurement using three-dimensional transesophageal echocardiography in assessing the severity of aortic regurgitation. *Echocardiography.* 2021;**38**:1307–13.
16. Sato H, Ohta T, Hiroe K, *etal.* Severity of aortic regurgitation assessed by area of vena contracta: a clinical two-dimensional and three-dimensional color Doppler imaging study. *Cardiovasc Ultrasound.*2015;**13**:24–30.
17. Sato Y, Kawazoe K, Nasu M, Hiramori K. Clinical usefulness of the proximal isovelocity surface area method using echocardiography in patients with eccentric aortic regurgitation. *J Heart Valve Dis.*1999;**8**:104–11.
18. Devabhaktuni SR, Chakfeh E, Malik AO, *et al.* Subvalvular aortic stenosis: a review of current literature. *Clin Cardiol.* 2018;**41**:131–6

11

Aortic valve repair

For decades, AV replacement with mechanical or biological valve prostheses was the standard of care for all types of severe AV pathology. More recently, AV repair has become increasingly common for treating selected patients with AR and/or aortic root aneurysm. This development was driven by the potential advantages of AV repair over replacement. Valve repair usually obviates the need for lifelong anticoagulation, which makes the procedure attractive for young patients with physically active lifestyles. Compared to bioprosthetic valve replacement, valve repair potentially affords greater freedom from reoperation, especially in young patients, as degeneration of bioprosthetic valves is strongly age-related. For instance, in one series, freedom from reoperation due to structural deterioration of the Carpentier–Edwards pericardial bioprosthesis at 15 years was 89.4% for patients aged 65–75 years, but only 34.7% for patients aged <65 years.[1] By contrast, long-term outcome data for tricuspid AV repair showed freedom from reoperation rates of 88% after 5 years and of 73% after 10 years, with survival of 77% after 10 years and 57% after 15 years, respectively.[2] Additional potential benefits of AV repair are low rates of endocarditis, low thromboembolic risk, and the potential for the repaired valve to grow with the patient. There are also downsides to AV repair. Repair procedures are much more technically demanding than conventional AV replacement, and careful patient selection based on a thorough understanding of valvular morphology is essential for superior patient outcome. Echocardiography in general—and TOE in particular—plays an essential role in the preoperative evaluation of suitability for AV repair. Following surgery, TOE is also very important for assessing the reconstructed valve.

Patient selection for AV repair

Indications for surgical intervention for AR are discussed in Chapter 10. Published guidelines include AV repair as an alternative, when performed by experienced surgeons, in specialized centres and in selected patients, although it is noted that valve replacement remains the standard procedure in the majority of patients with AR.[3] While AV repair is occasionally performed for mixed stenosis and regurgitation, the great majority of AV repair procedures are performed in patients with severe AR, alone or in combination with aortic aneurysm surgery. AV repair is included in surgical procedures addressing aneurysms of the aortic root and ascending aorta, as valve-sparing root replacement is recommended for AR with significant aortic root dilatation and normal cusp motion.[3] Guidelines recommend surgery for asymptomatic aneurysms of the ascending thoracic aorta if the dimension of the aorta or sinuses of Valsalva measures ≥5.5 cm, but this is lowered to ≥5.0 cm in patients undergoing cardiac surgery for other indications, including AV surgery, and to ≥4.5 cm with experienced surgeons in a multidisciplinary aortic team.[4]

The most common causes of AR amenable to repair include aortic root dilatation, AV cusp prolapse, bicuspid AV, and endocarditis. Successful AV repair requires sufficient valve cusp tissue to achieve leaflet coaptation and/or a correctable pathology of the aortic root. More details can be found in these recent reviews.[5,6]

Anatomical considerations

The anatomy of the aortic root is outlined in Chapter 10 and illustrated in Figures 10.1 and 10.2. The plane connecting the nadirs of this crown-shaped line marks the basal aortic annulus, which is not an anatomical structure per se and is not synonymous with the ventriculo-aortic junction (VAJ).[7] The term 'functional aortic annulus' is used by some authors to encompass the VAJ, sinotubular junction (STJ), and anatomic crown-shaped leaflet insertion.[8] AR results from either dilatation of the functional aortic annulus or from abnormal AV cusp function.

Mechanisms of AR

Two systems of classifying AR are commonly used to help guide AV repair: (1) the 'functional' classification introduced

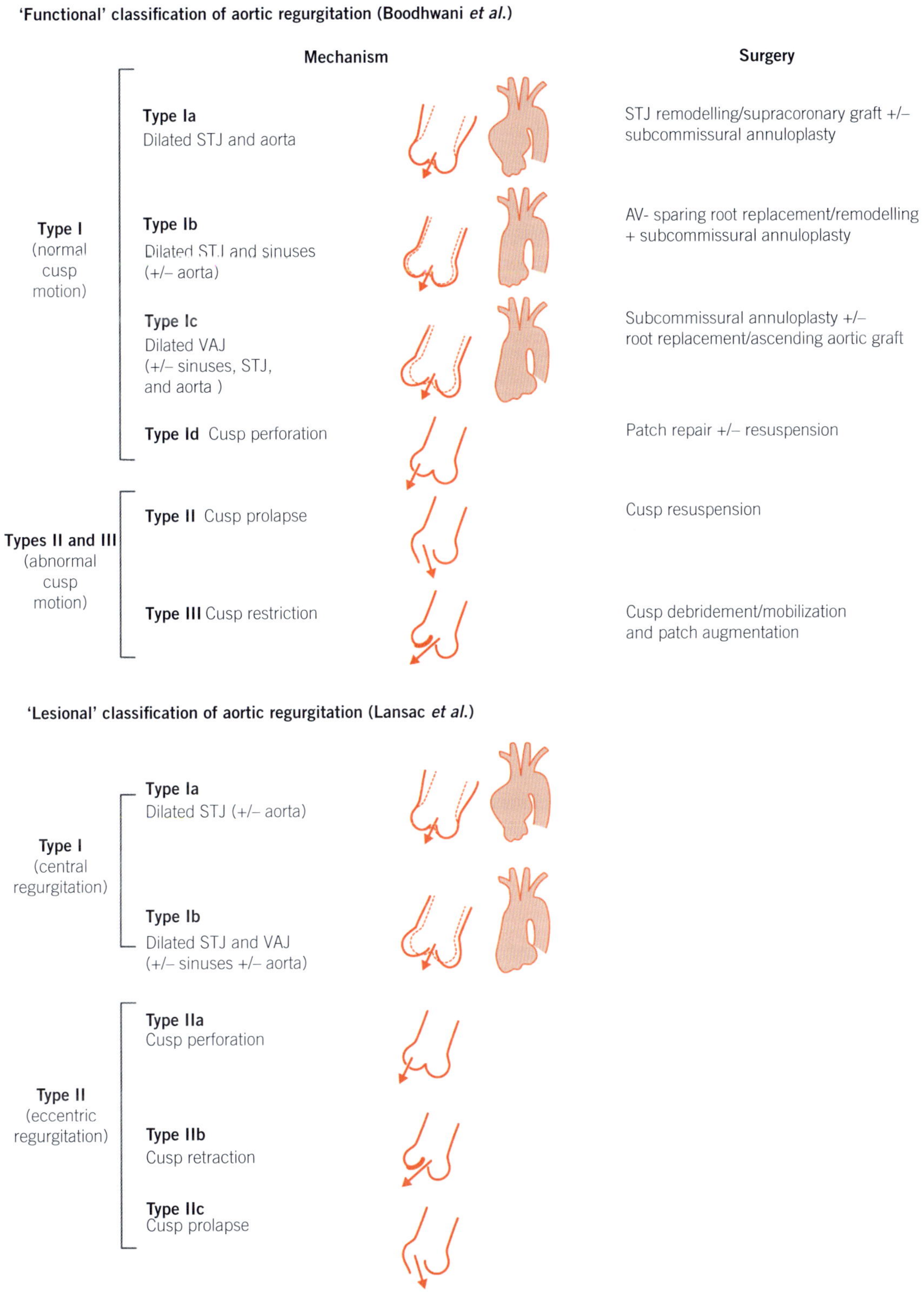

Figure 11.1 Classifications of AR.

Data from Boodhwani M, de Kerchove L, Glineur D, Poncelet A, Rubay J, Astarci P, *et al.* Repair-oriented classification of aortic insufficiency: impact on surgical techniques and clinical outcomes. *J Thorac Cardiovasc Surg.* 2009;**137**:286–94; Data from Lansac E, Di Centa I, Raoux F, Al Attar N, Acar C, Joudinaud T, *et al.* A lesional classification to standardize surgical management of aortic insufficiency towards valve repair, *European Journal of Cardiothoracic Surgery.* 2008;**33**:872–78.

by Boodhwani and colleagues;[9] and (2) the 'lesional' classification introduced by Lansac and colleagues.[10] The functional system is loosely based on the Carpentier classification used for MR, and the regurgitation mechanism is classified according to leaflet motion: normal (type I); prolapsing (type II); or restricted (type III). Type I (normal motion) is further divided into four subgroups, based on pathology of the aortic root. Specific primary and secondary repair techniques are assigned to each type. With the lesional system, the regurgitation mechanism is classified according to jet direction, as central (type I) or eccentric (type II). Again, each group is subclassified and specific surgical strategies are assigned to each subgroup. Both classifications are illustrated in Figure 11.1.

While distinct, the two classifications describe similar mechanisms of AR. Thus, *central* AR tends to be associated with normal leaflet motion and arises due to dilatation of the aortic root. Repair usually involves surgical remodelling to restore normal aortic root geometry. By contrast, *eccentric* regurgitation is usually associated with abnormal leaflet motion and arises due to cusp abnormalities (prolapse, restriction/retraction, perforation). Surgical repair is directed at restoration of normal cusp motion and function. Not infrequently, more than one mechanism of regurgitation is present in a given patient. In particular, asymmetric aortic root aneurysms frequently cause single-leaflet strain, causing tears of the free leaflet margin, with resulting leaflet prolapse.

In addition to determining the repair technique, these classification systems facilitate explicit communication between the echocardiographer and the surgeon, and they help to stratify the likelihood of a successful outcome. For instance, in one study, reparability was >90% in patients with functional type I (dilated aortic root) and type II (cusp prolapse) defects, but only 50% in patients with functional type III (restricted motion) defects.[11] Restricted cusp motion, along with a bicuspid anatomy, are consistently associated with lower rates of successful repair, compared to other pathologies.[9,12]

The functional classification, being more commonly used, will be used throughout the remainder of this chapter.

Examination of the AV prior to repair

A comprehensive TOE examination should be performed on all patients, with a special focus on the anatomic structure, dimensions, and function of the entire aortic root and each valve cusp.[13] All components of the AV function as one unit, and each one must be evaluated for its contribution to the overall valve dysfunction and its consideration in the surgical repair. The goal is to accurately characterize the mechanism, location, and severity of the regurgitation and to obtain precise measurements that will assist the surgeon in repairing the valve. Specific questions that must be addressed on the pre-repair examination are presented in Table 11.1.

The short- and long-axis views of the AV are the primary 2D imaging planes, and measurements are generally acquired from leading edge to leading edge. One major limitation of 2D imaging lies in the risk of inadvertently measuring oblique planes, with consequent under- or overestimation of dimensions. Another limitation of 2D imaging is

Table 11.1 Pre-repair 2D and 3D TOE examination

Value structure and function	Findings
Aortic root geometry	• Normal • Dilated (location) • Measurements (VAJ, sinuses of Valsalva, STJ, ascending aorta)
Number of cusps	• Tricuspid • Bicuspid • (Unicuspid, quadricuspid)
Cusp morphology	• Normal • Thickened • Calcified • Free margin (pliable or stiff) • Perforation (precise location) • Vegetation(s) (number, precise location, extension, leaflet destruction)
Cusp mobility	• Normal • Prolapsing (flail, complete, partial, precise location) • Restricted (systole, diastole, precise location)
Cusp coaptation	• Coaptation height • Effective height • Geometric height • Precise location of reduced or absent coaptation
Regurgitation	• Number of jets • Jet direction (central, eccentric) • Jet origin(s) • Severity
Systolic flow pattern	• Laminar • Turbulent • Flow convergence zone • Transvalvular gradients/AV area (continuity method)

that, because of the fixed position of the transducer in the oesophagus, only two of the three coaptation lines can be evaluated (RCC-LCC and RCC-NCC). The LCC-NCC coaptation line can never be seen with 2D imaging (only with 3D).

3D TOE has now become a standard in many centres around the world and 3D is a key imaging modality in AV repair. Simultaneous orthogonal (biplane) views help to distinguish the left (LCC) and non-coronary cusp (NCC) in the long-axis AV view. With dynamic 3D imaging and multi-planar reconstruction, a 3D data set can be cropped and imaging planes can be freely oriented in an orthogonal relationship for optimal visualization and measurement of all valve components. The entire AV complex can then be viewed from all aspects, which is crucial to obtaining reliable measurements of the functional aortic annulus and to identifying the exact position, size, and morphology of each cusp. A recent expert opinion recommends inner edge to inner edge measurements for 3D images, based on superior border demarcation.[7]

Some limitations remain with 3D TOE, compared to 2D, as spatial and temporal resolution is lower with 3D imaging. Even with optimal image settings, artificial 'holes' sometimes can appear at the base of the thin AV cusps in diastole, caused by inadequate lateral and elevational plane resolution.

Adding colour Doppler not only provides essential information on regurgitant jet severity and jet anatomy, including its precise origin and extent, but it also shows the relationship of the AR jet to the anatomical structures of the AV complex, thus adding a functional correlation to the structural examination of the valve components. As indicated earlier, jet direction (central vs eccentric) is important. Vena contracta width (in 2D) and area (in 3D), as well as the proximal isovelocity surface area (PISA) method (if it can be obtained), are used for quantification. PW Doppler is used to assess aortic diastolic flow reversal and can be used to compare RV and LV stroke volumes (thereby estimating the AR volume). CW Doppler allows the estimation of AR severity by pressure half-time (see Chapter 10).

Aortic root

As discussed in Chapter 10, the dimensions of the aortic root (VAJ, sinuses of Valsalva (SoV), STJ) can be measured in the mid-oesophageal AV long-axis view or with a 3D data set. The VAJ is measured in mid systole, and all other measurements are made at end-diastole (see Figures 10.4 and 10.6, and Online appendix 7.3.13).[7]

In a normal-size aortic root, the STJ is 15–20% larger in diameter than the VAJ. A VAJ dimension of >25 mm and an STJ dimension of >30 mm may be used to define dilatation.[10] As noted earlier, the LVOT is not circular—being smaller in the anterior–posterior dimension than in the medial–lateral dimension. Thus, slightly larger values for the VAJ will be obtained with quantitative 3D imaging, compared to standard 2D imaging (see Figure 10.7).

Type I aortic regurgitation: dilatation of the functional aortic annulus

Type I AR results from dilatation of the functional aortic annulus. **Type Ia** involves dilatation of the STJ and ascending aorta (Figure 11.2); **type Ib** involves the SoV

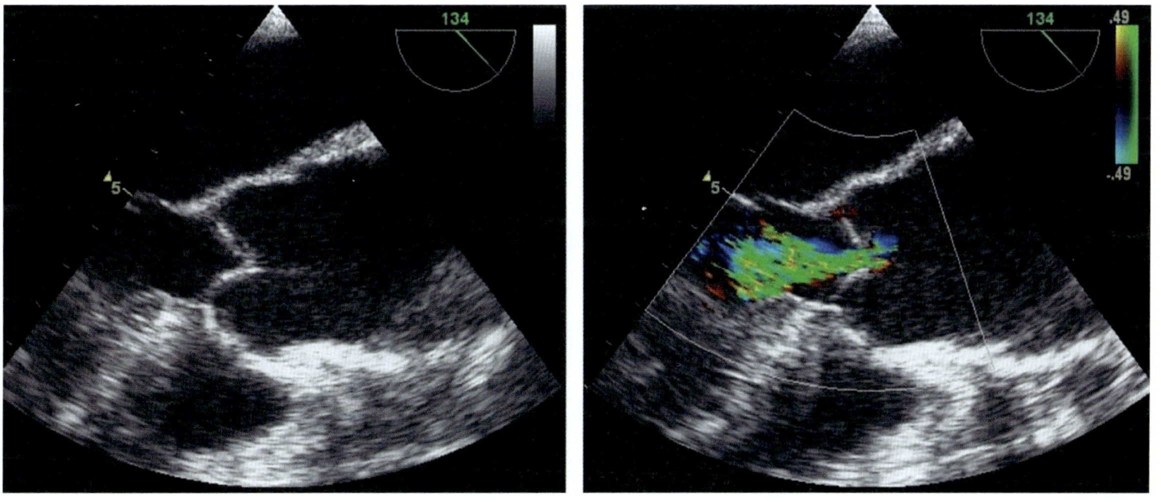

Figure 11.2 Type 1a aortic regurgitation. In this mid-oesophageal AV long-axis view, dilatation of the ascending aorta and STJ can be seen leading to reduced coaptation length and a centrally directed regurgitant jet. The dimensions of the SoV and VAJ are normal.

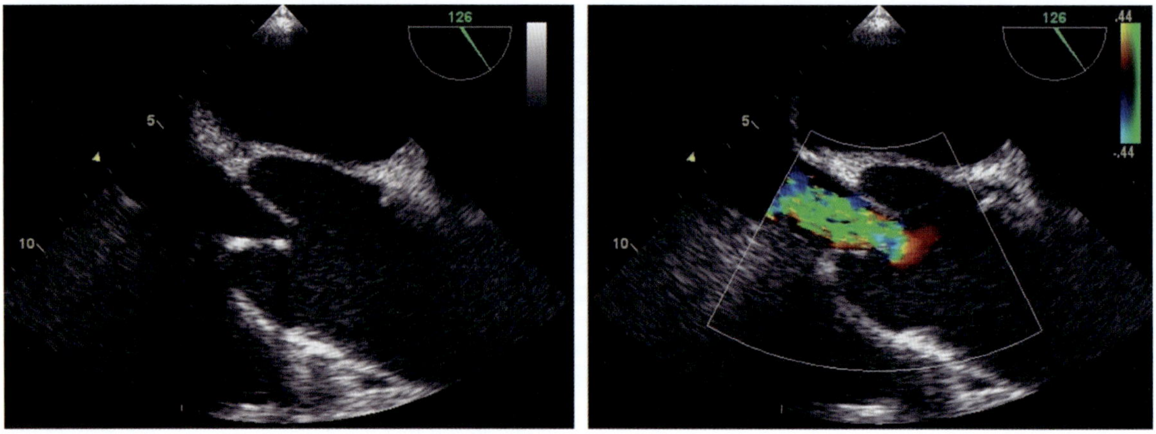

Figure 11.3 Type 1b aortic regurgitation. In this mid-oesophageal AV long-axis view, dilatation of the SoV and STJ can be seen, leading to a central coaptation deficit and a centrally directed regurgitant jet. The dimension of the VAJ is normal.

and STJ (±the ascending aorta) (Figure 11.3; see Online appendix 7.6); and **type Ic** involves dilatation of the VAJ (Figure 11.4) (±the sinuses, STJ, and ascending aorta). In all cases, the *morphology and motion of the leaflets are normal*, but they are pulled apart, resulting in a central coaptation defect, which is best seen in short axis (Figure 11.4). The regurgitant jet is usually central.

Leaflets

When assessing the AV leaflets, several factors should be considered. First, the *number of cusps* should be confirmed (see Figure 10.8 and Online appendix 7.1). Normally, a trileaflet AV is present; however, bicuspid aortic valves (BAV) can be repaired, especially in young patients. AR due to BAV frequently involves dilatation of the aortic root and ascending aorta, in addition to leaflet abnormalities. Quadricuspid and unicuspid AVs are rare, with the latter being typically unsuitable for repair.

Second, *cusp morphology* should be assessed with respect to the thickness of each cusp, abnormalities of the free margins, the presence of leaflet fenestrations or perforations, and the location and severity of any calcifications, vegetations, or thrombotic adhesions. Measuring the **geometric height** (gH) of each cusp helps to identify cusp retraction, which is an important determinant of reparability. Also called cusp height, gH is defined as the curved length of the cusp in diastole, from the aortic insertion to the central part of the free margin (Figure 11.5). It is a measure of the length of the leaflet body and the amount of tissue available for repair. The gH is

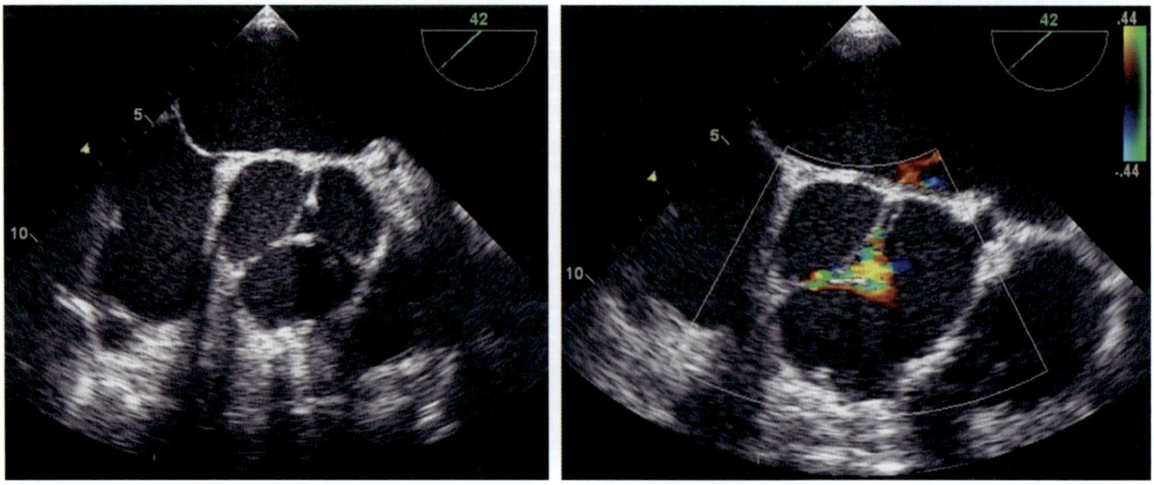

Figure 11.4 Type 1c aortic regurgitation. In this mid-oesophageal AV short-axis view, dilatation of the VAJ has resulted in a central coaptation deficit.

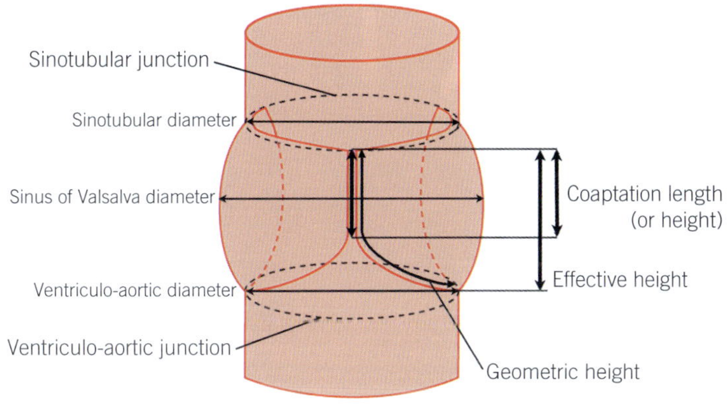

Figure 11.5 Diagram showing the various measurements made in the assessment of AV repair: coaptation length, effective height, and geometric height, as well as the various aortic root diameters.

measured directly by the surgeon at the time of the procedure, and because it is a curved measurement, it is not always easy to measure by echocardiography, but it can be done on some machines. A cusp is considered retracted when the gH is ≤16 mm in tricuspid aortic valves and ≤19 mm in the bicuspid non-fused cusp.[14]

When describing bicuspid leaflet morphology, it is useful to use standard nomenclature, such as described by Sievers and Schmidtke (see Figure 10.9).[15] It is important to assess the relative size and spatial position of the cusps, the number and location of raphes, and the origin of the coronary ostia in relation to the cusps.

Third, *cusp mobility* should be evaluated. Normal leaflet function must be distinguished from restricted motion and diastolic prolapse. M-mode imaging is useful for assessing the timing of abnormal leaflet motion.

Fourth, *cusp coaptation* should be evaluated by measuring the effective height and coaptation length. **Effective height** (eH) is defined as the orthogonal distance from the annulus (VAJ) to the middle of the free margin of the cusp, which normally measures 8–10 mm. **Coaptation length**, also called **coaptation height**, is defined as the length of cusp apposition in diastole, with a normal range of 4–5 mm[14] (Figure 11.5; see Online appendix 7.3.13).

Type Id aortic regurgitation: cusp perforation

With cusp perforation, an interruption in tissue continuity can often be detected with 2D or 3D imaging (Figure 11.6); it is possible, however, that the leaflets appear normal and the diagnosis is only confirmed when colour Doppler is

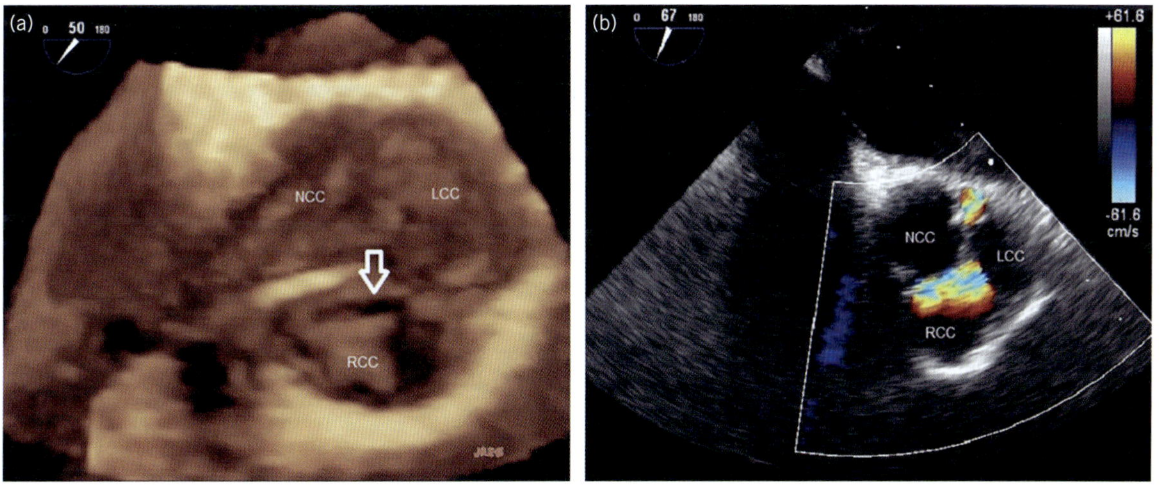

Figure 11.6 Cusp perforation (type Id AR). In (a), a 3D view of the AV is shown from the aortic aspect. A slit-like opening (arrow) can be seen close to the free margin of the RCC. In (b), colour Doppler imaging shows the regurgitant jet originating from within the RCC. In this short-axis view, it is not possible to say if the jet direction is central or eccentric. There is an additional small jet originating from the commissure between the NCC and the LCC. See also Online appendices 7.3.1–7.3.13.

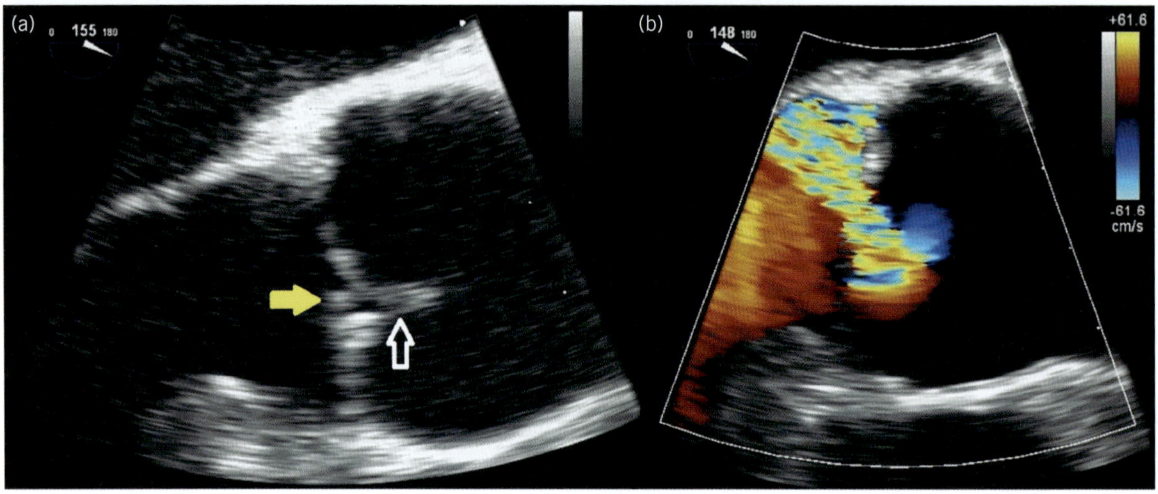

Figure 11.7 Free-edge perforation of the RCC. In these mid-oesophageal AV long-axis views, the RCC is seen at the bottom of the screen (i.e. anteriorly). The other visible cusp is either the NCC or the LCC. (a) A small defect (open white arrow) can be seen at the free edge of the RCC. A small strand of cusp tissue is seen prolapsing back into the LVOT (solid arrow). (b) Colour Doppler imaging shows a highly eccentric jet directed posteriorly.

applied. In the mid-oesophageal 2D AV short-axis view, as well as in the 3D en-face view of the AV, a diastolic regurgitant jet may be seen originating from *within* a cusp (i.e. away from the coaptation line). If the perforation involves the base of a leaflet, the jet is usually directed relatively centrally, whereas if the perforation involves the free edge of the cusp, the direction of the jet is usually eccentric (Figure 11.7; see Online appendices 7.3.1–7.3.4).

Type II aortic regurgitation: cusp prolapse

With cusp prolapse, the coaptation surface of the affected cusp(s) lies *below* that of the neighbouring cusps, resulting in a reduced or absent coaptation. The regurgitant jet is typically eccentric, directed *away from the prolapsing cusp*. If more than one cusp is prolapsing, the jet is usually orientated towards the non-prolapsing or the least prolapsing cusp. Cusp prolapse is best appreciated at end-diastole.

Three types of prolapse are recognized: flail cusp; whole cusp; and partial cusp.[11,16] With *flail cusp prolapse* (Figure 11.8), the cusp is everted, and the body and free margin of the cusp are seen in the LVOT at end-diastole. AR is usually eccentric and severe. With *whole cusp prolapse* (Figure 11.9), the cusp maintains its semicircular shape, but the entire body of the cusp lies below the VAJ in diastole. At end-diastole, the tip of the free margin of the cusp lies at the level of the aortic annulus and may be in contact with the body of the other leaflets. Regurgitation is usually eccentric and severe. With a *partial (or free margin) cusp prolapse* (Figure 11.10), the free margin of the cusp bends down towards the LVOT from the body of the leaflet, which, in short-axis view, appears as a linear fold across the body of the leaflet. The regurgitant jet tends to be less eccentric and less severe than with flail cusp or whole cusp prolapse (see Online appendices 7.3.5–7.3.12).

Type III aortic regurgitation: cusp restriction

Cusp thickening or commissural fusion leads to cusp retraction and reduced mobility. Coaptation is reduced and moved towards the STJ (i.e. the eH is increased, whereas the coaptation length is decreased). Cusp motion is typically restricted in systole and diastole, and there may be diastolic bending of the body of the cusp

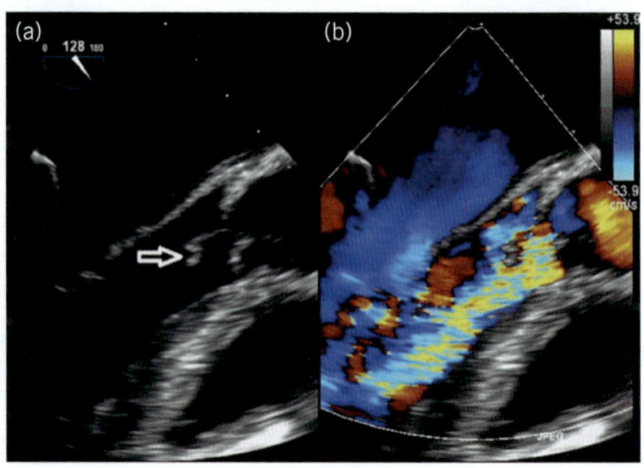

Figure 11.8 Cusp flail. In this mid-oesophageal AV view, flail of one of the posterior cusps—NCC or LCC—can be seen in (a) (arrow), resulting in severe AR directed away from the affected cusp, shown in (b).

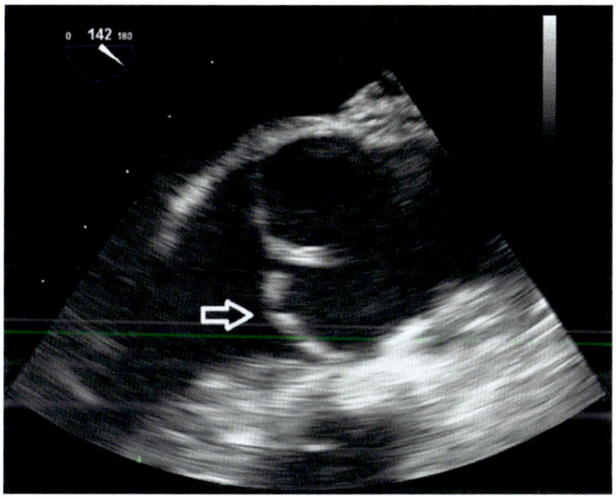

Figure 11.9 Whole cusp prolapse. In this mid-oesophageal AV long-axis view, the body and free margin of the RCC (arrow) lie below the VAJ. The cusp retains its semicircular shape, which distinguishes whole cusp prolapse from cusp flail. See Online appendices 7.3.9–7.3.12.

(Figure 11.11) (analogous to diastolic doming seen with rheumatic MV disease). The resultant jet originates from the distal end of the coaptation line and its direction is usually eccentric, towards the affected cusp, but it may also be central (see Online appendix 7.4).

Doppler assessment of valvular flow

The flow pattern across the valve should be assessed carefully by using colour and spectral Doppler imaging. During diastole, the size and direction of each individual regurgitant jet should be assessed in relation to adjacent anatomic structures, as more than one pathological process may be present. As noted previously, leaflet prolapse typically results in a regurgitant jet that is directed away from the affected cusp, whereas leaflet restriction typically results in a regurgitant jet that is directed towards the affected cusp. The severity of AR should be assessed by using techniques described in Chapter 10. Note that one should also look for systolic gradients across the valve, as the presence of concurrent stenosis makes the prospect of a successful AV repair much less likely.

Surgical techniques

Echocardiographers should have a general understanding of surgical techniques in order to interpret post-repair TOE images. However, the scope of this chapter does not allow more than a brief overview. Readers are referred to recent reviews on surgical approaches to AV repair.[8,14,17,18,19]

With type I defects, the primary problem is reduced leaflet coaptation due to dilatation of the functional aortic annulus. The goal of surgery therefore is to restore the anatomy of the aortic root and normalizing aortic root dimensions. With type Ia defects, where the STJ and ascending aorta are dilated, replacement of the ascending aorta with an appropriately sized tube graft is performed. Subcommissural annuloplasty can be added to further reduce the STJ diameter.[14] With type Ib defects, where there is dilatation of the SoV and STJ, surgical repair involves a valve-sparing root replacement with a graft and reimplantation of the coronary ostia. In type Ic defects, where dilatation of the VAJ is the primary problem,

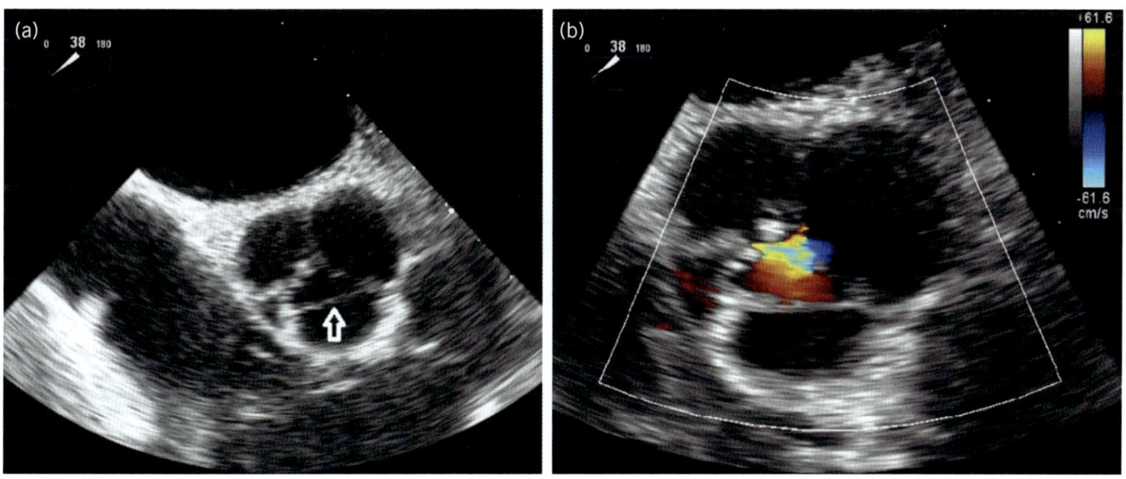

Figure 11.10 Partial cusp prolapse. In these mid-oesophageal AV short-axis views, a fold, or ridge, can be seen in (a) (arrow) along the free margin of the RCC, indicating partial cusp prolapse. In (b), the regurgitant jet is seen to originate between the fold and the free margins of the neighbouring cusps. See online appendices 7.3.5 -7.3.8 S.

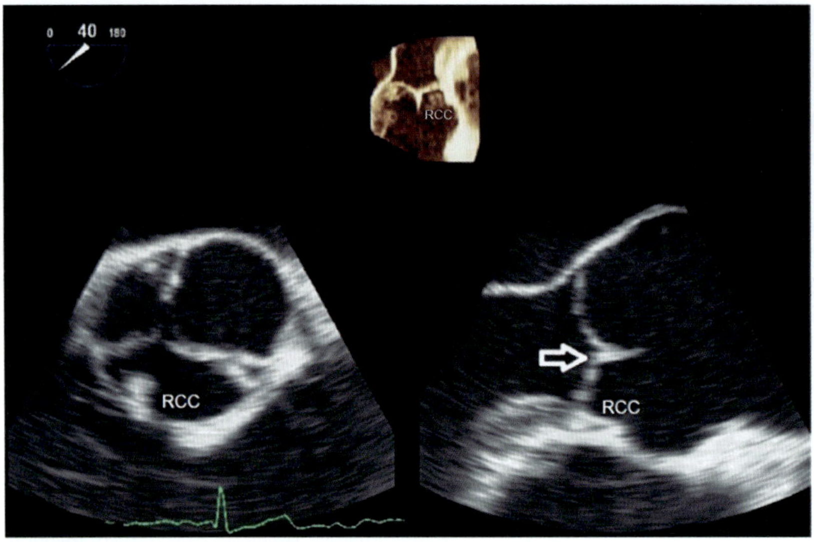

Figure 11.11 Cusp restriction. In this simultaneous multi-plane image, orthogonal views of the AV are shown. The RCC is pulled towards the STJ, creating a knee-like bend in the body of the cusp (arrow). The coaptation length is reduced, which has resulted in AR. See Online appendix 7.4.

annuloplasty is the surgical technique of choice (in the form of subcommissural sutures, suture annuloplasty, and external or internal rings). Depending on the involvement of the rest of the root and aorta, a full root replacement and/or ascending aortic graft may also be required.

In type Id defects, where AR results from cusp perforation, surgical correction involves a pericardial patch repair (Figure 11.12).

For type II regurgitation, in which there is prolapse of one or more cusps, the goal is to reduce the excess length of the free margin of the affected cusp(s) and to restore the cusp's effective height, thereby increasing the coaptation length. Appropriate techniques include central free margin plication, free margin resuspension, or triangular resection with or without patch repair. Surgical techniques to deal with restricted cusps causing type III AR involve shaving or decalcification of leaflets and/or patch repair to augment the free margin, thus restoring the geometric height of the respective cusp. Recently, the AV neocuspidization technique, initially developed as an alternative

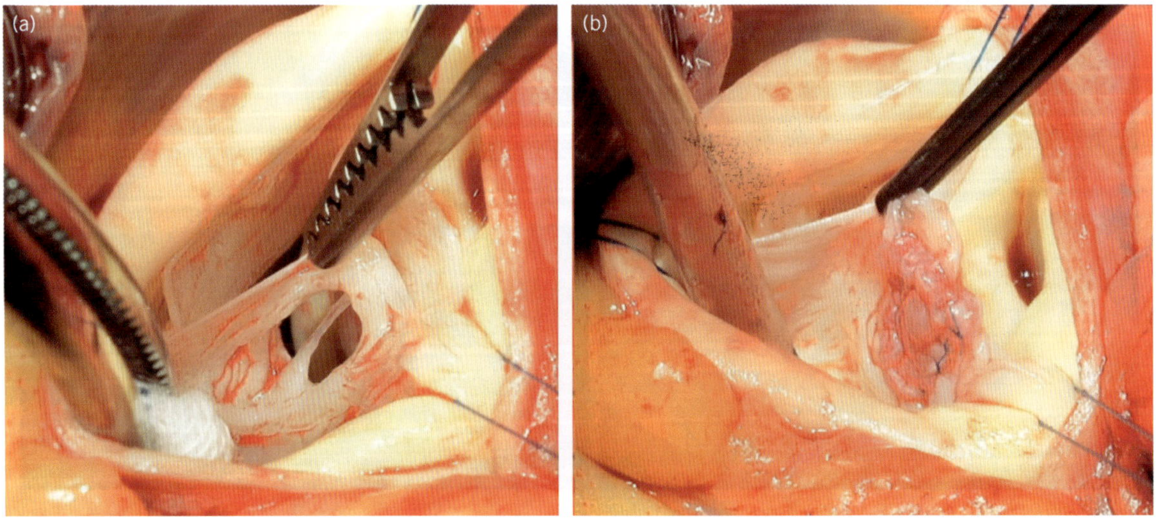

Figure 11.12 Surgical repair of cusp perforation. (a) shows a perforation near the free edge of the RCC. (b) shows repair of the defect with a pericardial patch.

to AV replacement by using autologous pericardium to construct AV cusps, has been used in AV reconstruction for single cusp pathologies. It may be potentially suitable in type Id, II, and III lesions.[20,21] It is important to remember that thickened, retracted aortic cusps are much more difficult to repair, and that both the success rate and durability of such repair are lower.

Examination following repair

A valid, definitive, and complete echocardiographic assessment of a valve repair can only be performed once the patient is completely weaned from CPB with stable haemodynamics, including normal loading conditions, cardiac output, and blood pressure. That being said, it is sometimes possible to get an echocardiographic 'glimpse' of the repaired valve at an earlier stage of the operation, to get a preliminary idea of the success of the repair. This is done by looking at the repaired AV with colour Doppler, while cardioplegia is given in a clamped and pressurized aortic root or graft. Imaging may be poor with a collapsed heart, but significant valvular regurgitation can sometimes be detected and immediately addressed prior to closing the distal aortic anastomosis. Beware that quantification of regurgitation in this setting depends on cardioplegia pressure in the root and vent uptake, which should be kept to institutional standard in order to make examinations comparable and interpretable.

The general goals of surgical AV repair are to: (1) restore coaptation; (2) maintain or restore the geometry and symmetry of the valve; and (3) avoid creating stenosis of the valve. Consequently, the post-repair examination should focus on all of the following elements: the diameter of the aortic root at all levels; the achieved coaptation length and effective height; and the presence and severity of any residual AR (Table 11.2). In addition, valve stenosis and coronary insufficiency should be excluded (see example in Online appendix 9.4).

Table 11.2 Post-repair 2D and 3D TOE examination

Value structure and function	Findings
Root geometry	• Measurements (VAJ, sinuses of Valsalva, STJ, ascending aorta)
Leaflets	• Morphology • Mobility • Effective height (above or below the VAJ) • Coaptation height (> or <4 mm) • Geometric height
Aortic regurgitation	• Any residual regurgitation? • Number of jets • Central versus eccentric • Jet origin (central, coaptation zone between two cusps, through cusp) • Severity
Systolic flow	• Proximal flow convergence zone? • Mean gradient (<15 mmHg) • Peak gradient (<30 mmHg) • AV area by continuity if gradients high
Coronary artery flow	• Flow in proximal left and right coronary arteries • New wall motion abnormalities?

Effective height and coaptation length

Effective height refers to the height above the VAJ at which coaptation occurs, and it is measured from the plane of the VAJ to the highest central coaptation point (Figure 11.5; see Online appendix 7.3.13). Ideally, the coaptation should be well above the VAJ in the central portion of the aortic root, with a minimum **effective height of >8 mm**. A low effective height, particularly if the entire coaptation surface lies below the VAJ (negative effective height with persisting cusp prolapse below the basal annulus) is predictive of recurrence of AR.[11,15,22,23] In one study, the presence of the coaptation surface below the VAJ following repair was associated with a recurrence rate of severe AR of 71% at a median follow-up of 18 months.[11] Coaptation length (or height) refers to the extent of the coaptation surface (Figure 11.5) and ideally should be **>4 mm**. In the same study, a coaptation length of <4 mm, in combination with residual AR, was associated with the development of severe regurgitation at follow-up in 47% of patients.[11] With 2D TOE, effective height and coaptation length are measured in the mid-oesophageal AV long-axis view at end-diastole. This view makes it possible to assess the coaptation between the right coronary cusp (RCC) (anteriorly) and the NCC or LCC (posteriorly). Coaptation length should be measured for all three pairs of cusps (RCC/LCC, RCC/NCC, NCC/LCC). Only with 3D multiplanar reconstruction can the coaptation between the LCC and the NCC be visualized (Figure 11.13).

Residual regurgitation

Residual AR should be described in terms of location, mechanism, and severity, using a combination of 2D, 3D, and colour Doppler imaging.

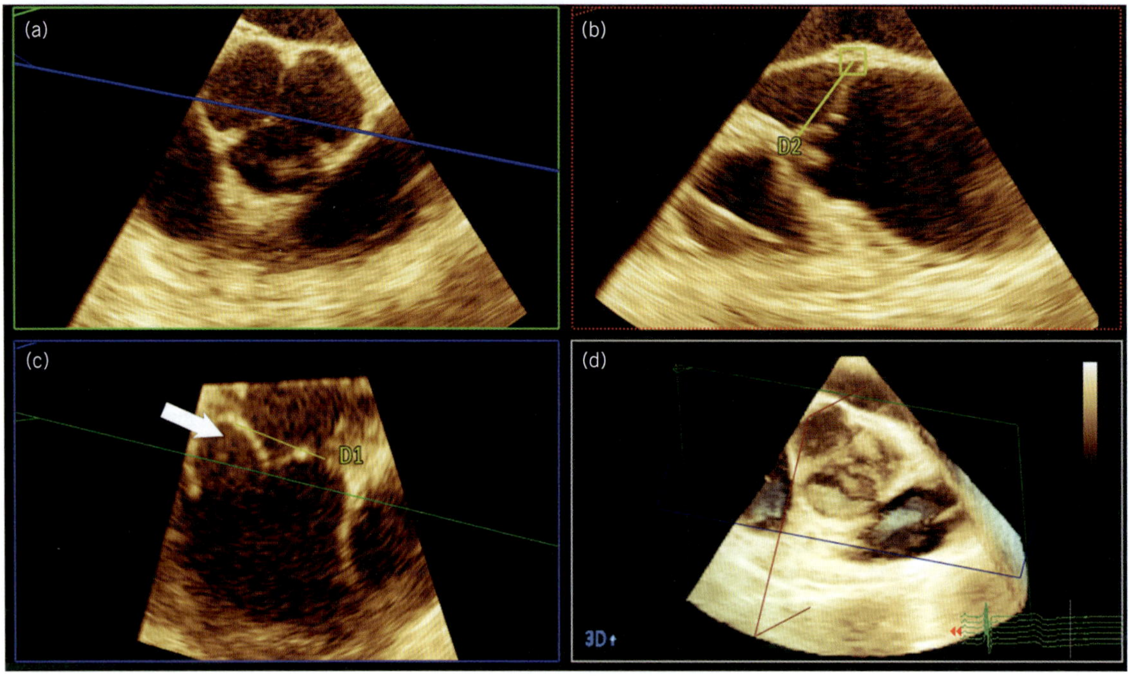

Figure 11.13 3D assessment of LCC/NCC coaptation. This is a 3D MPR of the aortic valve. In this example, the blue line is set to pass across the LCC–NCC coaptation (a), and the two cusps are visible in the blue box (c). Note that because of the position of the TOE probe inside the oesophagus, (b) this view is impossible to get with 2D imaging and can only be obtained with 3D MPR (d).

With colour Doppler imaging, the number, direction, and origin of regurgitant jet(s) should be noted. Jets may originate from the commissure or along the coaptation between two cusps; they can occur through a cusp (e.g. leakage through a patch repair), or they can originate centrally. Once the origin of residual regurgitation has been determined with colour Doppler imaging, the mechanism of the regurgitation should be assessed with 2D and 3D imaging. Root geometry should be assessed by measuring the VAJ dimension, sinuses, STJ dimension, effective height, coaptation length, and geometric height (Figure 11.5). Leaflet restriction, prolapse, or the presence of a central coaptation defect should be noted. If patch repair of a leaflet has been performed, careful inspection of the repair looking for a residual defect is also indicated.

Finally, the severity of AR should be assessed, using the methods outlined in Chapter 10. Although a fully competent AV is the ultimate goal after AV repair, mild residual AR (central AR $\leq$ grade I, <3 mm vena contracta at jet origin) does not preclude a satisfactory repair and, if not associated with other abnormalities (specifically a negative effective height with coaptation below the VAJ and coaptation height <4 mm), may be considered acceptable, as progression after surgery is unlikely.[19,24]

If moderate AR is identified, a thorough evaluation of the AV looking for a surgically correctable mechanism is indicated. In the absence of a correctable problem, the decision to leave moderate AR must take into account the overall clinical situation, including the patient's age, ventricular function, and comorbidities. Severe residual AR should never be accepted.

Aortic stenosis

Overcorrection of cusp pathology or undersizing the functional aortic annulus can lead to increased gradients across the AV, particularly in the presence of a BAV. In one study, 5/41 (12%) patients undergoing repair for bicuspid AR were classified as overcorrected, defined as a mean gradient >15 mmHg or a peak gradient >30 mmHg, on pre-discharge TTE.[12] Thus, careful assessment of transvalvular pressure gradients is important following repair, particularly for patients with a BAV. If spectral Doppler assessment suggests the presence of haemodynamically significant AS, careful inspection of the valve with 2D, 3D, and colour Doppler imaging is warranted, looking for a mechanism and site of obstruction. The haemodynamic state must be considered, as transvalvular velocities are strongly influenced by stroke volume and heart rate. Calculation of the AV area by the continuity method is less affected by the patient's haemodynamic state than transvalvular pressure gradients.

Coronary insufficiency

The qualitative presence of flow in the proximal coronary arteries should be assessed by colour Doppler (see Figure 10.3) and the absence of new RWMAs should be confirmed, especially after root replacement and coronary reimplantation. Coronary insufficiency can arise from direct injury, dissection, distortion, or haematoma causing compression.

Multiple choice questions

Discover interactive multiple choice questions to test your knowledge on this chapter by searching for this book's title or ISBN (9780198873686) at **https://academic.oup.com/** and going to the online appendix at the end of the book. Use your scratch-off code on the inside cover to access the material.

References

1. McClure RS, Narayanasamy N, Wiegerinck E, *et al.* Late outcomes for aortic valve replacement with the Carpentier–Edwards pericardial bioprosthesis: up to 17-year follow-up in 1,000 patients. *Ann Thorac Surg.* 2010;**89**(5):1410–16.
2. Anand J, Schafstedde M, Giebels C, Schafers HJ. Significance of effective height and mechanism of regurgitation in tricuspid aortic valve repair. *Ann Thorac Surg.* 2023;**115**(2):429–35.
3. Vahanian A, Beyersdorf F, Praz F, *et al.* 2021 ESC/EACTS Guidelines for the management of valvular heart disease. *Eur J Cardiothorac Surg.* 2021;**60**(4):727–800.
4. Isselbacher EM, Preventza O, Hamilton Black III J, *et al.* 2022 ACC/AHA Guideline for the diagnosis and management of aortic disease: a report of the American Heart Association/American College of Cardiology Joint Committee on Clinical Practice Guidelines. *Circulation.* 2022;**146**(24):e334–482.
5. Abeln KB, Giebels C, Ehrlich T, Federspiel JM, Schafers HJ. Which aortic valve can be surgically reconstructed? *Curr Cardiol Rep.* 2021;23(8):108.
6. Schafers HJ. The 10 commandments for aortic valve repair. *Innovations (Phila).* 2019;**14**(3):188–98.
7. Hagendorff A, Evangelista A, Fehske W, Schafers HJ. Improvement in the assessment of aortic valve and aortic aneurysm repair by 3-dimensional echocardiography. *JACC Cardiovasc Imaging.* 2019;**12**(11 Pt 1):2225–44.
8. El Khoury G, de Kerchove L. Principles of aortic valve repair. *J Thorac Cardiovasc Surg.* 2013;**145**(3 Suppl): S26–9.
9. Boodhwani M, de Kerchove L, Glineur D, *et al.* Repair-oriented classification of aortic insufficiency: impact on surgical techniques and clinical outcomes. *J Thorac Cardiovasc Surg.* 2009;**137**(2):286–94.
10. Lansac E, Di Centa I, Raoux F, *et al.* A lesional classification to standardize surgical management of aortic insufficiency towards valve repair. *Eur J Cardiothorac Surg.* 2008;**33**(5):872–8; discussion 878–80.
11. Le Polain de Waroux JB, Pouleur AC, Goffinet C, *et al.* Functional anatomy of aortic regurgitation: accuracy, prediction of surgical repairability, and outcome implications of transesophageal echocardiography. *Circulation.* 2007;**116**(11 Suppl):I264–9.
12. Pettersson GB, Crucean AC, Savage R, *et al.* Toward predictable repair of regurgitant aortic valves: a systematic morphology-directed approach to bicommissural repair. *J Am Coll Cardiol.* 2008;**52**(1):40–9.
13. Hahn RT, Abraham T, Adams MS, *et al.* Guidelines for performing a comprehensive transesophageal echocardiographic examination: recommendations from the American Society of Echocardiography and the Society of Cardiovascular Anesthesiologists. *J Am Soc Echocardiogr.* 2013;**26**(9):921–64.
14. Lansac E, de Kerchove L. Aortic valve repair techniques: state of the art. *Eur J Cardiothorac Surg.* 2018;**53**(6):1101–7.
15. Sievers HH, Schmidtke C. A classification system for the bicuspid aortic valve from 304 surgical specimens. *J Thorac Cardiovasc Surg.* 2007;**133**(5):1226–33.
16. Van Dyck MJ, Watremez C, Boodhwani M, Vanoverschelde JL, El Khoury G. Transesophageal echocardiographic evaluation during aortic valve repair surgery. *Anesth Analg.* 2010;**111**(1):59–70.
17. De Kerchove L, Boodhwani M, Glineur D, *et al.* Cusp prolapse repair in trileaflet aortic valves: free margin plication and free margin resuspension techniques. *Ann Thorac Surg.* 2009;**88**(2):455–61; discussion 461.
18. Boodhwani M, El Khoury G. Aortic valve repair: indications and outcomes. *Curr Cardiol Rep.* 2014;**16**(6):490.
19. Ehrlich T, de Kerchove L, Vojacek J, *et al.* State-of-the art bicuspid aortic valve repair in 2020. *Prog Cardiovasc Dis.* 2020;**63**(4):457–64.
20. Amabile A, Krane M, Dufendach K, *et al.* Standardized aortic valve neocuspidization for treatment of aortic valve diseases. *Ann Thorac Surg.* 2022;**114**(4):1108–17.
21. Rios-Ortega JC, Rodriguez-Urteaga Z, Carrasco-Rueda J, Talledo-Paredes L. Attached right aortic valve leaflet causing ischemia and severe regurgitation: successful repair with Ozaki technique. *J Card Surg.* 2022;**37**(9):2916–19.
22. Le Polain de Waroux JB, Pouleur AC, Robert A, *et al.* Mechanisms of recurrent aortic regurgitation after aortic valve repair: predictive value of intraoperative transesophageal echocardiography. *JACC Cardiovasc Imaging.* 2009;**2**(8):931–9.
23. Pethig K, Milz A, Hagl C, Harringer W, Haverich A. Aortic valve reimplantation in ascending aortic aneurysm: risk factors for early valve failure. *Ann Thorac Surg.* 2002;**73**(1):29–33.
24. Stephens EH, Liang DH, Kvitting JP, *et al.* Incidence and progression of mild aortic regurgitation after Tirone David reimplantation valve-sparing aortic root replacement. *J Thorac Cardiovasc Surg.* 2014;**147**(1):169–77, 178.e1–3.
25. Schafers HJ, Schmied W, Marom G, Aicher D. Cusp height in aortic valves. *J Thorac Cardiovasc Surg.* 2013;**146**(2):269–74.

12

The thoracic aorta

Thoracic aortic pathologies often present acutely and require urgent diagnosis and management. Reliable and timely information can be obtained by TOE without the risks of radiation exposure or contrast administration, thanks to multi-plane transducers and the proximity of the oesophagus to the thoracic aorta.[1] Thus, the diagnosis and management of thoracic aortic pathologies often rely heavily upon TOE guidance. This chapter reviews the clinically relevant anatomy of the thoracic aorta, as well as the echocardiographic features and the challenges associated with image acquisition and interpretation by TOE. It also addresses the fundamental role of TOE in the prompt recognition and management of various acute aortic syndromes (AAS), including aortic dissection, intramural haematoma (IMH), ruptured ascending aortic aneurysm, penetrating ulcer, and aortic trauma.

Anatomy and echocardiographic classification

The aortic wall is composed of three layers—the **tunica intima**, **media**, and **adventitia**—and it functions both as a conduit and as a reservoir.[2] The tensile strength and distensibility of its wall accommodate the systolic pulsatile output, while its elasticity maintains the continuous diastolic forward flow. The smooth muscle cells and multiple layers of elastic lamina composing the media contribute to these aortic wall properties. The age-related decrease in the amount of elastin within the tunica media reduces the elastic properties of the aorta and increases its susceptibility to shear forces.

The thoracic aorta is divided into the aortic root, ascending aorta, aortic arch, and descending thoracic aorta (Figure 12.1).[3] The aorta originates at the bulb-shaped

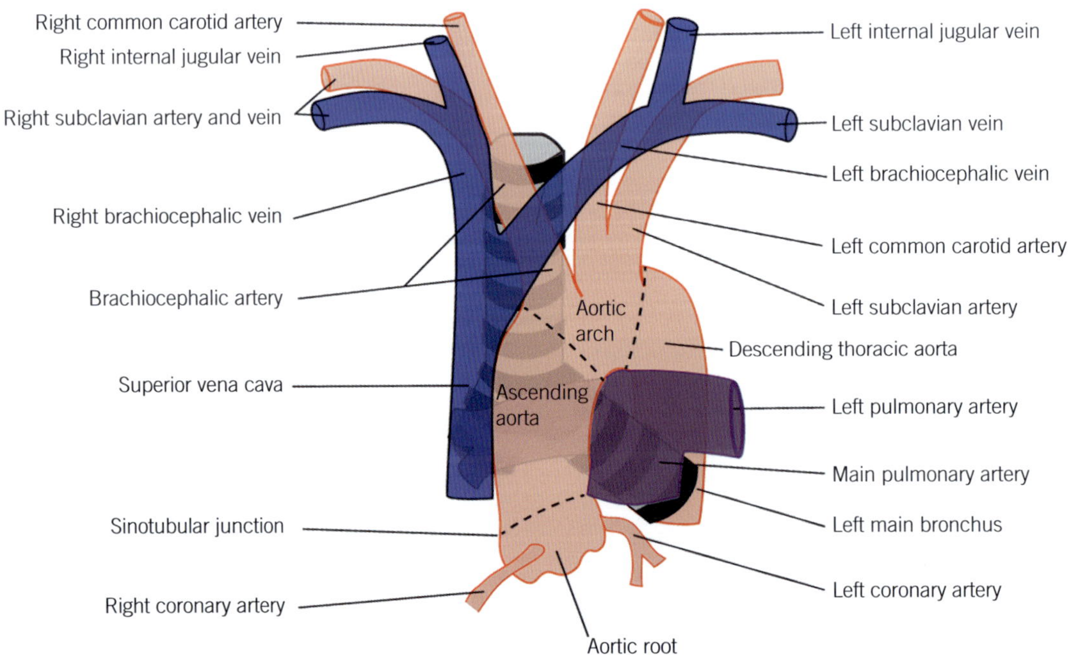

Figure 12.1 Anatomy of the thoracic aorta and related mediastinal structures.

aortic root, which includes the aortic valve (AV) annulus, cusps, coronary ostia, and sinuses of Valsalva (see Chapter 10). The **ascending aorta** begins at the sinotubular junction (STJ), passes superiorly and rightward, crosses the right pulmonary artery anteriorly, and ends just prior to the origin of the brachiocephalic (innominate) artery. The **aortic arch** includes the origin of the brachiocephalic artery and extends past the left carotid artery to include the origin of the left subclavian artery. The aortic arch lies anterior to the trachea, superior to the left pulmonary artery, and to the left of the oesophagus. The **descending thoracic aorta** may be subdivided into a proximal portion extending from the subclavian artery to the level of the pulmonary artery and a distal portion extending from the pulmonary artery to the diaphragm.

Excluding the aortic root, the thoracic aorta can be divided into six zones, corresponding to regions of potential manipulation during cardiac surgery. The ascending aorta contains **zones 1–3** (proximal, mid, and distal thirds); the arch contains **zones 4** and **5** (proximal and distal halves), and the entire descending thoracic aorta forms **zone 6**. Zone 1 is the site of aortotomy for AV replacement, zone 2 that of proximal anastomoses of coronary grafts, and zone 3 that of aortic cross-clamping, antegrade cardioplegia cannulation, and aortic cannulation. Zone 4 may also be used for aortic cannulation. Finally, the tip of a correctly positioned intra-aortic balloon pump (IABP) should be in the proximal portion of zone 6.

TOE views and thoracic aortic examination

Aortic root and ascending aorta

The aortic root and ascending aorta are best visualized with TOE in the mid-oesophageal long-axis view between 100° and 140° of transducer rotation. The image obtained corresponds to the parasternal long-axis view in TTE. The mid-oesophageal short-axis view of the aortic root is obtained between 45° and 60°, usually with some anteflexion of the probe. When evaluating the aortic root and ascending aorta, these two views are considered the most important.

Ascending aortic pathology is frequently associated with abnormalities of the aortic root. The presence of a bicuspid AV (associated with aortopathy and/or coarctation) or a dilated aortic root, and the severity of any AR should be noted. In the long-axis view, the dimensions of the LVOT, aortic annulus, sinuses, and STJ should also be measured, as described in Chapter 10. The ascending aortic short- and long-axis views are useful for identifying aortic atheroma and dissection, and measurement of the ascending aortic diameter, which should approximate that of the main pulmonary artery.[4]

Descending thoracic aorta

The descending thoracic aorta can also be visualized in both short- and long-axis views, to identify aortic atheroma, aortic aneurysms or dissections, coarctation, and left pleural effusions. From a mid-oesophageal four-chamber view at 0°, the probe is turned to the left until the descending thoracic aorta is seen in short axis as a hypocchoic circular structure. While keeping the thoracic aorta in view, the probe is withdrawn to image the upper thoracic levels of the descending aorta, and then advanced with some clockwise rotation, to image the more distal segments of the descending aorta. Visualization is possible until the probe is advanced into the stomach, at which point image degradation often occurs due to the presence of gastric air. With 3D multi-plane imaging (x-plane), the short- and long-axis views of the descending aorta can be looked at simultaneously. When using 2D, long-axis views of the descending aorta can be obtained at any of these levels by rotating the transducer 90° from the short axis. Of note, if the circular descending aorta suddenly becomes non-circular or 'oval-shaped' on short axis, this may indicate an ectatic or unfolded aorta.

Aortic arch

To obtain views of the aortic arch, the TOE probe is withdrawn from the mid to the upper oesophagus and turned clockwise to the patient's right to obtain the upper oesophageal long-axis view of the aortic arch. From this position, rotating the multi-plane angle to 90° will demonstrate the upper oesophageal short-axis view of the aortic arch. It is usually possible to visualize the take-off of the left subclavian artery, whereas the left common carotid and brachiocephalic arteries may be difficult to image. Note that the distal portion of the ascending thoracic aorta and the proximal aortic arch are usually impossible to visualize with TOE, due to a blind spot created by the interposition of the trachea (remember that air is a poor transmitter of ultrasounds and the air-filled trachea acts as a barrier).

The left subclavian artery is an important landmark that has implications in a number of clinical situations. An IABP is properly positioned when its tip is just distal to the left subclavian artery. The origin of a patent ductus arteriosus between the descending aorta and the pulmonary artery may be demonstrated by turning the probe clockwise from the origin of the left subclavian artery. In addition, the most common site for aortic coarctation and traumatic aortic injury is at the level of, or just distal to, the left subclavian artery. Finally, whether the origin of a descending thoracic aneurysm is proximal or distal to the left subclavian artery usually determines the surgical technique to repair it.

It is important to follow a systematic approach to ensure visualization of as much of the aorta as possible. When imaging the distal aortic arch and the descending thoracic aorta, it is helpful to reduce the sector depth to 5–6 cm and to carefully adjust the gain settings (gain and time-gain compensation (TGC) controls; see Chapter 2) in order to maximize resolution.

Note that although 3D TOE generally offers many advantages compared to 2D, there is currently no evidence supporting the added advantage of 3D versus 2D in the assessment of the thoracic aorta.

Normal aortic dimensions

Accurate and reproducible measurements of the various aortic dimensions are of paramount importance in establishing diagnoses and treatment strategies. In 2015, the American Society of Echocardiography published guidelines for the measurement of thoracic aortic dimensions using TOE to ensure intra- and inter-modality uniformity.[2]

Techniques for the measurement of the aortic root are described in detail in Chapter 10, and illustrated in Figures 10.4, 10.5, and 10.6. All measurements should be made from leading edge to leading edge at *end-diastole*, except for the ventriculo-aortic junction (VAJ), which should be measured in systole.

For the rest of the thoracic aorta, measurements should also be leading edge to leading edge, and the specific location of each measurement should be described in relation to other anatomic structures to facilitate subsequent comparison.[5] For example, the location of the maximum diameter of the ascending aorta can be reported with a distance from the STJ or in relation to the right pulmonary artery.

Overestimation of the aortic arch and descending thoracic aortic diameters may occur if the structures are imaged *obliquely* rather than in true cross-section. Reliability and accuracy of thoracic aortic measurements can be increased by recording three short-axis values of the segment and reporting the largest. The normal dimensions of the thoracic aorta are listed in Table 12.1.[6]

Acute aortic syndromes

TOE has several advantages over other imaging modalities in the diagnosis, clinical decision-making, and management of acute aortic syndromes (AAS). It is readily available in most centres and often less time-consuming than computed tomography angiography (CTA) or MRI when performed at the bedside. It is more invasive than TTE, CTA, or MRI, but it does not involve the use of radiation or iodinated contrast. Diagnostically, TOE has better sensitivity and specificity than TTE, but lower than CTA or MRI, especially in the detection of IMH or the location of intimal tears; on the other hand, TOE is highly effective at detecting and quantifying associated findings such as AV function, regional wall motion abnormalities (RWMAs), and the presence of pericardial/pleural effusions. Moreover, TOE provides a structural and functional assessment of the rest of the heart, which may also influence the clinical decision-making process.[7,8]

Table 12.1 Normal thoracic aortic dimensions

	Male	**Female**
Aortic annulus (ventriculo-aortic junction)	2.3–2.9 cm	2.1–2.5 cm
Sinuses of Valsalva	3.4–4.0 cm	3.0–3.6 cm
Sinotubular junction	2.9–3.6 cm	2.6–3.2 cm
Ascending aorta	3.0 cm	2.7 cm
Proximal descending thoracic aorta	2.1 cm	1.9 cm
Mid-descending thoracic aorta	2.4–3.0 cm	2.5–2.6 cm

Values for the aortic annulus: Data from Lang RM, Badano LP, Mor-Avi V, Afilalo J, Armstrong A, Ernande L, *et al.* Recommendations for cardiac chamber quantification by echocardiography in adults: an update from the American Society of Echocardiography and the European Association of Cardiovascular Imaging. *J Am Soc Echocardiogr.* 2015;**28**:1–39 e14. All other values: Data from Goldfinger JZ, Halperin JL, Marin ML, Stewart AS, Eagle KA, Fuster V. Thoracic aortic aneurysm and dissection. *J Am Coll Cardiol.* 2014;**64**:1725–39.

AAS encompass a spectrum of aortic pathologies that includes aortic dissection, IMH, penetrating aortic ulcer, and aortic aneurysm (contained or non-contained). Although these conditions share many similarities in symptoms and presentation, they vary in their pathophysiology and will be discussed separately.

Aortic dissection

Aortic dissection occurs when blood enters the media through an intimal tear, creating a false lumen and allowing blood to propagate proximally and distally. This may compromise blood flow to vital organs, including the heart.[3] Risk factors for aortic dissection are listed in Table 12.2. Two popular classification systems are the **Stanford classification** (types A and B) and the **Debakey classification** (types I, II, and III).[9] The Stanford classification is more commonly used, as it is based on the treatment strategy.[10] Stanford type A includes all dissections that involve the ascending aorta and arch, regardless of the site of origin, and such dissections require immediate surgical intervention. Stanford type B includes all dissections distal to the take-off of the left subclavian artery and most are managed medically.

Table 12.2 Risk factors for thoracic aortic aneurysm and dissection

Conditions associated with degeneration of the media	
Genetic diseases	**Inflammatory and infectious conditions**
• Bicuspid AV	• Takayasu arteritis
• Marfan syndrome	• Giant cell arteritis
• Ehlers–Danlos syndrome	• Behçet disease
• Turner syndrome	• Syphilitic aortitis
• Loeys–Dietz syndrome	• Infectious aortitis (mycotic syndrome)
• Familial thoracic aortic aneurysm dissection syndrome	
Conditions associated with increased wall stress	
• Hypertension	
• Smoking	
• Coarctation	
• Weightlifting	
• Trauma	

Data from Goldfinger JZ, Halperin JL, Marin ML, Stewart AS, Eagle KA, Fuster V. Thoracic aortic aneurysm and dissection. *J Am Coll Cardiol.* 2014;**64**:1725–39.

Apart from the obvious risk of rupture, the main complications of aortic dissection include AR, myocardial ischaemia, and cardiac tamponade when the ascending thoracic aorta is involved. In addition, distal organ malperfusion may occur at any level due to the obstruction of aortic branches by the expanding false lumen. The initial 24 hours of a type A dissection are considered the 'hyperacute' phase and represent a surgical emergency, because the risk of rupture approaches 1% per hour. If the patient survives without surgery, the mortality rate declines significantly after the first 2 weeks.[3] Therefore, the distinction between acute and subacute/chronic is based primarily on the time frame from initial symptoms to diagnosis rather than on specific echocardiographic findings, although some imaging differences exist and are discussed below.

Uncomplicated type B dissections are managed medically, but endovascular stent grafting is performed in cases where aneurysmal expansion of the aorta, contained rupture, or distal organ malperfusion are noted.

Echocardiography

TOE was shown in multicentre studies to have a high sensitivity (86–100%), specificity (90–100%), and negative predictive value (86–100%) for the diagnosis of aortic dissection.[11] Still, reported false positive rates of up to 3.5% underscore the importance of a careful, systematic TOE examination whenever aortic dissection is suspected. If the diagnosis of type A dissection was made with other imaging modalities, a detailed intraoperative TOE examination should confirm the diagnosis and carefully document the features of the dissection: origin and extent of the dissection flap, aortic dimensions, involvement of the AV, and other physical impacts of the dissection (coronary involvement, pericardial effusion, etc.).

The TOE appearance of an aortic dissection is often dramatic—the diagnostic hallmark is the presence of an oscillating intimal flap within the aorta. In the case of an ascending aortic dissection, the flap can be seen moving freely within the proximal ascending aorta and may sometimes prolapse through the AV into the LVOT, resulting in AR (Figure 12.2; see Online appendices 7.7.6–7.7.11). Such a flap usually moves towards the false lumen in systole and towards the true lumen in diastole. Of note, in chronic dissections, the dissection flap tends to be thicker, echo-dense, and less mobile. Note that reverberations and secondary lobe artefacts (see Chapter 2) may

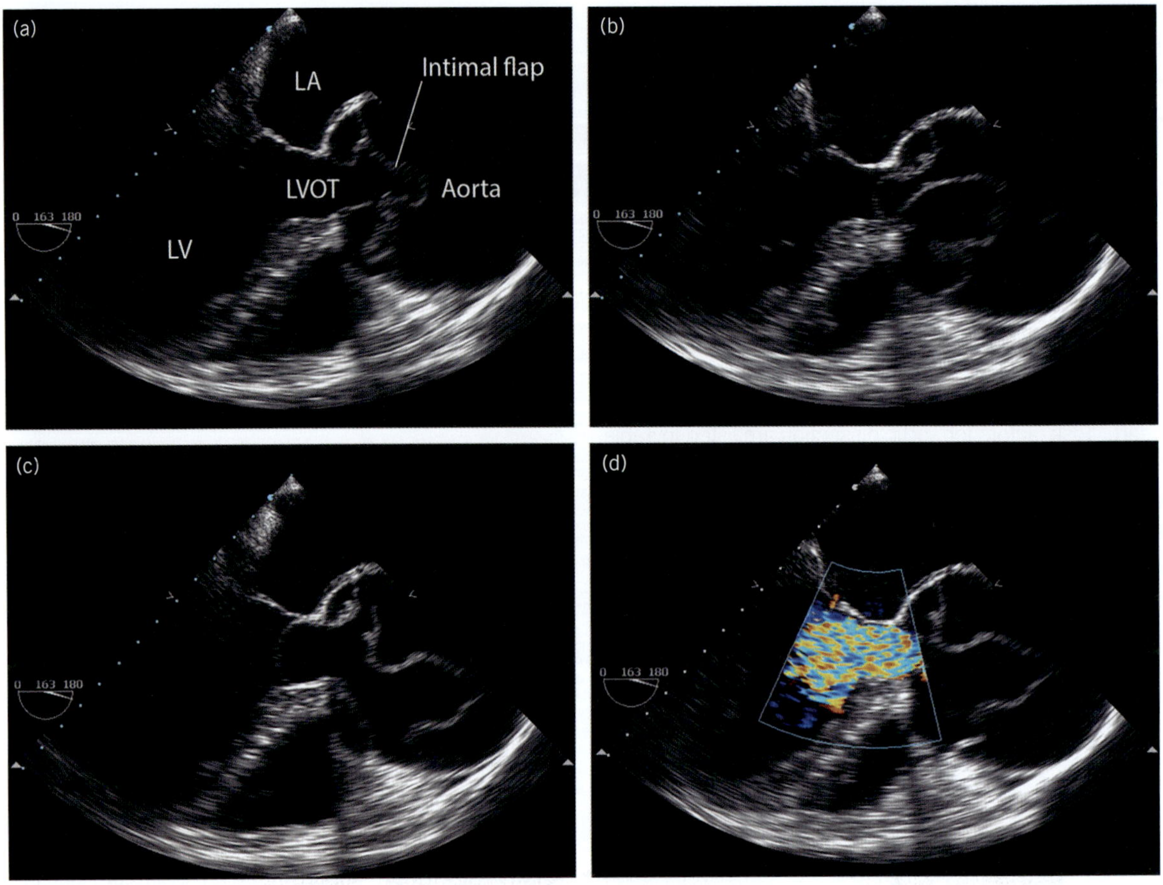

Figure 12.2 Type A aortic dissection. Frames (a) to (d) are mid-oesophageal AV long-axis views. Note the severely dilated ascending aorta with an intimal flap originating in the aortic root. The flap prolapses into the AV, causing torrential AR, shown in (d). See also Online appendices 7.7.6–7.7.11 S.

also cause linear shadows over the aorta resembling an intimal flap, and it is imperative that they be distinguished from a true dissection flap (Figure 12.3).[11]

When in doubt, a suspected dissection flap should be imaged in multiple different views, and 3D TOE can be used to further define the flap as a segment of tissue of variable thickness in the long, short, or oblique axis. A true dissection can often be distinguished from an artefact by the independent motion of the flap relative to the aortic walls (by contrast, the motion of an artefact tends to be synchronized with that of the surrounding structures causing it). Also, contrary to artefacts, true dissection flaps do not appear to pass through the aortic wall in any view.

In a true dissection, there is usually a difference in blood flow on both sides of the intimal flap demonstrated by colour Doppler, with flow usually greater in the true lumen (Figure 12.4). Finally, M-mode imaging can also be used to differentiate between true dissection flap and reverberation artefact (see Chapter 2). Salient diagnostic TOE examination criteria for the diagnosis of acute aortic dissection are listed in Table 12.3.

The primary intimal tear in aortic dissection most often occurs in one of two locations: the proximal ascending aorta (type A—most common) and the descending aorta, just distal to the left subclavian artery (type B). In the case of the ascending aorta, the tear usually originates just distal to the STJ but may originate in the root or more distally, including in the aortic arch. From its origin, the intimal flap frequently extends distally into the aortic arch and beyond into the descending thoracic aorta. The aorta should be carefully interrogated using colour Doppler to locate the site of the intimal tear, which may appear as a break in the intima with blood flow passing from the true to the false lumen. Secondary tears or fenestrations are common, resulting in multiple communications between the true and false lumen of the descending aorta (Figure 12.5; see Online appendix 7.7.15 S).

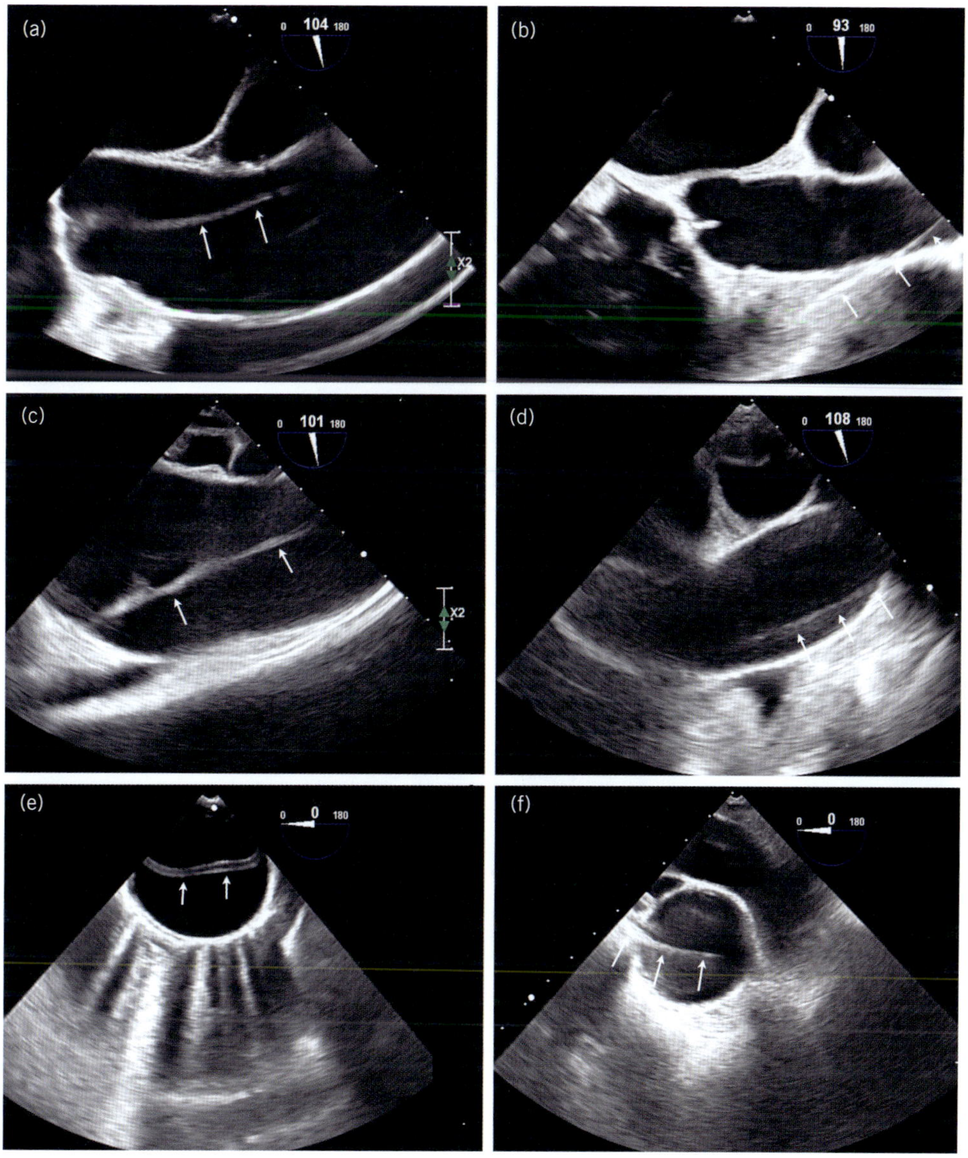

Figure 12.3 Dissection or artefact? This composite image shows three real dissections on the left (a, c, e) and three artefacts on the right (b, d, f). Panels (a) to (d) are mid-oesophageal long-axis views of the ascending aorta. Panels (a) and (c) show real dissection flaps, whereas panels (b) and (d) demonstrate artefacts that could be misinterpreted as aortic dissections. Panel (e) is a short-axis view of the descending aorta showing a real dissection flap. Panel (f) is an upper oesophageal short-axis view of the ascending aorta, showing a sidelobe artefact across the aorta. Note how in panels (b) and (f), the artefact seems to pass *through* the aortic wall, which is a clue to the artefactual nature of the image.

If the false lumen extends back into the pericardium, a pericardial effusion with some degree of cardiac tamponade may be present and is associated with a worse prognosis. Even small pericardial collections may quickly result in tamponade physiology and cause marked haemodynamic compromise. Thus, echocardiographic signs of cardiac tamponade should be sought whenever a pericardial collection is detected, regardless of its size.

AR is present in up to 50% of patients with type A dissections, and common mechanisms of AR are summarized in Figure 12.6. More than one mechanism may contribute to AR, necessitating a comprehensive assessment.

AV regurgitation secondary to prolapse of the type A dissection flap may resolve with surgical repair of the dissection, without any intervention to the valve. By

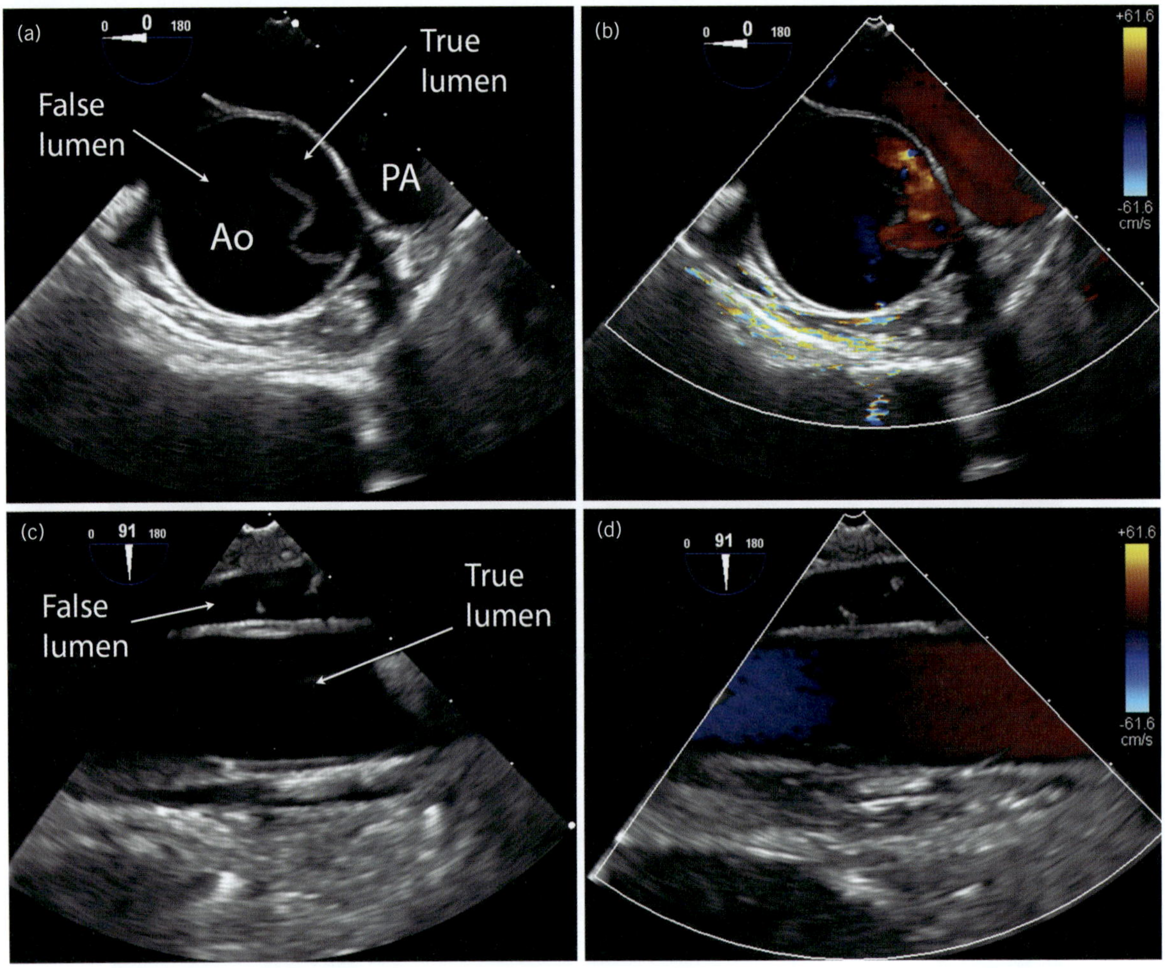

Figure 12.4 Type A aortic dissection. (a) and (b) are mid-oesophageal short-axis views of the ascending aorta, with and without colour, in mid systole. (c) and (d) are mid-oesophageal long-axis views of the descending aorta, with and without colour, also in systole. Note that in this example, the systolic flow is predominantly in the true lumen.

contrast, AR that occurs in association with pre-existing annular dilatation, morphologic leaflet pathology (e.g. bicuspid AV, calcified degeneration, prolapsed leaflets), or connective tissue disease typically necessitates a valve repair or replacement. The decision to repair or replace the AV is dictated by the AV pathology rather than by the severity of AR, and it necessitates a careful inspection of the valve and root to determine the mechanism of regurgitation. Other factors such as age and general condition of the patient also play a role in the decision.

In a minority of cases, myocardial ischaemia may occur due to the obstruction of a coronary ostium by the dissection flap or if the coronary ostium originates from the false lumen. This typically presents as a new RWMA on TOE. The coronary ostia and proximal coronary arteries can be visualized with TOE (see Figure 10.3), and the presence or absence of colour over the proximal coronaries should be documented with colour Doppler. Note that the presence of colour flow in the coronary arteries does not guarantee adequate blood flow, but it is reassuring in the absence of significant RWMAs.

Distinguishing between true and false lumen, particularly in the descending aorta, can be challenging, and Box 12.1 lists a number of features that help with this distinction. Note that none of these signs should be relied upon individually, but a combination of features will help make the correct diagnosis. This is especially critical during arterial cannulation for CPB, as inadvertent cannulation of the false lumen may result in expansion or rupture of the dissection. Thus, confirmation of the location of a guidewire in the true lumen prior to femoral or axillary cannulation is critical in patients with suspected or confirmed aortic dissection.

Table 12.3 TOE examination in acute aortic dissection

Diagnostic elements	Echocardiographic appearance
Identify dissection flap	• Intimal flap dividing true/false lumen
Identify true lumen	• Usually expands in systole • Absence of spontaneous contrast
Identify false lumen	• Often expands in diastole due to drop in true lumen pressure • Spontaneous contrast and/or thrombus formation • Reverse/delayed or absent flow
Define extent of dissection	• Extension of flap and true/false lumen in the aortic root, ascending aorta, arch, and descending aorta
Identify presence of false lumen thrombosis	• Mass inside the false lumen distinct from the intimal flap and aortic wall
Localize entry tear	• Fluttering or ruptured intimal borders • Demonstration of flow through the tear by colour Doppler
Look for presence, severity, and mechanism of AR	• Morphology of the valve (normal, bicuspid, degenerative) • Valve function o Malcoaptation (prolapse or flail) due to aortic root dilation and/or loss of annular support o Flap prolapsing into the LVOT during diastole o Severity of AR by classic TOE criteria
Assess coronary circulation	• Flap obstructing coronary ostia • Absence of coronary flow by colour Doppler • New RWMA
Assess great vessel involvement	• Flap obstructing/invaginated into great vessels
Pericardial and/or pleural effusion	• Echo-free space in the pericardial/pleural cavity • Standard echocardiographic and Doppler signs of tamponade

Adapted from *Journal of the American Society of Echocardiography*, 28, 2, Goldstein SA *et al.*, 'Multimodality imaging of diseases of the thoracic aorta in adults: from the American Society of Echocardiography and the European Association of Cardiovascular Imaging: endorsed by the Society of Cardiovascular Computed Tomography and Society for Cardiovascular Magnetic Resonance', pp.119–182, Copyright 2015, with permission from the American Society of Echocardiography.[2]

Following surgical repair, TOE examination should carefully assess: (1) the proximal and distal anastomoses of the aortic graft for leaks and patency; (2) the presence, severity, and mechanism of any residual AR (or prosthetic AV function if the valve was replaced); (3) the presence of myocardial dysfunction, including RWMAs; and (4) flow in the true and false lumen.

Repair of a type A dissection involves replacing the portion of the aorta containing the intimal tear and ensuring that there is continuous blood flow between the heart and the true lumen of the aorta distally. That usually requires an ascending aortic replacement and/or a hemi-/total arch replacement. Post-repair, secondary tears or fenestrations in the descending aorta may persist, and if flow to the splanchnic or renal vessels is compromised, further interventions (e.g. endovascular stenting) may be required.

The approach to the echocardiographic evaluation of a type A dissection can also be applied to the endovascular stent grafting of a type B dissection (see Online appendices 7.7.12–7.7.16).

Aortic intramural haematoma

Aortic IMH occurs when the vasa vasorum ruptures within the aortic media without an intimal tear (Figure 12.7; see Online appendices 7.7.1–7.7.6). Given the similarities in clinical presentation, especially when an aortic wall infarction causes a secondary intimal tear/dissection, IMH is considered a variant of, or a precursor to, aortic dissection, with similar prognosis and management.[1] TOE is superior to TTE in diagnosing IMH, which should be suspected when a circular or crescent-shaped thickening (>5 mm) of the aortic wall is visualized without

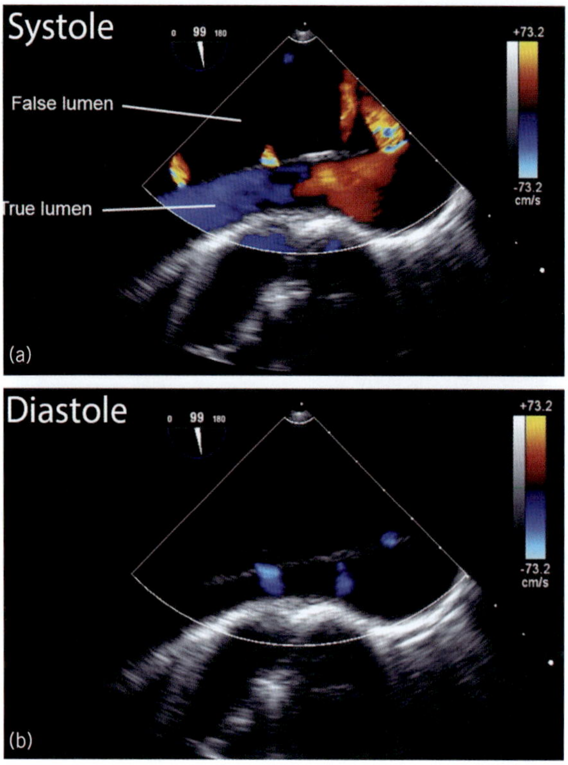

Figure 12.5 Type B aortic dissection. This is a long-axis view of the descending aorta with colour Doppler. Note the multiple colour jets representing fenestrations across the dissection flap. These jets appear red going *towards* the transducer from true to false lumen in systole (a), and blue going *away* from the transducer from false to true lumen in diastole (b). See also Online appendix 7.7.15.

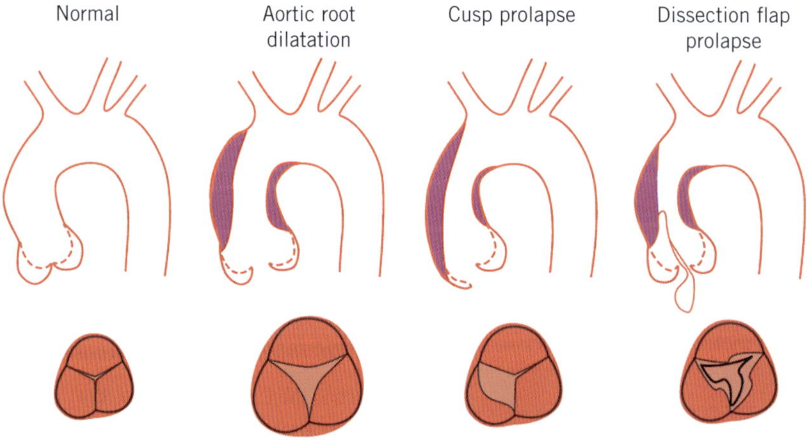

Figure 12.6 Mechanisms of AR in aortic dissection. Normally the leaflet tips coapt fully in diastole and the diameter of the STJ is similar to that of the VAJ (see Chapter 10). Dilatation of the STJ relative to the aortic annulus results in incomplete leaflet closure and a central coaptation defect with central AR. Cusp prolapse occurs when the dissection extends into the aortic root and disrupts the normal attachment of one or more of the leaflets. The resulting AR is usually eccentric. Diastolic prolapse of the intimal flap through the AV can also result in AR, which varies, depending on how the flap interferes with the normal function of the valve (see Figure 12.2).

Box 12.1 Echocardiographic features of true and false lumen in aortic dissection

True lumen

- The LV usually ejects into the true lumen
- Often circular in short axis during systole
- Usually expands in systole and contracts in diastole
- Often smaller than the false lumen
- Often normal flow pattern on colour Doppler imaging

False lumen

- Often crescent-shaped in short axis
- The intimal flap curves towards the false lumen in systole
- Usually contracts in systole and expands in diastole
- Spontaneous echo contrast or thrombus formation may be present in 2D imaging
- Reduced or sluggish flow on colour Doppler imaging

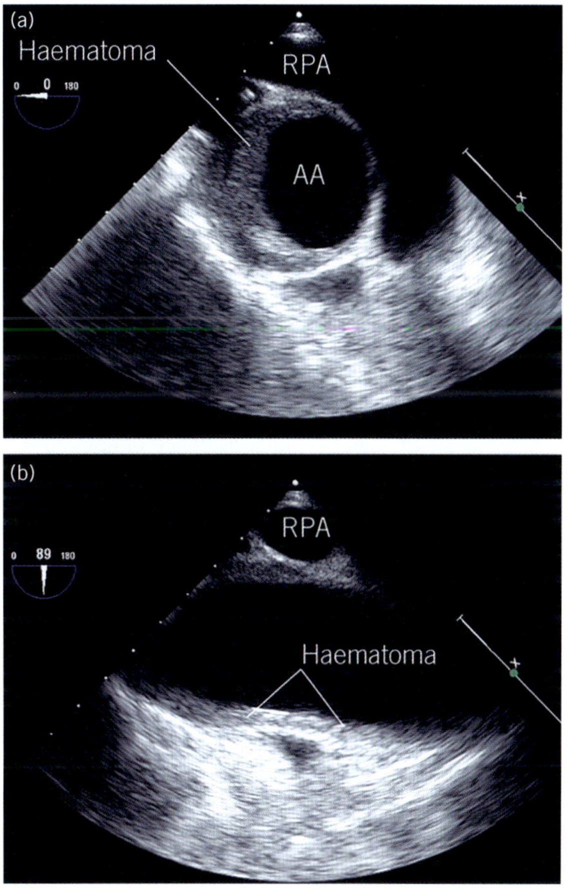

Figure 12.7 Intramural haematoma of the ascending aorta in short-axis (a) and long-axis views (b) of the ascending aorta. Note the crescent-shaped thickening of the aortic wall in the short-axis view, and the corresponding linear thickening in the long-axis view, but no intimal flap. AA, ascending aorta; RPA, right pulmonary artery. See also Online appendices 7.7.1–7.7.5 S.

blood flow.[3] IMH may be differentiated from intraluminal thrombus or dissection with a thrombosed false lumen by using the imaging features listed in Box 12.2.

Often, initial imaging yields false negative results for IMH, so if the diagnosis is suspected, serial imaging to note the progression of IMH is critical to the management strategy. Although contrast-enhanced CT scan is considered the initial diagnostic modality of choice, MRI can establish the diagnosis in acute settings when TOE or CT scan results are equivocal.[12,13]

Surgical decision-making is dictated by the major predictors of complications, including the type of IMH (type A vs type B), maximal aortic diameter in the acute phase, wall thickness, and presence of periaortic haemorrhage. In one case series, up to 34% of IMH resolved completely on serial imaging with medical management alone.[14]

Penetrating atherosclerotic ulcer

A penetrating atherosclerotic ulcer (PAU) occurs when an aortic atherosclerotic plaque ulcerates from the intima into the media.[13] A PAU is considered a disease of the intima, unlike aortic dissection and IMH, which also involve the media. It occurs predominantly in the mid to distal descending aorta, may be multifocal, and occurs more often in dilated aortas. A PAU may progress to IMH, aortic dissection, embolization of atherosclerotic debris, or aneurysmal rupture if the adventitia is breached. Depending on the location, a symptomatic PAU is managed similarly to dissection. Although TOE is not the diagnostic modality of choice for PAU, it can demonstrate an atheromatous aorta with a jagged focal ulcer, often with outpouching of the aortic wall (Figure 12.8; see Online appendix 7.7.17 S). The TOE report should include the following parameters: (1) the maximum depth of the PAU measured from the aortic lumen; (2) the width of the ulcer at the entry site; and (3) the axial length of the contained medial haematoma, if seen with TOE.

Box 12.2 Features of an intramural haematoma

1. Focal wall thickening (usually crescentic rather than concentric)
2. Preserved luminal shape
3. Smooth luminal border (contrary to irregular margins seen with atherosclerosis and penetrating ulcer)
4. Absence of dissection flap and/or false lumen
5. Presence of echolucent regions in the aortic wall
6. Central displacement of intimal calcium
7. Absence of colour Doppler evidence of communication between haematoma and true lumen
8. Usually a localized process
9. The diameter of IMH is usually smaller than the diameter of thrombosed false lumen of an aortic dissection
(often difficult to distinguish)

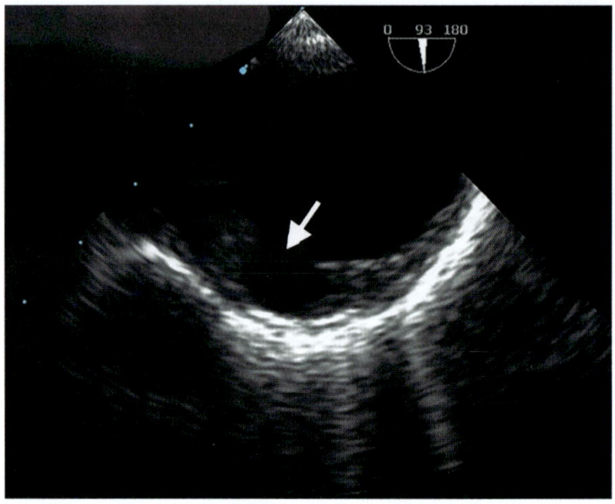

Figure 12.8 Penetrating atherosclerotic ulcer. Short-axis view of the descending aorta showing an ulcerated atherosclerotic plaque (arrow). Note the loss of the media, leaving the adventitia exposed. See also Online appendices 7.7.15–7.7.16 S.

Thoracic aortic aneurysm

Thoracic aortic aneurysms (TAAs) may involve one or more segments of the thoracic aorta, with up to 60% involving the aortic root and ascending thoracic aorta. Despite common risk factors (Table 12.2), aortic aneurysm is a pathologic entity distinct from aortic dissection, with most dissections occuring in the absence of an aneurysm.

A **true aneurysm** is defined as a focal or diffuse dilation of *all three layers* of the aorta (intima, media, and adventitia) to 50% or greater above the normal size, whereas a **false aneurysm** or **pseudoaneurysm** is a dilatation of the adventitia only, following a breach of the intima and media (in other words, it is a *contained aortic rupture*). The echocardiographic report should include diameters of the affected segments, which should be compared to threshold values and any available previous studies. Aortic diameter is the principal predictor of dissection or rupture, and at sizes ≥6.0 cm, the risk of aortic rupture or dissection approaches 7% per year versus 2% per year if <5.0 cm in diameter (see Online appendix 7.6).

Prophylactic surgical repair is based on the rate of expansion of a TAA, and contrast-enhanced CT scan provides more accurate measurements for staging and surveillance. Echocardiography can be used for routine screening of family members, serial follow-up post-diagnosis, and assessment of the presence and mechanism of AR, and to confirm suspected complications such as rupture, dissection, and thrombus formation. Ideally, serial measurements should be made by the same observer whenever possible and/or use the same anatomic references. TOE may be of particular value when surgical repair is being considered, although it may not adequately image the distal ascending aorta, proximal arch, or tortuous segments. Aside from the diagnosis of a dilated aorta, perioperative TOE is ideal to define the anatomy and function of the AV and to identify associated pathology (e.g. AR and LV dilatation).

Ascending aortic aneurysms

Aneurysms of the aortic root and ascending aorta require open surgical repair. Indications include an ascending aortic/sinus of Valsalva diameter ≥5.5 cm or a growth rate >0.5 cm/year.[15,16] Patients with connective tissue disease (e.g. Marfan syndrome) or other genetic disorders (e.g. bicuspid AV, Turner syndrome) should undergo repair at smaller diameters (4.0–5.0 cm). Concomitant thoracic aortic replacement should also be considered in patients undergoing AV surgery if the ascending aorta/aortic root diameter is >4.5 cm.

The echocardiographic assessment and surgical treatment of aortic aneurysms associated with aortic root pathology are discussed in Chapters 10 and 11. Large aneurysms of the ascending aorta typically distort the position of the heart in the chest cavity, resulting in non-standard mid-oesophageal views. While the dimensions and morphology of the aortic root can usually be accurately assessed with TOE, ascending aortic measurements are frequently unreliable due to poor image quality and oblique imaging. As previously noted, off-axis imaging in the ascending aortic long-axis view can lead to the aortic diameter being underestimated. Additionally, as the aortic root is not directly aligned with the ascending aorta (which curves superiorly and rightwards), the optimal long-axis views to measure the ascending aortic root dimensions may differ and 3D multi-plane imaging may be of benefit.

Following surgical repair, it is important to carefully assess AV function (particularly if the AV has been resuspended), ventricular function, and RWMAs, particularly if the coronary arteries were reimplanted as part of a Bentall procedure.

Sinus of Valsalva aneurysm

Sinus of Valsalva aneurysms are rare, most commonly affecting the right coronary sinus, and manifest as a saccular dilatation projecting into the RA or RVOT. Aetiology is often congenital but can also be acquired through medial degeneration of the aortic wall (e.g. due to connective tissue disease), endocarditis, or penetrating injury.

The aneurysm is best appreciated in the mid-oesophageal AV short- or long-axis views. Associated findings may include AR, VSD, valvular or subvalvular pulmonary stenosis, and compression of the RVOT. If a rupture occurs, it is most commonly into the RA or RVOT, producing a left-to-right shunt (Figure 12.9; see Online appendices 7.6.5–7.6.9).

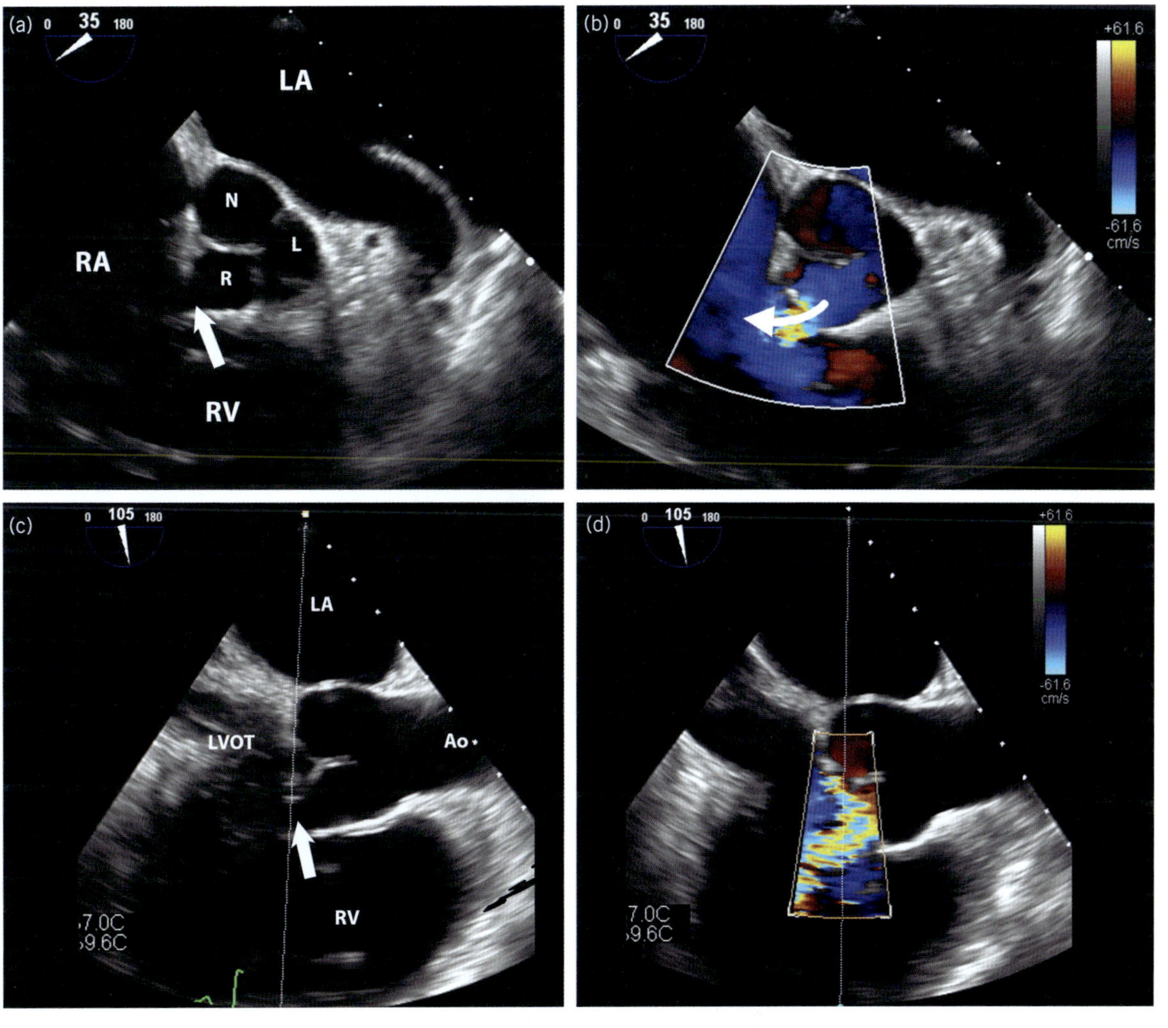

Figure 12.9 Sinus of Valsalva aneurysm with a fistula to the RA. In this composite image, frames (a) and (b) are mid-oesophageal short-axis views, and frames (c) and (d) are modified mid-oesophageal inflow–outflow views. 2D frames are shown in (a) and (c), and colour Doppler frames in (b) and (d). A large defect (fistula) can be seen between the dilated right sinus of Valsalva and the RA (arrows). The colour Doppler frames (b) and (d) show a large turbulent jet through the fistula.

Images courtesy of Dr A. Dryden.

Aortic arch and descending thoracic aortic aneurysm

In asymptomatic patients, elective repair of the aortic arch and descending thoracic aortic aneurysms is indicated for an aortic diameter >5.5 cm. Aneurysms involving the proximal aortic arch are typically repaired as an open procedure, whereas aneurysms of the distal arch and descending thoracic aorta are increasingly being treated with endovascular stent grafting. Complex thoracoabdominal aneurysms may be treated by open surgical repair or by a hybrid technique involving both open repair and endovascular stent grafting. Repairs of the proximal arch are approached through a standard sternotomy, while open repairs of the descending thoracic aorta are approached through a left thoracotomy.

For open repair, cannulation for CPB is often performed via the femoral vessels and TOE can confirm the correct positioning of the tip of the venous cannula in the RA and arterial guidewire in the true lumen of the descending aorta. For procedures performed via a left thoracotomy, the heart cannot be seen during CPB, and one important use of TOE is to detect LV dilatation due to AR. If blood is drained from the LA and returned to the femoral artery or descending aorta via partial left heart bypass, TOE can confirm the position of the LA cannula within the LA (rather than across the MV), as well as monitor LV volume status and RV function.

Endovascular approaches most commonly involve stent graft deployment from the femoral artery. Once the graft has been deployed, the proximal and distal ends of the stent graft are 'sealed' to the aortic wall by endoluminal balloon inflation. TOE is useful to verify an adequate proximal (and sometimes distal) landing zone for the stent graft seal (e.g. distal to the left subclavian artery) and to confirm the absence of excessive thrombus, calcification, or atheroma at the landing zone. The stent graft system should be visualized in the distal arch or descending aorta throughout the procedure, including during guidewire insertion, balloon inflation, and stent expansion.

Following the deployment of the stent, TOE can confirm that the aneurysmal sac has been excluded from the aorta (Figure 12.10; see Online appendices 7.9.3 and 7.9.4) and that there is no endoleak. An **endoleak** is defined as blood flow outside the stent graft, but within a vascular segment or an aneurysm sac. The most common type of endoleak involves incomplete sealing of the graft at the proximal or distal attachment site and usually requires further balloon inflation or additional stent graft deployment. The presence on TOE of swirling spontaneous echo contrast within the aneurysmal sac after stent graft deployment is suggestive of an endoleak. The distinction should be made between *swirling* echo contrast (suggestive of an endoleak) versus *static* contrast, suggesting the aneurysmal sac has been excluded.

Traumatic injury to the thoracic aorta

Traumatic injuries to the thoracic aorta can result from blunt or penetrating trauma. Penetrating injuries are usually the result of stab or bullet injuries and are often fatal, irrespective of the site of injury. Blunt traumas are far

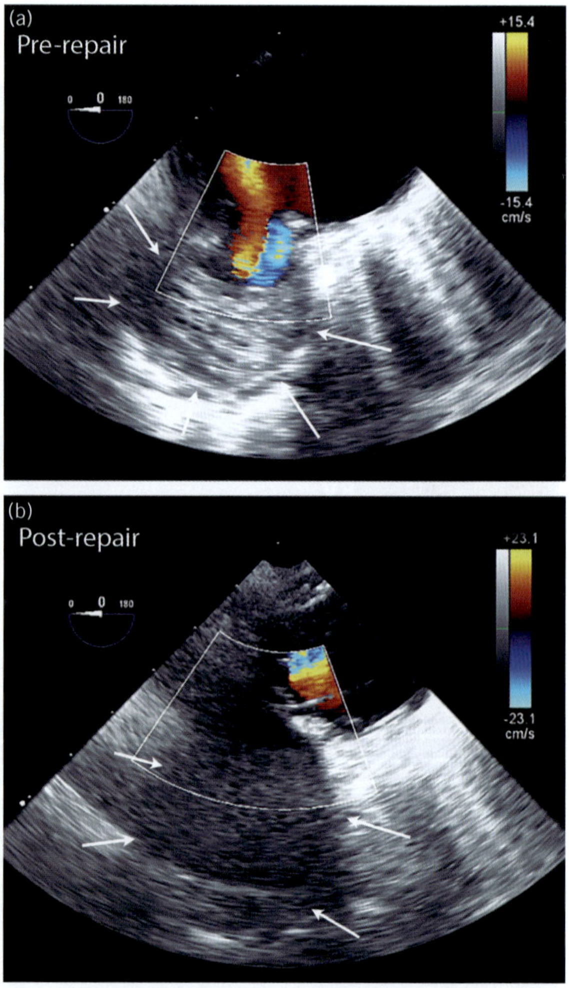

Figure 12.10 Endovascular stent grafting of a saccular descending aortic aneurysm. Frames (a) and (b) are short-axis views of the descending aorta with colour Doppler. (a) shows flow into a large saccular aneurysm (arrows). (b) shows the same aorta after endovascular stenting and exclusion of the aneurysm. Note that the colour is restricted to the aorta and there is no flow into the aneurysm.

more common, and motor vehicle accidents account for the majority of those injuries.[17]

Blunt aortic injuries involve rapid deceleration (e.g. motor vehicle accidents and/or falls) and patients typically have multi-system trauma. The most common location of blunt injuries is at the aortic isthmus, just distal to the left subclavian artery, where the aorta is tethered by the ligamentum arteriosum. A second common location is the supravalvular ascending aorta where the aortic root is fixed to the heart.[18] These two regions are vulnerable to deceleration injuries because they are transition points between relatively fixed and more mobile segments of the thoracic aorta.

Patients with complete aortic transection invariably die at the scene of injury. Those who survive transfer to a hospital usually have a partial rupture involving the intima and media, rather than a complete rupture. The diagnosis may be suspected if a widened mediastinum is noted on chest radiography and can be confirmed with a CT scan. Surgical treatment usually involves endoluminal stent grafting, with the proximal landing zone placed across the left subclavian artery. Cerebral CTA is usually performed to ensure sufficient collateral flow once occlusion of the left vertebral artery occurs (which originates from the left subclavian artery) or concurrent carotid to subclavian bypass can be considered.

TOE is of particular value in traumatic aortic injuries where urgent assessment of a suspected or impending rupture of the great vessels is required, as it is readily available and portable. One must remember that the blind spot in the distal ascending aorta may result in inadequate imaging and that the diagnostic yield is dependent on the proficiency of the operator.

The TOE examination should include all visible parts of the aorta. The site of injury is best imaged in the upper oesophageal aortic arch short-axis view or the proximal descending aorta short-axis view (Figure 12.11;

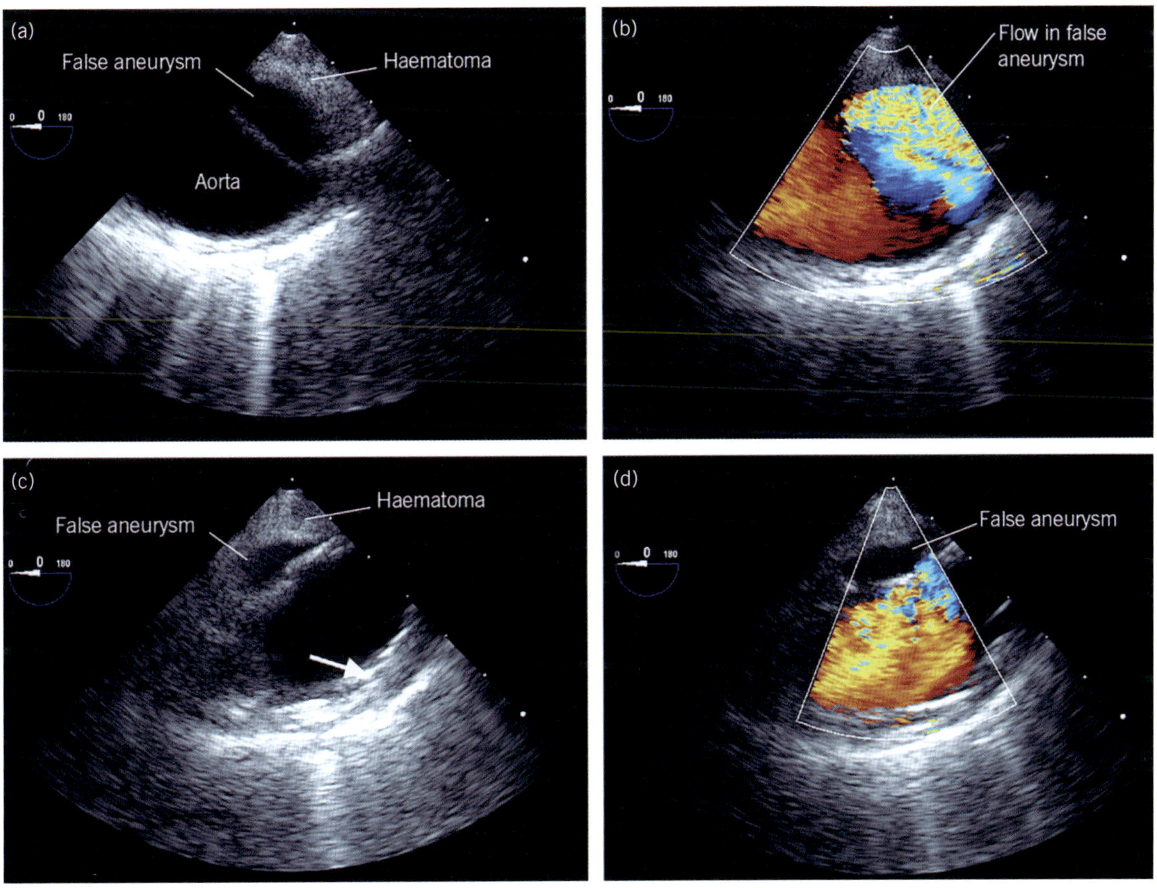

Figure 12.11 Traumatic aortic injury. All views are short-axis images of the proximal descending thoracic aorta. (a) demonstrates an intimal flap and a false aneurysm with surrounding haematoma. Colour Doppler imaging in (b) shows turbulent flow in the false aneurysm. (c) and (d) were obtained after stent graft placement. In (c), the stent is identified with an arrow. There has been a reduction in size of the false aneurysm. In (d), colour Doppler demonstrates the false aneurysm has been excluded from the aortic lumen. See also Online appendix 7.9.

Table 12.4 Aortic injuries resulting from blunt injury

Subadventitial aortic rupture with incomplete circumferential extension	Most frequent; protrusion of the disrupted aortic wall with saccular false aneurysm formation. Protrusion of aortic wall into the lumen can cause luminal stenosis with gradient
Subadventitial aortic rupture with complete circumferential extension	Fusiform pseudoaneurysm; circumferential tears do not cause luminal narrowing
Intramural haematoma	Localized, crescentic thickening (usually >5 mm); inner aortic surface smooth, lumen partially reduced, outer contour unaltered
Traumatic aortic dissection	May mimic spontaneous aortic dissection; unlike spontaneous aortic dissection, usually does not propagate distally; often thicker and less mobile dissection flap
Lesions of the aortic branches (great vessels)	Partial or total avulsion, pseudoaneurysm, dissection, thrombosis
Minimal aortic injuries	Often involves only the intima; low risk of rupture and heals spontaneously

see Online appendix 7.9.2 S), although the long-axis or oblique view may help to further define the pathology. Findings may include an intimal flap, a false aneurysm, or an associated haematoma. A greater distance between the TOE probe and the aorta due to mediastinal haematoma may degrade the image quality. Colour Doppler imaging may demonstrate turbulent flow into the false aneurysm. Following stent graft deployment, it is important to confirm that the false aneurysm has been excluded from circulation.

If TOE is used as the initial modality to diagnose and report such injuries, the description of the images should include the site of the lesion (ascending aorta, descending aorta), the distance of the lesion from a specific anatomic reference (e.g. the AV or the origin of the left subclavian artery), the size of the lesion, and the maximum aortic dimensions at the site of the lesion. Aortic lesions that result from blunt aortic injuries are listed in Table 12.4.

In addition to the assessment of a traumatic rupture, TOE is useful in identifying other cardiovascular injuries associated with severe trauma, including pericardial and pleural blood collections, valvular damage, and RWMAs secondary to cardiac contusions.

Depending on the clinical presentation, the following findings on a TOE examination can indicate a possible traumatic aortic injury: dilatation at the region of the isthmus; abnormal aortic contour; intraluminal medial flap; pseudoaneurysm; crescentic or circumferential thickening of the aortic wall; and intraluminal stenosis/gradient. Traumatic injuries tend to be confined to the isthmus and seldom propagate.

Aortic atheroma

Surgical manipulation may dislodge or fragment atheromatous plaques, leading to post-operative neurocognitive dysfunction and/or perioperative stroke.[4] The atheroma burden increases along the length of the aorta from lowest in the ascending aorta to highest in the distal descending aorta. The incidence is higher in older patients, with nearly one-third of those aged over 70 years having moderate or severe atheroma in the ascending aorta and proximal arch.[19] Additional factors associated with aortic atheroma include coronary artery disease, peripheral vascular disease, cerebral vascular disease, renal impairment, calcific aortic stenosis, and mitral annular calcification.

Several classification systems have been developed for grading the severity of aortic atheroma with either TOE or epiaortic ultrasound.[20] Atheroma that is >3 mm in height has a mobile component, or that is present in the aortic arch is associated with an increased risk of post-operative neurologic injury (Figure 12.12).[2,21] A major limitation of TOE is the fact that aortic atheroma tends to be poorly visible in the ascending aorta and proximal aortic arch. Nevertheless, the absence of significant atheroma in the visible aorta is associated with a very low risk of perioperative stroke.[22] If severe atheroma is identified in the descending aorta, careful imaging of the ascending aorta and aortic arch with epiaortic ultrasound is appropriate.

The presence of severe atheroma in the descending aorta is a contraindication to using an IABP.

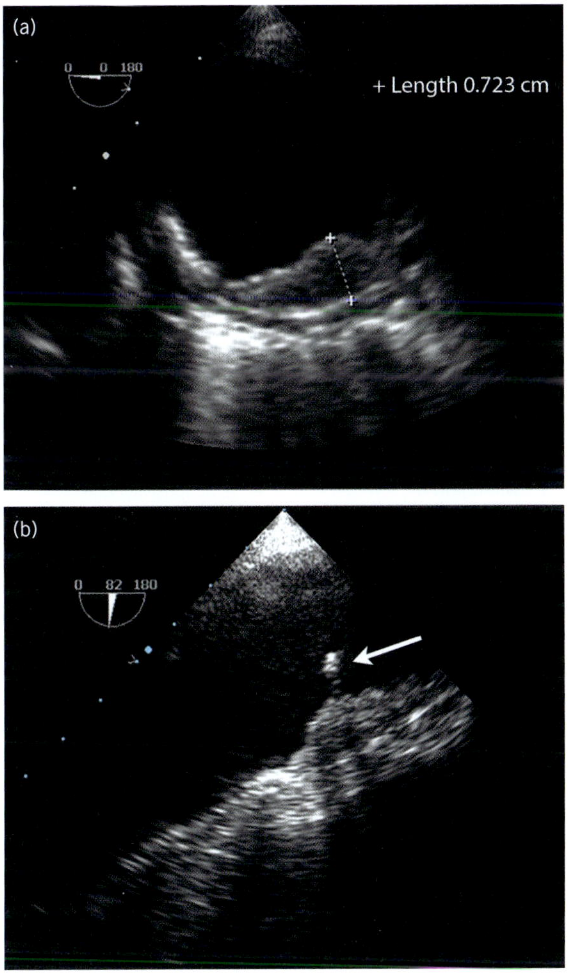

Figure 12.12 Severe aortic atheroma. (a) is a short-axis view of the descending aorta at the mid-thoracic level. Atheroma >7 mm is seen protruding into the aortic lumen. (b) is an upper oesophageal aortic arch long-axis view showing a mobile atheroma (arrow) in the distal aortic arch. See also Online appendix 7.8.

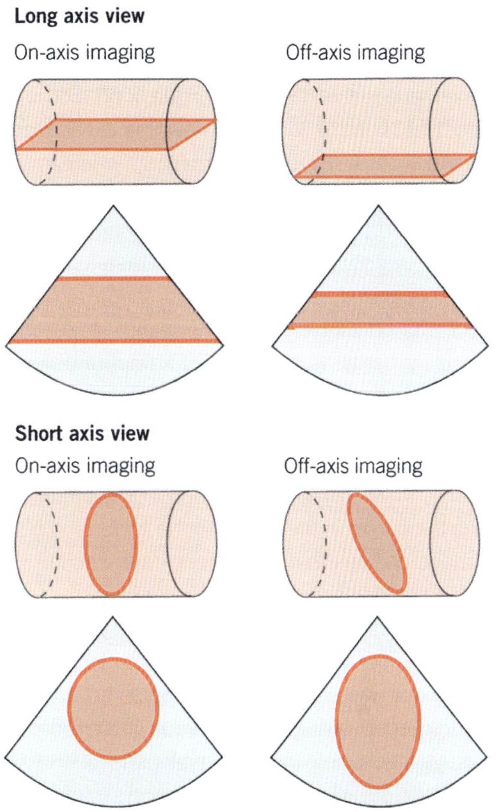

Figure 12.13 Schematic demonstration of the effects of off-axis and oblique imaging of the aorta. In long axis, off-axis imaging results in underestimation of the aortic diameter. In short axis, oblique imaging results in overestimation of the aortic dimension. Note that off-axis imaging in long axis does not distort the shape of the aorta, whereas oblique imaging in short axis results in the aorta appearing oval-shaped. Off-axis or oblique imaging can also make the aortic walls appear thickened.

Limitations of TOE for assessing the thoracic aorta

Interposition of the airways and distance from the transducer

The short segments of the distal ascending aorta (zone 3) and proximal arch (zone 4) just before the brachiocephalic artery are separated from the oesophagus by the trachea and left main bronchus (Figure 12.1), and may be impossible to image.[11] The proximal ascending aorta (zone 2) is an anterior structure and it may also be difficult to image, as calcification in the posterior aortic wall may cause ultrasound dropout, degrading the image quality of the anterior aortic wall. For these reasons, epiaortic ultrasound should be considered for patients at increased risk of embolic stroke.[20]

Reverberation artefacts

As discussed in Chapter 2, TOE examination of the thoracic aorta is affected by artefacts that arise due to calcification of the aortic wall. Reverberation or secondary lobe artefacts from the posterior aortic wall or the right pulmonary artery can appear as mobile, linear echo densities within the aortic lumen and can create a false impression of an aortic dissection. They tend to move in parallel with the reverberating structures and can be misdiagnosed as an intimal flap (Figure 12.3). In the descending aorta, a duplication of the whole aorta is often visible, termed 'double-barrel' or pseudo-aorta. Colour Doppler is often seen within the artefact, although with less intensity than in the true image (see Figure 2.14).

Oblique and off-axis imaging

Inaccuracies in the measurements of aortic dimensions can arise, due to the effects of oblique or off-axis imaging (Figure 12.13). In the long-axis view, the aortic diameter is underestimated by off-axis imaging, whereas in the short-axis view, oblique imaging leads to an overestimation of the aortic diameter. Oblique imaging in short axis confers an oval shape to the aorta and therefore can usually be recognized. By contrast, no shape distortion is present with off-axis imaging in long-axis views, making the problem harder to recognize. To avoid underestimating the aortic diameter with long-axis imaging, the probe should be turned left and right until the largest diameter is obtained. 3D imaging can also help to solve this problem—when using simultaneous orthogonal views, placing the cursor in the centre of the aorta on the short-axis image ensures that the proper cross-section is displayed in the long-axis view for measurement.

Oblique or tangential imaging is particularly problematic in the upper oesophageal aortic arch long-axis view where the curving arch may make the aortic wall appear falsely thickened, giving the erroneous impression of atheromatous thickening in the lateral parts of the sector scan. Finally, the aorta expands slightly in systole, causing a small increase in its diameter.

Multiple choice questions

Discover interactive multiple choice questions to test your knowledge on this chapter by searching for this book's title or ISBN (9780198873686) at **https://academic.oup.com/** and going to the online appendix at the end of the book. Use your scratch-off code on the inside cover to access the material.

References

1. Tsai TT, Nienaber CA, Eagle KA. Acute aortic syndromes. *Circulation*. 2005;**112**(24):3802–13.
2. Goldstein SA, Evangelista A, Abbara S, *et al.* Multimodality imaging of diseases of the thoracic aorta in adults: from the American Society of Echocardiography and the European Association of Cardiovascular Imaging: endorsed by the Society of Cardiovascular Computed Tomography and Society for Cardiovascular Magnetic Resonance. *J Am Soc Echocardiogr*. 2015;**28**(2):119–82.
3. Isselbacher EM, Preventza O, Hamilton Black J 3rd, *et al.* 2022 ACC/AHA Guideline for the diagnosis and management of aortic disease: a report of the American Heart Association/American College of Cardiology Joint Committee on Clinical Practice Guidelines. *Circulation*. 2022;**146**(24):e334–482.
4. Evangelista A, Flachskampf FA, Erbel R, *et al.* Echocardiography in aortic diseases: EAE recommendations for clinical practice. *Eur J Echocardiogr.* 2010;**11**(8):645–58 [published correction appears in *Eur J Echocardiogr.* 2011;**12**(8):642].
5. Asch FM, Yuriditsky E, Prakash SK, *et al.* The need for standardized methods for measuring the aorta: multimodality core lab experience from the GenTAC Registry. *JACC Cardiovasc Imaging*. 2016;**9**(3):219–26.
6. Goldfinger JZ, Halperin JL, Marin ML, Stewart AS, Eagle KA, Fuster V. Thoracic aortic aneurysm and dissection. *J Am Coll Cardiol*. 2014;**64**(16):1725–39.
7. Cigarroa JE, Isselbacher EM, DeSanctis RW, Eagle KA. Diagnostic imaging in the evaluation of suspected aortic dissection. Old standards and new directions. *N Engl J Med*. 1993;**328**(1):35–43.
8. Isselbacher EM. Thoracic and abdominal aortic aneurysms. *Circulation*. 2005;**111**(6):816–28.
9. Weintraub AR, Erbel R, Görge G, *et al.* Intravascular ultrasound imaging in acute aortic dissection. *J Am Coll Cardiol*. 1994;**24**(2):495–503.
10. Yamada E, Matsumura M, Kyo S, Omoto R. Usefulness of a prototype intravascular ultrasound imaging in evaluation of aortic dissection and comparison with angiographic study, transesophageal echocardiography, computed tomography, and magnetic resonance imaging. *Am J Cardiol*. 1995;**75**(2):161–5.
11. Appelbe AF, Walker PG, Yeoh JK, Bonitatibus A, Yoganathan AP, Martin RP. Clinical significance and origin of artifacts in transesophageal echocardiography of the thoracic aorta. *J Am Coll Cardiol*. 1993;**21**(3):754–60.
12. Mussa FF, Horton JD, Moridzadeh R, Nicholson J, Trimarchi S, Eagle KA. Acute aortic dissection and intramural hematoma: a systematic review. *JAMA*. 2016;**316**(7):754–63.
13. Oderich GS, Kärkkäinen JM, Reed NR, Tenorio ER, Sandri GA. Penetrating aortic ulcer and intramural hematoma. *Cardiovasc Intervent Radiol*. 2019;**42**(3):321–34.
14. Nauta F, deBeaufort H, Mussa FF, *et al.* Management of retrograde type A IMH with acute arch tear/type B dissection. *Ann Cardiothorac Surg*. 2019;**8**(5): 531–9.
15. Erbel R, Aboyans V, Boileau C, *et al.* 2014 ESC Guidelines on the diagnosis and treatment of aortic diseases: document covering acute and chronic aortic diseases of the thoracic and abdominal aorta of the adult. The Task Force for the Diagnosis and Treatment of Aortic Diseases of the European Society of Cardiology (ESC). *Eur Heart J*. 2014;**35**(41):2873–926 [published correction appears in *Eur Heart J*. 2015;**36**(41):2779].
16. Hiratzka LF, Bakris GL, Beckman JA, *et al.* 2010 ACCF/AHA/AATS/ACR/ASA/SCA/SCAI/SIR/STS/SVM guidelines for the diagnosis and management of patients with thoracic aortic disease: a report of the American College of Cardiology Foundation/American Heart Association Task Force on Practice Guidelines, American Association for Thoracic Surgery, American College of Radiology, American Stroke Association, Society of Cardiovascular Anesthesiologists, Society for Cardiovascular Angiography and Interventions, Society of Interventional Radiology, Society of Thoracic Surgeons, and Society for Vascular Medicine. *Circulation*. 2010;**121**(13):e266–369 [published correction appears in *Circulation*. 2010;**122**(4):e410].

17. Mutsuga M. Traumatic thoracic injury. *Kyobu Geka*. 2022;**75**(10):759–62.
18. Mouawad NJ, Paulisin J, Hofmeister S, Thomas MB. Blunt thoracic aortic injury—concepts and management. *J Cardiothorac Surg*. 2020;**15**(1):62.
19. Royse A, Royse C. A standardised intraoperative ultrasound examination of the aorta and proximal coronary arteries. *Interact Cardiovasc Thorac Surg*. 2006;**5**(6):701–4.
20. Glas KE, Swaminathan M, Reeves ST, *et al*. Guidelines for the performance of a comprehensive intraoperative epiaortic ultrasonographic examination: recommendations of the American Society of Echocardiography and the Society of Cardiovascular Anesthesiologists; endorsed by the Society of Thoracic Surgeons. *Anesth Analg*. 2008;**106**(5):1376–84.
21. Van der Linden J, Hadjinikolaou L, Bergman P, Lindblom D. Postoperative stroke in cardiac surgery is related to the location and extent of atherosclerotic disease in the ascending aorta. *J Am Coll Cardiol*. 2001;**38**(1):131–5.
22. Wilson MJ, Boyd SY, Lisagor PG, Rubal BJ, Cohen DJ. Ascending aortic atheroma assessed intraoperatively by epiaortic and transesophageal echocardiography. *Ann Thorac Surg*. 2000;**70**(1):25–30.

13 Prosthetic valves

Valvular heart disease is common, due to age-related degeneration and to a high incidence of rheumatic disease in developing countries. In 2017, the Centers for Disease Control and Prevention (CDC) reported approximately 3000 deaths due to rheumatic valvular heart disease and 25000 deaths due to non-rheumatic valvular heart disease in the United States.

The number of valve replacements performed yearly worldwide is around 300000, and it is projected to increase to 850000 per year by 2050.[1]

Perioperative TOE is invaluable in evaluating the nature and severity of lesions in both native and prosthetic valves, identifying related complications (e.g. atrial thrombus, chamber dilatation) and confirming the adequacy of prosthetic function following valve replacement. The introduction of 3D has been a significant advance, particularly in the identification of paravalvular leak (PVL) location.

Guideline recommendations for surgical prosthetic valvular assessment are applied throughout this chapter.[1,2] Percutaneous prosthetic valves are discussed in Chapter 17.

Approach to imaging prosthetic valves

It is essential to conduct a systematic and comprehensive TOE examination in all patients presenting with prosthetic valves by using approaches and techniques described for native valves. The findings are interpreted in the context of the patient's clinical history, prior echocardiograms, and haemodynamic loading conditions if the examination is performed under general anaesthesia.[3] Knowledge of the type, size, and documented pressure gradients of previously implanted prosthetics is also helpful.

The comprehensive TOE evaluation of prosthetic valves begins with an understanding of the type and size of prosthesis and the timing and clinical context within which it was inserted. Like any other cardiac structure, the TOE evaluation includes a structural and functional assessment of the prosthetic valve: morphology, motion of the occluders/leaflets, and integrity/motion of the sewing ring. Colour and spectral Doppler analyses include gradients, VTI, and calculation of the effective orifice area (EOA) of the valve. The presence, severity, and precise location of any intra- and peri-valvular regurgitation are noted. Finally, adjacent and remote cardiac structures should also be evaluated: chamber dilatation, ventricular

Box 13.1 Intraoperative TOE assessment of prosthetic valves

Pre-CPB

- Confirm the indications for surgery by assessing the aetiology and severity of valve dysfunction
- Measure appropriate dimensions
- Assess the risk of patient– prosthesis mismatch
- Identify any associated pathology that may alter surgical plan (root dilation, valvular calcification, presence of clots, vegetations, abscesses, risk of SAM)
- Assess biventricular size and function

Post-CPB

- Assess prosthetic function (with consideration of loading conditions)
- Ensure correct seating of prosthesis
- Assess leaflet motion
- Assess forward flow (velocity, pressure gradients, EOA, PHT)
- Assess for abnormal regurgitant jets (transvalvular, paravalvular)
- Rule out associated complications (e.g. damage to circumflex coronary artery, coronary ostium obstruction)
- Assess adequacy of de-airing
- Assessment of biventricular function

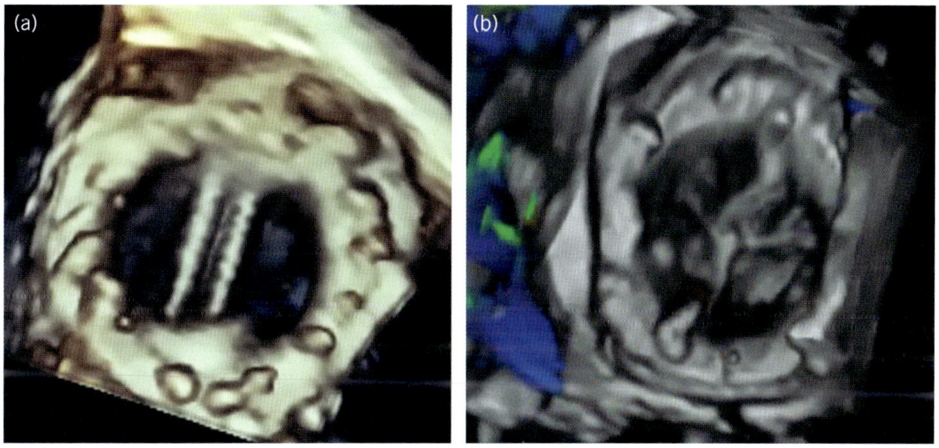

Figure 13.1 3D images of mitral prostheses from the LA aspect. (a) shows a mechanical valve in diastole (leaflets open). (b) shows a stented bioprosthesis in systole (leaflets closed). See Online appendix 9.1.1 for more examples.

hypertrophy and systolic function, and estimation of PA pressures.[1,2]

Prosthetic valves, particularly mechanical prostheses, are strong ultrasound reflectors and the source of many 2D and 3D imaging artefacts. Pitfalls associated with imaging these structures can be avoided by understanding how artefacts complicate echocardiographic interpretation. Acoustic shadowing is particularly problematic and imaging should be performed in multiple views. In addition, the intense echo reflections from artificial surfaces often lead to reverberations that make interpretation difficult and may be reduced by decreasing the 2D gain setting. Artefacts are discussed in Chapter 2.

Specific issues to address during the intraoperative TOE examination are summarized in Box 13.1.

Mitral prosthetic valves

TOE is superior to TTE for assessing prosthetic valves in the mitral position, because acoustic shadowing does not obscure the LA aspect of the prosthesis. Both 2D and 3D imaging from the atrial aspect provide information on leaflet integrity and motion, dehiscence of the sewing ring, thrombus or vegetations, and the presence and anatomical location of any PVLs (Figure 13.1; see Online appendix 9.1.1 S).[4]

Aortic prosthetic valves

Prosthetic valves in the aortic position are not as easy to visualize as those in the mitral position. While important information may be obtained from the mid-oesophageal AV views, acoustic shadowing from the posterior sewing ring often masks anterior PVLs and complicates the assessment of leaflet motion.

> ***Expert tip: Aortic prosthetic leaflet motion and paravalvular leaks may be better demonstrated in deep transgastric views. This is also true of transvalvular flow patterns, as the Doppler beam is usually well aligned with the direction of blood flow.***

Types of prosthetic valves

More than 100 types of prosthetic valves are in clinical use today.[4] Familiarity with the echocardiographic features and transvalvular blood flow of those in widespread use is essential to differentiate normal from abnormal function (Figure 13.2; Table 13.1). Currently, the most commonly used valves are either bileaflet mechanical or stented bioprosthetic, and may be used in all valve positions. Stentless bioprosthetic and homograft valves, however, may only be used in the aortic and pulmonary positions.

Most adults receive a 19- to 25-mm valve in the aortic position (the largest available being 29 mm) and a 27- to 33-mm valve in the mitral position. The echocardiographic features of the new sutureless bioprosthetic valves will be discussed later in this chapter.

Bileaflet mechanical valves

Bileaflet mechanical valves consist of two semicircular leaflets (or 'occluders') attached to a pyrolytic carbon ring, which is, in turn, enclosed in a sewing ring. The leaflets pivot at two recessed hinges located slightly lateral

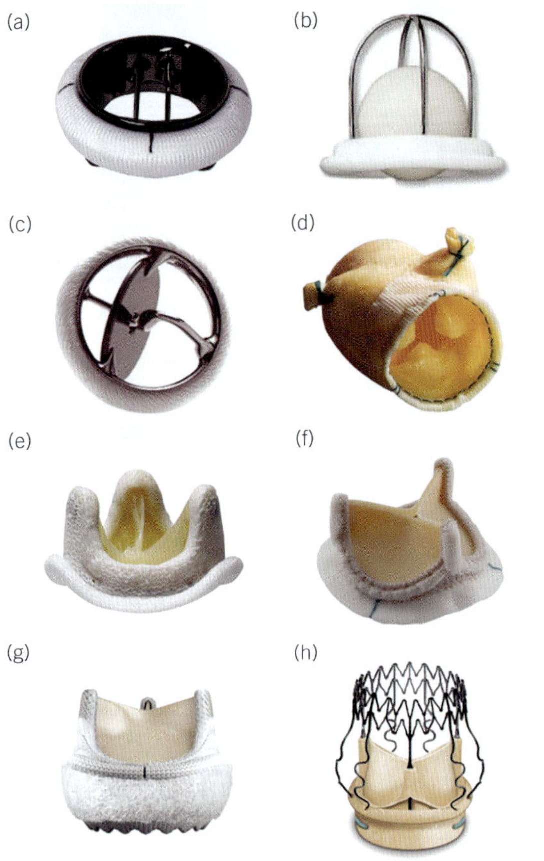

Figure 13.2 Different types of prosthetic valves. (a) Bileaflet valve (On-X valve shown). (b) Ball-and-cage valve (Starr–Edwards shown). (c) Tilting disc valve (Medtronic Hall shown). (d) Stentless tissue valve (Medtronic Freestyle shown). (e) Stented porcine aortic valve (Carpentier Edwards shown). (f) Stented bovine pericardial valve (Medtronic valve shown). (g) Stented sutureless aortic valve (Edwards Intuity valve shown). (h) Stented sutureless aortic valve (Corcym Perceval PLUS valve shown).

(a) Courtesy of On-X. (b), (e), and (g) Courtesy of Edwards. (c), (d), and (f) With kind permission from Medtronic. (h) Courtesy of Corcym Group.

to the central axis of the valve, and the valve mechanism can be rotated within the sewing ring. Two large lateral semicircular orifices and a narrow rectangular central orifice permit symmetrical flow. The leaflets' opening angle (Figure 13.3) ranges from 75° to 90°, depending on the specific valve. Compared to older mechanical valves, the large opening angle provides relatively unobstructed forward flow but results in a somewhat larger regurgitant volume (because the leaflets must swing through a large arc to close). The closing angle of most bileaflet valves is approximately 25°, with the exception of the On-X® valve (Artivion, Kennesaw, GA, USA) that has a closing angle of 43°—this should not be misinterpreted as incomplete closure. Following leaflet closure, characteristic regurgitant jets help 'wash' the leaflet surfaces and reduce the risk of thrombus formation. The On-X® valve has larger washing jets than other commonly used bileaflet valves.

Echocardiographic appearances

With 2D imaging, the echogenic sewing ring is easily seen as two bright spots on the edges of the prosthesis (Figure 13.4; see Online appendix 9.1.1.1). In the mitral position, the leaflets are well seen in the mid-oesophageal views. If the mechanical prosthesis is interrogated through the centre of the valve and **perpendicular** to the leaflets, two leaflets are seen opening and closing symmetrically in a characteristic 'bat wing appearance'. If the image plane passes through the centre of the valve and **parallel** to the leaflets, a single flat disc is seen in systole and no leaflet is seen in diastole. If the image plane does not pass through the centre of the valve or is **oblique** to the leaflets, they may appear asymmetric or to have a reduced range of motion (Figure 13.3). In this case, they may be mistakenly identified as immobile or 'stuck'. Note that when the metal leaflets close in systole, they block the transmission of ultrasound and cause complete shadowing of all structures distal to the valve.

The degree to which the leaflet mechanism is manually rotated within the sewing ring at the time of implantation dictates the angle at which the image plane is perpendicular or parallel to the leaflets. In the mitral position, the valve is usually implanted with the leaflets *perpendicular* to the original leaflets' orientation (also called *anti-anatomic* position) to prevent impingement of the subvalvular apparatus and to maintain left ventricular function and geometry.[4,5] Thus, it is essential to interrogate the prosthesis fully from 0° to 180° to find the two orthogonal views in which the ultrasound beam is perpendicular and parallel to the leaflets. 3D imaging from the LA aspect demonstrates the entire valve and sewing ring (Figure 13.5; see Online appendix 9.1.1).

Colour Doppler imaging of a mechanical bileaflet valve in the mitral position usually displays two or more characteristic 'washing jets' (Figure 13.4; see Online appendix 9.1.1.2) originating within the sewing ring (i.e. transvalvular jets). When the image plane is parallel to the leaflets, there will usually be two peripheral jets originating at the pivot points. When the image plane is perpendicular to the leaflets, a central jet (originating from the space between the occluders) and two peripheral jets (originating from the space between the valve leaflets and the ring) are usually seen.

In the aortic position, the leaflets and washing jets are typically incompletely visualized in the mid-oesophageal

Table 13.1 Transvalvular velocities, pressure gradients, and effective orifice areas for some commonly used prosthetic valves (readers should be familiar with valves commonly used in their own centres/countries)

Valve	Position	Size	Peak gradient (mmHg)	Mean gradient (mmHg)	EOA (cm^2)	Pressure half-time (ms)
St Jude (bileaflet)	Aortic	21	25.7±9.5	15±5.0	1.4±0.4	
		27	13.7±4.2	8.4±3.4	2.5±0.4	
	Mitral	27	11.0±4.0	5±1.8		75±10
		31	12.0±6.0	4.5±2.2		74±13
On-X (bileaflet)	Aortic	21	16.4±5.9	9.9±3.6	1.7±0.4	
		25	16.5±10.2	6.9±4.3	2.4±0.6	
	Mitral	25	11.5±3.2	5.3±2.1		
		31–33	9.8±3.8	4.8±2.4		
Starr–Edwards (ball-and-cage)	Aortic	23	32.6±12.8	22.0±9.0	1.1±0.2	
		27	30.8±6.3	18.5±3.7		
	Mitral	30	12.2±4.6	6.9±2.5		125±25
		32	11.5 ± 4.2	5.1±2.5		110±25
Baxter Perimount (stented bovine)	Aortic	21	24.9±7.7	13.8±4.0	1.3±0.3	
		27	12.8±5.4	4.8±2.2	2.0±0.4	
Carpentier–Edwards (stented bovine)	Mitral	29		5.2±2.3		110±15
		33		1.0		80
Medtronic Intact (stented porcine)	Aortic	21	40.9±15.6	19.6±8.1	1.6±0.4	
		27	25.0±7.6	15.0±4.5		
	Mitral	29	3.5±0.5			
		35	3.2±1.7			
Medtronic Freestyle (stentless)	Aortic	21		9.1±5.1	1.4±0.3	
		27		4.6±3.1	2.5±0.1	

Data from Zoghbi WA, *et al.* Recommendations for Noninvasive Evaluation of Native Valvular Regurgitation. A Report from the American Society of Echocardiography Developed in Collaboration with the Society for Cardiovascular Magnetic Resonance. *J Am Soc Echocardiogr.* 2017;**30**(4):303–371.

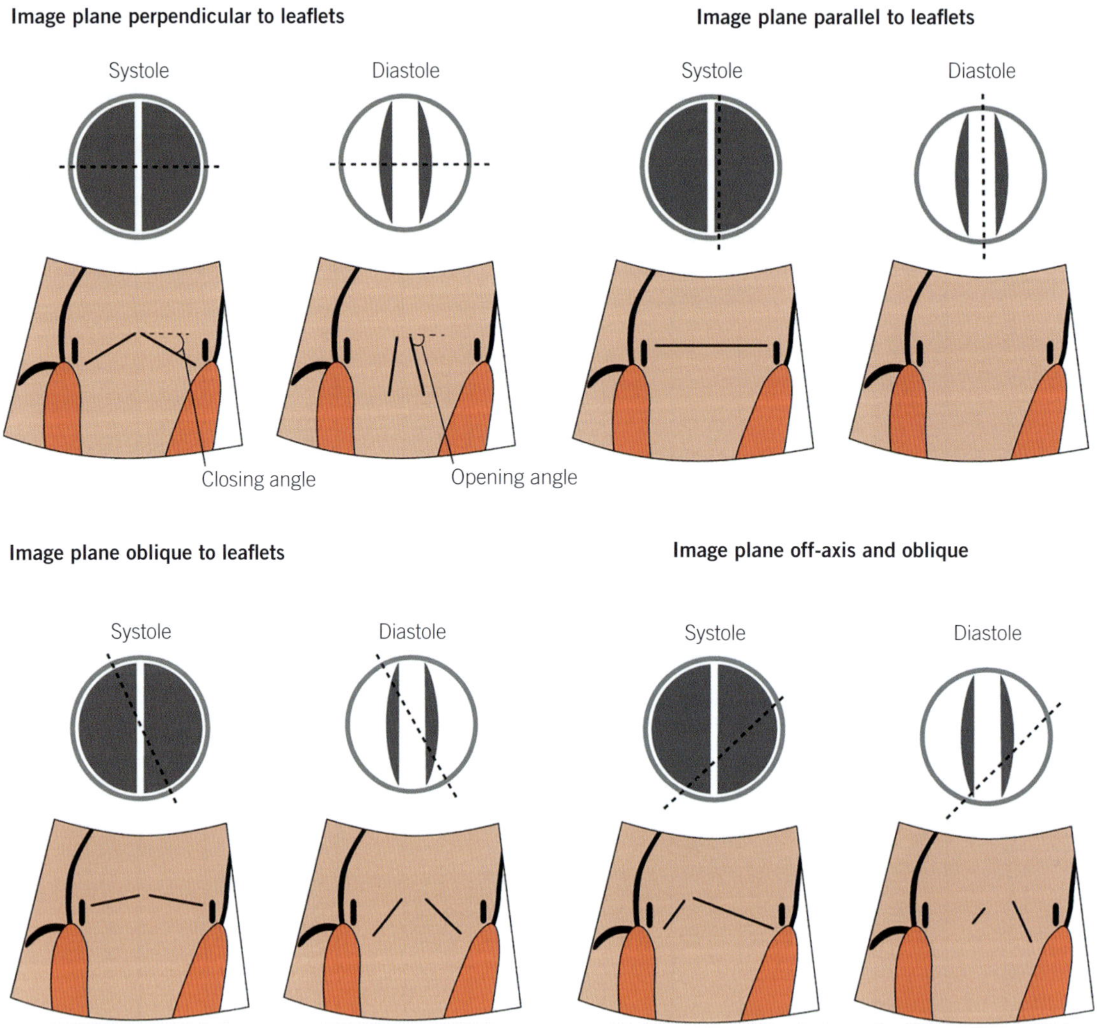

Figure 13.3 Schematic showing the appearances of a bileaflet prosthesis in the mitral position with different imaging planes. The opening and closing angles of the valve, relative to the annular plane, are shown. See text for details.

views due to acoustic shadowing from the sewing ring (Figure 13.6; see Online appendix 9.1.5.4). Leaflet motion and washing jets are better appreciated in the deep transgastric views (Figure 13.7; see Online appendix 9.1.5.5).

> ***Expert tip:*** *Normal washing jets tend to be small and short-lived (only a few frames), and they always originate within the sewing ring.*

Tilting disc valves

Tilting disc valves are no longer implanted but may be encountered in patients presenting for redo surgery. Tilting disc valves consist of a single circular disc suspended from a sewing ring by a single strut. The strut attaches to the disc eccentrically, resulting in a complex flow pattern, with approximately 70% of flow passing through the major orifice and 30% through the minor orifice.

Echocardiographic appearances

The strut can be seen in a central position above the sewing ring. Motion of the single leaflet is best visualized by imaging the valve in a scan plane that passes through the hinge point perpendicular to the axis of disc motion. Tilting disc valves are much easier to see in the mitral position than in the aortic position. Small transvalvular jets between the disc and the sewing ring are common. The Medtronic–Hall valve was a widely used tilting disc valve with a long central jet originating between the disc and the strut.

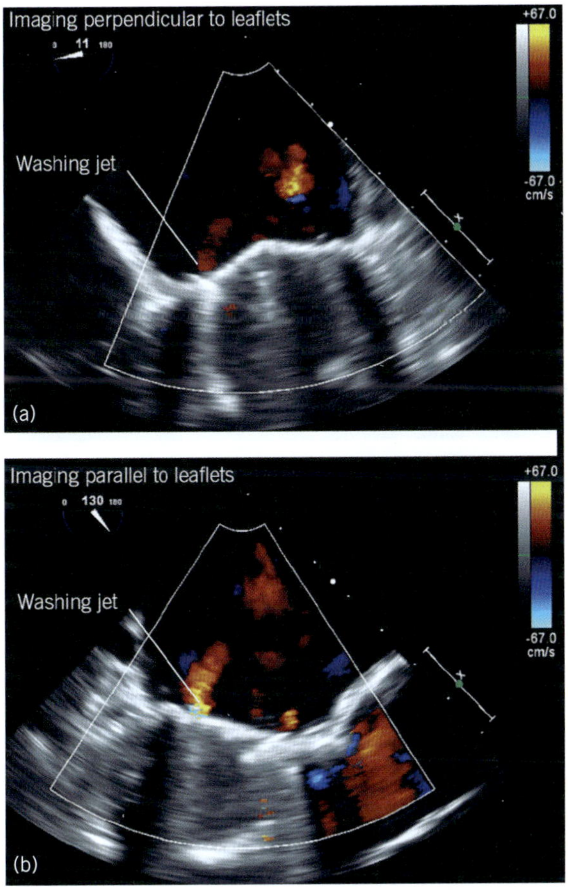

Figure 13.4 Normal bileaflet mechanical MV in mid-oesophageal views. Both frames (a) and (b) are in systole (leaflets closed), and imaging is shown perpendicular and parallel to the leaflets. See also Online appendix 9.1.1.

Ball-and-cage valves

Ball-and-cage valves are no longer implanted but may be encountered in patients presenting for redo surgery. Ball-and-cage valves consist of a sewing ring and a cage containing a silastic ball. The cage comprises three struts for aortic prostheses and four struts for mitral prostheses. Ball-and-cage valves, of which the Starr–Edwards valve was the most common, have a high profile that intrudes into the LVOT (mitral position) and into the sinuses of Valsalva (aortic position).

Echocardiographic appearances

It is usually possible to see parts of the metallic cage and a partial outline of the edge of the ball, particularly in the mitral position (see Online appendix 9.1.2). Colour Doppler displays the laterally directed forward flow and the low-velocity closure backflow around the ball. Transvalvular velocity measurements should be performed with the ultrasound beam aligned with the laterally directed forward flow.

Stented bioprosthetic valves and sutureless aortic valves

Stented bioprosthetic valves are either porcine AVs or valves fashioned from bovine or equine pericardium and suspended in a frame (the 'stent'). Three stent posts extend beyond the plane of the annulus to support the leaflet commissures. In the mitral position, the stent posts extend into the LV; in the aortic position, the stent posts extend into the sinuses of Valsalva. Note that prosthetic leaflets are stiffer than native valve leaflets as a result of the preservation technique, and they tend to soften over time. For this reason, forward gradients often improve between separation from CPB and sternal closure.

> ***Expert tip: The stents of a mitral bioprosthetic valve may extend into the LVOT, especially if the LV cavity is small. This may cause flow obstruction and should be carefully ruled out.***

Due to a growing interest in minimally invasive procedures and shorter operating times, manufacturers have developed expanding, self-anchoring pericardial stented valves for treating aortic stenosis, termed 'sutureless' or 'rapid deployment' aortic valves. These bioprosthetic valves leverage the technology of intravascular stents and transcatheter valves, and are inserted under direct vision after excision of the diseased native valve and debridement of the aortic annulus.[6]

These valves are inserted in a compressed state, using only 1–3 sutures, and then expanded to normal size when correctly positioned. The smaller profile of sutureless valves, compared to traditional stented valves, allows for easier insertion during minimally invasive surgery and in patients with small aortic roots.

Two different types of sutureless valves are currently available: Perceval® (LivaNova, London, UK) and Intuity® (Edwards Lifesciences, Irvine, CA, USA) (Figure 13.2). The Perceval® bioprosthetic valve is constructed from bovine pericardium mounted on a nitinol frame (Figure 13.2). Three intercommissural sutures are used to guide the valve to the annulus, and these sutures are removed after valve deployment.[7] The Intuity® is also a bovine pericardial valve but is mounted on a short balloon-expandable stainless steel frame coated with a

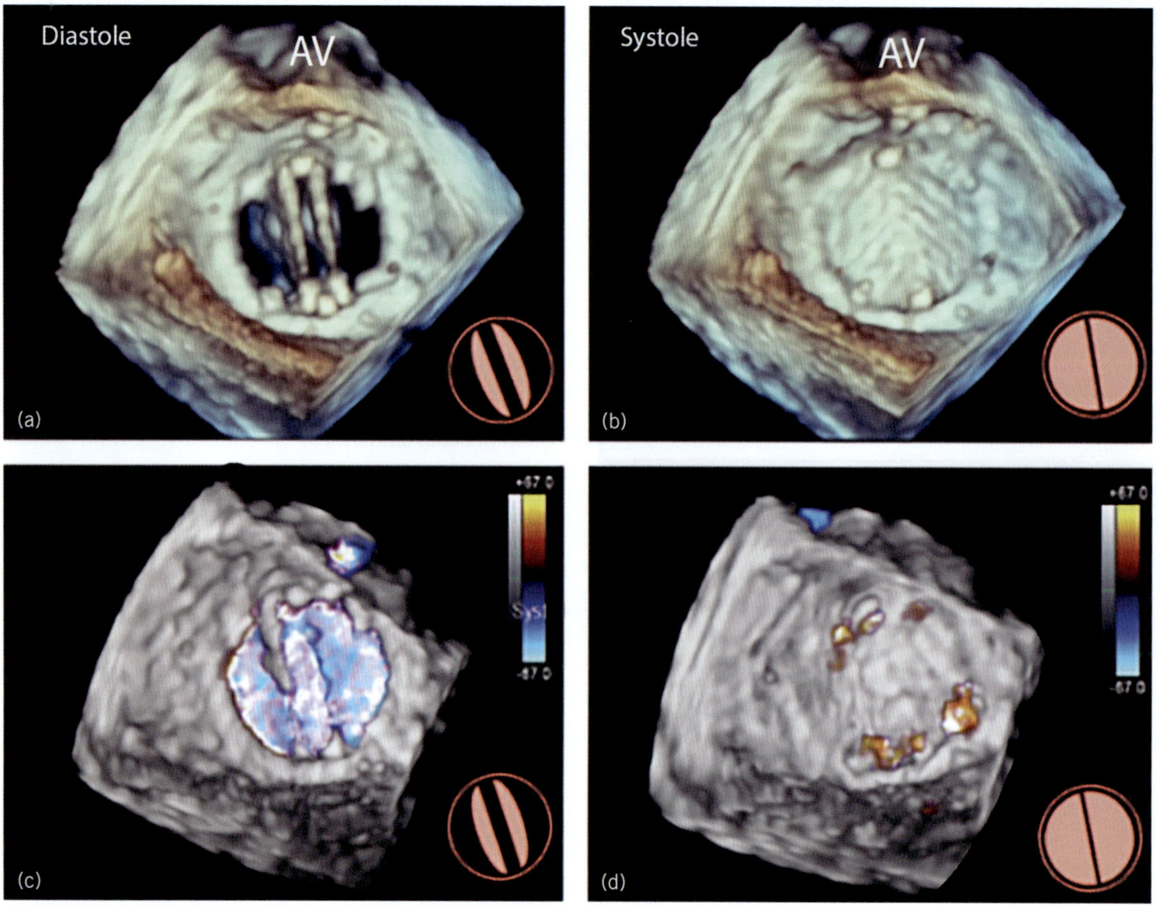

Figure 13.5 3D imaging of a normal bileaflet mechanical MV. The valve is shown from the atrial aspect in the surgical orientation (note the aortic valve at 12 o'clock). Frames (a) and (c) show the valve in diastole, and frames (b) and (d) in systole. (c) and (d) are with colour Doppler. Note the washing jets in the systolic colour Doppler frame (d). See also Online appendix 9.1.1.

textured cloth to provide a good annular seal and reduce the incidence of PVL. The valve is seated within the annulus using three guide sutures, which are tied after the stent deployment.[7] Sizing correlates with the annular diameter as shown in Table 13.2.

The clinical indications for sutureless valve implant are:[9,10]

- Patients requiring concomitant procedures (reducing total CPB time)
- Small, calcified roots (to reduce patient–prosthesis mismatch)
- Redo AV replacement
- Prior implantation of an aortic homograft or stentless prosthesis

Contraindications to sutureless AVs include isolated AR, recent endocarditis, or aortic root dilatation. There are currently no clinical data demonstrating the safe use of sutureless valves in patients with congenital bicuspid AV.[7,10] Asymmetry of the sinuses of Valsalva due to bicuspid AV or aortic root dilatation can prevent correct seating and anchoring of the device. Compared with conventional AV replacement, sutureless valves are associated with a higher incidence of PVLs and requirement for pacemaker implants.[11]

Echocardiographic appearances

All traditional stented bioprosthetic valves display an echo-dense sewing ring, which appears as two bright spots on the edges of the valve. Parts of the stent posts may be seen within the ring. In the mitral position, the sewing ring and two of the three leaflets can usually be seen from the mid-oesophageal views (Figure 13.8; see Online appendix 9.1.3). One or two stent posts may be seen extending into the LV. All three leaflets and stent posts can sometimes be seen in the transgastric basal short-axis view.

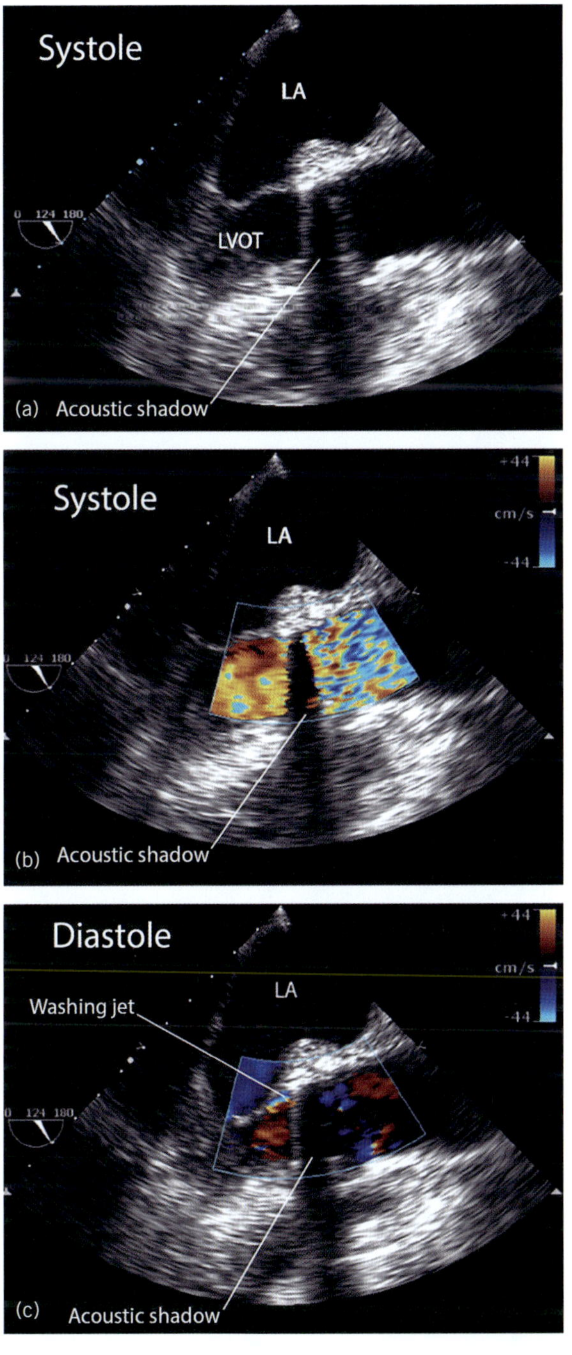

Figure 13.6 Normal bileaflet mechanical AV in the mid-oesophageal long-axis view. (a) Acoustic shadowing from the posterior sewing ring obscures the valve leaflets. The aortic root is slightly thickened, which is a normal finding after AV replacement. In (b) (systole), aortic ejection is seen with colour Doppler imaging. A mosaic colour pattern is seen in the ascending aorta, indicating turbulent flow. In (c) (diastole), a single washing jet can be seen. Other washing jets may be present but are obscured by acoustic shadowing. See also Online appendix 9.1.5.

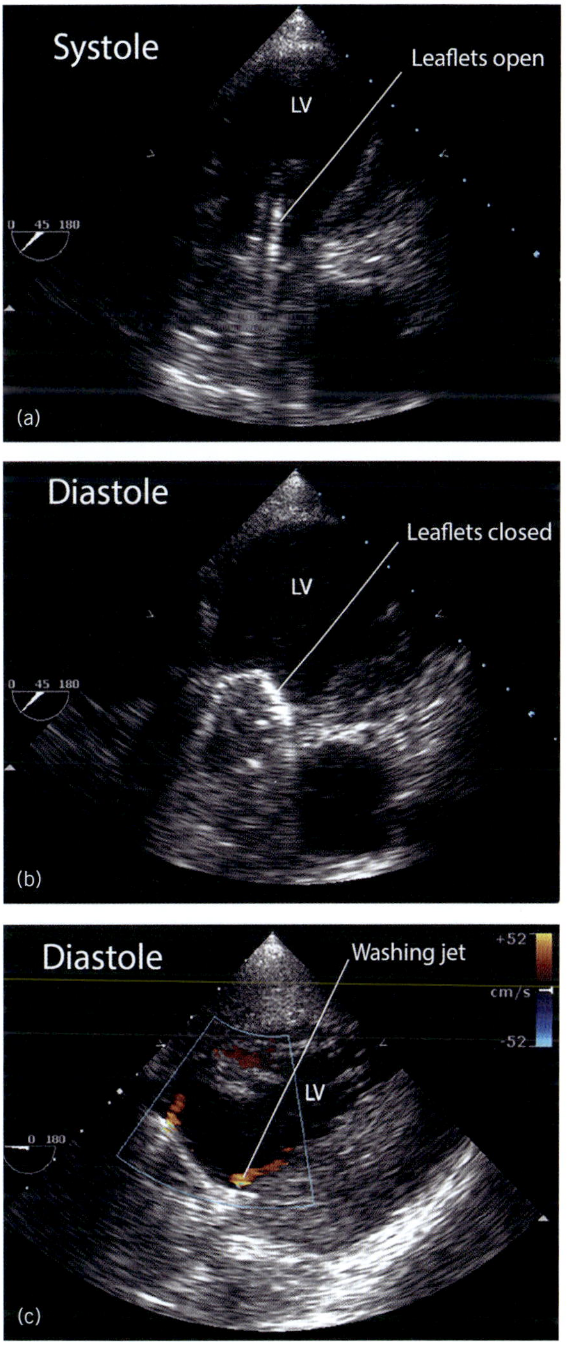

Figure 13.7 Normal bileaflet mechanical AV in the deep transgastric five-chamber view. In (a) (systole), the leaflets are in the open position. In (b) (diastole), the leaflets are in the closed position. In (c) (diastole), the valve leaflets are closed and two peripheral washing jets can be seen. Note that in the transgastric view, visualization of the AV prosthesis is not impeded by acoustic shadowing. See also Online appendix 9.1.5.

Table 13.2 Sizing for Perceval® sutureless aortic valve[8]

Size	Aortic annulus diameter (mm)
S	19–21
M	21–23
L	23–25
XL	25–27

Data from Glauber M, Miceli A, di Bacco L. Sutureless and rapid deployment valves: implantation technique from A to Z—the Perceval valve. *Ann Cardiothorac Surg* 2020;**9**(4):330–340.

In the aortic position, the leaflets and stent posts of a bioprosthetic valve can usually be seen in the mid-oesophageal short-axis views with either 2D or 3D imaging (Figure 13.9; see Online appendix 9.1.6). In long-axis views, acoustic shadowing from the sewing ring may impair visualization of the leaflets and stent posts. When the valve is implanted into a dilated aortic root, a hypoechoic space may be noted between the sewing ring and the sinuses of Valsalva in the mid-oesophageal AV short-axis view. This is a normal finding and must not be mistaken for a pathologic space (e.g. abscess) that may be associated with a PVL.

Colour Doppler imaging of bioprosthetic valves typically shows a small central regurgitant jet (Figure 13.8). Immediately after separation from CPB, 1–3 small peripheral transvalvular jets may also be seen originating at the commissures, especially with pericardial valves. Both these types of regurgitant jet typically decrease in size or disappear within the first hour following separation from CPB, as the leaflets soften.

Because sutureless aortic valves are contraindicated in patients with asymmetric sinuses of Valsalva, the morphology and dimensions of the aortic root must be carefully assessed prior to implantation of these devices. For the Perceval S® valve, implantation is not recommended when the aortic annulus is >25 mm and the ratio of sinotubular junction diameter-to-annular diameter (ventriculo-aortic junction) is ≤1.3 (Box 13.2).[5] Following implantation, it is important to confirm correct seating of the valve and to rule out significant paravalvular regurgitation (see Online appendices 9.1.6.4–9.1.6.7). Although the risk of PVL is higher with sutureless AVs than with traditional stented valves, the goal is always to achieve zero or trivial paravalvular regurgitation (Figure 13.10).

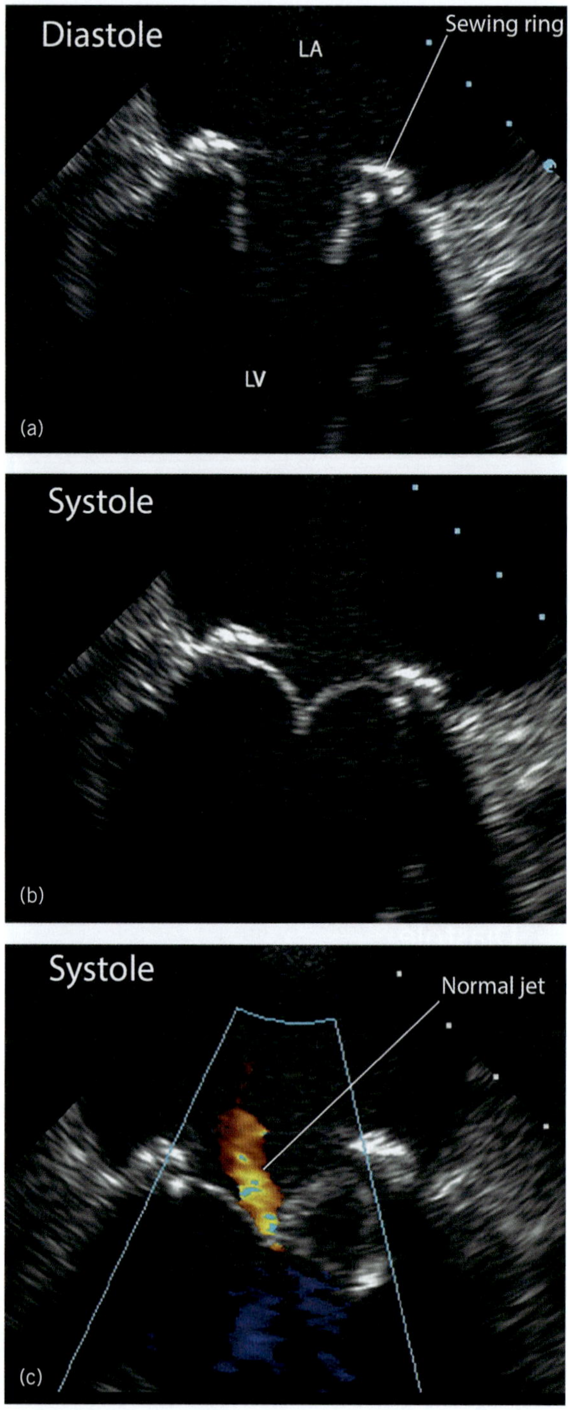

Figure 13.8 Normal stented bioprosthetic MV in the mid-oesophageal two-chamber view. In (a) (diastole), the leaflets are open. In (b) and (c) (systole), the leaflets are closed. The sewing ring is identified. With colour Doppler imaging, a small central jet of MR can be seen, which is a normal finding. See also Online appendix 9.1.3.

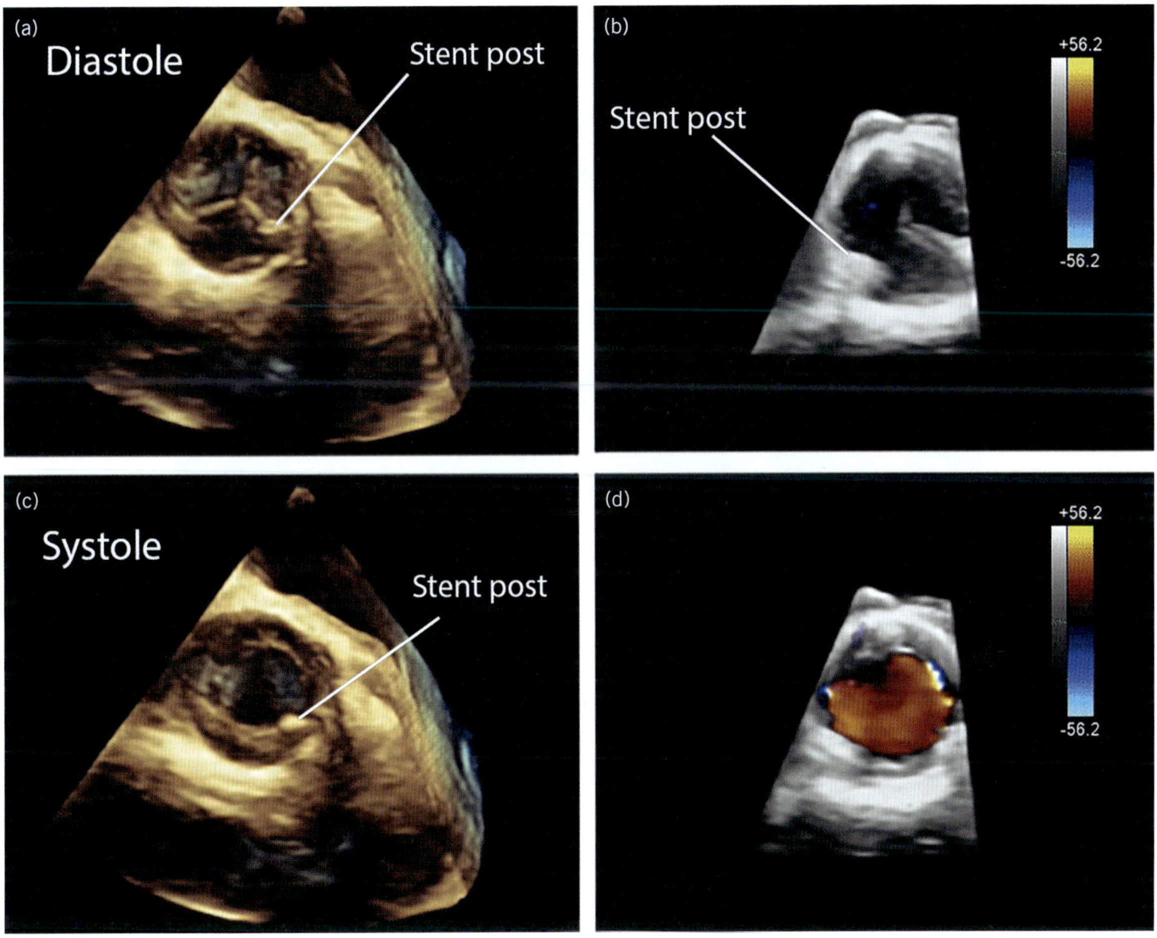

Figure 13.9 3D imaging of a normal stented bioprosthetic AV. The images were obtained using the narrow sector (3D live) mode. The AV is viewed from the aortic perspective at the level of the annulus in the normal orientation (i.e. the RVOT is at the bottom of the screen). (a) and (b) are in diastole, and (c) and (d) are in systole. The leaflets and stent posts can be seen. The leaflets open widely in systole, and there is no transvalvular or paravalvular regurgitation in diastole (b). See also Online appendix 9.1.6.

Stentless porcine and homograft valves

Stentless bioprosthetic valves are preserved porcine AVs, whereas homograft valves are preserved human cadaveric valves. Both types of valves are designed to be used in the aortic or pulmonary positions and may be used as subcoronary implants or—more commonly—as valve/root replacements. The main advantage of stentless valves is a greater EOA and lower transvalvular pressure gradients, compared to stented valves; however, they are technically more difficult to implant than stented valves. The valves must be sized to the patient's ventriculo-aortic junction and sinotubular junction; therefore, these dimensions must be measured accurately prior to implantation (see Chapter 10). For subcoronary implantation, if the sinotubular junction is significantly larger than the aortic annulus, a sinotubuloplasty may be required to prevent post-operative AR.

Echocardiographic appearances

Stentless valves have similar echocardiographic appearances to native aortic valves. The only distinguishing feature is slightly increased tissue thickness around the aortic root. Trivial central AR is common.

Assessment of prosthetic valve function

TOE assessment of prosthetic valves is performed in three clinical situations: (1) during the immediate post-CPB period following valve implantation; (2) when there is suspected dysfunction of a previously implanted valve; and (3) prior to CPB in a patient undergoing redo valve surgery.

The objectives of the echocardiographic assessment are to measure the haemodynamics of forward flow

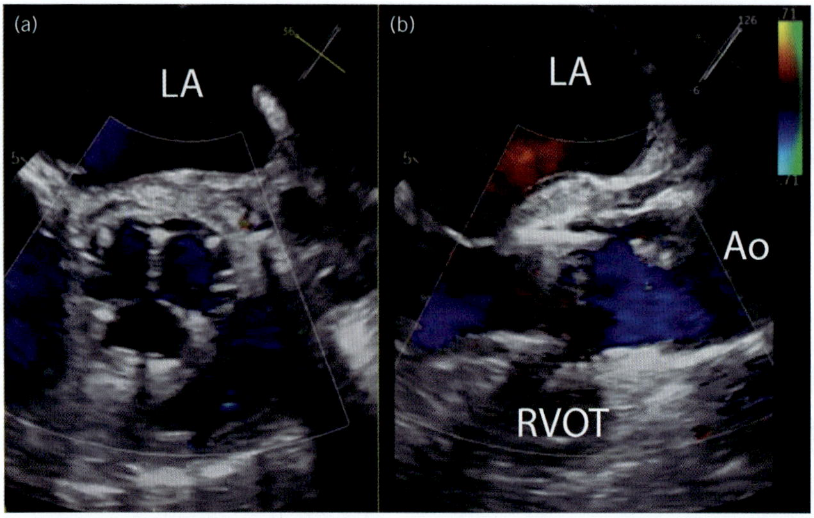

Figure 13.10 Sutureless aortic valve. (a) is a mid-oesophageal AV short-axis view, and (b) is a corresponding mid-oesophageal AV long-axis view, both with colour Doppler, showing a sutureless AV in diastole (leaflets closed). There is no evidence of diastolic transvalvular or paravalvular leak.

Box 13.2 Summary of TOE requirements for peri-operative assessment of Perceval® implantation[11]

Pre-implant assessment

- Number of valve leaflets
- Measure diameter of aortic annulus
- Measure diameter of sinotubular junction
- Ratio of STJ:annulus <1.3

Post-implant assessment

- Perceval® valve appearance on TOE (coaptation line)
- Evaluation of valve seating
- No infolding of frames or leaflets
- Full stent expansion
- PVL and central leak less than mild
- Evaluation of peak/mean gradient

Data from Vasanthan V, *et al. Ann Thorac Surg.* 2019;**107**(3):e223–e225.

(velocity, pressure gradients, EOA), to determine the presence and severity of any pathological regurgitant jets (trans- or paravalvular), to diagnose valve-related pathology (structural degeneration, thrombus, endocarditis, abscess, etc.), and to assess the secondary consequences of valve-related pathology (e.g. ventricular dysfunction, atrial thrombus, etc.).

Haemodynamic assessment

The haemodynamic measurements of prosthetic valves depend on the valve position. For the aortic position, recommended measurements include peak velocity, peak and mean pressure gradients, EOA, and Doppler velocity index (DVI); for the mitral and tricuspid positions, recommended measurements include peak velocity, peak and mean pressure gradients, and PHT.[12] For the MV, good alignment between blood flow and a spectral Doppler beam is usually easily obtained in mid-oesophageal views. For the TV, a modified four-chamber view, RV inflow–outflow view, or modified bicaval view is usually satisfactory, but alignment may be challenging if the heart is distorted. For the aortic position, a deep transgastric five-chamber view or transgastric long-axis view is required. To avoid underestimation of velocities and gradients, it is essential to keep the angle between the ultrasound beam and the blood flow across the valve to <20° (see cosine effect, Chapter 1).

Velocities and gradients

In routine practice, the modified Bernoulli equation (see Equation 3.29 and Chapter 3) is used to estimate gradients across valve prostheses. All prosthetic valves, whether mechanical or bioprosthetic, cause some degree of flow obstruction and thus generate higher pressure gradients than native valves. Depending on the type and size of the valve and the patient's body surface area (BSA), normal pressure gradients across prosthetic valves may approach values similar to those seen in mild to moderate native valve stenosis, especially in the aortic position. A selected range of normal velocities, pressure gradients, and EOAs for different valves in the aortic and mitral positions is provided in Table 13.1; a more complete list is published in the 2009 ASE[13] and 2016 EACVI guidelines.[1]

Like any other parameter in the heart, prosthetic valve gradients should be evaluated in light of the prevailing haemodynamics, and high flow states will produce higher gradients through any given valve orifice. The operator should also be aware of specific situations that can lead to under- or overestimation of prosthetic valve gradients. Underestimation is most often due to poor alignment of the Doppler signal with blood flow, but it may also be caused by low transvalvular flow or by elevated blood pressure.

Overestimation of prosthetic valve gradients can occur in the aortic position, when the LVOT velocity is >1.5 m/s (as seen in hyperdynamic states or narrow LVOT due to LV hypertrophy or a sub-aortic membrane) and when the simplified Bernouilli equation is used (remember: unless $V_2 >>> V_1$, V_1 *cannot* be ignored and one should use Equation 3.28 instead of Equation 3.29). The presence of marked colour aliasing in the LVOT points to an increased LVOT velocity. Likewise, if a large bioprosthetic valve is used in the aortic position, V_2 may be low, leading to a similar situation (where V_2 is not much greater than V_1).

Other causes of false measurements include significant tachycardia (the effect is most marked with prosthetic valves in the mitral and tricuspid positions due to the shorter diastolic time), use of angle correction (not recommended—see Chapter 1), and the phenomenon of **pressure recovery** (Figure 13.11). This effect is most marked for small valves (19–21 mm) in the aortic position, particularly when cardiac output is high.

Finally, for bileaflet mechanical valves, CW Doppler interrogation through the smaller central orifice typically measures a higher transvalvular velocity (and hence a higher calculated pressure gradient) than that measured through the lateral orifices or obtained from invasive catheterization. This is most relevant for bileaflet valves in the aortic position. For this reason, the Doppler beam should be directed across one of the two lateral orifices.

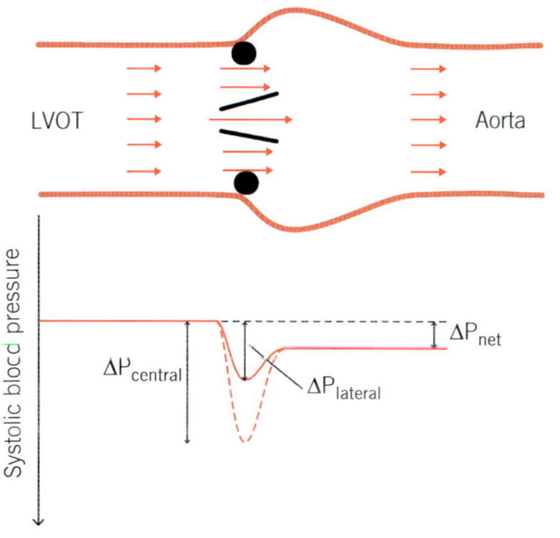

Figure 13.11 Schematic demonstration of pressure recovery across a bileaflet mechanical valve. Velocity is represented by arrow length, and pressure is shown graphically. As blood flows through a narrowed orifice, its velocity increases. Thus, the velocity through the valve is higher than in the LVOT or the aorta, and higher through the smaller central orifice than through either lateral orifice. Because of the law of conservation of energy, any increase in velocity is associated with a drop in pressure, as potential (pressure) energy is converted to kinetic (velocity) energy. Thus, the drop in pressure through the central valvular orifice (dotted line) is greater than the drop in pressure through either lateral orifice (solid line). Distal to the valve, some of the kinetic energy is converted back to potential energy, and the pressure partially recovers. The degree of pressure recovery depends on how much energy was lost due to viscous and turbulent energy losses at the site of stenosis. Doppler measurements are based on the highest velocities through the valve (i.e. before pressure recovery has occurred), whereas catheter-based measurements are obtained by comparing the difference in pressure proximally and distally across the valve (i.e. ΔP_{net}). The distal pressure is measured after pressure recovery has occurred. The difference in Doppler-derived and catheter-derived pressure gradients is shown diagrammatically in Figure 3.6. Thus, Doppler-derived pressures across a narrowed orifice are typically higher than catheter-derived pressures through the same orifice. Additionally, Doppler-derived pressures through the central orifice of a bileaflet mechanical valve are higher than Doppler-derived pressures through a lateral orifice.

Adapted from *Journal of the American Society of Echocardiography*, 22, 9, Zoghbi WA, Chambers JB, Dumesnil JG, *et al.*, Recommendations for evaluation of prosthetic valves with echocardiography and Doppler ultrasound, pp. 975–1014, pp. 981, Figure 3, Copyright 2009, with permission from the American Society of Echocardiography

Effective orifice area

Using the continuity equation, one can calculate the EOA of a prosthetic valve. The EOA is a measure that evaluates the cross-sectional area of the transprosthetic systolic jet. In theory, this should be relatively independent of flow (cardiac output) when compared to transvalvular velocities and gradients, making it a more reliable measure of prosthetic valvular haemodynamic performance. In practice, EOA is still subject to error and technical pitfalls. Ideally, stroke volume should be measured at the LVOT. For aortic prostheses, the equation takes the form (Equation 13.1):

$$EOA = \frac{VTI_{LVOT} \times CSA_{LVOT}}{VTI_{AV}} \qquad \text{Equation 13.1}$$

Or (Equation 13.2):

$$EOA = \frac{SV}{VTI_{AV}} \qquad \text{Equation 13.2}$$

where VTI_{LVOT} is the VTI across the LVOT (measured with PW Doppler); VTI_{AV} is the VTI across the AV (measured with CW Doppler); CSA_{LVOT} is the cross-sectional area of the LVOT measured just proximal to the valve; and *SV* is the stroke volume.

To obtain a reliable measurement, the PW Doppler sample volume must be positioned about 0.5 cm from the prosthetic valve (ideally the same anatomical site for obtaining the LVOT diameter), and a clear envelope must be obtained. Proper measurement of the LVOT diameter is essential, since a 0.2 cm error translates to an approximately 20% change in EOA value. When using the continuity equation, peak velocity may be substituted for VTI in the above equations (see Chapter 3 for details). Measurement of the LVOT-CSA may be difficult due to its non-circular nature, as well as acoustic shadowing (see Chapter 10). Note that the labelled size of the prosthetic valve is not a reliable surrogate for LVOT area.[13] Also, for reasons described above, EOA is underestimated if the smaller central orifice of a bileaflet valve is used to measure the AV velocity or AV-VTI.

For serial studies performed over time, the DVI or dimensionless index is widely used to monitor prosthetic AV function (see Chapter 10). The advantage of DVI, compared to EOA, is that LVOT diameter is not required. Like EOA, DVI is minimally affected by cardiac output. DVI is always <1, as the velocity across the AV is always greater than that across the LVOT. A DVI <0.25 is highly suggestive of significant prosthetic valve stenosis.[13]

Calculation of EOA or DVI is less suited to prosthetic valves in the mitral position due to difficulty in measuring a velocity proximal to the valve. PHT may be used to assess the severity of prosthetic MV stenosis (see Chapter 8). It is important to note that the empiric formula for MV area (220/PHT) is not valid for assessing prosthetic valve EOA unless there is significant stenosis. This is because when EOA exceeds 1.5 cm^2, the PHT is more dependent on LA and LV compliance than on valve area.[13]

Patient–prosthesis mismatch

When a prosthetic valve with normal structure and function is too small for a patient's body size and/or cardiac output requirements, patient–prosthesis mismatch (PPM) may result. PPM is most often seen in young patients with small annular dimensions undergoing AV replacement. As a result, high transvalvular gradients may be measured, representing a true increase in transvalvular gradient over and above the effects of pressure recovery. In addition to a worse functional class and exercise capacity, patients with PPM are at risk of higher rates of heart failure, reduced regression of ventricular remodelling, accelerated structural prosthetic degeneration, and lower survival. The risk of developing PPM may be assessed prior to the surgery, by referencing tables of type-specific predicted EOA values and dividing the EOA by the patient's BSA.[14,15] One should be aware that the valve orifice diameter provided by the manufacturer may not exactly correspond to the actual EOA of the prosthesis. Pre-procedural imaging can estimate the annular size, but ultimately the annulus is measured by the surgeon at the time of insertion after debridement of the annulus. Knowing the model of the prosthetic valve and the patient's BSA, as demonstrated in Table 13.1, one can quickly calculate the predicted indexed EOA and estimate the risk of post-operative PPM. If there is moderate or severe risk of PPM, it may be appropriate to use a stentless prosthesis or to perform an aortic root enlargement. Table 13.3 shows the threshold values of indexed prosthetic valve EOA for quantification of PPM. Note that the indexed EOA may overestimate the severity of PPM in obese patients (body mass index >30 kg/m^2), and the EACVI and Valve Academic Research Consortium recommend using an alternative definition of PPM severity based on indexed EOA in obese patients (i.e. <0.70 cm^2/m^2 for moderate PPM and <0.55 cm^2/m^2 for severe PPM, instead of <0.85 and <0.65 cm^2/m^2, respectively).[15]

Diagnosis of prosthetic valve stenosis

As previously discussed, numerous factors influence the measured pressure gradients and EOA of prosthetic valves, and elevated transvalvular pressures can occur in the absence of valvular pathology. Careful assessment of prosthetic valve function using a combination of 2D, 3D, colour Doppler, and spectral Doppler imaging should be performed. Velocities, pressure gradients, and EOAs should be reported and compared to the valve type- and size-specific normal range. The patient's haemodynamic state, particularly an increased cardiac output and/or heart rate, may increase velocities and gradients. Ideally, the haemodynamic diagnosis of prosthetic stenosis should be accompanied by evidence of pathology on 2D or 3D imaging (e.g. vegetations, thrombus, pannus, calcific degeneration, restricted leaflet opening;

Table 13.3 Threshold values of indexed prosthetic valve effective orifice area for quantification of patient–prosthesis mismatch risk

	Mild or not clinically significant	Moderate	Severe
Aortic	>0.85 cm^2/m^2	0.65–0.85 cm^2/m^2	<0.65 cm^2/m^2
Mitral	>1.2 cm^2/m^2	0.9–1.2 cm^2/m^2	<0.9 cm^2/m^2

Data from Zoghbi WA, *et al.*, *J Am Soc Echocardiogr.* 2009;**22**:975–1014.

see Online appendices 9.2.1.3–9.2.1.7). It is also important to remember that in many reported series of Doppler-derived pressure gradients across clinically *normal* prosthetic valves, there are outliers with abnormally high measured gradients, possibly due to the effects of pressure recovery. Thus, measurement of EOA and DVI (for the AV) and PHT (for the MV) provides a more reliable indication of prosthetic valve stenosis than pressure gradients and velocities.

Suicide left ventricle

The term '**suicide left ventricle**' has been used in the recent literature to refer to haemodynamic instability, due to an acute lowering of LV afterload resulting in dynamic LVOT and/or intracavitary obstruction. It has been described upon separation from CPB after surgical AV replacement and post-deployment of transcatheter aortic valve implantation (TAVI) valves, and it is probably more common than reported. Echocardiographically, the LV cavity is small (sometimes apparently collapsed in systole) and in some cases, MV systolic anterior motion (SAM) can contribute to the obstruction. Asymmetric septal hypertrophy is reported to be a predisposing factor, but any patient with chronic concentric LV remodelling is at risk of developing this condition. The management involves restoring LV cavity volumes with judicious fluid administration and pharmacologic afterload support.

Pathological valvular regurgitation

Pathological prosthetic regurgitation may be transvalvular (within the sewing ring) or paravalvular (outside the sewing ring).

Transvalvular

As discussed previously, trivial transvalvular regurgitation is a normal finding for many prosthetic valves. Pathological transvalvular regurgitation is usually associated with an identifiable pathology (see Online appendix 9.2.1), as described later. The severity of transvalvular regurgitation should be assessed using standard techniques (vena contracta, flow convergence, etc.).

Paravalvular

Persistent paravalvular regurgitation is never normal. Trivial paravalvular jets seen immediately after separation

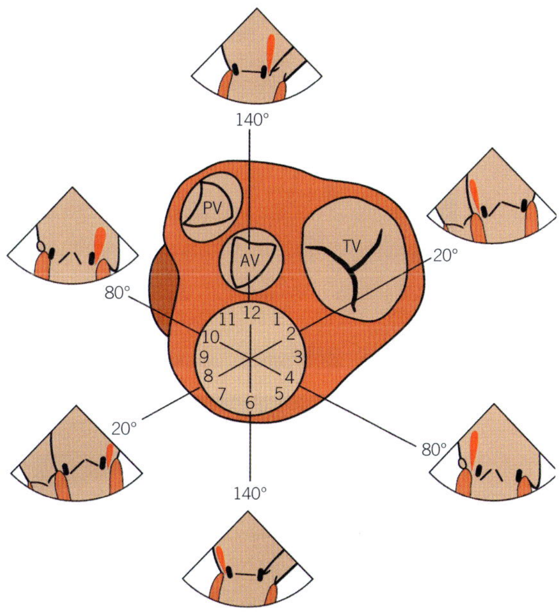

Figure 13.12 Technique for describing the location of paravalvular MR with 2D imaging. The MV and surrounding structures are shown in the surgical orientation. A clock face is superimposed on the MV, with the AV defined as the 12 o'clock position, the centre of the posterior leaflet as the 6 o'clock position, and the LA appendage as the 9 to 10 o'clock position. The positions of the standard mid-oesophageal views are shown with respect to the clock face. For example, the mid-oesophageal long-axis view (approximately 140°) passes through the 12 and 6 o'clock positions. The extent and location of any paravalvular regurgitation are reported with respect to the clock face (e.g. '*from 2 to 6 o'clock*').

from bypass are relatively common and usually resolve following protamine administration or in the first few post-operative weeks as the sewing ring becomes covered with endothelium. The presence of more than trivial paravalvular regurgitation in the post-CPB period is usually an indication for immediate revision. An exception is a mild PVL in a patient with a severely calcified annulus, in which case the leak may not be repairable.

The distinction between trivial and mild paravalvular regurgitation can be difficult, particularly for jets that are markedly eccentric. For aortic prostheses, eccentric jets that are directed obliquely across the LVOT may lead to overestimation of severity, as it is easy to confuse jet length with jet width. Conversely, some very eccentric jets may be hidden by acoustic shadowing from the posterior sewing ring.

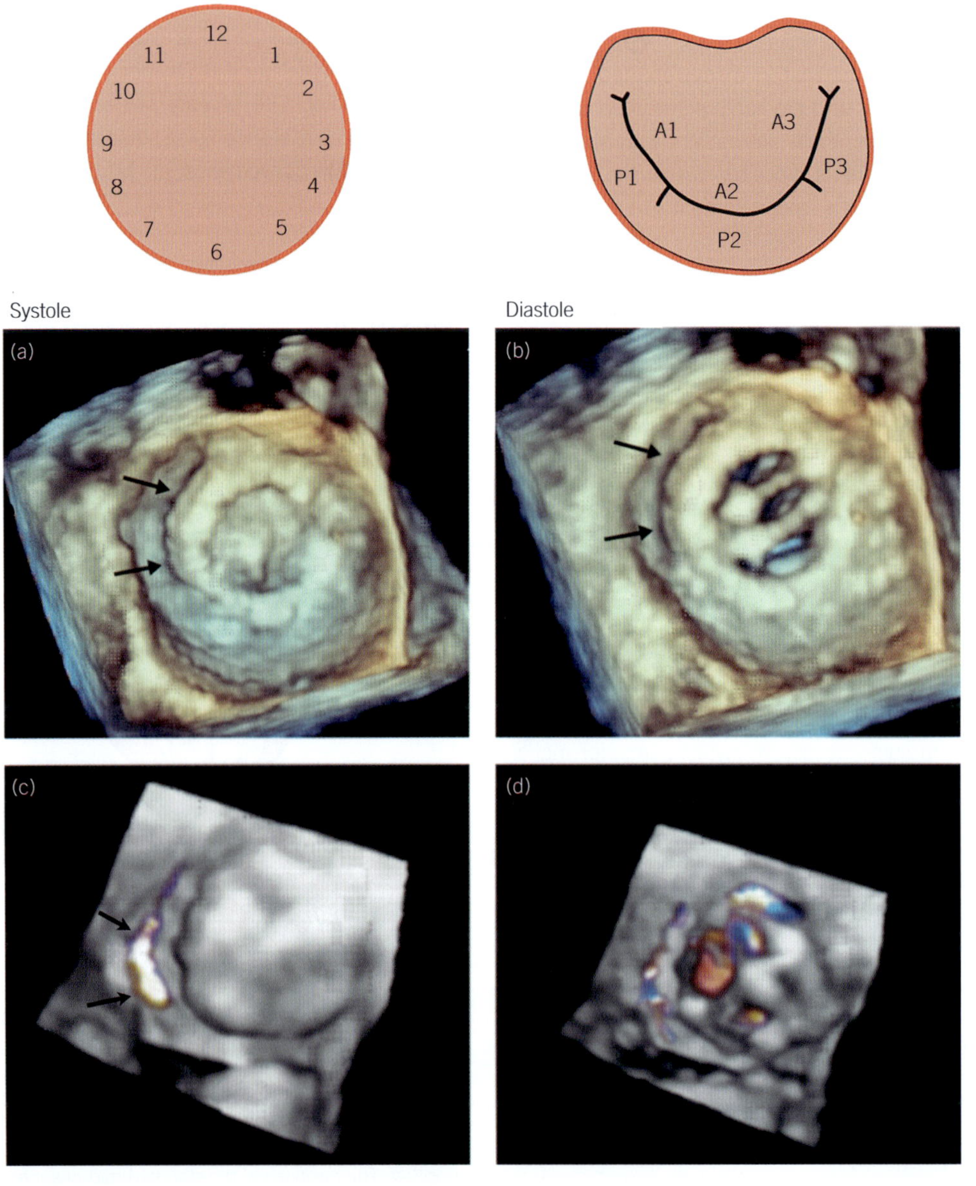

Figure 13.13 Alternative ways to describe the location of an MV paravalvular leak. A bileaflet mechanical MV is shown in 3D, from the atrial aspect in the surgical orientation. With standard 3D imaging (a) and (b), a visible defect (arrows) can be seen between the valve and the annulus. With 3D colour Doppler (c), an abnormal jet can be seen in the same location. The location of the defect can be reported using a clock face, as explained in Figure 13.12 ('the leak is located at 9 to 10 o'clock, assuming the aortic valve is at 12 o'clock'), or in relation to the location of the corresponding (excised) native mitral segments ('the leak is located laterally, in the area of the native P1 scallop').

> ***Expert tip:*** ***Jets from aortic prostheses usually appear larger with deep transgastric imaging (when the ultrasound beam is aligned with blood flow) than with mid-oesophageal imaging (when the ultrasound beam is typically perpendicular to blood flow—see Chapter 1 for details).***

PVLs can be difficult to find surgically and it is essential to accurately describe the precise location of the defect to facilitate surgical repair. In the case of the MV, it is usually possible to determine the anatomical location of a PVL using colour Doppler imaging in the standard mid-oesophageal views. However, this approach requires a thorough knowledge of the anatomic–echocardiographic relationships for the mid-oesophageal views (Figure 13.12), and it is easy to misdiagnose the location and extent of the jet. 3D imaging with colour Doppler is much more intuitive and allows the location and extent of PVLs to be accurately determined. The MV should be displayed in the surgical orientation from the LA aspect, with the AV at 12 o'clock, and the location of the defect reported in relation to either the (excised) native mitral segments or a clock face (Figures 13.12 and 13.13; see Online appendices 9.2.2 and 9.2.3).

In the case of the AV, it is usually possible to determine the location of the jet with colour Doppler imaging in the mid-oesophageal AV short-axis view. The location of the jet can be reported with respect to the location of the (excised) native AV cusps (Figure 13.14; see Online appendix 9.3.3). 3D colour Doppler imaging is also helpful in determining the location of prosthetic AV leaks but does not offer the same advantage over 2D colour

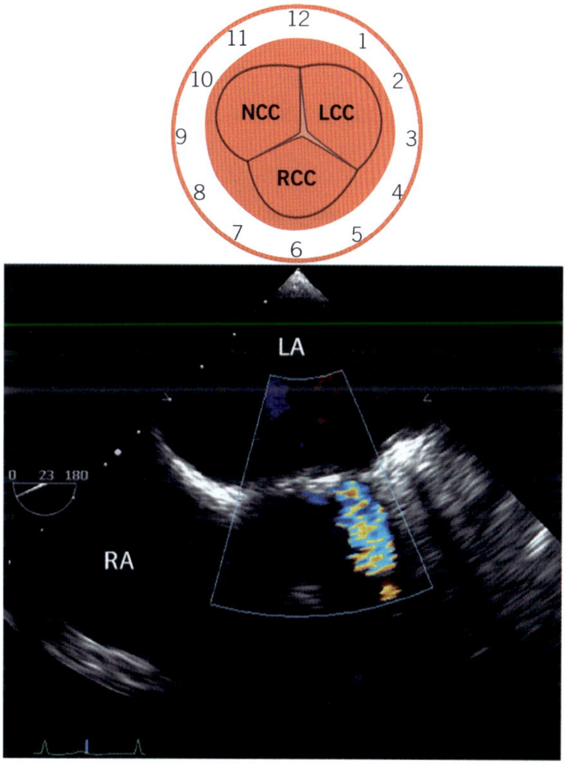

Figure 13.14 Describing the location of aortic paravalvular regurgitation. In this mid-oesophageal AV short-axis view from a patient with a bileaflet mechanical AV, the probe was advanced slightly to visualize the LVOT. A diastolic jet of AR can be seen. The location of the jet can be reported in relation to the location of the (excised) native AV leaflets. In this example, the jet is in the region of the (excised) LCC. The leak can also be described in reference to a clock where the centre of the RCC is at 6 o'clock and the commissure between the NCC and the LCC is at 12 o'clock. See also Online appendix 9.3.3.

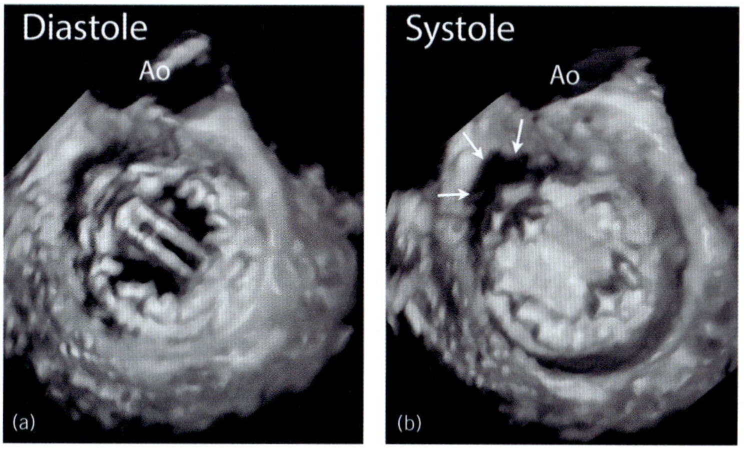

Figure 13.15 Dehiscence of part of the sewing ring. (a) This is a zoomed 3D *en face* view of a mechanical MV prosthesis from the surgeon's perspective, with the aorta (Ao) at the top. The systolic frame (b) shows a large gap anteriorly, between the sewing ring and the annulus (arrows), representing a dehiscence of the sewing ring. A colour Doppler of the same valve would show a large paravalvular leak.

Doppler, as is seen in the mitral position, because 3D is subject to the same acoustic shadowing from the posterior sewing ring as 2D. The 3D data set should be orientated to display the AV prosthesis from the LVOT aspect, with the (excised) right coronary cusp at the bottom of the screen.

Severe paravalvular regurgitation often implies dehiscence of part of the sewing ring (Figure 13.15; see Online appendix 9.3.2–9.3.3). The defect may be visible on 2D or 3D imaging, and the valve may demonstrate a rocking motion with the cardiac cycle. A broad turbulent regurgitant jet is typically seen with colour Doppler. The severity of paravalvular regurgitation should be assessed using standard grading techniques (vena contracta, flow convergence, etc.). It is important to note that even haemodynamically insignificant paravalvular regurgitation can cause clinically significant haemolysis. 3D multiplanar reconstruction at the level of the vena contracta can add information regarding the severity of a PVL with the measurement of the vena contracta area.[16]

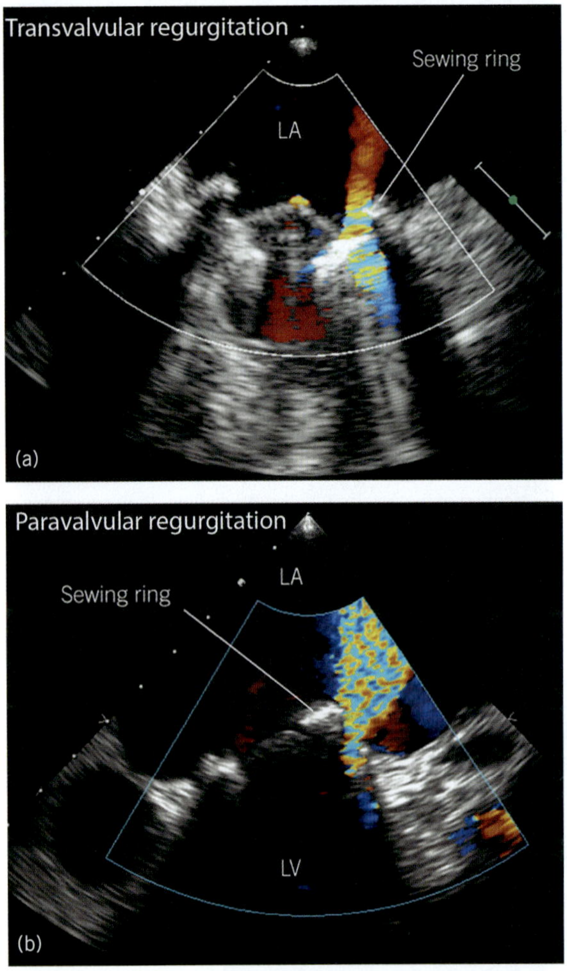

Figure 13.16 Transvalvular versus paravalvular MR. Both images show a bileaflet mechanical MV in mid-to-late systole. In (a), the regurgitant jet originates *inside* the sewing ring, indicating the regurgitation is *trans*valvular. In this case, the cause of the regurgitation was an entangled subvalvular apparatus preventing proper leaflet closure. In (b), the regurgitant jet originates *outside* the sewing ring, indicating the regurgitation is *para*valvular. In this case, the cause of the paravalvular regurgitation was partial dehiscence of the sewing ring due to torn annular sutures. See also Online appendix 9.2.1.

Transvalvular versus paravalvular

Differentiating transvalvular regurgitation from paravalvular regurgitation is not always straightforward, especially when transvalvular jets are close to the sewing ring (Figure 13.16). The distinction between paravalvular and transvalvular jets is particularly problematic for AV prostheses, because acoustic shadowing and reverberation artefact from the posterior aortic sewing ring can make it difficult to visualize the origin of regurgitant jets in the mid-oesophageal aortic views (Figure 13.17). This difficulty is compounded when there is also a mitral prosthesis *in situ* or significant mitral annular calcification, which causes even more acoustic shadowing of the LVOT in the mid-oesophageal AV long-axis view. Transgastric imaging is helpful in this situation where the origin of regurgitant jets is not masked by acoustic shadowing (Figure 13.18). As a rule of thumb, markedly eccentric jets are usually paravalvular. Finally, with stented bioprostheses, the location of paravalvular leaks in relation to the stent posts can provide a clue to the nature of the leak.

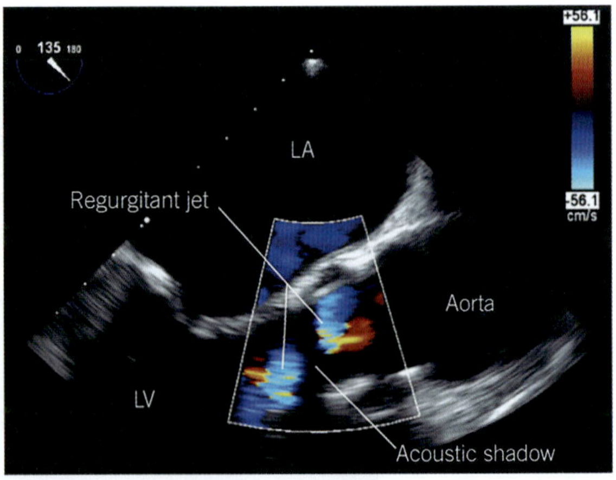

Figure 13.17 Bioprosthetic AV regurgitation. In this mid-oesophageal AV long-axis view, a regurgitant jet is seen. Acoustic shadowing from the prosthesis limits visualization of the jet origin, making it hard to determine in this view whether the jet is transvalvular or paravalvular. See Online appendices 9.3.3 and 9.3.4.

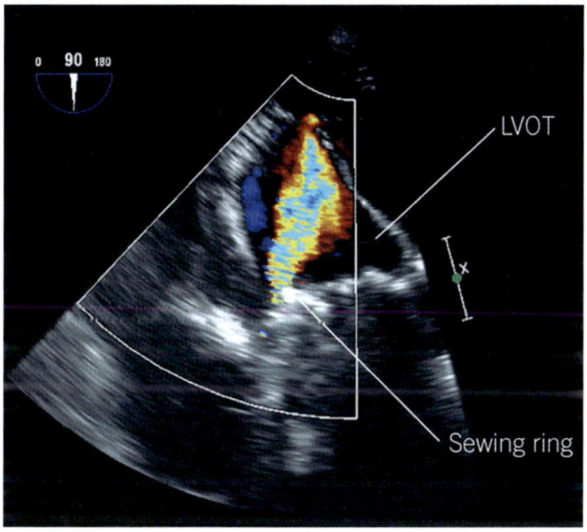

Figure 13.18 Paravalvular regurgitation across a bileaflet mechanical AV. In this deep transgastric view, the jet can be clearly seen to arise from outside the sewing ring, indicating the AR is paravalvular. See also Online appendix 9.3.2.

Expert tip: A commissural transvalvular leak can only, by definition, occur at the site of a commissure. If a leak appears to be located between two stent posts, it has to be paravalvular.

Valve-related pathology

Valve-related pathology can be categorized as early, occurring in the immediate or early post-CPB period, or late, occurring in the days, months, or years following surgery. Early complications are usually a manifestation of technical problems at the time of insertion, whereas late complications relate to valve degeneration and other pathological processes.

Early

Following MV replacement with a bileaflet mechanical valve, the preserved subvalvular apparatus can become entangled in the prosthetic leaflets, with several possible effects. One or both leaflets may be stuck in an open, closed, or partially open position, resulting in transvalvular regurgitation, valvular stenosis, or mixed stenosis/regurgitation. One example of both leaflets stuck in a partially open position is shown in Figure 13.19 and Online appendix 9.2.1. A single leaflet that is stuck in a closed position in the immediate post-CPB period may spontaneously start moving normally in the first few minutes following separation from CPB. However, an entangled subvalvular apparatus resulting in valve dysfunction usually necessitates revision, usually by rotating the valve mechanism within the sewing ring.

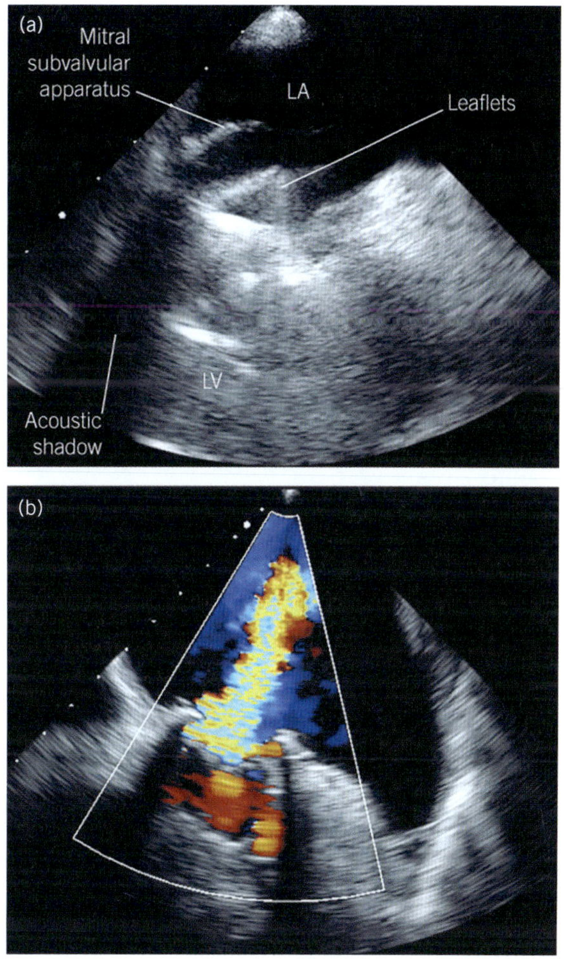

Figure 13.19 Stuck leaflets causing severe transvalvular regurgitation across a bileaflet mechanical MV. Both frames (a) and (b) are in mid systole. With 2D imaging, the leaflets appear to be incompletely closed, and an entangled mitral subvalvular apparatus can be seen in the LA. Colour Doppler imaging demonstrates severe MR. See Online appendix 9.2.1.

Note that a bileaflet mechanical valve may appear to have abnormal leaflet motion if the imaging plane is oblique or off-axis. The presence of normal-flow patterns on colour Doppler imaging helps to distinguish this problem from true valvular pathology.

Leaflet impingement by a suture can result in restricted motion of a bioprosthetic valve, resulting in transvalvular regurgitation and/or valvular stenosis.

Significant paravalvular regurgitation in the immediate post-CPB period is usually the result of broken/loose sutures or annular calcification preventing close approximation of

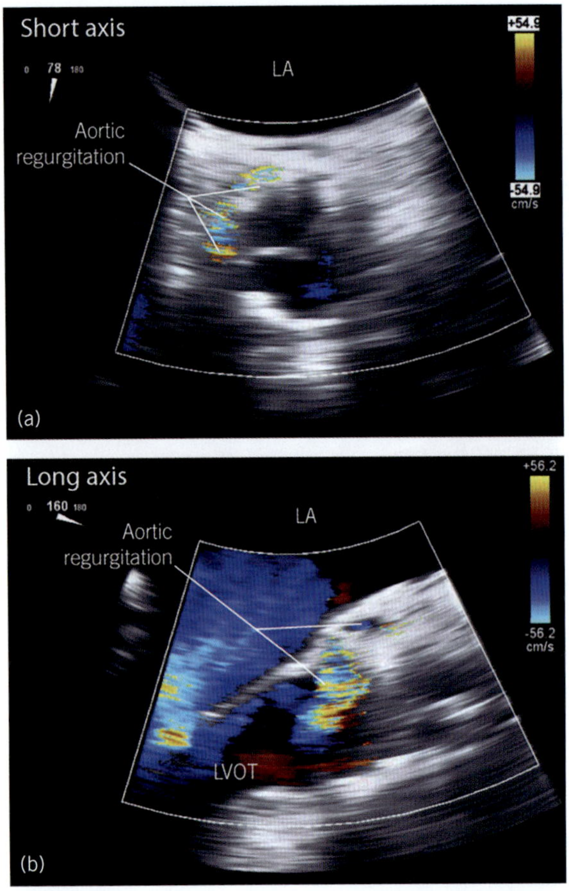

Figure 13.20 Paravalvular regurgitation across a sutureless AV prosthesis. (a) In the mid-oesophageal short-axis view, a jet of regurgitation can be seen in the region of the (excised) non-coronary cusp. (b) In the long-axis view, the jet can be seen to originate around the valve, in the non-coronary sinus of Valsalva. See Online appendices 9.3.3.6–9.3.3.9.

the sewing ring with the annulus. Paravalvular regurgitation noted with sutureless valve implantation may be due to incorrect sizing or improper seating of the valve (Figure 13.20; see Online appendices 9.3.3.6–9.3.3.9). If paravalvular AR is seen following sutureless AV replacement, return to CPB and further balloon inflation of the valve may be indicated.[10,12]

Damage to adjacent cardiac structures can also occur. A misplaced mitral annular suture can disrupt flow in the circumflex coronary artery (see Figure 8.1). Sutures or an incorrectly positioned prosthesis may obstruct the coronary ostia during AV replacement and result in significant regional wall motion abnormality (RWMA) in the immediate post-CPB period. LVOT obstruction can occur from both an annular suture (see Online appendix 9.2.7) or the stent post of a mitral bioprosthesis, especially in a small heart.

Finally, dynamic intracavity or LVOT obstruction with SAM may occur after AV replacement for AS. SAM is precipitated by the reduced LV afterload associated with the relief of AS in the context of marked LV hypertrophy. The problem is exacerbated by hypovolaemia, tachycardia, and increased contractility. The TOE features of SAM are described in Chapters 6 and 8. LVOT obstruction can also occur after placement of MV prostheses with preservation of the subvalvular apparatus.

Late

Bioprosthetic valves are subject to structural deterioration, which is usually progressive over time. Structural deterioration is typically more rapid for bioprosthetic valves in the mitral position than in the aortic position and is more common in younger patients. In one study, the rate of reoperation following bioprosthetic AV replacement due to structural deterioration was 60% at 10 years in patients aged 16–39, compared to <15% at 15 years in patients aged over 70.[17] The mechanism of failure is usually calcification with leaflet thickening and immobility, resulting in progressive stenosis and/or regurgitation (typically transvalvular). Occasionally, a calcified bioprosthetic leaflet may fracture, causing acute transvalvular regurgitation in the absence of widespread leaflet deterioration. Mechanical valves are extremely durable, but very occasionally, structural failure can occur, causing acute severe regurgitation.

Other late causes of valve dysfunction include endocarditis, thrombus formation (Figure 13.21), and the development of pannus (fibrous ingrowth from the sewing ring). These conditions can be difficult to distinguish echocardiographically.

Vegetations from endocarditis usually appear as irregular, echogenic masses attached to valve components, most often in the clinical context of infection and/or positive blood cultures. Small vegetations may be hard to see or to distinguish from suture material, valve strands, thrombi, or the irregular surface of a degenerating bioprosthetic valve.

Expert tip: It is important to obtain and store detailed images of a valve prosthesis in the immediate post-operative period, so that when patients return at a later date, these images can be used as a reference to help differentiate between pre-existing and new, potentially pathologic, appearance of their valves.

Endocarditis of bioprosthetic valves usually results in leaflet destruction, which leads to transvalvular

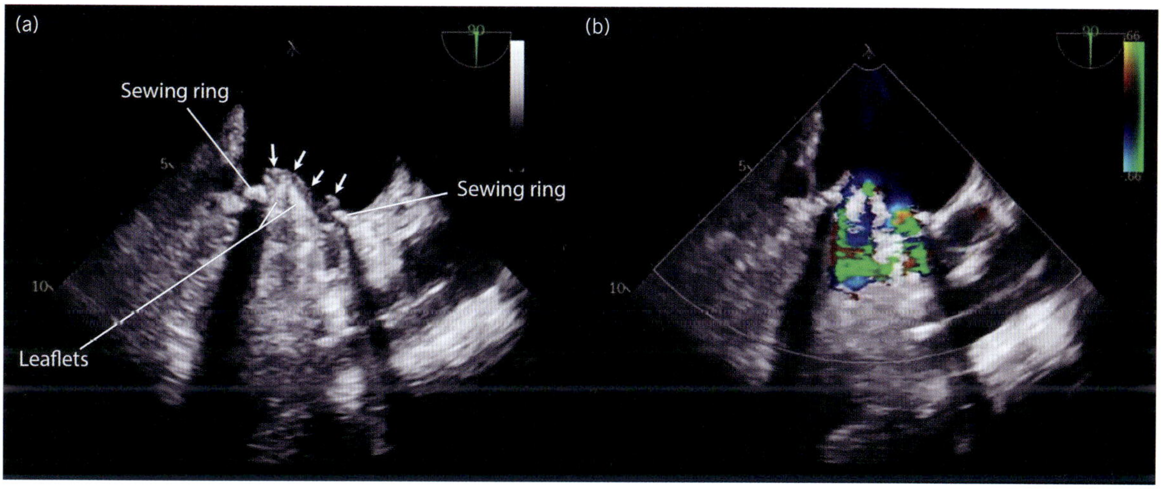

Figure 13.21 Thrombosed bileaflet mechanical MV. This is a mid-oesophageal two-chamber view showing an MV prosthesis in 2D (a) and with colour Doppler (b). Both frames (a) and (b) are taken in early diastole (leaflets open). (a) shows a large thrombus attached to the atrial side of the valve (arrows). (b) shows diastolic aliasing (the colour green represents high variance—see Chapter 2), consistent with diastolic obstruction of the valve.

regurgitation. With mechanical valves, vegetations may interfere with leaflet motion, resulting in either stenosis or regurgitation. For both types of valves, endocarditis may also cause dehiscence of the sewing ring, resulting in severe paravalvular regurgitation and a characteristic 'rocking' motion of the prosthesis on imaging. Endocarditis may also result in a paravalvular abscess or fistula formation (see Online appendix 9.3.1), particularly with valves in the aortic position.

Thrombus formation may result in stenosis and/or transvalvular regurgitation. It occurs most often in inadequately anticoagulated patients with mechanical valves and is more common in the mitral position. On TOE, thrombus is easily visualized on mitral prostheses (see Online appendix 9.2.4) but can be difficult to see on aortic valves. Echocardiographic evaluation of pannus can be challenging, as it is often small (compared to thrombus), lies within the plane of the valve, and grows inwards from the sewing ring. The only clue to pannus formation may be abnormal valve function on Doppler assessment. Pannus is less common than thrombus, occurs on both mechanical and bioprosthetic valves, and is more common in the aortic than in the mitral position.

Valve strands are commonly seen on prosthetic valves and have no functional significance.

Multiple choice questions

Discover interactive multiple choice questions to test your knowledge on this chapter by searching for this book's title or ISBN (9780198873686) at **https://academic.oup.com/** and going to the online appendix at the end of the book. Use your scratch-off code on the inside cover to access the material.

References

1. Lancellotti P, Pibarot P, Chambers J, *et al.* Recommendations for the imaging assessment of prosthetic heart valves: a report from the European Association of Cardiovascular Imaging endorsed by the Chinese Society of Echocardiography, the Inter-American Society of Echocardiography, and the Brazilian Department of Cardiovascular Imaging. *Eur Heart J Cardiovasc Imaging.* 2016;**17**(6):589–95.
2. Otto CM, Nishimura RA, Bonow RO, *et al.* 2020 ACC/AHA Guideline for the management of patients with valvular heart disease: executive summary: a report of the American College of Cardiology/American Heart Association Joint Committee on Clinical Practice Guidelines. *Circulation.* 2021;**143**(5):e35–71.
3. Zoghbi WA, Adams D, Bonow RO, *et al.* Recommendations for noninvasive evaluation of native valvular regurgitation. *J Am Soc Echocardiogr.* 2017;**30**(4):303–71.
4. Mahmood F, Matyal R, Mahmood F, Sheu RD, Feng R, Khabbaz KR. Intraoperative echocardiographic assessment of prosthetic valves: a practical approach. *J Cardiothorac Vasc Anesth.* 2018;**32**(2):823–37.
5. Sotiropoulos F, Le TB, Gilmanov A. Fluid mechanics of heart valves and their replacements. *Annual Review of Fluid Mechanics.* 2016;**48**(1):259–83.
6. Schaff HV. Sutureless prostheses for aortic valve replacement: quicker may not be better. *J Am Coll Cardiol.* 2018;**71**(13):1429–31.
7. Bilkhu R, Borger MA, Briffa NP, Jahangiri M. Sutureless aortic valve prostheses. *Heart.* 2019;**105**(Suppl 2):s16–20.

8. Glauber M, Miceli A, di Bacco L. Sutureless and rapid deployment valves: implantation technique from A to Z—the Perceval valve. *Ann Cardiothorac Surg*. 2020;**9**(4):330–40.
9. Gersak B, Fischlein T, Folliguet TA, *et al*. Sutureless, rapid deployment valves and stented bioprosthesis in aortic valve replacement: recommendations of an International Expert Consensus Panel. *Eur J Cardiothorac Surg*. 2016;**49**(3):709–18.
10. Mazine A, Bonneau C, Karangelis D, Yanagawa B, Verma S, Bonneau D. Sutureless aortic valves: who is the right patient? *Curr Opin Cardiol*. 2017;**32**(2):130–6.
11. Phan K, Tsai Y, Niranjan N, *et al*. Sutureless aortic valve replacement: a systematic review and meta-analysis. *Ann Cardiothorac Surg*. 2015;**4**(2):100–11.
12. Vasanthan V, Kent W, Gregory A, *et al*. Perceval valve implantation: technical details and echocardiographic assessment. *Ann Thorac Surg*. 2019;**107**(3):e223–5.
13. Zoghbi WA, Chambers JB, Dumesnil JG, *et al*. Recommendations for evaluation of prosthetic valves with echocardiography and Doppler ultrasound. *J Am Soc Echocardiogr*. 2009;**22**(9):975–1014.
14. Pibarot P, Dumesnil JG. Prosthesis–patient mismatch: definition, clinical impact, and prevention. *Heart*. 2006;**92**(8):1022–9.
15. Pibarot P, Magne J, Leipsic J, *et al*. Imaging for predicting and assessing prosthesis–patient mismatch after aortic valve replacement. *JACC Cardiovasc Imaging*. 2019;**12**(1):149–62.
16. Konoske R, Whitener G, Nicoara A. Intraoperative evaluation of paravalvular regurgitation by transesophageal echocardiography. *Anesth Analg*. 2015;**121**(2):329–36.
17. Rahimtoola SH. Choice of prosthetic heart valve for adult patients. *J Am Coll Cardiol*. 2003;**41**(6):893–904.

14
The right ventricle

Right ventricular (RV) failure is an important cause of morbidity and mortality in cardiac surgical patients, with a 0.1% incidence of severe acute perioperative RV failure after cardiotomy. Furthermore, acute refractory RV failure is associated with a 22–90% risk of hospital mortality. Thus, careful assessment of RV function is essential when performing TOE to assess for haemodynamic instability. Patients with pre-existing RV dysfunction or severe pulmonary hypertension (e.g. secondary to MV disease), and those undergoing heart or lung transplantation or requiring LV assist device implantation are at highest risk of developing post-operative RV failure. This chapter outlines an approach to imaging the RV with TOE, along with the echocardiographic features of the different mechanisms of RV dysfunction.

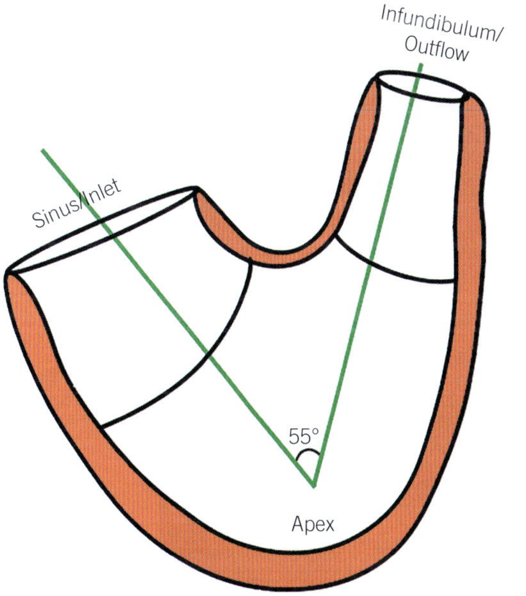

Figure 14.1 RV chamber geometry and angle of blood flow.

Anatomical chambers and walls

The RV can be described as having three main segments: the **sinus or inlet portion**, the **infundibulum or outflow portion**, and an **apical trabecular component** (Figure 14.1). The RV is an anterior mediastinal cardiac structure, which has a crescentic shape in cross-section when viewed using TOE (Figure 14.2d) and a triangular appearance when viewed *en face* (Figure 14.2a). Four distinct RV wall segments can be seen: the **lateral or free wall**, the **anterior wall**, the **infundibulum**, and the **inferior wall** (Figure 14.2a–f). Contrary to the LV where inflow and outflow are nearly parallel, the inflow and outflow are at approximately 55° to each other (Figure 14.1). Compared to the LV, the RV has coarser trabeculae, a **moderator band**, and a tricuspid annular plane that is more apical than that of the MV. The RV wall is thinner than that of the LV and yet presents a complex three-dimensional muscular arrangement: a *subepicardial circumferential* to oblique layer with superficial fibres shared with the LV, and a predominantly *subendocardial longitudinal* layer with septal fibres shared with the LV.[1,2] Contraction is peristaltic in nature, progressing from the apex to the infundibulum. It comprises three separate motions: inward free wall motion, longitudinal motion towards the apex, and free wall traction resulting from LV contraction.[3,4] The sinus portion contributes the bulk of the work performed by the RV, although the LV may contribute up to 40% of RV pressure generation.[5]

Coronary blood supply

The RV is largely supplied by the right coronary artery (RCA) (Figure 14.2). A right dominant circulation is present when the RCA supplies the posterior descending artery (PDA). The anterior wall and the infundibulum are supplied by both the RCA and the left anterior descending artery (LAD). The lateral wall of the RV is supplied exclusively by the RCA (acute marginal branch), whereas the inferior wall of the RV and the posterior third of the septum are supplied by the PDA.[6,7,8]

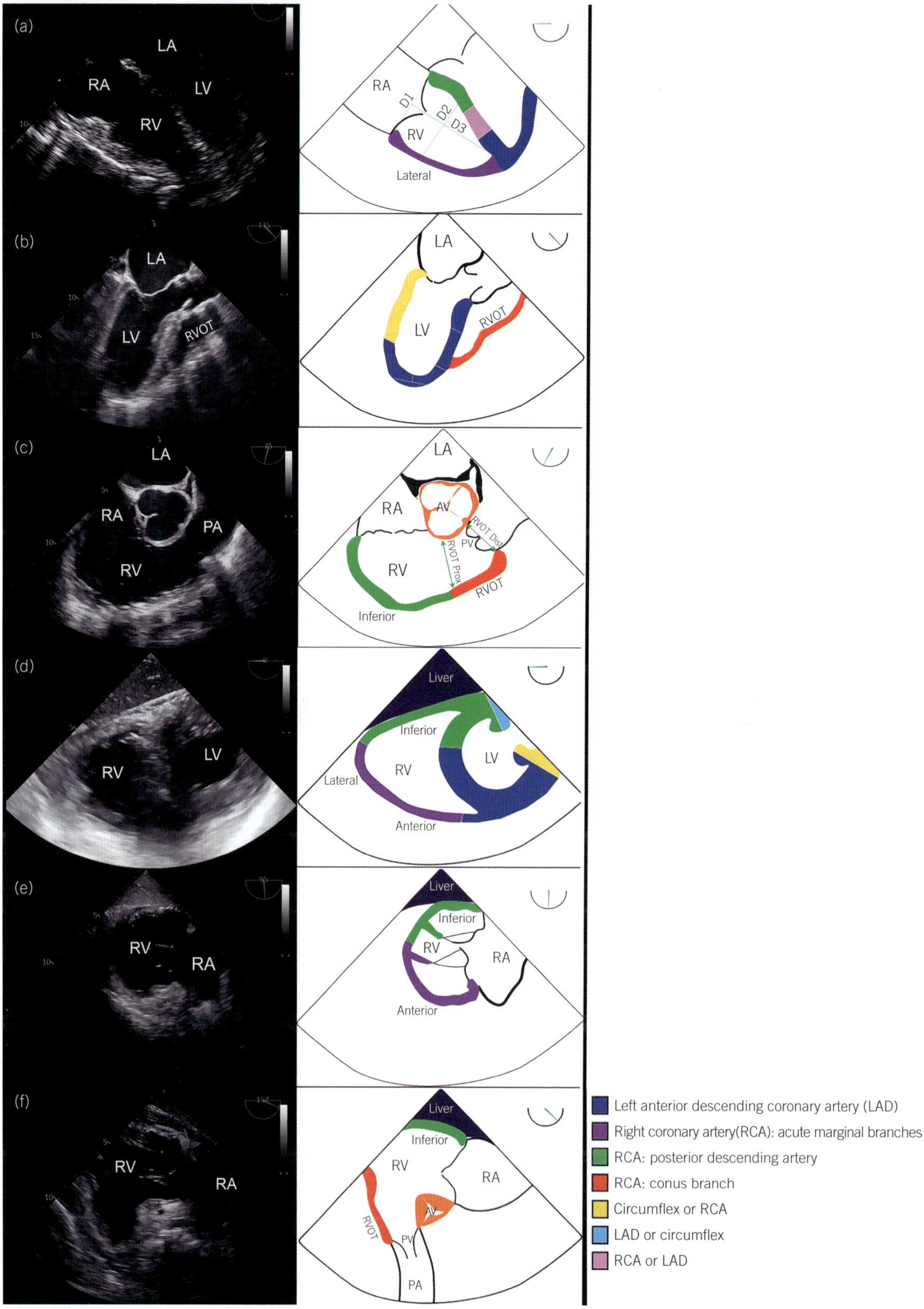

Figure 14.2 TOE views of the RV with coronary blood flow distribution. See text for details.

Physiology and pathophysiology

In the perioperative period, the RV may fail due to pre-existing conditions such as pulmonary hypertension, volume overload, or myocardial infarction. Furthermore, poor myocardial protection during cardiopulmonary bypass (CPB), ischaemia, or previously unrecognized dysfunction may occur independently or exacerbate pre-existing disease. A good understanding of RV physiology and a thorough examination are critical to the recognition and anticipation of RV dysfunction.

RV ejection is uniquely dependent on the low hydraulic impedance of the normal pulmonary circulation. Increased resistance, and reduced compliance and capacitance, as well as pressure wave reflections, may collectively impede RV ejection and performance. RV adaptability is better suited to gradual increases in impedance, and thus acute changes, such as increases in pulmonary artery pressure, may result in RV distension and catastrophic RV failure.[2] In cases of chronic pressure overload, the RV may become hypertrophied and a flat or 'D-shaped' interventricular septum (IVS) may be noted in systole (Figure 14.3).

As a result of RV geometry and distensibility, the volume to surface area relationship is relatively stable during normal changes in preload.[3] Thus, the Frank–Starling recruitment through RV stretch will only occur at larger RV volumes, at which point RV distension results in a leftward diastolic IVS shift and impaired LV filling.

Echocardiographic views

The RV is directly visible to the surgeon and anesthesiologist due to its anterior mediastinal position. Although gross disruptions in RV function and size are readily observable, subtler changes may not be visible. Standard echocardiographic images used to examine the RV are discussed in Figure 14.2.[6]

Standard TOE views with anatomical markers

Mid-oesophageal (RV-focused) four-chamber view (Figure 14.2a): in this view, the RV sinus, the apex, and the more apical position of the tricuspid

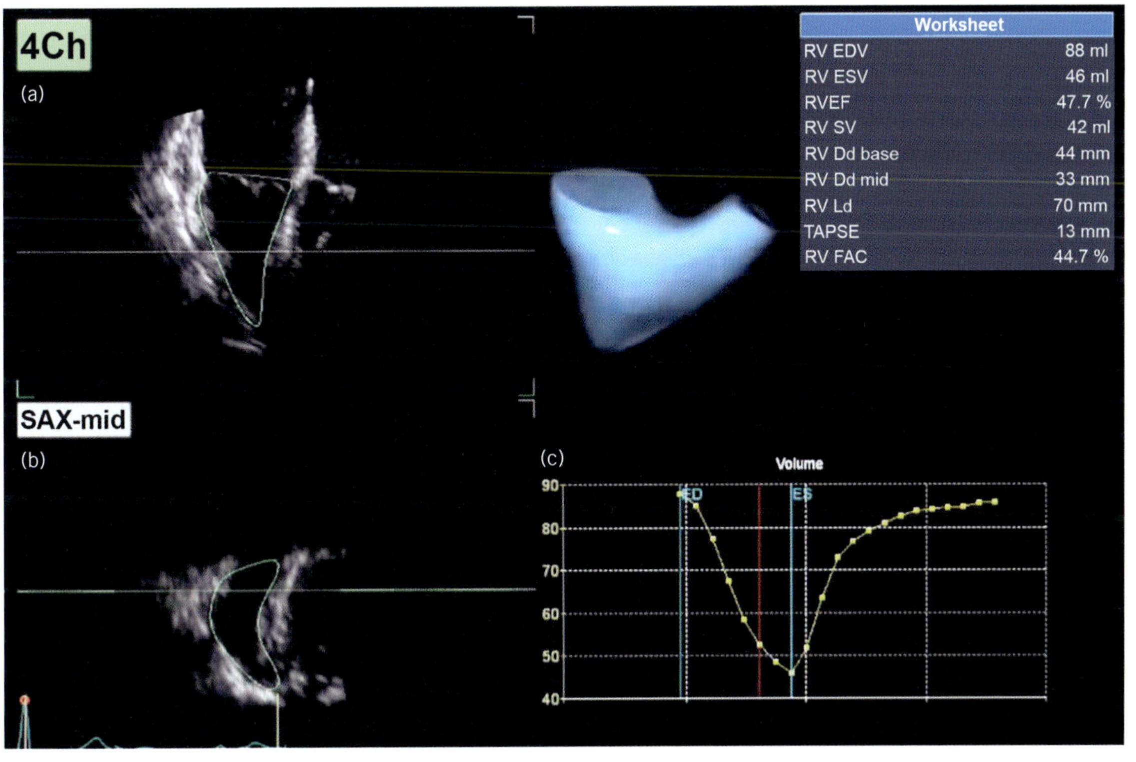

Figure 14.3 Calculation of RV ejection fraction using 3D imaging. After obtaining a 3D data set of the RV, the operator places six landmarks on the image—tricuspid annular points and RV apex in the four-chamber view (a), and anterior/posterior LV–RV junctions and free wall in the short-axis view (b). The machine then automatically detects the RV borders and calculates RV volumes and parameters of global systolic function. The information is displayed graphically and numerically (c). See Online appendix 8.9.1b.

annular plane are demonstrated. The lateral (or free) wall of the RV is identified, along with the IVS.

Mid-oesophageal long-axis view (Figure 14.2b): this view demonstrates the infundibular portion of the RV as it appears anterior to the LV septum.

Mid-oesophageal RV inflow–outflow view (Figure 14.2c): this view demonstrates the portion of the RV that wraps around the AV. The lateral, anterior, and infundibular portions of the RV wall are also seen.

Transgastric short-axis view (Figure 14.2d): this transgastric view focuses on the distinctive crescentic shape of the RV as it wraps around the LV. The inferior and anterior walls of the RV can be identified.

Transgastric RV inflow view (Figure 14.2e): the scanning angle is rotated 90° from the transgastric short-axis view to show the inferior and anterior walls of the RV.

Transgastric RV basal view (Figure 14.2f): rotating the probe slightly clockwise from the transgastric RV inflow view will demonstrate the RV outflow, with a focus on the infundibulum and the PV.

Assessment of RV size and systolic function

The echocardiographic assessment of RV function may be achieved using either geometric markers such as ejection fraction (EF), fractional area of change (FAC), and tricuspid annular plane systolic excursion (TAPSE), or non-geometric markers such as the RV myocardial performance index (MPI). Each method has advantages and limitations, which will be discussed below.

Geometric markers

RV size

The RV has a complex geometric shape and is heavily trabeculated, which makes it difficult both to model and to detect endocardial borders. As a result, there are no reliable 2D-based geometric and volumetric RV measurements.[6,8] RV volumetric measurements are best determined using 3D echocardiography and will be discussed later in this chapter, along with volumetric-based measures of function.

Linear assessments of size offer quick and easy ways to assess RV dimensions in TOE. In the perioperative setting, RV size is assessed by measuring major and minor axes of the sinus portion of the RV in the mid-oesophageal four-chamber view. The RV-focused modification of the mid-oesophageal four-chamber view allows for minimization of apical foreshortening while simultaneously optimizing the size of the TV annulus. It may be necessary to adjust the depth of the probe and rotate the scanning plane slightly forward (10–15°) to maximize the basal diameter. Diameters are measured at the base (D1) and the mid portion (D2) of the RV at end-diastole (Figure 14.2a). D1 measurements >41 mm and D2 measurements >35 mm are considered abnormal (Table 14.1).[8] When the basal or D1 measurement is enlarged, TV coaptation may be decreased and result in TR. This may result in a vicious cycle where volume overload and dilatation secondary to TR compromise TV coaptation even further, resulting in worsening TR. RV outflow dimensions are measured in the mid-oesophageal RV inflow–outflow view (Figure 14.2c). Care must be taken to avoid foreshortening the outflow tract. The RV proximal diameter is measured from the anterior wall to the ventricular septal–aortic junction. The RVOT distal measurement is made at the level of the PV. Both measurements are made at end-diastole. RVOT proximal diameters >35 mm and RVOT distal diameters >27 mm are considered abnormal (Table 14.1).

Expert tip: The RV is very sensitive to volume overload, and RV enlargement is an important clinical sign. The cause of RV enlargement should never remain unexplained, and it should never be assumed to be due to LV dysfunction until an intracardiac shunt or other primary cause has been ruled out.

The presence of epicardial fat and endocardial trabeculations may make the true measurement of RV wall thickness difficult. In TTE, RV wall thickness is measured at the midpoint of the wall in the subcostal view at end-diastole. In TOE, RV wall thickness can be measured in the transgastric RV inflow view at the diaphragmatic surface, with care taken to exclude epicardial fat, trabeculations, and papillary muscles (Figure 14.2e). Values above 5 mm are considered abnormal (Table 14.1).

Fractional area change and ejection fraction

Global geometric assessments of RV function include surface area change during the cardiac cycle such as FAC, or volumetric changes such as EF, based on 3D volumetric measures. The FAC is measured in the mid-oesophageal four-chamber RV-focused view by tracing the endocardial border to obtain the area at end-systole (RVESA) and diastole (RVEDA). The chordae tendineae, papillary muscles, and trabeculations are included as part of the

Table 14.1 Measures of RV systolic function

Parameter		Normal value	Limitations	Advantages	Measurement
Longitudinal	**TAPSE**	>1.6cm	Single-segment displacement (basal) may not reflect entire RV Load-dependent Regional measurement Angle-dependent Not reliable post-cardiopulmonary bypass	Reproducible Can be acquired from low-quality images	**View for simple caliper measurement: ME-4CH** Advance frame by frame, and caliper the extremes of annular displacement **View for M-mode:** Anatomical M-mode can be used with **ME-4CH** **View for TDI:** **Deep TG** with anteflexion and clockwise rotation
	S'	>9.5cm/s	Regional measurement (inferior wall function) Angle-dependent Not validated with TOE	Reproducible Simple to execute Good discrimination with TTE	**View:** **Deep TG long-axis** Record TDI of free wall Offline software to map velocity of tissue movement and measure S' based on colour coding Pulsed TDI of free wall in real time
	Longitudinal strain: RVFWS, RVGLS	<–20%	Regional measurement Relatively angle-dependent May require offline analysis (depending on vendor software) High variability	Less load-dependent	**View:** **ME-4CH view** with real-time autostrain (depending on vendor software) **Deep TG** recording for offline analysis. Narrow sector to keep frame rates >150; keep Doppler angle <15° from line of tissue movement
Global	**FAC**	>35%	2D estimate of RVEF RV inflow measurement only	Angle-independent	**View: ME-4CH** Trace endocardium from annulus to apex in systole and diastole (chordae and trabeculations are included as part of the cavity)
	MPI: PWD MPI, TDI MPI	<0.43, <0.54	PWD imaging requires multiple views TDI requires high-quality signal Unreliable if R–R intervals differ (arrhythmia) Load-dependent Unreliable with high RA pressures	Does not require geometric assumptions Reproducible TDI can measure S', E', and A' on one image	**Equation: MPI = IVCT + IVRT/ET** **PWD view:** **IVRT/IVCT**—ME modified bicaval, PWD through TV **ET**—UE Ao in short axis or deep TG. PWD through RVOT **TDI view:** Deep TG—pulsed TDI through TV annulus
	3D RVEF	>45%	Software mostly offline Can underestimate RV volumes Reduced accuracy in dilated or dysfunctional ventricles	Most accurate measurement of ejection fraction	**Views: ME inflow–outflow and associated orthogonal view** 3D software required

(*continued*)

Table 14.1 Continued

Parameter		Normal value	Limitations	Advantages	Measurement
IVS	**Pressure/ volume overload**		Limited if septal ischaemia or pacing	Easy to visualize Quick qualitative assessment	**View: LV SAX TG** Pressure overload—septal shift towards LV/D shape at end-systole Volume overload—septal shift towards LV/D shape at end-diastole
	Eccentricity index (EI)	<1	Interaction/interpretation complicated by concomitant RV systolic pressure overload and LV diastolic pressure overload	Quantitative measure of septal shift	**View: LV short-axis TG** EI = LV AP dimension/LV septolateral dimension

TAPSE, tricuspid annular plane systolic excursion; ME-4CH, mid-oesophageal four-chamber view; TDI, tissue Doppler imaging; TG, transgastric; RVFWS, right ventricular free wall strain; RVGLS, right ventricular global longitudinal strain; RVEF, right ventricular ejection fraction; MPI, myocardial perfusion index; PWD, pulsed-wave Doppler; ET, ejection time; UE, upper oesophageal; Ao, aorta; RVOT, right ventricular outflow tract; AP, anteroposterior.

RV cavity. The FAC is then calculated using a modification of Equation 6.6, where (Equation 14.1):

$$FAC = \frac{RVEDA - RVESA}{RVEDA} \quad \text{Equation 14.1}$$

FAC values <35% are considered abnormal (Table 14.1).[8]

TTE-derived 3D RV assessments correlate well with the gold standard cardiac MRI imaging.[9] TOE-derived 3D assessments of right ventricular ejection fraction (RVEF) have correlated well with TTE-derived values and with thermodilution.[6] Analysis software specifically designed for the RV is now available on some echo machines, as well as offline software (Figure 14.4; see Online appendix 8.9.1).

Basic principles affecting 3D image quality include: (1) temporal resolution (i.e. frame rate); and (2) spatial resolution (affected by the number of scanning lines and sector size—see Chapter 2). Altering one parameter will invariably affect the other, so a compromise between

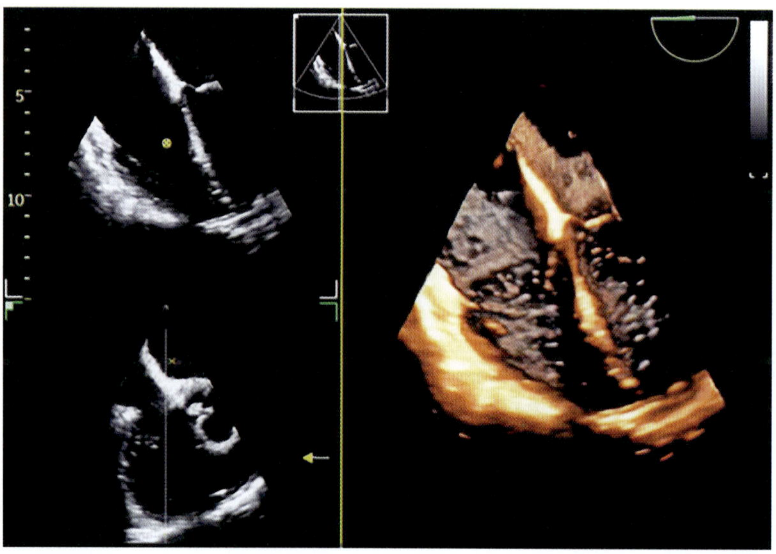

Figure 14.4 3D TOE full-volume reconstruction of the RV. See Online appendix 8.9.1a.

spatial and temporal resolution is often necessary. A 'live' 3D data set may be acquired or alternatively, a full-volume data set with improved resolution can be obtained by using ECG-gated multi-beat acquisition.[10] This may be challenging in the presence of arrhythmia or electrocautery and requires a pause in mechanical ventilation (see Chapter 2).

TOE examination of the RV can be challenging, because its location in the far field results in poorer resolution and shadowing from proximal structures like the AV. Still, 3D rendering is possible in most circumstances but requires a minimum frame rate of 25 Hz.[10] The distal position and width of the RV with TOE may require the use of ECG-gated multi-beat loops to achieve adequate spatial and temporal resolution (see Online appendix 8.9.1).

Examples of 3D TOE rendering of the RV is demonstrated in Figures 14.3 and 14.4. Segmentation and calculation of RV volume and surface areas will yield end-systolic and end-diastolic volumes, EF, and FAC. EF values above 45% and FAC values above 35% are considered normal (Table 14.1).

2D-based annular displacement

Tricuspid annular plane systolic excursion (TAPSE) is commonly used as a simple and fast method to assess RV function. Apical TV annular displacement is assumed to correlate with the systolic function of the RV. Using TTE, it is measured by aligning an M-mode cursor with tricuspid annular motion. Excursion values above 16 mm are considered normal (Table 14.1).[8]

With TOE, however, the annular motion often does not align with the M-mode cursor in the mid-oesophageal four-chamber view, and TAPSE may be underestimated unless an anatomical cursor is utilized (Figure 14.5). Anatomical M-mode is a post-processing modality that corrects the alignment of the M-mode cursor, thereby overcoming its natural limitations (note that this has nothing to do with the Doppler angle correction discussed in Chapter 2).

The deep transgastric RV inflow view provides better alignment for TAPSE measurement (Figure 14.2e). Although the measurement may be more difficult to obtain, it correlates well with TTE-derived TAPSE.[6] Alternatively, apical displacement of the annulus may also be measured directly on the 2D image. Angle-independent measures are preferred when measuring TAPSE using TOE. Speckle tracking technology (discussed later in this chapter and in Chapter 6) can also be used to track the annulus and measure TAPSE (see Online appendix 8.9.2). Overall, TAPSE has shown poor correlation with MRI-derived RVEF, but good sensitivity in predicting RV dysfunction after left ventricular assist device (LVAD) implantation.[6] Furthermore, the value for TAPSE may be partly dependent on LV function due to shared fibres with the LV and ventricular interdependence.[11]

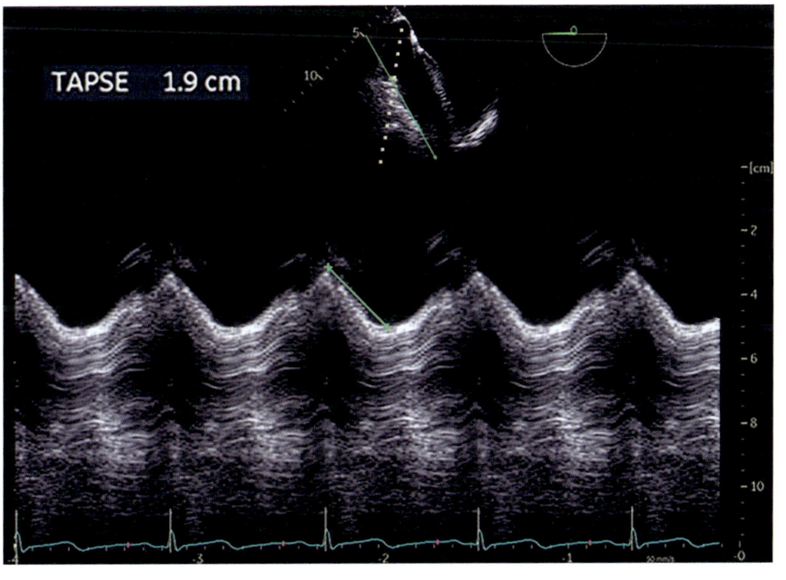

Figure 14.5 Measuring TAPSE with the anatomical M-mode. From a mid-oesophageal four-chamber view, the M-mode is placed across the tricuspid annulus to display the TAPSE. Since the tricuspid annular motion is not aligned with the M-mode cursor in this view (yellow dotted line on the 2D image), the anatomical correction (green cursor on the 2D image) is used. Proper alignment of the M-mode cursor with the motion allows for a more accurate measurement of TAPSE.

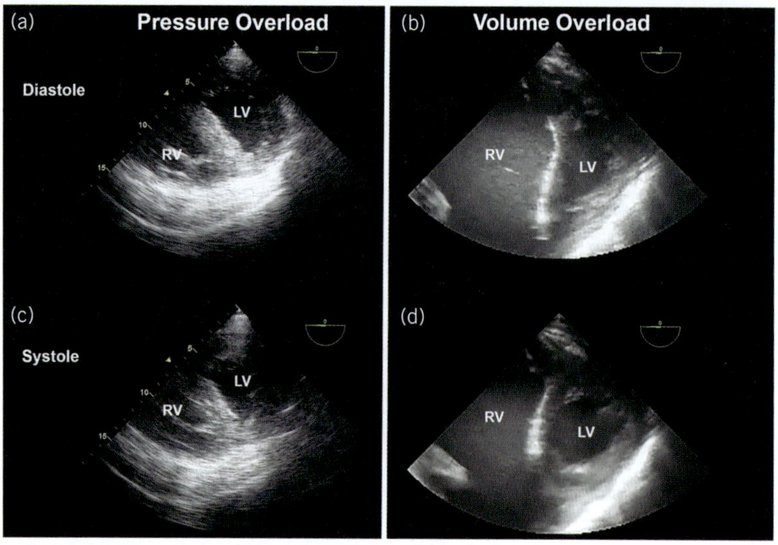

Figure 14.6 Effect of RV pressure and volume overload on the interventricular septum. All frames in this composite image are transgastric short-axis views. (a) and (b) are taken at end-diastole, and (c) and (d) at end-systole. (a) and (c) demonstrate a patient with RV pressure overload. Note the hypertrophied RV and the D shape of the LV in *both* diastole and systole. (b) and (d) depict a patient with severe volume overload. In diastole (b), the massively dilated RV pushes the IVS towards the LV, leading to a D shape of the LV and a consequent decrease in LV filling. In systole (d), the LV regains its normal shape.

The interventricular and inter-atrial septa

The IVS is an important contributor to RV function, and its impairment may result in significant reduction in RV performance in the setting of RV sinus dysfunction. On 2D examination, the IVS has a convex shape towards the RV.

Under conditions of *volume overload*, the IVS will be shifted towards the LV in diastole. This will give the LV a D-shaped appearance in the transgastric short-axis view in *diastole*. Leftward septal shifting will also impair diastolic LV filling. Under conditions of *pressure* overload such as pulmonary hypertension, the IVS will also flatten in systole, giving the LV a D-shaped appearance in *both systole and diastole* (Figure 14.6; see Online appendices 8.1.3 and 8.1.5). Septal shifting can be quantified using the **eccentricity index (EI)**.[6] This is a ratio of the LV diameter measured in a plane parallel to the IVS (D1) divided by its perpendicular plane (D2) measured both in systole and diastole. A normal ratio in both systole and diastole is approximately 1, while a systolic value above 1.08 is a good predictor of pulmonary hypertension.[6]

Expert tip: RV volume overload causes an increase in EI in diastole, but not in systole. RV pressure overload causes an increase in EI in both systole and diastole.

In cases where RV dysfunction has led to an increase in the RA pressure, a leftward shift of the inter-atrial septum (IAS) will occur. This can be seen in the mid-oesophageal four-chamber view (Figure 14.7; see Online appendices 8.1.3 and 8.1.6) and should prompt further examination of RV function in the intraoperative period.

Non-geometric measures

Non-geometric measures of RV function are the simplest and fastest RV assessment methods in the perioperative setting. These measurements are based on the longitudinal analysis of the RV free wall through either velocity or deformation, with the assumption that the free wall

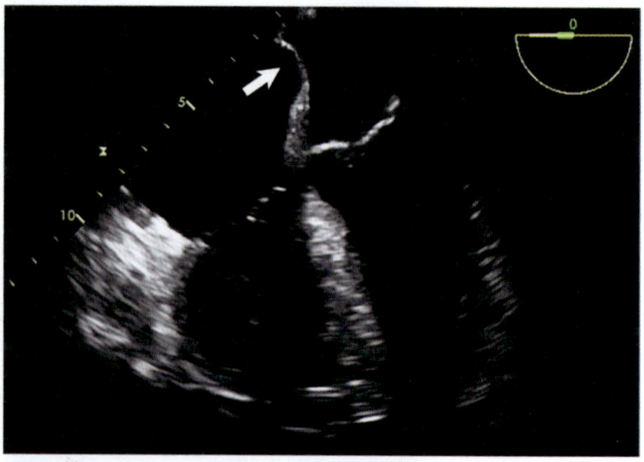

Figure 14.7 Leftward shift of the IAS from high RA pressure. In this mid-oesophageal four-chamber view in systole, RA is large and the IAS is shifted leftwards, indicating high RA pressure, most likely due to RV dysfunction. Note also the enlarged spherical RV.

function can be extrapolated to reflect global RV function. Care should be taken to align the TOE Doppler plane with the motion of the RV annulus and free wall.

Annular velocity-based measures

Similar to the LV (see Chapter 6), the systolic annular velocity, or S', is a measure of load-dependent RV systolic function and can be measured with TTE (post-processed) using PW or colour tissue Doppler imaging. The two methods are not interchangeable and yield different cut-off values—normal values for PW tissue Doppler (PWTD) by TTE are ≥9.5 cm/s or and ≥6.0 cm/s for colour tissue Doppler (Table 14.1).[8] The mathematical integration of velocity over systolic time will yield a value for TAPSE. With TOE, the tricuspid annular motion aligns most reliably with the Doppler plane in the deep transgastric RV inflow view (Figure 14.2e). However, systolic annular velocities have not been validated for this TOE view and cannot be extrapolated from those using the TTE apical four-chamber view.

Speckle tracking utilizes brightness or B-mode image markers to track tissue movement via frame-by-frame mapping of speckle patterns. It has the distinct advantage of being independent of Doppler angle, but it is dependent on 2D image quality and an adequate frame rate of >40 frames per second (FPS). When the frame rate is too low, speckle pattern variation tracking and measurement reliability are impaired. S' and TAPSE measurements using speckle tracking compare favourably with traditional methods using this technique (see Online appendix 8.9.2).[6]

Tissue deformation indices

Tissue Doppler may be used to measure velocity gradient-based deformation (Eulerian) indices such as strain and strain rate. However, when using TOE, the difficulty in aligning RV tissue motion with the Doppler plane limits its usefulness.

Speckle tracking, however, measures the distance separating B-mode markers—or speckles—over time and permits the direct measurement of deformation indices such as strain and strain rate (Lagrangian). RV strain is calculated in the mid-oesophageal four-chamber view using dedicated software (Figure 14.8a, b). RV strain can

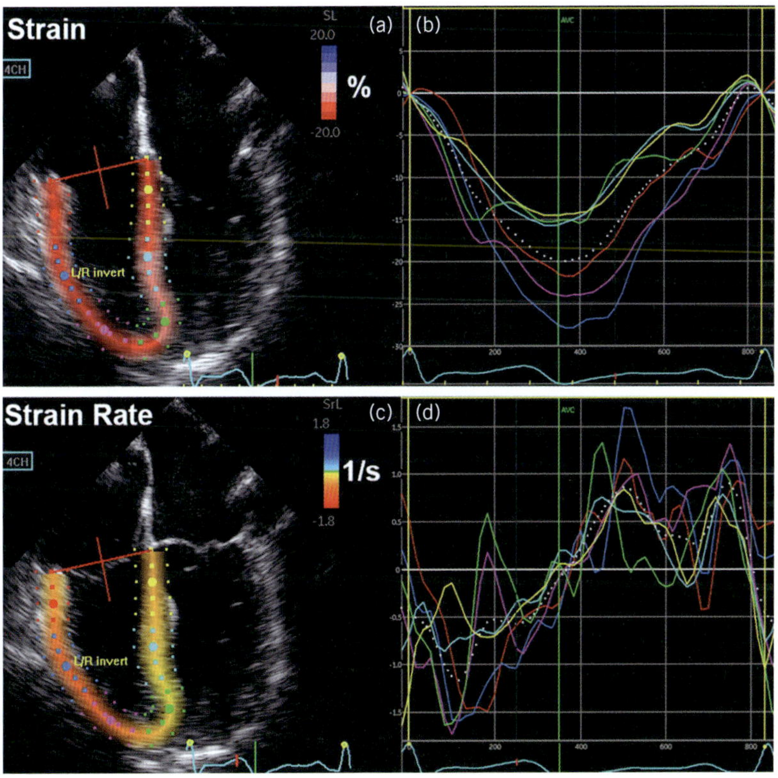

Figure 14.8 RV strain and strain rate measurement using speckle tracking. (a) and (b) demonstrate strain measurement for six segments of the RV in a mid-oesophageal four-chamber view. (a) shows the six colour-coded RV segments analysed. (b) graphically depicts the strain, with each line corresponding to the RV segment of the same colour. The dotted line represents global strain. Strain is expressed in percentage change in myocardial fibre length on the *y*-axis. (c) and (d) demonstrate strain rate of the same six RV segments during the same cardiac cycle. Again the dotted line represents global SR. SR is the slope of strain and is expressed as 1/s. See Online appendix 8.9.2.

be calculated for the entire RV or the free wall only. Free wall strain values may be calculated for individual segments such as the base, mid wall, and apex. As systolic strain describes longitudinal *shortening*, a negative value is assigned. The following relationship is used to calculate strain (Equation 14.2):

$$Strain = \frac{L_{systole} - L_{diastole}}{L_{diastole}} X100 \qquad \text{Equation 14.2}$$

where L is the distance between two points within the myocardium.

Global free wall strain values 'more negative' than –20% are considered normal. Strain rate (SR) is a dimensionless value per second that represents the rate of shortening in systole (Figure 14.8c, d). No normal cut-off values are currently available.

In summary, most non-geometric-based values have been validated using TTE, in the apical four-chamber view. RV free wall assessment by TOE using tissue Doppler in the mid-oesophageal four-chamber view is extremely limited because of poor alignment. If image quality and frame rate can be optimized, angle-independent speckle tracking-derived measures of annular displacement and velocity (TAPSE, S'), as well as free wall deformation and deformation rate (strain and strain rate), are better suited to TOE.

The myocardial performance index

The **myocardial performance index (MPI)**, also referred to as **RV index of myocardial performance** (RIMP) or Tei index, is a non-geometric flow- or tissue Doppler-based measure of global RV function. It is calculated as the ratio of the sum of the isovolumic contraction and relaxation times divided by the ejection time, as described by the following relationship (Equation 14.3):

$$MPI = \frac{IVRT + IVCT}{ET} \qquad \text{Equation 14.3}$$

where $IVCT$ is isovolumic contraction time, $IVRT$ is isovolumic relaxation time, and ET is ejection time.

These time intervals are calculated from PW Doppler (PWD) assessment of the onset and termination of tricuspid inflow and pulmonic outflow velocities. As these are not measured simultaneously, a regular heart rate is required. A transgastric TOE approach may be required for optimal alignment with the pulmonic valve. Single-beat, simultaneous measures can be made using PWTD at the tricuspid annulus in the mid-oesophageal four-chamber view. An increased IVRT versus ET, and thus a higher MPI, correlates with poorer RV function. However, increased preload may shorten the IVRT and thus spuriously improve the MPI. Normal values of <0.43 for PWD and <0.54 for PWTD, respectively, are noted in Table 14.1.

Post-operative RV dysfunction

RV dysfunction may be present prior to weaning from CPB in patients with pulmonary hypertension, valvular disease such as TR/MR or MS, and/or prior myocardial infarction. The most common cause of acute RV dysfunction during weaning from CPB is air embolization to the RCA and/or grafts supplying the RV (see discussion in Chapter 6 and Figure 6.15). Of note, the native contraction pattern of the RV may be altered post-CPB. Longitudinal parameters of RV function are reduced, and parameters of circumferential contraction are increased—this may persist for up to 1 year post-bypass despite preserved global function, as measured by 3D RVEF.[12,13] For this reason, post-bypass longitudinal parameters must be interpreted with caution and ideally, global volumetric modalities such as 3D RVEF should be used.[6,8]

Assessment of RV diastolic function

Diastolic assessment using echocardiography is complex and frequently overlooked, and a comprehensive review is beyond the scope of this chapter. In addition, it is limited to patients without valvular abnormalities, such as moderate to severe TR, and with regular rhythms. Briefly, diastolic performance impacts the RA pressure (RAP), which, when elevated, will impact hepatic and renal function. Several factors contribute to increases in RAP, including myocardial relaxation rate, RV compliance, and systolic function. To assess diastolic function, a PWD sample is placed at the tip of the tricuspid leaflets in the mid-oesophageal four-chamber view. Care must be taken to align tricuspid inflow with the Doppler beam. Similar to MV assessment (see Chapter 7), tricuspid E and A velocities and deceleration time (DT) are measured on the PWD trace, where the DT is the time taken from peak E velocity to return to baseline. Tissue Doppler is sampled at the lateral wall of the RV, and E' and A' measurements are made at the lateral wall annulus. As RV relaxation becomes impaired, the pressure gradient between the RA and RV will drop, resulting in a reduced E velocity. As the disease process advances and ventricular compliance decreases, RAP rises to maintain RV filling, cardiac output, and homeostasis. Additionally, deteriorating systolic function increases end-systolic, and consequently early diastolic, volumes, further escalating RAP. An increase in RA size due to the rise in RAP reflects the time–pressure burden on the RA. The E velocity is dependent on the diastolic RA to RV pressure gradient, and a low gradient will result in a lower E velocity. Normal RV E velocities range from 35 cm/s to 73 cm/s.[5] The E/A ratio is normally 0.8–2.1. A reduction in relaxation will decrease the E/A ratio, and an increase in RAP will restore the ratio to normal values (pseudo-normalization), which signifies advanced diastolic disease. It is therefore important to try to estimate the RAP to fully assess diastolic dysfunction. Although the E and E' velocities are preload-dependent, the E' is reduced when relaxation is impaired and becomes preload-independent. Under these circumstances, the E velocity will rise in the presence of a more fixed E' and the E/E' ratio will become a better gauge of RAP. A normal E' value ranges from 0.08 to 0.20 m/s. A normal E/E' ratio ranges from 2 to 6, and values above this represent an elevated RAP. The DT, or time from peak inflow velocity to the end of diastolic flow, may also be used to assess diastolic function. Prolonged relaxation will result in a long DT, whereas poor compliance will result in a shortened DT due to rapid equalization of the RA and RV pressures with early cessation of diastolic flow.

Current guidelines separate diastolic function into three categories: **impaired relaxation** (decreased E velocity and reduced E/A ratio), **pseudo-normalization** (increased RAP with normalization of E velocity and E/A ratio), and **restrictive filling** (increased RAP with early arrest of RA–RV flow and short DT). In summary, an E/A ratio <0.8 suggests impaired relaxation. An E/A ratio of 0.8–2.1 associated with an E/E' of >6 suggests pseudo-normalization. An E/A ratio >2.1 with a DT of <120 ms suggests restrictive filling (Table 14.2).[8,14]

Extra-cardiac Doppler assessments

The venous system and organ perfusion

In the presence of significant RV dysfunction, the rise in RAP will affect the central venous system.[15,16,17] Elevation in central pressures will have a significant impact on venous drainage, and consequently on splanchnic perfusion. Normally, the compliance of the venous system means that distal Doppler flow patterns (such as the femoral veins) are more uniform and non-pulsatile. However, in the presence of RV failure and an elevated RAP, decreased central venous compliance results in increased transmission of pressure changes, as well as in pulsatile Doppler flow patterns.

Hepatic vein flow

The three major hepatic veins (right, middle, and left) can be imaged using TOE. The *right* hepatic vein is readily visible in nearly all patients as it enters the IVC, by advancing the probe below the diaphragm and turning it to the right at a transducer angle of 60–90° (Figure 14.9). The other

Table 14.2 Measures of RV filling and diastolic function

DIASTOLIC FUNCTION				
Parameter	**Normal value**	**Limitations**	**Advantages**	**Measurement**
E/e' **Deceleration time** **E/A**	<6.0 120–200 ms 0.8–2.1	Angle-dependent Load-dependent	Reproducible Easily obtained	**View:** **Mid-oesophageal modified bicaval** **Tricuspid inflow PW**
MARKERS OF VENOUS CONGESTION				
IVC size/ collapsibility	<2.1 cm/>50%	Not validated with TOE or PPV		**View:** **Deep TG**, probe rotated clockwise towards liver
Splenic/portal vein pulsatility index	<0.5	Not validated with TOE Can be challenging to visualize	Can give an indication of overall congestion	**View:** Portal: **deep TG** with probe anteflexed, rotated clockwise towards liver, and advanced just distal to IVC Splenic: **deep TG** with probe anteflexed and rotated counterclockwise
RRI	<0.7			

PW, pulsed wave; PPV, positive pressure ventilation; TG, transgastric; RRI, renal resistive index.

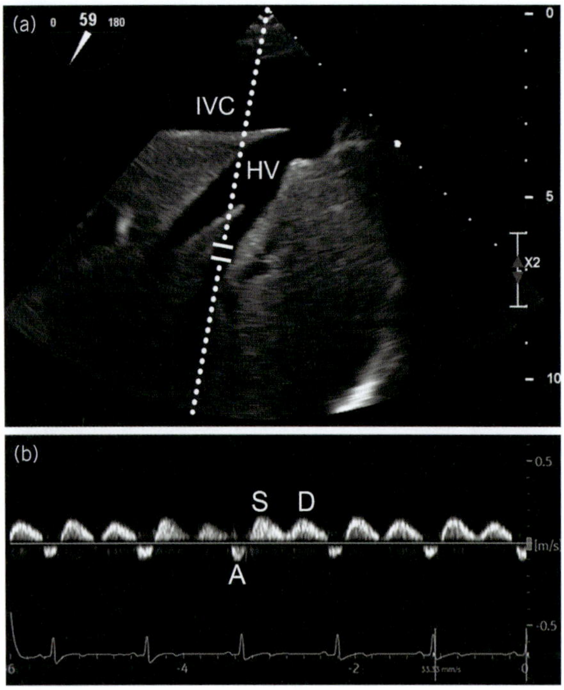

Figure 14.9 Hepatic vein flow. (a) is a 2D image showing the right hepatic vein (HV) as it enters the IVC, obtained by advancing the probe below the diaphragm and turning it to the right at a transducer angle of 60–90°. A PW Doppler cursor is positioned in a branch of the HV that is parallel to the Doppler beam. (b) shows the PW spectral Doppler signal of hepatic venous flow, demonstrating the A-, S-, and D-waves (V-wave is not visible in this example).

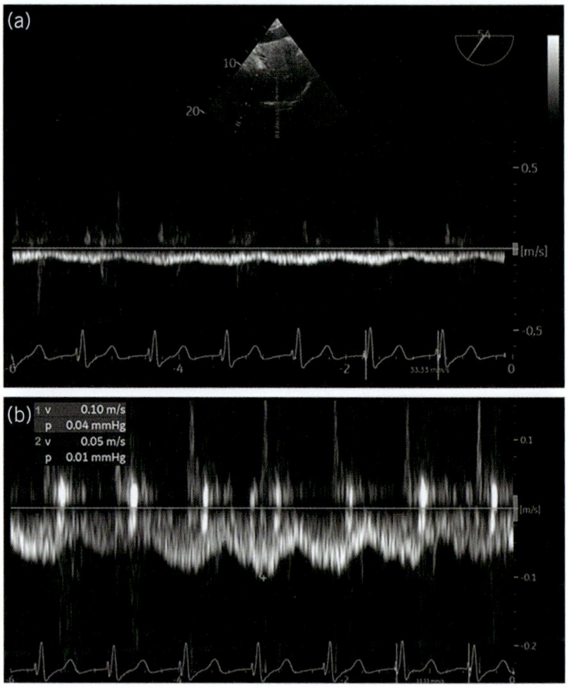

Figure 14.10 Portal vein flow. (a) demonstrates a normal spectral PW Doppler signal of portal vein flow, showing minimal pulsatility. (b) shows an abnormal pattern with significant pulsatility, consistent with venous congestion due to RV dysfunction.

hepatic veins are more difficult to visualize. A PWD sample placed within the hepatic vein demonstrates forward flow above the baseline. Four waves may be identified on spectral Doppler: **A-wave** (atrial contraction resulting in flow reversal below the baseline); **S-wave** (antegrade flow above the baseline due to RV annular descent); **V-wave** (retrograde flow from annular ascent at end-systole—not always visible); and **D-wave** (antegrade flow during tricuspid valve opening). These waves are altered by abnormalities in RV function, TV disease, or pericardial disease. In the presence of severe TR, for example, the S-wave will be blunted or reversed (analogous to S-wave reversal in the pulmonary veins seen with severe MR).

As RV dysfunction progresses, the RAP increases. The PWD profile in the hepatic veins will demonstrate an exaggerated A-wave due to increased flow reversal during atrial systole. Reduction in RVEF with incomplete ventricular emptying decreases annular descent, and thus the S-wave is decreased. If RV dysfunction becomes severe, the S-wave may be reversed.[15] There will also be a relative rise in the D-wave due to the increased atrioventricular pressure gradient.

Portal, splenic, and renal venous flow

TOE can be used to image and measure the Doppler velocity profiles of the portal or splenic veins. Under normal conditions, the flow velocity profile during the cardiac cycle is relatively flat. With increasing venous congestion, it will appear pulsatile. Higher RAP leads to more pronounced pulsatility. With further worsening of the RAP, the systolic portion of the Doppler profile will be reversed to produce a characteristic sinusoidal wave pattern (Figure 14.10).[15]

The left kidney can also be imaged using TOE, and the intra-renal veins (interlobar or arcuate) can be sampled using PWD. Here again, the normal Doppler tracing appears continuous or monophasic. Pulsatility will increase in the presence of RV failure and a rise in the RAP.[15]

A more detailed discussion of extra-cardiac venous flow is beyond the scope of this chapter.

Multiple choice questions

Discover interactive multiple choice questions to test your knowledge on this chapter by searching for this book's title or ISBN (9780198873686) at **https://academic.oup.com/** and going to the online appendix at the end of the book. Use your scratch-off code on the inside cover to access the material.

References

1. Ho SY. Anatomy, echocardiography, and normal right ventricular dimensions. *Heart.* 2006;**92**(Suppl 1):i2–13.
2. Sheehan F, Redington A. The right ventricle: anatomy, physiology and clinical imaging. *Heart.* 2008;**94**(11):1510–15.
3. Greyson CR. Pathophysiology of right ventricular failure: *Crit Care Med.* 2008;**36**(Suppl):S57–65.
4. Haddad F, Hunt SA, Rosenthal DN, Murphy DJ. Right ventricular function in cardiovascular disease, Part I: anatomy, physiology, aging, and functional assessment of the right ventricle. *Circulation.* 2008;**117**(11):1436–48.
5. Konstam MA, Kiernan MS, Bernstein D, *et al.* Evaluation and management of right-sided heart failure: a scientific statement from the American Heart Association. *Circulation.* 2018;**137**(20) e578–622.
6. Silverton NA, Gebhardt BR, Maslow A. The intraoperative assessment of right ventricular function during cardiac surgery. *J Cardiothor Vasc Anesth.* 2022;**36**(10):3904–15.
7. Crystal GJ, Pagel PS. Right ventricular perfusion. *Anesthesiology.* 2018;**128**(1):202–18.
8. Rudski LG, Lai WW, Afilalo J, *et al.* Guidelines for the echocardiographic assessment of the right heart in adults: a report from the American Society of Echocardiography. *J Am Soc Echocardiogr.* 2010;**23**(7):685–713.
9. Kwon A, Ahn HS, Kim GH, Cho JS, Park CS, Youn HJ. Right ventricular analysis using real-time three-dimensional echocardiography for preload dependency. *J Cardiovasc Imaging.* 2020;**28**(1):36.
10. Vegas A. Three-dimensional transesophageal echocardiography: principles and clinical applications. *Ann Card Anaesth.* 2016;**19**(5):35.
11. López-Candales A, Rajagopalan N, Saxena N, Gulyasy B, Edelman K, Bazaz R. Right ventricular systolic function is not the sole determinant of tricuspid annular motion. *Am J Cardiol.* 2006;**98**(7):973–7.
12. Hedman A, Alam M, Zuber E, Nordlander R, Samad BA. Decreased right ventricular function after coronary artery bypass grafting and its relation to exercise capacity: a tricuspid annular motion-based study. *J Am Soc Echocardiogr.* 2004;**17**(2):126–31.
13. Mandoli GE, Cameli M, Novo G, *et al.* Right ventricular function after cardiac surgery: the diagnostic and prognostic role of echocardiography. *Heart Fail Rev.* 2019;**24**(5):625–35.
14. Jung YH, Ren X, Suffredini G, Dodd-o JM, Gao WD. Right ventricular diastolic dysfunction and failure: a review. *Heart Fail Rev.* 2022;**27**(4):1077–90.
15. Rola P, Miralles-Aguiar F, Argaiz E, *et al.* Clinical applications of the venous excess ultrasound (VExUS) score: conceptual review and case series. *Ultrasound J.* 2021;**13**(1):32.
16. Denault AY, Haddad F, Jacobsohn E, Deschamps A. Perioperative right ventricular dysfunction. *Curr Opin Anesthesiol.* 2013;**26**(1):71–81.
17. Torres-Arrese M, García de Casasola-Sánchez G, Méndez-Bailón M, *et al.* Usefulness of serial multiorgan point-of-care ultrasound in acute heart failure: results from a prospective observational cohort. *Medicina.* 2022;**58**(1):124.

15

The tricuspid and pulmonary valves

The tricuspid valve complex

The tricuspid valve (TV) is the largest and most apical of the four cardiac valves. In addition, it has the most variable anatomy. It comprises the annulus, leaflets, papillary muscles, chordae tendinae, and associated ventricular myocardium.[1] Though its name suggests the presence of three well-defined leaflets, a trileaflet configuration is present in only 54–57% of patients. In another 40% of patients, the TV has four (or rarely five) leaflets in various configurations.[2,3] The **anterior leaflet** has the largest radial area, extending from the infundibular region anteriorly to the posterolateral annulus, and is the most mobile. The **septal leaflet** has the shortest radial area, is directly attached to the annulus above the ventricular septum, and is the least mobile. The **posterior leaflet** typically has numerous small scallops and extends from the ventricular septum to the posterolateral annulus. There are two papillary muscles—the larger **anterior** papillary muscle subtends chordae to the *anterior* and *posterior* leaflets, while the **posterior** papillary muscle subtends chordae to the *posterior* and *septal* leaflets. The **ventricular septum** provides chordae directly to the *anterior* and *septal* leaflets.

The TV annulus is a complex D-shaped dynamic three-dimensional structure, with major (long) and minor (short) axes, and a *semi-saddle* shape with high (atrial) and low (ventricular) points (Figure 15.1).[4,5] Unlike the mitral annulus, the high and low points do not align directly with either the major or the minor axes; rather the major dimension is orientated in an anterior–posterior direction, and the minor dimension is orientated in a septal–lateral direction. The high points are in the anteroseptal (close to the AV) and posterolateral positions, and the low points are in the anterolateral and posteroseptal positions.

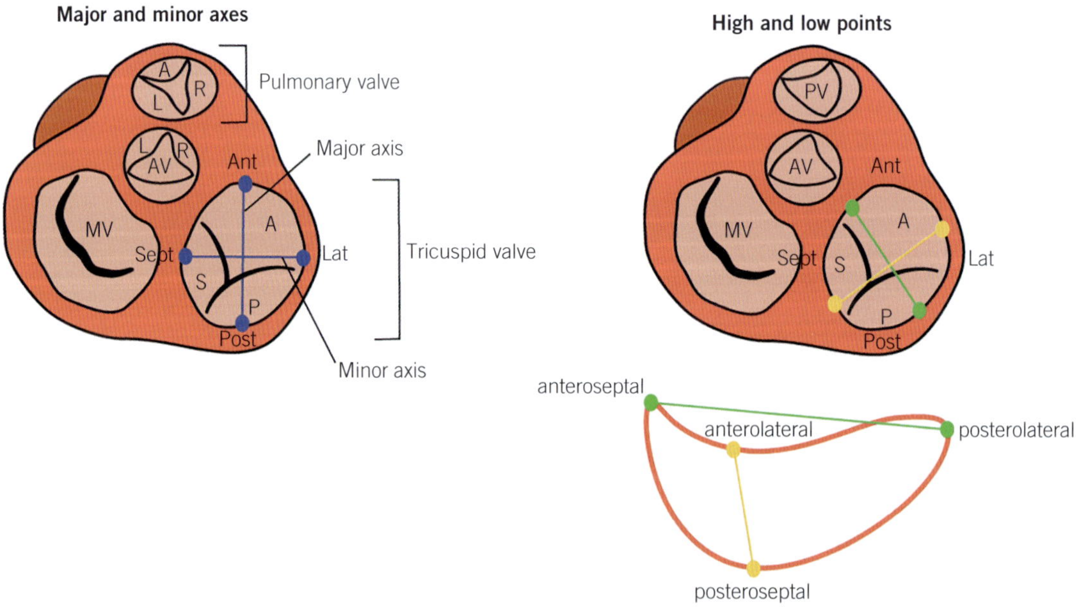

Figure 15.1 Tricuspid valve annulus and leaflets. The tricuspid annulus has a complex 3D shape, with major and minor axes and high and low points. During systole, the annulus descends towards the RV apex and contracts, resulting in a 30% reduction in annular area. This schematic representation shows the heart from the base, with the atria removed. The anterior is at the top of the image. The patient's left side is on the left of the image.

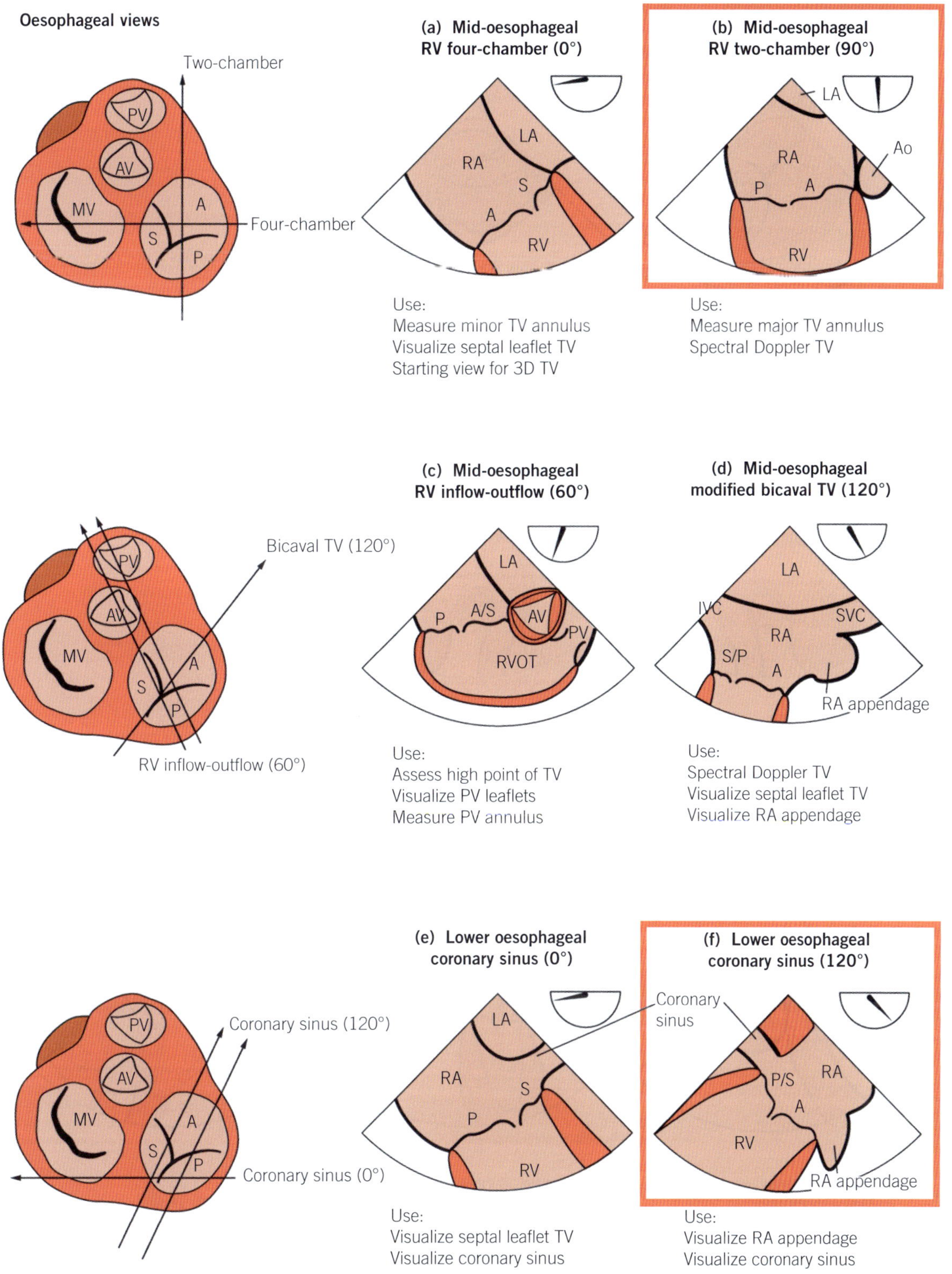

Figure 15.2 TOE views of the tricuspid and pulmonary valves. Standard ASE/SCA views, introduced in Chapter 4, are illustrated. Additional 'non-standard' views of the TV, not discussed in Chapter 4, are indicated by being boxed and are discussed in the text. The letters A, P, and S refer to the anterior, posterior, and septal leaflets, respectively, of the TV. In Figure 15.2L, the letters A, L, and R refer to the anterior, left, and right leaflets, respectively, of the PV. See Online appendix 1.7.

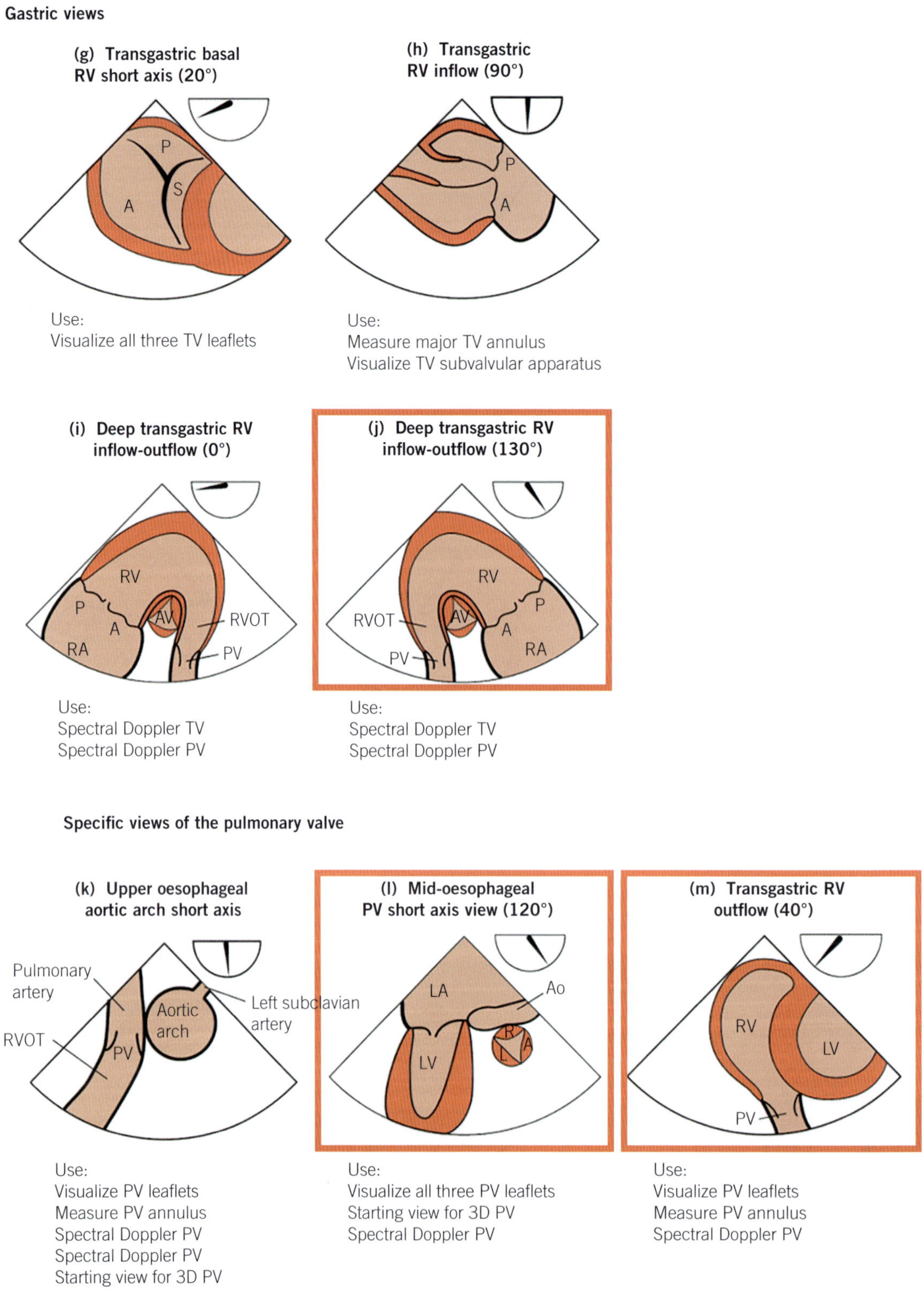

Figure 15.2 *Continued*

Imaging the tricuspid valve complex

An in-depth understanding of the TV anatomy, particularly the number and location of supernumerary leaflets or scallops, is essential for peri-procedural planning. TV imaging can be challenging due to the location of the TV in the far field, distant from the oesophageal echo transducer. Image quality can also be reduced by the oblique angle of the ultrasound beam with the thinner and less distinct TV leaflets (compared to the MV), as well as reflectors from the AV or MV (e.g. calcifications or valve prostheses) obstructing the view. Finally, views of the right heart tend to be more variable than those of the left heart, with fewer landmarks.

TOE views of the right heart are demonstrated in Figure 15.2 and Online Appendix 1.7, including 'standard' views outlined in the ASE/Society of Cardiovascular Anesthesiologists SCA guidelines[6] and some 'non-standard views'.

Among the standard views, the mid-oesophageal RV inflow–outflow view (Figure 15.2c) is aligned with the high (more basal) axis of the TV and is a good view to assess prolapse, especially when biplane imaging is used (discussed later). 'Non-standard' views of the TV are often used in procedural TV echocardiography to measure leaflet length;[7] these include the mid-oesophageal RV two-chamber view (Figure 15.2b), the deep oesophageal 120° coronary sinus view (Figure 15.2f), and the deep transgastric 130° RV inflow–outflow view (Figure 15.2j).

The RV inflow–outflow view is particularly important in the assessment of the TV, especially when used with biplane (x-plane) imaging. By 'sweeping' the biplane cursor from the antero-septal commissure, through the centre of the TV and towards the posterior–septal commissure, the entire valve is visualized, allowing one to determine the origin and extent of leaflet pathology or TR jets (Figure 15.3).

Non-standard TOE TV views

From the mid-oesophageal four-chamber view centred on the RV (0–20°), the sector scan is forward-rotated to 70–100° to obtain the mid-oesophageal RV two-chamber view. This view passes through the major axis of the annulus, and at this angle, a Doppler beam is usually well aligned with blood flow through the TV.

From the lower oesophageal coronary sinus view (0°), the sector scan is forward-rotated to 110–130° to obtain the lower oesophageal coronary sinus 120° view. This usually provides a clear view of the right atrial appendage.

From the deep transgastric five-chamber view, the sector scan is forward-rotated to 90–140° and the probe turned to the right to obtain the deep transgastric 130° RV inflow–outflow view. This view is almost a mirror image of the 'standard' deep transgastric RV inflow–outflow view obtained at 0° but is often more easily obtained.

Simultaneous 2D visualization of all TV leaflets can only be obtained by using the transgastric basal RV short-axis view (Figure 15.4) or by using 3D imaging (Figure 15.5).

> ***Expert tip: In the mid-oesophageal four-chamber view, advancing the probe until the aortic valve disappears should demonstrate the anterior and septal leaflets. If the probe is withdrawn slightly from the coronary sinus view, the posterior and septal leaflets are usually visualized.***

3D imaging

The thin leaflets and the distance from the transducer often make it more challenging to image the TV with 3D TOE than the MV or AV. 3D datasets should be acquired using zoom or full-volume modes from the mid-oesophageal RV four-chamber view, RV inflow–outflow view, or transgastric short-axis view. The sector should be wide enough to include the entire annulus and deep enough to include full leaflet excursion. As with all 3D imaging, increasing the sector size to include the surrounding structures (atrial septum, MV, AV) helps to orientate the dataset but reduces spatial and temporal resolution.

The orientation of the 3D dataset is an issue that has evolved over the past decade. The 2012 European Association of Echocardiography (EAE)/ASE recommendations for 3D image acquisition/display and the 2013 ASE/SCA guidelines for performing a comprehensive TOE examination both recommend displaying an *en face* view of the TV leaflets from the atrial perspective, with the septal leaflet at the bottom of the screen.[8] However, these recommendations were written when TV interventional procedures were not available, and the proposed orientation was aimed at replicating the surgical view. In recent years, numerous experts have proposed orienting the *en face* image with the inter-atrial septum oriented vertically with the AV at the 5 o'clock position (which puts the septal leaflet between 12 and 5 o'clock). The authors of this chapter believe that this is likely to be incorporated in future guidelines and this is the orientation that will be presented throughout this chapter (Figure 15.5).[3,9]

Quantitative measures

TV leaflet lengths can be measured by biplane TV imaging, using the technique described earlier of 'sweeping' the biplane cursor in the RV inflow–outflow view from the

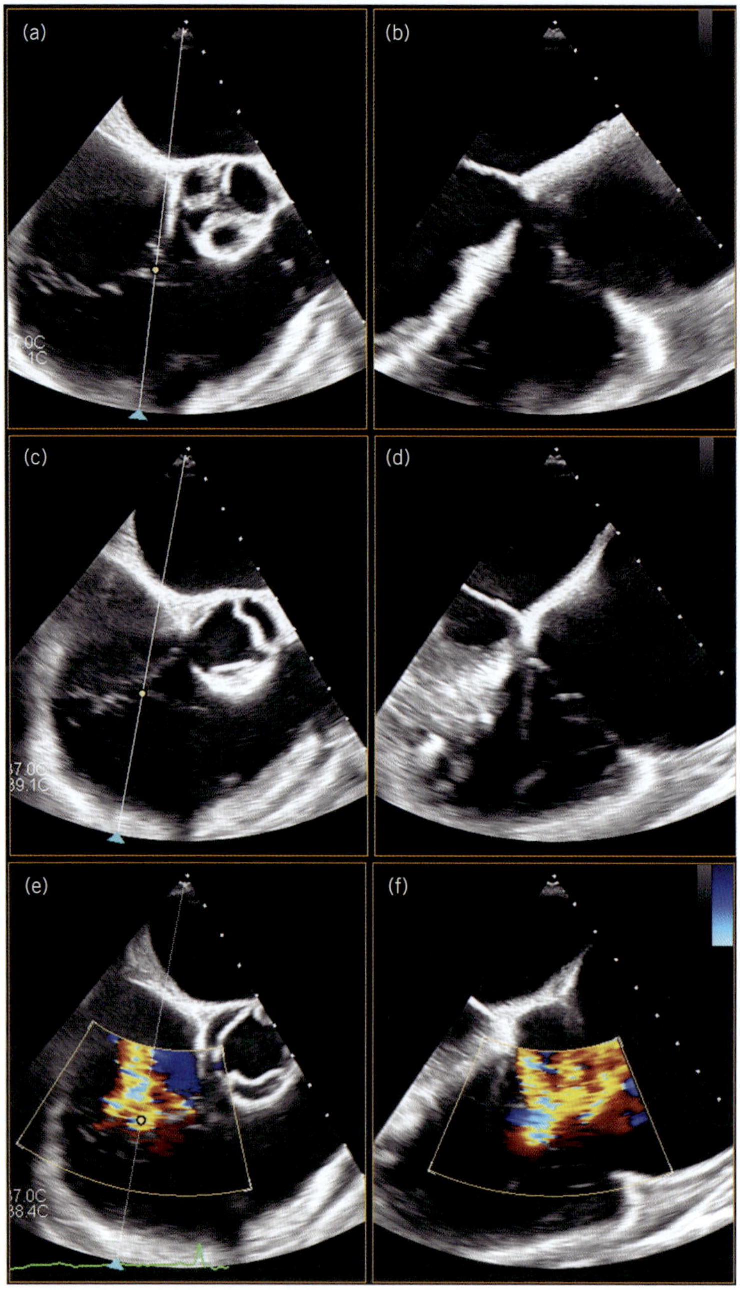

Figure 15.3 Biplane imaging of the TV. Frames (a) and (c) show the same mid-oesophageal RV inflow–outflow view. From that view, a biplane cursor is placed across the TV and moved across the valve from one end to the other, producing a series of corresponding orthogonal views. All coaptation planes can be visualized in this fashion. In this example, the cursor was moved to the left between frames (a) and (c), producing different orthogonal images of the TV (frames (b) and (d)). The same process can also be with colour Doppler (frames (e) and (f)) to determine the extent and severity of a TR jet.

anterior–septal commissure to the posterior–septal commissure (Figure 15.3). A transgastric basal RV short-axis view also permits measurement of the coaptation gaps between the leaflets if present (Figure 15.4).

Quantitative assessment of the TV annular anatomy can be performed using multi-planar reconstruction of 3D datasets,[4] but this is often impractical during the intraoperative period. The mid-oesophageal RV four-chamber view (Figure 15.2a) is usually aligned with the minor axis of the valve, and the mid-oesophageal RV two-chamber view (Figure 15.2b) and transgastric RV inflow view (Figure 15.2h) with the major axis of the valve.

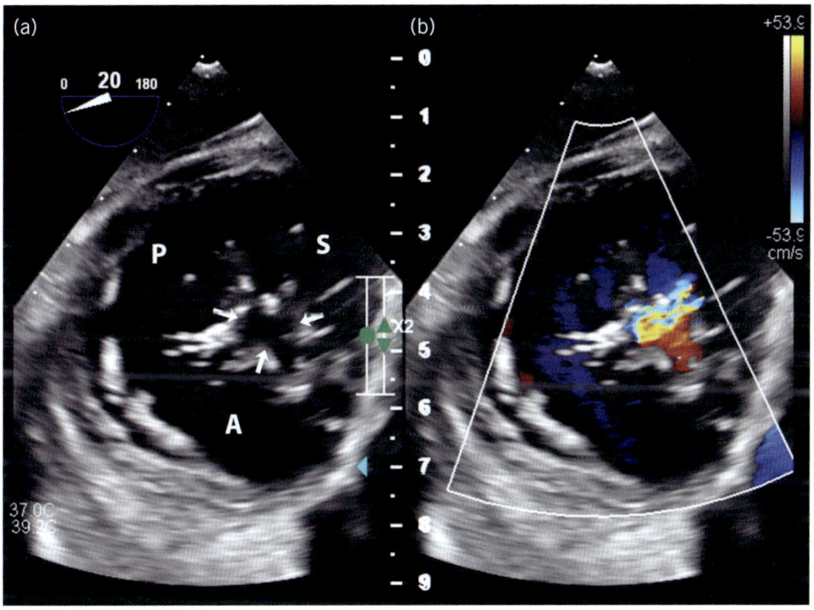

Figure 15.4 Two-dimensional short axis-view of the TV. This is a transgastric basal RV short-axis view in dual display (a, b), frozen in mid systole. A large coaptation gap (a, arrows) is seen between the anterior (A), posterior (P), and septal (S) leaflets, measuring approximately 1.4 × 1.0 cm in diameter. The corresponding colour Doppler image (b) shows a large regurgitant jet in the centre of the valve.

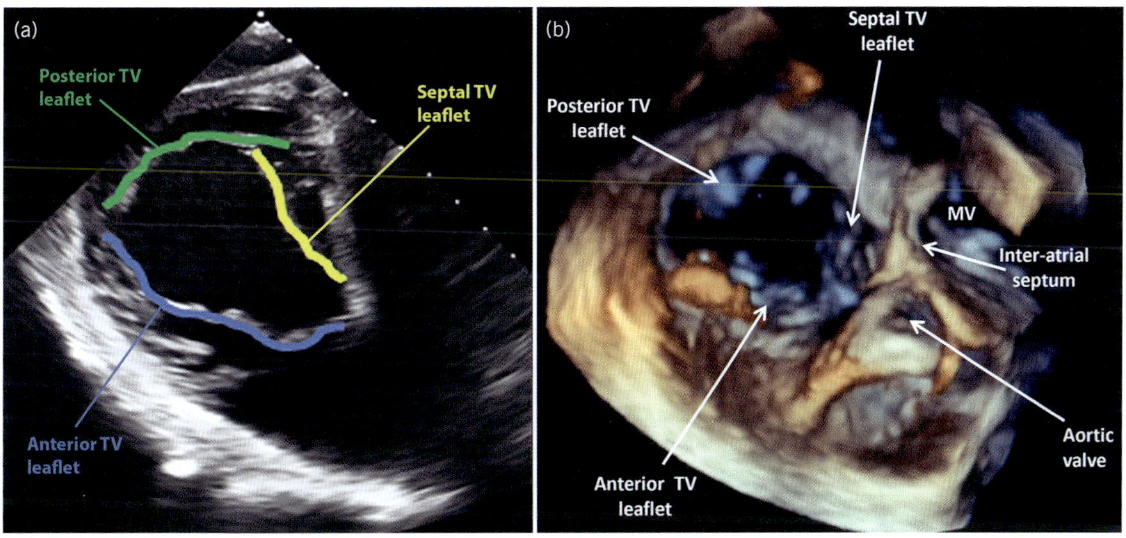

Figure 15.5 3D imaging of the TV. (a) is a 2D transgastric basal RV short-axis view showing the three TV leaflets. (b) is an *en face* 3D view of the TV from the right atrium, oriented with the AV at the 5 o'clock position (see text for details).

However, since there are no anatomical landmarks to confirm the correct positioning, it can be difficult to accurately identify the axes.

The 2017 ASE guidelines define 'significant' TV annular dilatation as an *end-diastolic* diameter >40 mm or >21 mm/m^2 in the apical four-chamber TTE view. The 2013 EACVI recommendations define significant dilatation as an end-diastolic diameter of >35 mm or >21 mm/m^2. Of note, normal values for 2D TOE annular dimensions have not been validated and are not mentioned in TOE guidelines. Until future guidelines dictate otherwise, it is reasonable to apply these numbers to TOE, at end-diastole (or the greatest possible opening) in the mid-oesophageal four-chamber view. It is important to remember that, while reasonably reproducible, the mid-oesophageal four-chamber view does not represent the long axis of the TV, and much larger values for annular dimension have been reported from quantitative 3D measurements (which measures the true long axis of the valve).[10,11,12]

Spectral Doppler imaging

Spectral Doppler interrogation of the TV involves assessing diastolic RV filling (looking for tricuspid stenosis), measuring TR jet velocity (to evaluate RV systolic pressure and systolic pulmonary artery pressure (SPAP))(Figure 15.6), and measuring the velocity of the lateral tricuspid annulus by tissue Doppler as part of the evaluation of RV systolic function (see Chapter 14). Although the incident angle for Doppler interrogation of the TV is variable, the mid-oesophageal modified bicaval and RV two-chamber views tend to yield the best alignment. For eccentric jets directed over the septal leaflet, the mid-oesophageal RV four-chamber view may be useful.

Tricuspid regurgitation

Trivial TR is normal, occurring in two-thirds of healthy subjects.[11] Such physiological regurgitation is associated with structurally normal TV components and no RV dilatation.

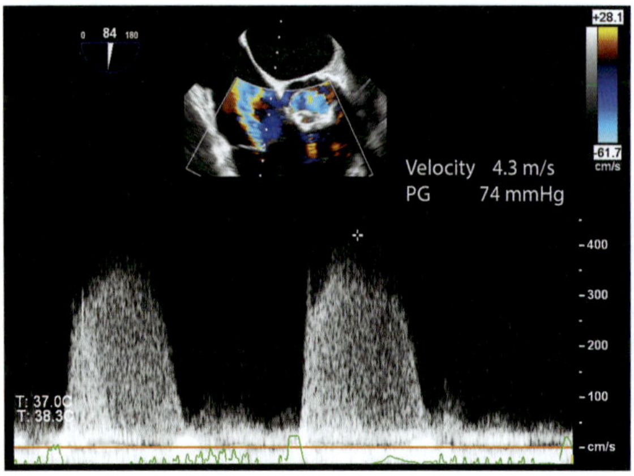

Figure 15.6 Estimating the RV systolic pressure using the TR jet. A CW Doppler cursor was placed across the TR jet in the mid-oesophageal inflow–outflow view. Note the dense spectral Doppler signal, consistent with significant TR. The peak TR velocity of 4.3 m/s translates into an estimated RV systolic pressure of 74 mmHg, consistent with severe pulmonary hypertension. Note that the cursor is slightly off axis from the direction of the TR jet in this view, meaning that the velocity will be underestimated (see cosine effect in Chapter 1).

Physiological TR is central and does not extend throughout systole, and a peak velocity of <2.5 m/s is consistent with normal pulmonary pressures.

Classification of pathological tricuspid regurgitation

Evaluation of pathological TR must include an assessment of the mechanism and severity of TR, as well as of the impact on right heart function, which is intricately linked to clinical outcome. Accordingly, the PCR Tricuspid Valve Working Group recently proposed a new integrative classification of TR inspired by the Carpentier functional classification of MR, recognizing that the initial aetiology based on valve and chamber morphology/function may become more challenging to identify as TV disease progresses (Table 15.1).[13]

Primary tricuspid regurgitation

Primary TR is caused by a structural abnormality of the TV leaflets and is observed in only 8–10% of patients with TV disease. Causes include endocarditis, rheumatic disease, degenerative disease, trauma, carcinoid heart disease, myxomatous disease, endomyocardial fibrosis, congenital heart disease (e.g. Ebstein anomaly), thoracic trauma, and iatrogenic TV damage.

Endocarditis

TV vegetations typically occur on the RA (upstream) side of the valve (Figure 15.7; see Online appendix 8.5) and may be associated with leaflet perforation. Multiple/complex jets suggest significant leaflet destruction. Vegetations may be related to vascular catheters or pacing wires in the right heart, and it may be impossible to distinguish vegetation from thrombus (in such cases, the diagnosis relies on the clinical presentation).

Rheumatic TV disease

Rheumatic TV disease occurs in association with rheumatic disease of the aortic and mitral valves. The leaflets are typically thickened with restricted mobility (Figure 15.8; see Online appendix 8.3). Leaflet thickening may be subtle and is less obvious than in rheumatic MV disease. TR results from leaflet shortening and retraction or fusion, and from shortening and/or fusion of the TV chords and papillary muscles, so careful assessment of the subvalvular apparatus is important. TR is often eccentrically directed over the septal leaflet towards the atrial septum. The TR jet velocity is increased, reflecting elevated pulmonary pressures due to frequent concomitant

Table 15.1 Classification of tricuspid regurgitation

	Leaflet structure	Pathophysiology	Aetiology	Imaging
Primary (organic)				
	Abnormal	Lack of leaflet coaptation due to intrinsic changes leading to restrictive or excessive leaflet mobility or leaflet perforation	**Carpentier I:** Congenital, endocarditis **Carpentier II:** Myxomatous disease, trauma **Carpentier IIIA:** Carcinoid, rheumatic, radiotherapy, tumours	TV leaflet structurally abnormal TV leaflet mobility is variable TV annulus, RV, and RA typically dilated
Secondary (functional)				
Atrial	Normal	RA enlargement and dysfunction leading to significant isolated annular dilatation; RV often normal*	**Carpentier I:** Atrial fibrillation/flutter Age Heart failure with preserved ejection fraction	Marked TV annular dilatation Leaflet tethering absent/minimal (except late stages with secondary RV dysfunction) TV leaflet mobility typically normal RA significantly dilated RV volume typically normal (except late stages)
Ventricular	Normal	RV enlargement and/or dysfunction leading to significant leaflet tethering and annular dilatation	**Carpentier IIIB:** Left-sided LV or valve disease Pulmonary hypertension RV cardiomyopathy RV infarction	Marked TV leaflet tethering TV leaflet typically restricted in systole (Carpentier IIIB) TV annulus, RV and RA are dilated and/or dysfunctional
3-CIED-related	Normal/abnormal	Leaflet impingement Leaflet/chordal entanglement, chordal rupture Leaflet adherence Leaflet laceration/perforation Leaflet avulsion	Pacemaker ICD CRT	TV leaflet structural abnormalities may be present TV leaflet mobility is variable (all Carpentier types) TV annulus, RV, and RA typically dilated (except acute TR)

*Right ventricular basal diameter may appear abnormal due to the conical shape of the right ventricle.

CIED, cardiac implanted electronic device; CRT, cardiac resynchronization therapy; ICD, implantablecardioverter–defibrillator; LV, left ventricular; RA, right atrial; RV, right ventricular; TR, tricuspid regurgitation; TV, tricuspid valve.

Adapted with permission of Europa Group, from *EuroIntervention*, Praz F et al., Transcatheter treatment for tricuspid valve disease, 2021;17(10):791–808; permission conveyed through Copyright Clearance Center, Inc.

MV involvement. However, rheumatic TR in the absence of pulmonary hypertension from MV disease (rare) may be associated with normal TR jet velocity. There may be concomitant TV stenosis due to commissural fusion.

Degenerative disease

Degenerative TV disease is much less common than degenerative MV disease and it usually occurs in the presence of degenerative MV disease (Figure 15.9; see Online Appendices 8.4.7 and 8.4.8). The anterior TV leaflet is most frequently involved. Leaflet motion may demonstrate prolapse or flail, which should be evaluated relative to the *high axis* of the annulus (i.e. in the mid-oesophageal RV inflow–outflow view). 3D imaging from the atrial perspective readily demonstrates leaflet prolapse (Figure 15.9), and the presence of thickened diseased leaflets often improves 3D image quality. Leaflet flail can also occur with endocarditis and chest trauma. In cases of degenerative TV disease, TR is usually eccentric and directed *away from* the predominantly affected leaflet.

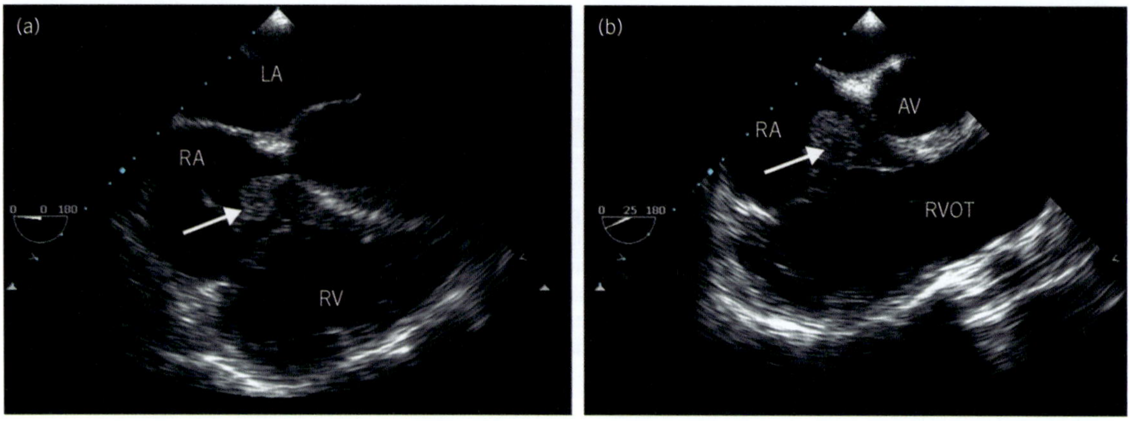

Figure 15.7 Tricuspid endocarditis. A large echogenic mass (arrow) is attached to the septal TV in the mid-oesophageal four-chamber (a) and RV inflow–outflow (b) views.

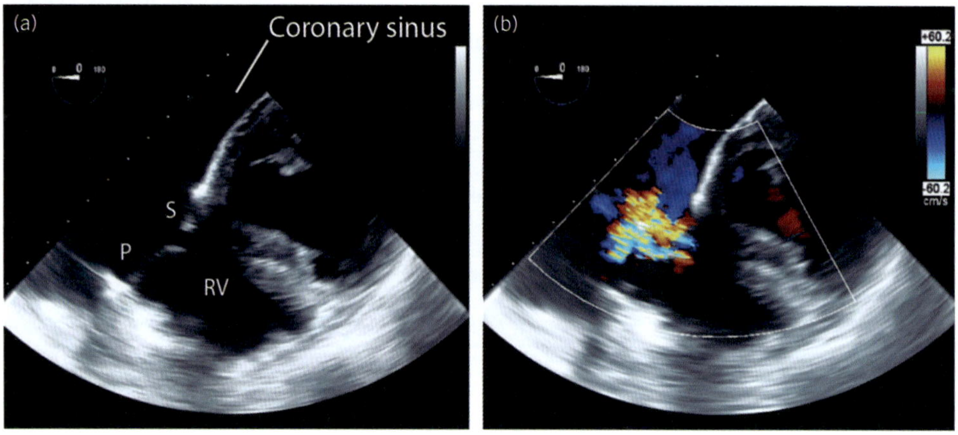

Figure 15.8 Rheumatic TV disease. The septal (S) and posterior (P) leaflets of the TV are demonstrated in the lower oesophageal coronary sinus view, without (a) and with (b) colour Doppler. In these late-systolic frames, thickening of both leaflets and a large coaptation defect can be seen. While not apparent in these still frames, leaflet motion was severely restricted in both systole and diastole. There is severe central TR on the colour Doppler image (b).

Trauma

Damage to the TV can result from blunt chest trauma (e.g. sudden deceleration injury) or from iatrogenic injury (e.g. cardiac biopsy, pacemaker leads). There may be leaflet perforation, or chordal or papillary muscle rupture, depending on the mechanism of injury. Chordal or papillary muscle rupture results in leaflet prolapse/flail and severe TR (see Online appendix 8.4).

Carcinoid disease

Carcinoid disease of the TV causes thickening and fibrosis of the leaflets, resulting in restricted motion (Figure 15.10; see Online appendix 8.6). In contrast to rheumatic disease, carcinoid is associated with a smoothly thickened appearance to the leaflets *without commisural fusion*. Concomitant pulmonary valve involvement is common. Left-sided valve involvement suggests lung metastasis of the tumour.

Secondary tricuspid regurgitation

Secondary TR is common and occurs in the context of relatively normal TV leaflets and TV annular dilatation. This can be due to RA dilatation, RV dilatation, or both. RA dilatation is frequent in patients with atrial fibrillation and results in TV annular dilatation and horizontal apposition of the TV leaflets. The causes of RV dilatation are discussed in Chapter 14 and include:(1) RV pressure overload due to elevated pulmonary vascular resistance (PVR) or PV stenosis; (2) primary RV volume overload (ASD, PV regurgitation); or (3) primary RV systolic dysfunction

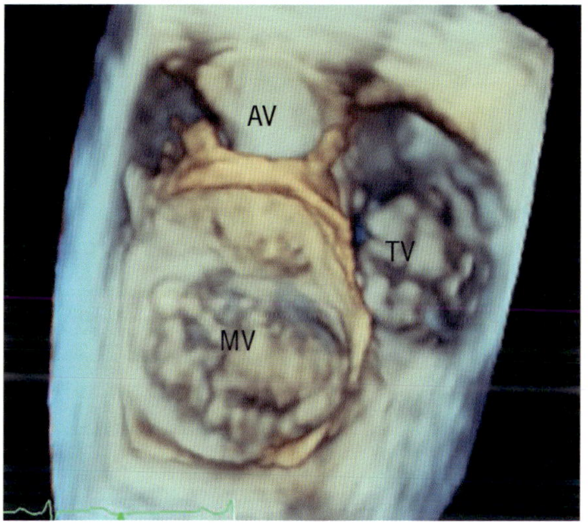

Figure 15.9 Myxomatous mitral and tricuspid valves. In this full-volume 3D view of the mitral, aortic, and tricuspid valves from the atrial perspective, widespread billowing of the mitral and tricuspid leaflets can be seen, consistent with Barlow disease (see Chapters 8 and 9). Because the diseased TV leaflets are thickened, they are easier to visualize than normal.

(ischaemia/infarction, cardiomyopathy). In the perioperative setting, RV systolic dysfunction may arise due to inadequate myocardial protection or gas embolus to the right coronary artery. Causes of acute increases in PVR during the perioperative period include hypoxia, hypercarbia, acidosis, atelectasis, the systemic inflammatory response to CPB, and protamine administration.

RV dilatation causes secondary TR due to the combined effects of annular dilatation, papillary muscle displacement, and leaflet tethering. With severe secondary TR, the tricuspid annulus dilates along the septal–lateral axis away from the interventricular septum. This pattern of dilatation results in decreased coaptation of the septal leaflet with the anterior and posterior leaflets.

Tricuspid regurgitation related to cardiac implantable electronic device

Implantation of permanent pacing leads is associated with significant TR in 20–30% of patients.[14] The pathophysiology of pacemaker-related TR includes leaflet/chordal entanglement, impingement, adherence, laceration, or avulsion (following lead extraction; see Chapter 17). In addition to TV leaflet structural abnormalities, leaflet mobility is variable, and the TV annulus, RA, and RV are typically dilated.[13]

Echocardiographic quantification of tricuspid regurgitation

The echocardiographic features of secondary TR are annular dilatation, leaflet tethering, and RA and RV dilatation in the context of structurally normal TV leaflets (Figure 15.11; see Online appendix 8.2). TR is mostly central. If the cause is elevated PVR, TR jet velocity is increased (>2.5 m/s) and there may be other signs of RV pressure overload (see Chapter 14). RV systolic function is variably affected. If the underlying cause of secondary TR is RV dysfunction, RV systolic function is typically severely impaired. For other causes of secondary TR, RV systolic function may be relatively preserved, at least initially. Eventually, severe TR from any cause leads to RV systolic dysfunction and right-sided failure.

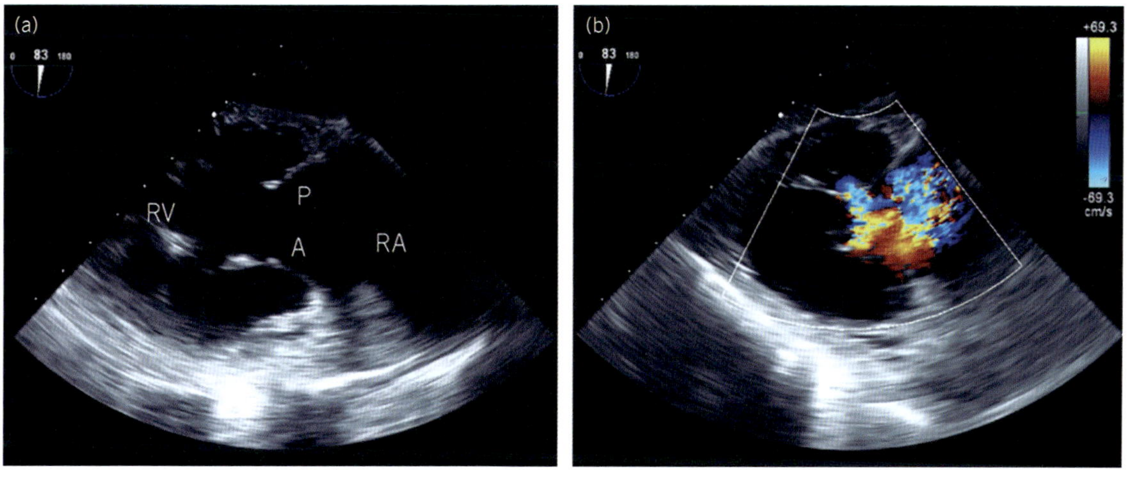

Figure 15.10 Carcinoid TV disease. The TV is shown from the transgastric RV inflow view. The 2D frame (a) shows marked thickening of the posterior (P) and anterior (A) leaflets. The colour Doppler frame (b) shows severe associated TR.

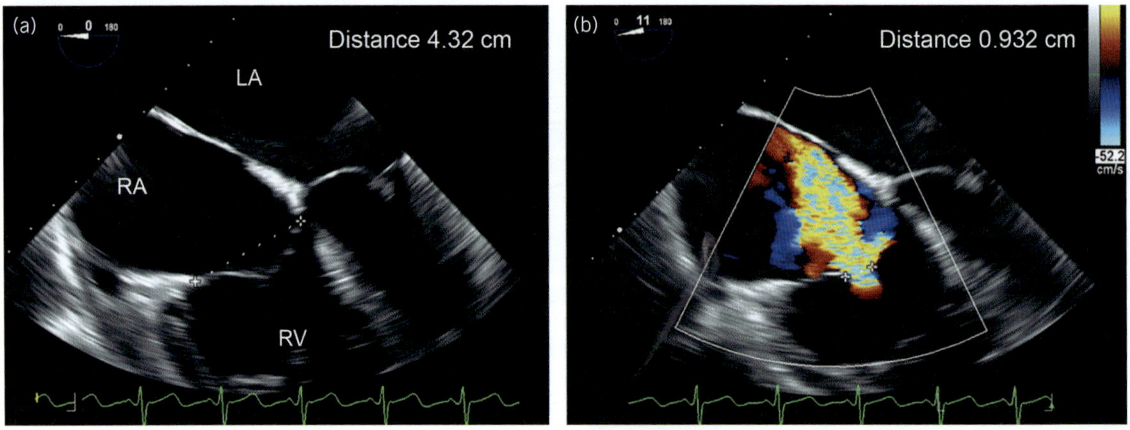

Figure 15.11 Torrential secondary TR. This mid-oesophageal four-chamber view shows the right heart in late systole. On the 2D image (a), the TV annulus is severely dilated (4.32 cm) and there is tenting of the TV leaflets, which are otherwise structurally normal. Note that the TV annulus is usually measured in late diastole, not systole, but this frame is also meant to demonstrate leaflet tenting. (b) shows a severe, mostly central, TR jet (vena contracta width 0.932 cm). Note also the dilated RA and RV (relative to the LV).

Like its mitral counterpart, the assessment of TR severity is based on several qualitative and quantitative parameters of 2D and 3D imaging, and colour and spectral Doppler.[8] Qualitative/semi-quantitative signs of significant TR include a visible systolic coaptation gap between the TV leaflets on 2D imaging, a large and broad-based aliasing systolic jet crossing the TV on colour Doppler imaging, and the presence of a zone of flow convergence on the ventricular side of the valve. Spectral Doppler usually demonstrates a dense and triangular (early peaking) CW Doppler signal across the TR jet. In addition, hepatic vein systolic flow reversal by PW Doppler may be demonstrated in the transgastric inferior vena cava view (Figure 15.12). It is important to note that the TR colour jet is not a measure of regurgitant volume and that there is no direct relationship between TR jet velocity and TR severity. However, similar to MR, the density of the TR jet by CW Doppler is proportional to the regurgitant volume, and a dense signal suggests more severe regurgitation.

Since none of the above signs is absolute, quantitative measures of TR are important to further define severity. This includes: (1) estimation of anatomical regurgitant orifice size by biplane vena contracta (VC) measurement; and (2) quantification of physiological effective regurgitant orifice area (EROA) and regurgitant volume (RVol), measured on the RV side of the TV in late systole in the mid-oesophageal RV four-chamber view. Current ASE/EACVI guidelines define severe TR as VC diameter ≥7 mm, EROA ≥0.40 cm^2, and RVol ≥45 mL.[11] However, much higher values for the VC width may be obtained in other views, particularly the mid-oesophageal RV inflow–outflow view (Figure 15.12), which may sample the jet along the coaptation line between the septal and anterior leaflets. Moreover, since patients undergoing transcatheter TV interventions frequently have anatomical regurgitant areas several times greater than EROA of 0.40 cm^2, an extension of the TR severity grading system has been proposed to include additional TR grades of 'massive' and 'torrential' TR (Figure 15.13), using greater EROA values derived from 3D vena contracta area measurements.[15] Table 15.2 summarizes the main quantitative parameters of TR severity.

Indications for TV intervention

Surgical TV intervention using TV annuloplasty is preferable to TV replacement, which should only be considered when the TV leaflets are severely tethered or damaged and the annulus is significantly dilated.

Patients with severe secondary TR should have a TV annuloplasty performed at the time of left-sided valve surgery, given that the additional operative risk is small.[16,17] When annular dilation is present, even in the absence of severe TR, this promotes reverse remodelling of the RV and improves functional status. In the latest European (European Society of Cardiology (ESC)/ European Association of Cardiovascular Imaging (EACVI)) and American (American College of Cardiology (ACC)/ American Heart Association (AHA)) valve guidelines,[16,17] TV annuloplasty is a **Class I** recommendation for patients with **severe secondary TR** undergoing left-sided valve surgery (Figure 15.14). The European guidelines also

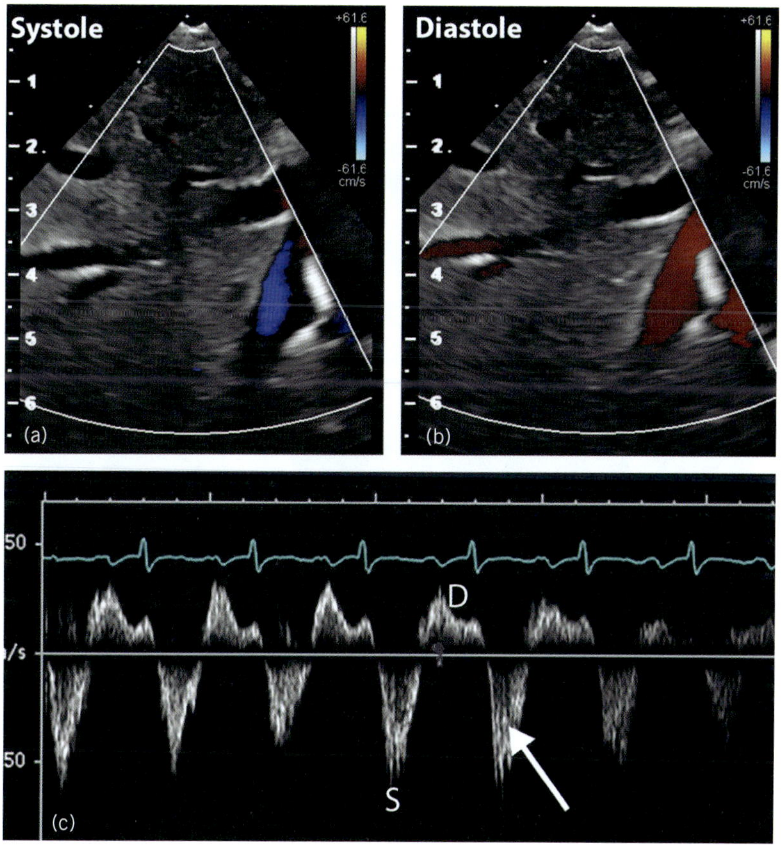

Figure 15.12 Hepatic venous flow reversal due to severe TR. (a) and (b) show colour Doppler images of the hepatic veins in systole (a) and diastole (b). Systolic flow reversal is away from the transducer (blue), and diastolic flow is towards the transducer (red). (c) demonstrates the PW Doppler pattern of hepatic venous flow in systole (S) and diastole (D). Note the reversed S-wave due to severe TR.

consider TV annuloplasty as a **Class IIa** recommendation for patients with **mild or moderate TR** undergoing left-sided valve surgery when the TV annulus dimension exceeds 40 mm or 21 mm/m^2 by 2D echocardiography in the mid-oesophageal four-chamber view.[16,18] It should also be considered in patients who are symptomatic or have RV dilatation in the absence of severe RV or LV dysfunction and severe raised PVR.[16]

Treatment of primary TR depends on the aetiology, severity, and symptomatology of the regurgitation. The European (ESC/EACVI) guidelines consider surgery a **Class I** recommendation for patients with **severe primary TR** undergoing left-sided valve surgery or for symptomatic patients with **isolated severe TR** without severe RV dysfunction.[16] Both the European and American guidelines consider TV surgery a **Class IIa** indication for patients with **moderate primary TR** undergoing left-sided valve surgery or for asymptomatic patients with **isolated severe TR** and RV dilatation.[16,17]

Tricuspid stenosis

Tricuspid stenosis (TS) is rare, almost always rheumatic in origin, and usually associated with left-sided valve lesions. TS results from leaflet immobility and commissural fusion. As with the MV, there is typically diastolic doming of the anterior, and occasionally the posterior, leaflet. Commissural fusion is best seen in the transgastric RV basal short-axis view and with *en face* 3D imaging. TS may also be secondary to congenital lesions, carcinoid disease, or cardiac masses (e.g. atrial myxoma), or following annuloplasty placement, particularly for correcting primary TR (Figure 15.14).

No universally accepted grading of TS exists, and evaluation can be challenging; the pressure half-time method is not validated for TS, and the continuity equation is rarely applicable because of concomitant valvular regurgitation. A mean diastolic gradient of >5 mmHg (in the absence of tachycardia) is usually used to define severe stenosis.

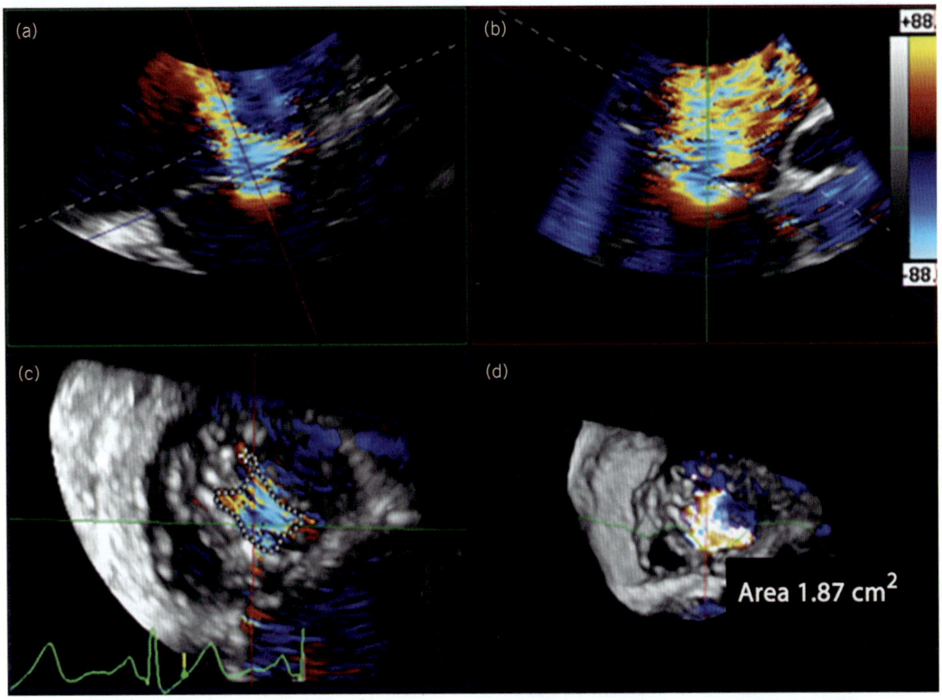

Figure 15.13 3D measurement of vena contracta area. This is a 3D multi-planar reconstruction of the TV. Similar to the MV and AV (see Chapters 8 and 10), the long axes of the valve are aligned with the centre of the TR jet, and the short-axis plane (blue) is adjusted to the level of the vena contracta (a, b). The vena contracta area is then measured by planimetry (c). Note that the calculated area of 1.87 cm^2 is consistent with 'torrential' TR (d).

Table 15.2 Extending grading scheme for tricuspid regurgitation

Variable	Mild	Moderate	Severe	Massive	Torrential
VC (biplane)	<3 mm	3–6.9 mm	7–13 mm	14–20 mm	≥21 mm
EROA (PISA)	<20 mm^2	20–39 mm^2	40–59 mm^2	60–79 mm^2	≥80 mm^2
3D VCA or quantitative EROA*			75–94 mm^2	95–114 mm^2	≥115 mm^2

* 3D VCA and quantitative Doppler EROA cut-offs may be larger than PISA EROA.

VC, vena contracta; EROA, effective regurgitant orifice area; 3D VCA, three-dimensional vena contracta area.

Adapted with permission of Europa Group, from *EuroIntervention*, Praz F et al., Transcatheter treatment for tricuspid valve disease, 2021;17(10):791–808; permission conveyed through Copyright Clearance Center, Inc.

Assessment of tricuspid valve repair

Secondary TR is usually repaired with an undersized annuloplasty. Annuloplasty may also be appropriate for primary TR, but if the TV anatomy is severely distorted (particularly severe leaflet restriction), valve replacement is usually necessary. The goal of TV repair is to achieve mild TR or less, while not inducing significant TS. However, what constitutes an acceptable result depends on the patient's clinical situation and haemodynamic state at the time of assessment (Figure 15.14). Hence, moderate TR may be acceptable in a young woman wishing to avoid valve replacement and warfarin anticoagulation. Elevated cardiac output and tachycardia in the early post-CPB period increase diastolic velocity across the TV. Seemingly 'severe' TS may decrease in the hours/days following surgery once the haemodynamic state stabilizes. Although commissurotomy and ring annuloplasty may provide an acceptable result in patients with TS, valve replacement is usually necessary.

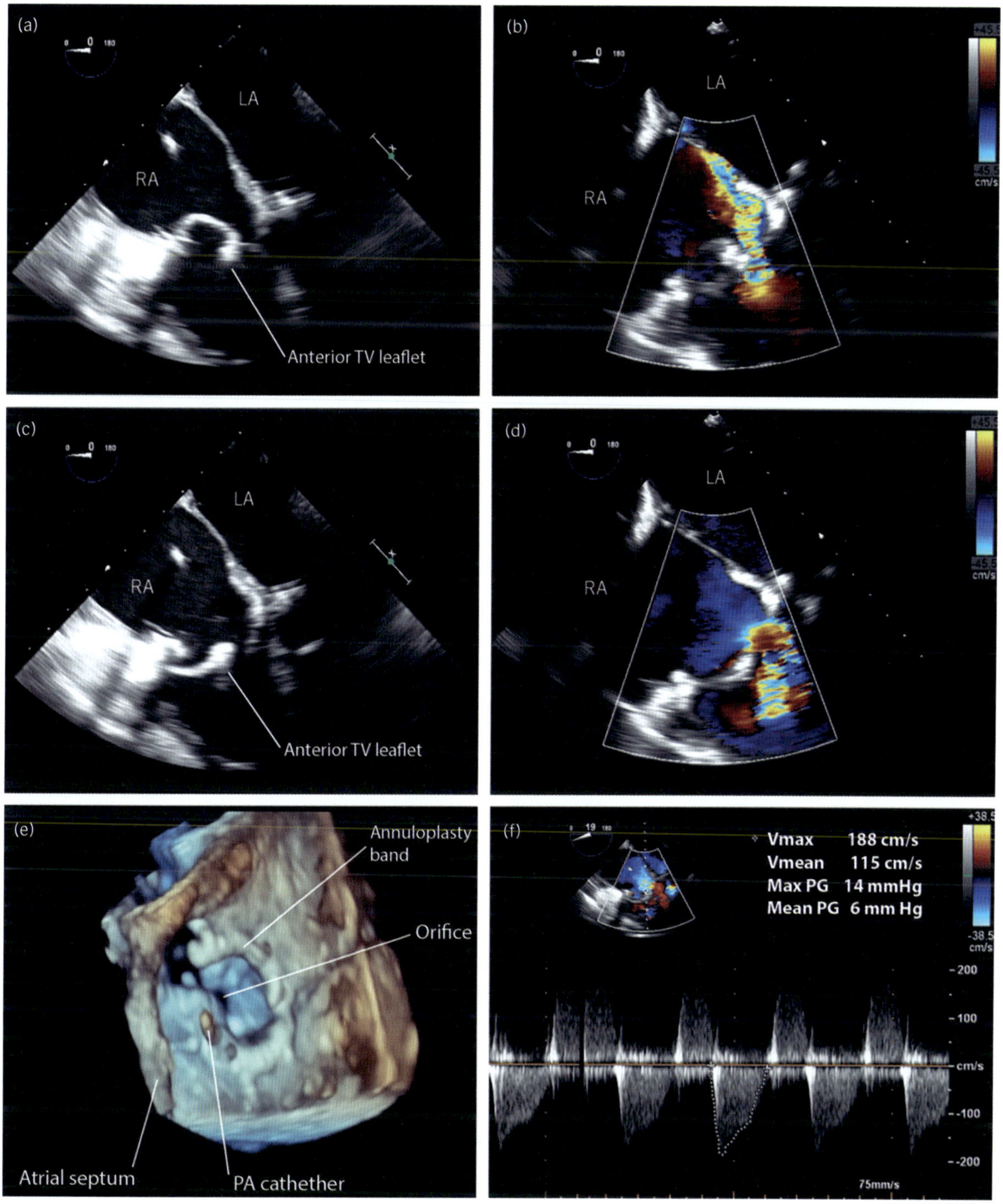

Figure 15.14 Effect of a restrictive annuloplasty band for treating severe rheumatic TR. (a) Systolic frame showing prolapse of the body of the anterior leaflet. (b) Systolic frame showing moderate residual TR, directed towards the inter-atrial septum. (c) Diastolic frame showing doming of the anterior tricuspid leaflet. (d) Diastolic frame showing diastolic aliasing with a zone of flow convergence on the RA side of the TV, suggesting stenosis. (e) 3D view of the TV from the RA aspect in the surgical orientation (here the septum is on the left-hand side) in diastole. The small tricuspid orifice with annuloplasty band is clearly seen. A pulmonary artery (PA) catheter can also be seen, positioned through the TV. (f) CW Doppler interrogation of tricuspid flow. The mean diastolic gradient is 6 mmHg, suggesting severe stenosis. These images were obtained immediately following repair of rheumatic mitral and tricuspid regurgitation. While the tricuspid repair could be considered inadequate, in this circumstance, it was accepted due to the condition of the patient. Follow-up echocardiography before discharge from hospital demonstrated mild TR and a mean diastolic gradient of 3 mmHg, suggesting moderate TS. The clips from which this composite image was made are in Online appendices 8.3.1–8.3.6.

The pulmonary valve

The pulmonary valve (PV) is a trileaflet valve with an oval annulus slightly larger than the AV. Unlike the AV, there are no coronary ostia or fibrous connection to the TV. The thinner PV leaflets are the **anterior** (furthest from the AV), **left**, and **right**. The left and right pulmonary leaflets are directly opposite the AV leaflets of the same name.

Imaging the pulmonary valve

As the PV is the most anterior of the heart valves and the furthest from the oesophagus, 2D TOE image quality is usually poor, and 3D imaging is usually of low quality and non-contributory. Views for imaging the PV are shown in Figure 15.2, along with two non-standard views of the PV (not discussed in Chapter 4): the mid-oesophageal PV short-axis view (Figure 15.2l) and the transgastric RV outflow view (Figure 15.2m). From the mid-oesophageal long-axis view, slightly withdrawing and turning the TOE probe to the left (away from the aorta) provides a short-axis view of the PV (Figure 15.2l). The transgastric RV outflow view is obtained by rotating the sector scan to 30–60° from a transgastric mid-papillary view that has been centred on the RV (see also Online appendix 1.7).

Pulmonary valve leaflets

Several TOE views display the PV leaflets, though it can be difficult to distinguish individual leaflets. The most reliable is the mid-oesophageal RV inflow–outflow view. The mid-oesophageal PV short-axis view and the uppero-esophageal aortic arch short-axis view may also be useful. Transgastric imaging is helpful when there are strong reflectors from the aortic and mitral valves that obscure the PV in the mid-oesophageal windows; however, the increased distance from the probe limits spatial resolution.

Pulmonary artery

The main pulmonary artery and right pulmonary artery can be visualized in the mid-oesophageal ascending aortic views (see Figures 4.4 and 4.8) and the upper oesophageal ascending aorta short-axis view.

Spectral Doppler

Gastric views of the PV usually provide good alignment between a Doppler beam and flow through the PV and can help to assess the severity of PS and/or RVOT conduit obstruction or stenosis.

Pulmonary regurgitation

Pulmonary regurgitation (PR) is often seen on colour Doppler, even when the PV itself is not visible. Trivial PR is normal. Such jets are usually small and central. Patients with pulmonary hypertension and associated pulmonary arterial dilatation frequently demonstrate mild or moderate PR. Severe PR is uncommon and usually seen in patients with congenital heart disease (see Chapter 18). Rarely, PR results from endocarditis, carcinoid heart disease, or rheumatic disease.

With severe PR, there is rapid equalization of the diastolic pulmonary arterial and RV pressures, resulting in a brief colour jet in early diastole. This phenomenon can lead to PR severity being underestimated. Instead, severity is usually estimated by the diameter of the jet origin, measured just below the PV. Although there is significant inter-observer variability in measurements, a jet occupying >50–65% of the RV outflow tract suggests PR is severe (Figure 15.15). Colour flow reversal in the pulmonary arteries is a specific sign of severe PR.

Pulmonary stenosis

Most cases of pulmonary stenosis (PS) relate to congenital heart disease and may be infundibular, subvalvular, valvular, and/or supravalvular (see Chapter 18). Additionally, carcinoid heart disease can cause PS and should always be considered when patients have concomitant TV involvement. The mechanism and site of stenosis should be assessed with 2D and colour Doppler imaging. With

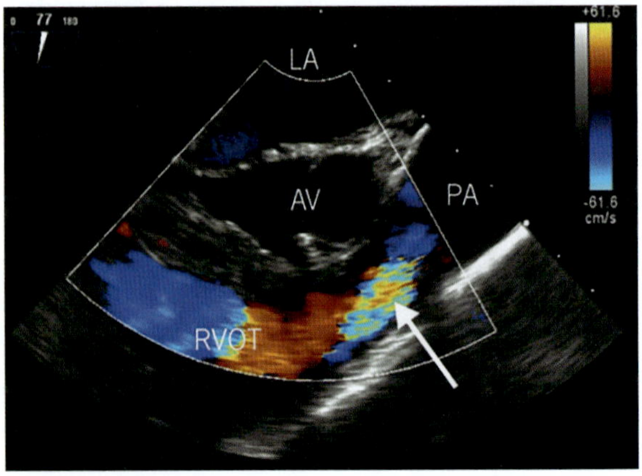

Figure 15.15 Severe pulmonary regurgitation. A mid-oesophageal RV inflow–outflow view showing a broad-based jet of PR in early systole. Additional examples in Online appendix 8.7.

CW Doppler imaging, PS is graded as mild (<3 m/s), moderate (3–4 m/s), or severe (>4 m/s).

Multiple choice questions

Discover interactive multiple choice questions to test your knowledge on this chapter by searching for this book's title or ISBN (9780198873686) at **https://academic.oup.com/** and going to the online appendix at the end of the book. Use your scratch-off code on the inside cover to access the material.

References

1. Rogers JH, Bolling SF. The tricuspid valve: current perspective and evolving management of tricuspid regurgitation. *Circulation.* 2009;**119**:2718–25.
2. Holda MK, Zhingre Sanchez JD, Bateman MG, Iaizzo PA. Right atrioventricular valve leaflet morphology redefined: implications for transcatheter repair procedures. *JACC Cardiovasc Interv.* 2019;**12**(2):169–78.
3. Hahn RT, Weckbach LT, Noack T, *et al.* Proposal for a standard echocardiographic tricuspid valve nomenclature. *JACC Cardiovasc Imaging.* 2021;**14**(7):1299–305.
4. Fukuda S, Saracino G, Matsumura Y, *et al.* Three-dimensional geometry of the tricuspid annulus in healthy subjects and in patients with functional tricuspid regurgitation: a real-time, 3-dimensional echocardiographic study. *Circulation.* 2006;**114**:I492–8.
5. Anwar AM, Geleijnse ML, Soliman OI, *et al.* Assessment of normal tricuspid valve anatomy in adults by real-time three-dimensional echocardiography. *Int J Cardiovasc Imaging.* 2007;**23**:717–24.
6. Hahn RT, Abraham T, Adams MS, *et al.* Guidelines for performing a comprehensive transesophageal echocardiographic examination: recommendations from the American Society of Echocardiography and the Society of Cardiovascular Anesthesiologists. *J Am Soc Echocardiogr.* 2013;**26**:921–64.
7. Tan CO, Harley I. Perioperative transesophageal echocardiographic assessment of the right heart and associated structures: a comprehensive update and technical report. *J CardiothoracVascAnesth.* 2014;**28**:1112–33.
8. Lang RM, Badano LP, Tsang W, *et al.* EAE/ASE recommendations for image acquisition and display using three-dimensional echocardiography. *J Am Soc Echocardiogr.* 2012;**25**:3–46.
9. Muraru D, Hahn RT, Soliman OI, Faletra FF, Basso C, Badano LP. 3-dimensional echocardiography in imaging the tricuspid valve. *JACC Cardiovasc Imaging.* 2019;**12**(3):500–15.
10. Montealegre-Gallegos M, Bergman R, Jiang L, Matyal R, Mahmood B, Mahmood F. Tricuspid valve: an intraoperative echocardiographic perspective. *J CardiothoracVascAnesth.* 2014;**28**:761–70.
11. Lancellotti P, Tribouilloy C, Hagendorf A, *et al.* Recommendations for the echocardiographic assessment of native valvular regurgitation: an executive summary from the European Association of Cardiovascular Imaging. *Eur Heart J Cardiovasc Imaging.* 2013;**14**:611–44.
12. Zoghbi WA, Adams D, Bonow RO. Recommendations for noninvasiveevaluation of native valvular regurgitation:areport from the American Society of Echocardiography Developed in Collaboration with the Society for Cardiovascular Magnetic Resonance. *J Am Soc Echocardiogr.* 2017;**30**(4):303–71
13. Praz F, Muraru D, Kreidel F, *et al.* Transcatheter treatment for tricuspid valve disease. *EuroIntervention.* 2021;**17**(10):791–808.
14. Anvardeen K, Rao R, Hazra S, *et al.* Prevalence and significance of tricuspid regurgitation post-endocardial lead placement. *JACC Cardiovasc Imaging.* 2019;**12**:562–4.
15. Hahn RT, Zamorano JL. The need for a new tricuspid regurgitation grading scheme. *Eur Heart J Cardiovasc Imaging.* 2017;**18**(12):1342–3.
16. Vahanian A, Beyersdorf F, Praz F, *et al.*;ESC/EACTS Scientific Document Group. 2021 ESC/EACTS Guidelines for the management of valvular heart disease. *Eur Heart J.* 2022;**43**(7):561–632.
17. Otto CM, Nishimura RA, Bonow RO, *et al.*2020 ACC/AHA Guideline for the management of patients with valvular heart disease: executive summary: areport of the American College of Cardiology/American Heart Association Joint Committee on Clinical Practice Guidelines. *Circulation.* 2021;**143**(5):e35–71.
18. Chikwe J, Itagaki S, Anyanwu A, Adams DH. Impact of concomitant tricuspid annuloplasty on tricuspid regurgitation, right ventricular function, and pulmonary artery hypertension after repair of mitral valve prolapse. *J Am Coll Cardiol.* 2015;**65**:1931–8.

16

The pericardium and pericardial disease

The pericardium is difficult to assess by any imaging modality. Normal pericardium is extremely thin and virtually invisible on cross-sectional imaging, and the pericardial space is a virtual space. The adverse effects of pericardial disease arise from the alterations in cardiac physiology, and assessment of pericardial pathology usually relies on the variation of physiological parameters with respiration rather than on anatomical appearances, which can be misleading. Echocardiography is the most useful non-invasive technique for assessing the pericardium, particularly for identifying pericardial collections and diagnosing pericardial tamponade and pericardial constriction. As the important echocardiographic parameters to be measured are physiological, not anatomical, pericardial pathology is better evaluated by imaging patients when they are awake and breathing spontaneously (i.e. with TTE). This is not always possible; hence this summary provides guidance for assessment with TOE in the mechanically ventilated patient.

Anatomy and function of the pericardium

The pericardium is a fibro-serous membranous structure containing the heart, the roots of the aorta and pulmonary artery, and the terminations of the venae cavae. It is composed of two layers: a tough, thicker outer layer—the fibrous pericardium; and a thin, membranous inner layer—the serous pericardium. The fibrous pericardium is anchored to the adventitia of the great vessels and the walls of the heart. The serous pericardium is composed of two layers: the outer parietal layer, fused to the fibrous pericardium; and the inner visceral layer, apposed to the myocardium. Where the visceral pericardium is in contact with the heart muscle, it is called the epicardium. The visceral pericardium extends to the roots of the great vessels where it becomes continuous with the parietal pericardium. Between the two layers of serous pericardium, there is a virtual space, which typically contains 20–30 mL of lubricating plasma ultrafiltrate.

Pericardial reflections

The pericardium surrounds the heart, except in two areas where the visceral and parietal pericardium form two blind pockets behind the heart—the pericardial reflections. The **transverse sinus** is a small, horizontal pocket, posterior to the ascending aorta and pulmonary trunk. The **oblique sinus** is a vertically orientated fold between the insertions of the pulmonary veins into the LA. The transverse sinus can often be visualized in the mid-oesophageal AV long-axis view (see Figure 4.4 and Online appendix 2.9). The oblique sinus is not usually seen, unless increased fluid is present, in which case it can be visualized posteriorly in the LA in any mid-oesophageal view (see Figure 4.4).

Expert tip: As a result of these reflections, pericardial fluid cannot track further posteriorly than the descending thoracic aorta. This landmark is useful in differentiating pericardial from pleural fluid.

Functions of the pericardium

The pericardium has four major functions: (1) to prevent overdistension of the heart; (2) to ensure the heart remains relatively fixed in the mediastinum; (3) to reduce contact with adjacent structures, particularly the lungs which could transmit infection; and (4) to reduce friction due to the constant motion of the heart. It also plays a minor role in neural modulation and in regulating the tone of the epicardial coronary arteries.

Pericardial pathology

The three most commonly encountered pathologies affecting the pericardium are acute pericarditis, constrictive pericarditis, and pericardial fluid collections, with or without tamponade. Other abnormalities are rare and may present as incidental findings.

Congenitally absent pericardium

Congenitally absent pericardium is very rare and may be complete or incomplete. Complete absence is usually asymptomatic, but partial absence (most commonly of the left pericardium) carries the risk of cardiac herniation. Coronary artery compression, pulmonary vein compression, and severe TR have been described as a consequence of partial herniation of the heart due to partially absent pericardium.[1] The condition is also associated with other congenital abnormalities, including bicuspid AV, patent ductus arteriosus, and ASDs.

During echocardiographic imaging, partially absent pericardium may result in exaggerated or 'hinge' motion of the posterior wall of the LV. The atria may appear compressed, and there may be interposition of lung tissue between the base of the heart and the diaphragm. Valvular abnormalities should be sought.

Pericardial cysts and tumours

Pericardial cysts are fluid-filled sacs adjacent to the heart. They rarely cause symptoms, unless very large. The most common sites are adjacent to the RA (in the right cardiophrenic angle on a chest radiograph) and adjacent to the LV (in the left cardiophrenic angle on a chest radiograph). Pericardial cysts can also occur in the posterior mediastinum adjacent to the LA, and in the anterior mediastinum adjacent to the RV and/or pulmonary artery (Figure 16.1; see Online appendix 3.2.1). The latter two sites are more likely to result in symptoms, due to compression of the heart or great vessels. Although benign, pericardial cysts can rupture, causing pericardial collection.

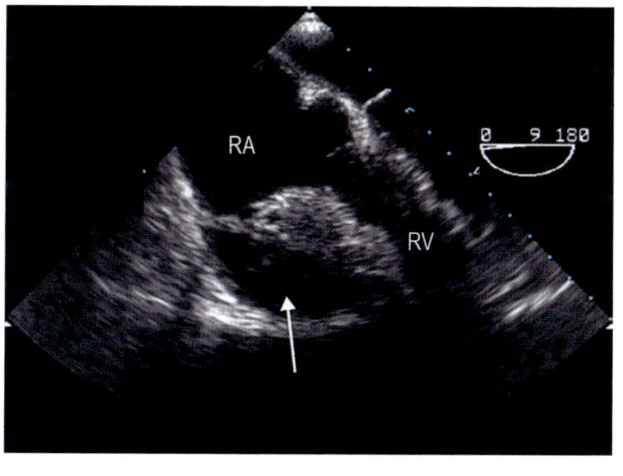

Figure 16.1 Pericardial cyst. In this mid-oesophageal four-chamber view, a fluid-filled space (arrow) due to a pericardial cyst can be seen overlying the RV. The clip related to this image appears in Online appendix 3.2.1.

On TOE, pericardial cysts appear as variably sized (2–15 cm in diameter), echolucent, unilocular cavities adjacent to the pericardium. Cyst cavities are devoid of blood flow. Cysts may be difficult to differentiate from other causes of mediastinal echolucencies such as pericardial effusion, pleural effusion, hiatal hernia, fluid in the pericardial sinuses, and aneurysms or pseudoaneurysms of the heart, great vessels, and coronary arteries. If symptomatic, treatment options include echocardiographically guided percutaneous aspiration, video-assisted thoracoscopic surgery (VATS), or open thoracotomy.

Most malignant pericardial disease is metastatic, commonly from breast or lung cancers or from lymphomas. Primary tumours are rare, and at least 50% are mesotheliomas. Tumour deposits may or may not be seen within the pericardium, but pericardial effusion is common.

Acute pericarditis

Acute pericarditis has a number of causes, the most common being viral infection and myocardial infarction. Less common causes are uraemia, autoimmune relapsing serositis, and cardiac trauma. Diagnosing acute pericarditis depends on a combination of clinical findings and imaging, but it is often a diagnosis of exclusion.

Echocardiographic findings are usually non-specific, consisting of increased echogenicity (brightness) of the pericardium and a small pericardial effusion. There may be fibrin strands in the pericardial fluid (again a non-specific finding). Notwithstanding these limitations, echocardiography is indicated if the diagnosis is suspected clinically to confirm or exclude specific pathologies such as myocardial ischaemia/infarction, endocarditis, or malignancy.

Constrictive pericarditis

Constrictive pericarditis is characterized by fibrous thickening of the pericardium, often with calcification. The diseased pericardium forms a rigid shell around the heart, preventing normal diastolic filling. Common causes of constrictive pericarditis include infection (particularly with tuberculosis and viruses), chronic haemopericardium, thoracic radiotherapy, chronic uraemia, and rheumatic heart disease. In >50% of cases, the cause is unknown.[2]

2D echocardiographic appearances

With 2D imaging, the pericardium may appear thickened (>3 mm) and demonstrate increased echogenicity (Figure 16.2). Calcification within the pericardium may be apparent. Chronically increased filling pressures result in atrial

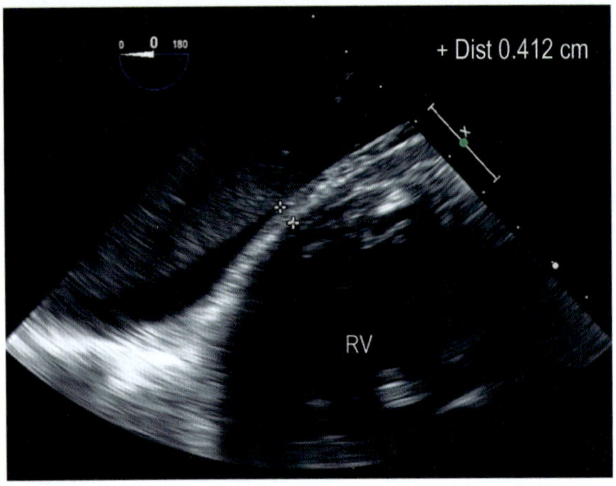

Figure 16.2 Thickened pericardium due to constrictive pericarditis. In this transgastric view, thickened pericardium (0.412 cm) can be seen overlying the RV. Normally, the pericardium is too thin to measure.

enlargement, which is usually mild. There may be leftward bowing of the atrial septum, indicating that RA pressure is higher than LA pressure (see Figure 21.1). Elevated systemic venous pressure causes marked dilatation of the extra-pericardial vena cavae and hepatic veins, with loss of normal respiratory variation in diameter. Ventricular size and systolic function are typically normal.

The motion of the ventricular septum is typically abnormal, displaying a characteristic *bouncing* motion in early diastole. RV diastolic filling normally begins before LV diastolic filling. In circumstances of increased ventricular interdependence (constrictive pericarditis, cardiac tamponade), RV pressure may transiently exceed LV pressure in early diastole, causing a brief leftward (i.e. paradoxical) shift of the ventricular septum.[3] With spontaneous breathing, septal bounce is augmented during inspiration, whereas during positive pressure ventilation, septal bounce is augmented during expiration. Septal bounce is best appreciated in the mid-oesophageal four-chamber view.

Spectral Doppler appearances

Constrictive pericarditis is associated with exaggerated inspiratory-to-expiratory variations in diastolic filling velocities across the mitral and tricuspid valves.

During spontaneous breathing in normal subjects, trans-tricuspid velocity increases by up to 20% during inspiration due to enhanced systemic venous return, while trans-mitral velocity decreases by up to 5% due to reduced pulmonary venous return. This normal cyclical variation with spontaneous breathing is enhanced by constrictive pericarditis, typically to >40% for trans-tricuspid flow and to >25% for trans-mitral flow.[4] Marked diuresis, which is common with constrictive pericarditis, reduces cardiac filling pressure and diminishes the cyclic variability in flow velocities.

The effects of constrictive pericarditis on diastolic filling velocities during positive pressure ventilation are less well understood. In one small study examining the effects of constrictive pericarditis on left heart filling velocities, maximal trans-mitral E-wave and pulmonary venous D-wave velocities were increased by 18% and 28%, respectively, during positive pressure inspiration, indicating that positive pressure ventilation reverses the inspiratory/expiratory pattern, at least for left heart filling (Figure 16.3).[5] In spontaneously breathing subjects, constrictive pericarditis is associated with restrictive diastolic filling. During positive pressure ventilation, an incomplete restrictive filling pattern was identified, with a very short E-wave deceleration velocity.[5]

In addition to constrictive pericarditis, several other conditions are associated with enhanced respiratory variability in diastolic filling velocities (Box 16.1).

The effects of constrictive pericarditis on mitral annular TDI velocities have been investigated in spontaneously breathing subjects.[4] TDI measurements demonstrate a normal or elevated e'-wave velocity, compared to normal (typically >7 cm/s). Despite an elevated LA pressure, the trans-mitral E-wave-to-mitral annular e'-wave (E/e') ratio remains low, a phenomenon termed annulus paradoxus.[4] TDI measurements in constrictive pericarditis have not been validated in ventilated patients.

Elevated systemic venous pressure may result in systolic flow reversal in the hepatic veins, despite the presence of only mild TR.

Intraoperative assessment during pericardiectomy

Pericardiectomy for constrictive pericarditis carries significant risk; in one series, perioperative mortality was 7%.[2] The pericardium is resected from the atria, ventricles, and the great vessels, as feasible. Resection can be guided by TOE, and transgastric views may be useful in identifying areas of thickened pericardium. TOE is also useful for identifying hypovolaemia and ventricular dysfunction, which may arise due to injury to a coronary artery or from repeated handling of the heart.

Spectral Doppler abnormalities (annulus paradoxus, enhanced respiratory variation in trans-mitral velocity) typically immediately improve with relief of constriction. Other parameters (septal bounce, dilated IVC, and reversed hepatic venous flow) may take months to normalize, if ever.

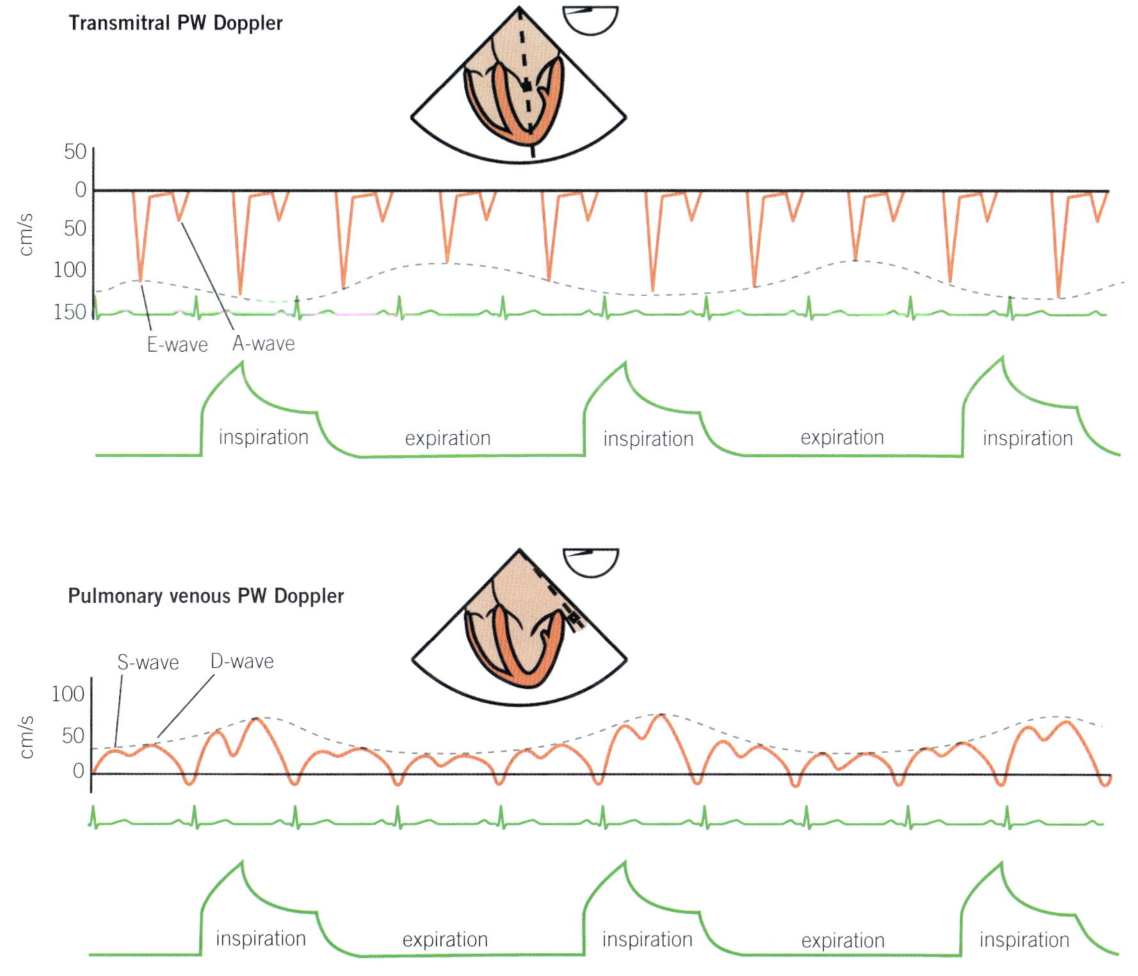

Figure 16.3 Respiratory variations in transmitral and pulmonary venous PW Doppler velocities with constrictive pericarditis during positive pressure ventilation. During inspiration, the transmitral E-wave velocity and pulmonary venous D-wave velocities both increase by 20–30%. This is opposite to the pattern seen with spontaneous breathing and much greater than occurs in normal subjects. In addition, an incomplete restrictive filling pattern (increased E/A, decreased S/D) is seen on both waveforms, maximal during positive pressure inspiration.

Differentiating pericardial constriction from myocardial restriction

Restrictive cardiomyopathy is a relatively rare myocardial abnormality characterized by normal-sized ventricles, marked atrial enlargement, and abnormal diastolic filling (see Chapter 7). Differentiating constrictive pericarditis from restrictive cardiomyopathy may be difficult, but several echocardiographic parameters are useful (Table 16.1).

Atrial enlargement is usually more marked with restrictive cardiomyopathy than with constrictive pericarditis (although patients with constrictive pericarditis may have other causes for LA enlargement). Pulmonary arterial pressure is usually significantly elevated with restrictive cardiomyopathy but is normal with constrictive pericarditis. Restrictive diastolic filling is typically more pronounced with restrictive cardiomyopathy than with constrictive pericarditis, but can occur in both conditions. Variations in ventricular inflow velocities with respiration tend to be less for restrictive cardiomyopathy than with constrictive pericarditis.

> ***Expert tip:** The two most reliable echocardiographic parameters for distinguishing constrictive pericarditis from restrictive cardiomyopathy are mitral annular TDI and septal bounce. Mitral annular e'-velocity is normal or increased (>7 cm/s) with constrictive pericarditis and significantly decreased with restrictive cardiomyopathy. Septal bounce is only present with constrictive pericarditis.*

Box 16.1 Conditions associated with enhanced respiratory variation in trans-mitral and trans-tricuspid Doppler velocities

The Doppler findings during positive pressure ventilation have not been validated for most of these conditions.

- Constrictive pericarditis
- Cardiac tamponade
- Restrictive cardiomyopathy
- Marked hypovolaemia
- RV infarction
- Tension pneumothorax
- Dynamic pulmonary hyperinflation (gas trapping during mechanical ventilation)
- Chronic obstructive pulmonary disease
- Asthma
- Sleep apnoea

Pericardial effusion and cardiac tamponade

Abnormal fluid collections around the heart can arise from bleeding or from effusions (e.g. inflammatory, malignant). The clinical condition wherein a pericardial fluid collection compromises the haemodynamic state is termed cardiac tamponade. Post-surgical bleeding into the pericardium causing cardiac tamponade is discussed in Chapter 21. The focus in this chapter is on pericardial effusion.

Malignancy and tuberculosis are the two most common causes of pericardial effusion. Other causes are similar to constrictive pericarditis. In contrast to post-surgical blood collections, non-surgical pericardial effusions typically develop slowly and tend *not* to be localized or loculated. If accumulation is slow (over weeks or months), large volumes of fluid (>500 mL) may be accommodated without causing much haemodynamic compromise (see Online appendices 4.1.5–4.1.7). Much smaller volumes cause cardiac tamponade if accumulation is rapid or the patient is hypovolaemic.

2D echocardiographic appearances

2D imaging shows an echolucent, fluid-filled space around (or adjacent to) the heart. Note that epicardial fat is also relatively echolucent and can be mistaken for fluid. In the supine position, small liquid collections (<1 cm) settle posteriorly, behind the LA and LV; larger collections are typically circumferential and involve the right heart. With

Table 16.1 Comparison of echocardiographic findings between constrictive pericarditis and restrictive cardiomyopathy
Several of these parameters have not been validated during positive pressure ventilation.

	Constriction	Restriction
2D imaging		
Pericardial thickening	Present	Absent
Atrial size	Normal or mildly increased	Markedly increased
LV and RV cavity size	Normal or reduced	Normal or reduced
LV hypertrophy	Absent	Present
LVEF	Normal	Normal
Septal bounce	Present	Absent
Trans-mitral PW Doppler		
Restrictive pattern	May be incomplete	Marked
Respiratory variation	>25%	≤10%
Mitral annular TDI		
e'- wave velocity	Normal or increased (>7 cm/s)	Decreased (<7 cm/s)
E/e' ratio	Normal	Increased
CW Doppler tricuspid regurgitation		
Jet velocity	Normal or mildly increased	Severely increased

Table 16.2 Volumes of pericardial effusion

Maximum circumferential dimension (cm)	Estimated volume (mL)
<1.5	<200
1.5–2.5	200–500
>2.6	>500

large effusions (>3 cm circumferentially), the whole heart may be seen to 'bob' within the fluid, a phenomenon termed 'swinging heart'. The volume of pericardial fluid cannot be directly measured by echocardiography but may be estimated with reasonable accuracy (Table 16.2).

Cyclical collapse of cardiac structures is common with large effusions. RV collapse occurs during ventricular diastole, when RV chamber pressure is lowest, and frequently accompanies the clinical features of cardiac tamponade. RA and LA collapse is typically maximal at end-diastole (see Chapter 21) and is less specific for cardiac tamponade. Collapse of the LV is very rare. As with constrictive pericarditis, septal bounce is usually apparent. The extra-pericardial venae cavae are typically distended, with loss of respiratory variation in dimension. The 'sniff' test (collapse of the IVC during inspiration), used for assessing central venous pressure with TTE, is obviously not applicable to ventilated patients.

Spectral Doppler appearances

As with constrictive pericarditis, cardiac tamponade exaggerates the normal inspiratory-to-expiratory variations in diastolic filling velocities associated with spontaneous breathing. During spontaneous inspiration, trans-tricuspid E-wave velocity can increase by as much as 50% and trans-mitral E-wave velocity can decrease by as much as 40%.[6] The effect of positive pressure ventilation on Doppler filling velocities is poorly defined. In an animal model of acute pericardial tamponade, positive pressure ventilation was associated with *reduced* transmitral E-wave velocity during both inspiration and expiration and with *reduced* cyclical variation in the presence of tamponade, compared to normal.[7] The European Society for Intensive Care Medicine 2021 guidelines for basic intensive care ultrasound made no recommendation regarding the use of TOE in the assessment of potential perioperative pericardial collections.[8] Consequently, the operator must interpret the TOE findings within the clinical context.

Multiple choice questions

Discover interactive multiple choice questions to test your knowledge on this chapter by searching for this book's title or ISBN (9780198873686) at **https://academic.oup.com/** and going to the online appendix at the end of the book. Use your scratch-off code on the inside cover to access the material.

References

1. Newman B. Congenital absence of the pericardium: pearls and pitfalls. *Semin Ultrasound CT MR*. 2022;**43**(1):47–50.
2. Szabo G, Schmack B, Bulut C, *et al.* Constrictive pericarditis: risks, aetiologies and outcomes after total pericardiectomy: 24 years of experience. *Eur J Cardiothorac Surg*. 2013;**44**(6):1023–8.
3. Walker CM, Chung JH, Reddy GP. 'Septal bounce'. *J Thorac Imaging*. 2012;**27**(1):W1.
4. Cosyns B, Plein S, Nihoyanopoulos P, *et al.* European Association of Cardiovascular Imaging (EACVI) position paper: multimodality imaging in pericardial disease. *Eur Heart J Cardiovasc Imaging*. 2015;**16**(1):12–31.
5. Abdalla IA, Murray RD, Awad HE, Stewart WJ, Thomas JD, Klein AL. Reversal of the pattern of respiratory variation of Doppler inflow velocities in constrictive pericarditis during mechanical ventilation. *J Am Soc Echocardiogr*. 2000;**13**(9):827–31.
6. Appleton CP, Hatle LK, Popp RL. Cardiac tamponade and pericardial effusion: respiratory variation in transvalvular flow velocities studied by Doppler echocardiography. *J Am Coll Cardiol*. 1988;**11**(5):1020–30.
7. Faehnrich JA, Noone RB Jr, White WD, *et al.* Effects of positive-pressure ventilation, pericardial effusion, and cardiac tamponade on respiratory variation in transmitral flow velocities. *J Cardiothorac Vasc Anesth*. 2003;**17**(1):45–50.
8. Robba C, Wong A, Poole D, *et al.* Basic ultrasound head-to-toe skills for intensivists in the general and neuro intensive care unit population: consensus and expert recommendations of the European Society of Intensive Care Medicine. *Intensive Care Med*. 2021;**47**(12):1347–67.

17

Transoesophageal echocardiography for interventional cardiology procedures

Percutaneous interventions for structural heart disease are expanding rapidly. To perform in this environment, echocardiographers require advanced imaging skills and experience, as well as a detailed understanding of cardiac anatomy and of the various devices and procedural steps involved. Recent guidelines outline the skill sets and training pathways required.[1] This chapter is intended to provide the reader with a sample of interventional procedures, and a brief overview of the ways in which expert TOE imaging contributes to successful outcomes. ***Interventional cardiology is a rapidly evolving field and at the time of writing these lines, devices discussed in this chapter are at various stages of approval in different parts of the world. Our goal is to describe TOE techniques to assist in the insertion, positioning, and evaluation of such devices, but the reader should refer to their own country's health regulators for specific devices***.

Safety

Radiation safety

Performing TOE for interventional cardiology procedures requires exposure to radiation. Because echocardiographers are positioned near the patient's head and receive both direct and scattered X-rays, data suggest that they can be exposed to up to 11.7 times more radiation than procedural cardiologists.[2] The workload should be divided to dilute exposure to radiation. Maximizing distance from the X-ray beam is not always possible when constant probe manipulation is required. Adjustable protection screens should be placed between the patient and the echocardiographer, and when TOE is not required, the operator should move away from the patient and stay behind the screen. Shielding with radioprotective aprons, thyroid shields, and goggles, in keeping with local practice standards, is essential.

TOE-related patient injury

Percutaneous procedures are associated with a higher risk of patient injury because these procedures are longer and require more probe manipulation than a standard examination. Major oesophageal injuries causing haemodynamic instability or requiring blood transfusion are significantly more common in structural cardiology cases, particularly transcatheter edge-to-edge MV repair.[3]

Inter-atrial septum and left atrial access

Trans-septal puncture (TSP) is a critical step in successful left-sided structural heart procedures. TOE-guided TSP reduces the risks of complications and sets up delivery systems for the best trajectory to position devices.

Inter-atrial septal anatomy

The inter-atrial septum (IAS) consists of the thin **fossa ovalis** (FOv) and the usually thicker **septum secundum** (SS). The FOv is derived from the embryonic septum primum and forms the central portion of the IAS. It represents the 'true' separation between the left and right atria.[4] The SS is a large muscular rim around the FOv, arising from an infolding of the atrial wall with adipose tissue epicardially (Figure 17.1a). While this 'false' septum may appear to separate the left and right atria, sometimes it may not, and if punctured, the needle may exit the heart and cause an inter-atrial dissection or haematoma (Figure 17.1b; see Online appendix 9.5.7). Puncture in the anterior–superior portion of the FOv also risks aortic root injury. A thickened or aneurysmal FOv may require radiofrequency or electrocautery applied to the TSP needle. Finally, TSP can be performed away from, or directly through, an implanted septal occluder if present.

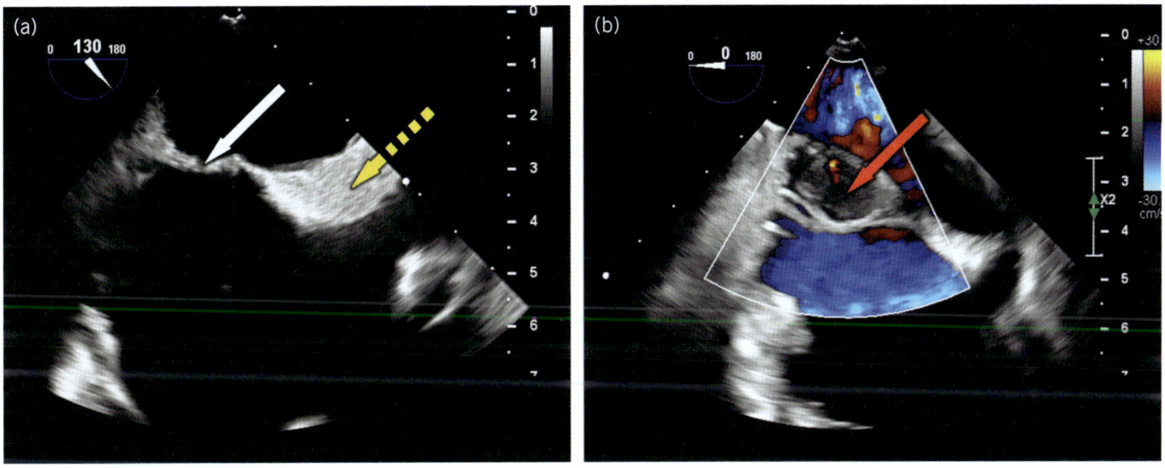

Figure 17.1 Interatrial septal anatomy. Frame (a) is a modified mid-oesophageal bicaval view, showing the FOv centrally (solid arrow) and adipose tissue in the inter-atrial groove (dotted arrow). Frame (b) is a mid-oesophageal four-chamber view, zoomed to demonstrate the inter-atrial septum. An inter-atrial dissection is visible (arrow), with echolucent blood accumulating between the brighter layers of the septum secundum. Note the difference in appearance between adipose tissue (a) and haematoma (b).

Imaging for trans-septal puncture

Relevant TSP anatomy and imaging planes are shown in Figure 17.2a.[5] The TSP needle tip should be visualized in the mid-oesophageal bicaval view and followed as it drops from the SVC to the FOv. The site of 'tenting' (a visible indentation) of the FOv by the needle is identified for the superior–inferior (cephalad–caudad) position (Figure 17.2b). Tenting is then assessed in the aortic short-axis view for the anterior–posterior position (Figure 17.2c). The four-chamber view is used to determine the height above the MV annulus for MV procedures (Figure 17.2d). Once the puncture site is chosen, the needle tip should be imaged while crossing the septum and its position should be confirmed in the LA.

Site-specific trans-septal puncture

The best location for TSP, while always within the FOv, depends on the procedure (Table 17.1). For left atrial appendage occluders (LAAOs), puncture of the inferior and posterior portion of the FOv is best for alignment with the left atrial appendage (LAA). For mitral repair, the optimal TSP site depends on the type of pathology (degenerative MR vs secondary MR) and the location of the pathology (central, lateral, or medial). The ideal TSP height is 4–5 cm above the target grasping zone of the MV. In general, a mid-to-superior and mid-to-posterior puncture site is used. A puncture further from the MV may be necessary for degenerative disease, and a lower puncture for secondary disease. A higher TSP is needed for medial pathology to allow enough height for the **steerable guide catheter** (SGC) to bend medially. To move further from the MV, a more posterior puncture is performed. For balloon mitral valvotomy and MV replacement, a mid-to-superior and mid-to-posterior puncture is used. For mitral paravalvular leaks, the optimal site depends on the location of the leak—medial leaks require a higher (more posterior) puncture. TSP for transcatheter electrophysiology ablation procedures is commonly performed in the centre of the IAS for safety, as procedural success does not depend on a specific TSP location.

Edge-to-edge mitral valve repair

Given the increased prevalence of MR with old age and the frailty of these patients, transcatheter techniques are desirable because they are less invasive and lead to quicker patient recovery. Percutaneous MV annuloplasty devices have been used to improve coaptation but have not yet had commercial or regulatory success and will not be discussed further in this chapter.[6]

The MitraClip™ (Abbott, Abbott Park, IL, USA) and PASCAL™ (Edwards Lifesciences, Irvine, CA, USA) are two commercially available devices used for the primary method of repair—**transcatheter edge-to-edge repair** (TEER) (Figure 17.3). TEER duplicates a surgical technique known as the 'Alfieri stitch' whereby a suture is used to approximate the anterior and posterior leaflets in the centre of the MV, creating a double orifice valve. In selected patients, TEER results in decreased MR, hospitalizations, and mortality.[7,8] TEER is recommended

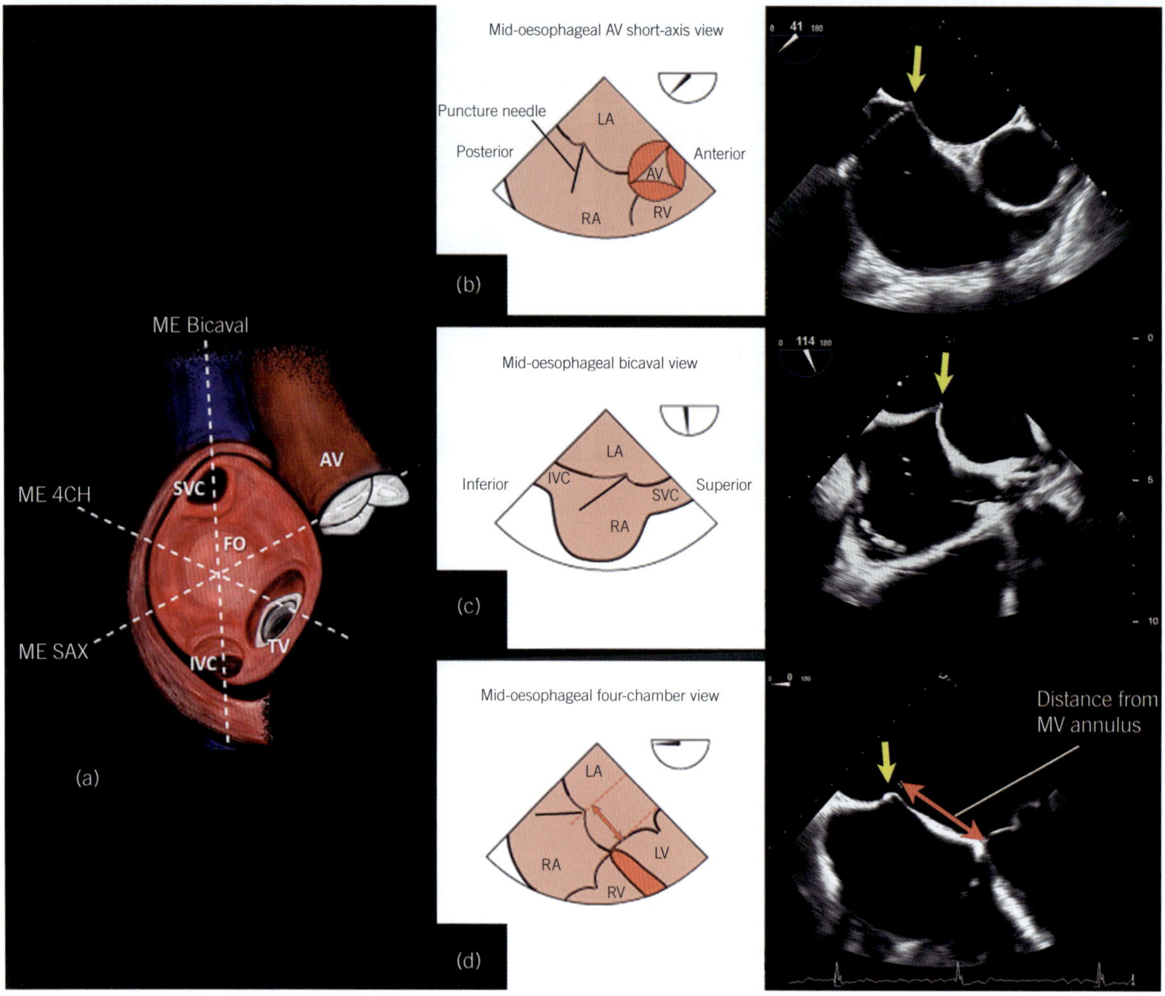

Figure 17.2 TOE imaging for trans-septal puncture. (a) Imaging planes for trans-septal puncture. (b) Mid-oesophageal AV short-axis view for the anterior–posterior position. (c) Mid-oesophageal bicaval view for the superior–inferior position. (d) Mid-oesophageal four-chamber view showing the height above the MV annulus (double-headed arrow). In all frames, note the tenting of the septum by the puncture needle (single-headed arrows).

Table 17.1 Location of trans-septal puncture based on procedure

Procedure	**Superior–inferior axis (bicaval view)**	**Anterior–posterior axis (AV short-axis view)**
TEER of MV	Mid to superior	Mid to posterior
TMVR	Mid to superior	Mid to posterior
MV balloon valvuloplasty	Mid to superior	Mid to posterior
Paravalvular leak closure	Mid to superior	Mid to posterior
LAA occlusion	Inferior	Posterior
PFO closure	Superior	Anterior
Ablation procedures	Middle	Middle

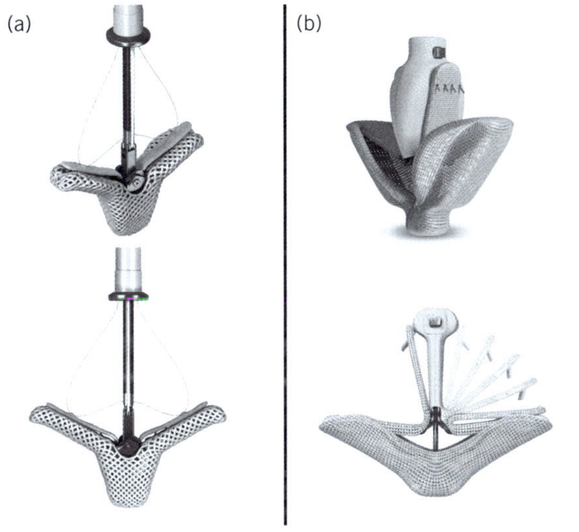

Figure 17.3 Images of the MitraClip™ (a) and PASCAL™ devices (b). The current generation of the MitraClip™ is available in four sizes, whereas the PASCAL™ device is available in two sizes.
Courtesy of Abbott and Edwards Lifesciences LLC, Irvine, CA with permission.

for patients with significant degenerative MR who are at moderate or higher surgical risk, or medically optimized patients with significant secondary MR.

Screening

A detailed pre-procedure screening TOE examination should demonstrate:

- Number, location, and severity of each MR jet
- Mechanism of each MR jet
- Leaflet mobility
- Length of mobile portions of each leaflet
- Number of scallops
- Presence of indentations and involvement in MR
- Thickening, sclerosis, or calcification of leaflets, the annulus, or the subvalvular apparatus
- Mitral valve area (MVA) by 3D planimetry
- Diastolic mitral gradients.

Candidacy for TEER has broadened over the years with increased experience. Relative contraindications to TEER are show in Table 17.2.

Procedure

The screening study should be repeated at the beginning of the procedure itself, to confirm pre-procedure findings and devise an appropriate clip strategy. The heart must also be examined in detail for thrombus, as this is a contraindication to TEER.

Table 17.2 Relative contraindications to TEER

Patient characteristics	Low surgical risk for open MV repair Long life expectancy (durability of TEER is not well demonstrated) Asymptomatic MR Secondary MR without medical optimization Active endocarditis
Valve features	Valve area ≤3 cm Leaflet length ≤6 mm Mean diastolic gradient ≥5 mmHg Calcification at intended grasping area Thrombus or mass on valve or annulus Valve perforation Leaflet cleft with significant regurgitation Regurgitation at commissure
Atrial access	Inability to achieve >35 mm above mitral valve for TSP Very small LA Thrombus in the LAA

Once a clip strategy is chosen, the TSP is performed as described earlier. A wire is first inserted into the LA to facilitate IAS balloon dilation. The dilating tip of the SGC is imaged carefully in long axis (often at 60°) as it enters the LA to ensure the SGC (not the dilator) is at least 2 cm across the IAS (Figure 17.4a). As the clip is introduced through the SGC, care is taken to prevent contact with the LA wall. Often the clip is directed into the left upper pulmonary vein.

Expert tip: Constant fine-tuning of the imaging plane and angle is essential to follow the SGC and clips throughout the procedure.

The clip is steered towards the MV using biplane imaging to give the operator both a 'medial/lateral' and an 'anterior/posterior' orientation (Figure 17.4b). Biplane imaging and a 3D *en face* view from the LA perspective are used to position the clip at its target location and to verify the orthogonal trajectory as it crosses the valve. Independent grasper position is checked. A 3D *en face* view is used to rotate the open clip arms perpendicular to the line of coaptation at the grasping site (Figure 17.4c).

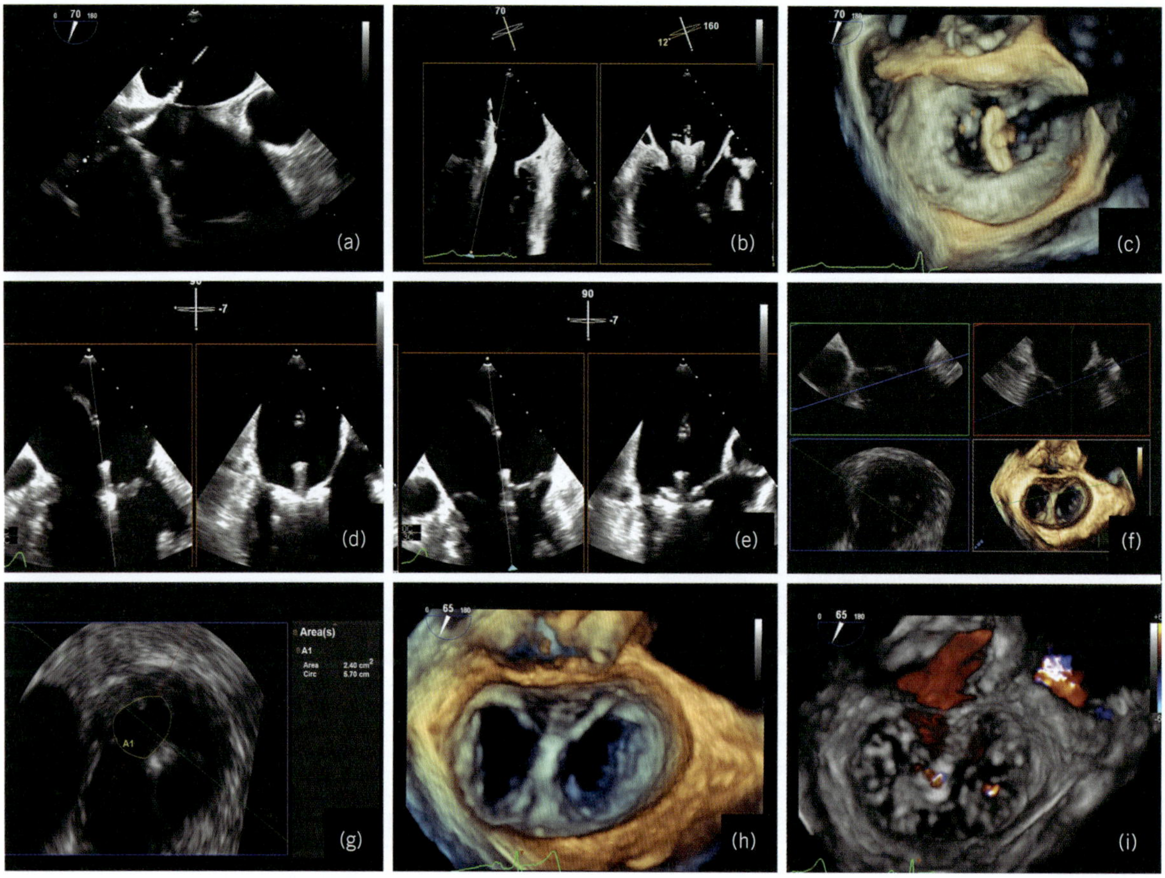

Figure 17.4 Imaging steps of MitraClip™ placement. (a) The delivery system is advanced 2 cm across the IAS. (b) The clip is opened and positioned above the mitral valve. (c) The clip is orientated perpendicular to the coaptation line; in this example, the clip should be rotated clockwise. (d, e) The leaflets are grasped in biplane views, and the grippers are seen bouncing on top of the mitral leaflets. (f, g) MVA is assessed with 3D multi-planar imaging. (h, i) Result with ideal tissue bridging and minimal residual MR. See Online appendix 9.5.1.

Biplane imaging is used to monitor trajectory changes and rotation, as the closed clip crosses the MV and opens in the LV. The positioning and rotation are re-examined prior to a grasping attempt.

Expert tips: Any time clip positioning or rotation is changed while in the LV, watch carefully on the biplane views for any interaction with the leaflets or chordal structures. Lower 3D gain is helpful to accentuate the clip when checking for subvalvular rotation.

Using the MV long-axis view, the leaflets are completely inserted along the entire length of the clip arms (Figure 17.4d). The grippers are dropped and can be seen 'bouncing' on the leaflet before clip closure (Figure 17.4e). As the clip is closed, leaflet slippage out of the clip is monitored for.

Using a combination of transgastric MV short axis, mid-oesophageal biplane, and 3D imaging, the grasp is examined for appropriate location, rotation, and proper leaflet insertion. The clip is closed while imaging the valve with colour Doppler to assess for MR reduction in real time. The valve is assessed for residual MR and stenosis prior to final clip release (Figure 17.4f–i). The clip is monitored during release for detachment. The clip delivery system is observed as it is pulled back into the LA until it is safely retracted into the SGC.

Post-procedure evaluation

After each clip deployment, the MV is evaluated for location and severity of residual MR, diastolic MV gradients, and surface area of each MV orifice, using planimetry with 3D multi-planar reconstruction (MPR) (Figure 17.4f, g). The procedure is completed when the overall residual MR is mild or less, or when there is concern about MS. The mean MV diastolic gradient should be ≤5 mmHg and MVA ≥2 cm^2. As with other MV repair procedures (see Chapter 9), the effects of general anaesthesia on MR and gradients should be considered, and haemodynamic manipulations may be required when assessing the results.

When the steerable guide is retracted into the RA, the IAS should be examined for shunting. A moderate amount of left-to-right shunting is acceptable. Although there is controversy in the literature on what size defect should be closed, device closure of the IAS should be considered if there is severe left-to-right shunting, a large defect, or right-to-left shunting. A complete TOE study should be performed at the conclusion of the procedure to rule out damage to other cardiac structures, pericardial effusions, or clip detachment.

Transcutaneous mitral valve replacement

Despite over 10 years of experience with transcutaneous MV replacement (TMVR), it is not yet a standard of care. The complex annular geometry and subvalvular support system of the MV (see Chapter 8) create design challenges. Valves must be delivered without entanglement and be seated well enough to prevent embolization and minimize paravalvular leaks. Additional challenges include displacement of the anterior mitral leaflet into the LVOT, causing systolic anterior motion (SAM) and subvalvular LVOT obstruction (LVOTO). The currently available devices were reviewed in a recent publication.[9] Early devices were delivered trans-apically (TA-TMVR) and remain the most commonly used. Complications seen in TA-trans-aortic valve replacement have furthered the desire to develop trans-septal (TS-TMVR) approaches. At the time of this publication, all devices are investigational.

Screening

High-resolution computerized tomography (CT) is used to screen patients and predict the impact of implantation on cardiac anatomy, particularly the LVOT, post-procedure. Screening TOE is required to assess the degree of MR or MS, the amount and location of mitral annular calcification (MAC), the quality of the leaflets and subvalvar apparatus, the presence of flail or prolapse, the length of the anterior leaflet, the size of the LVOT, and the thickness of the proximal interventricular septum.

Procedure

The implant and TOE procedure for each device are unique and the manufacturer's instructions for use (IFU) should be carefully reviewed. TSP is as described earlier, and TOE guidance is used to place wires and guide catheters, position the device, and confirm appropriate fixation. Assessing for proper valve positioning, function, and absence of LVOTO are essential.

Patients with degeneration of bioprosthetic MVs are candidates for TS valve-in-valve (TMVR ViV) with Edwards Sapien 3® or Sapien XT® balloon-expandable valves, using the same delivery system as a transcatheter aortic valve implantation (TAVI) and inverted valve loading. After TSP, balloon valvuloplasty of the degenerated valve is performed, and the new valve is positioned and deployed using fluoroscopy and TOE. Rapid ventricular pacing is required for both steps, to prevent movement of the valve during deployment. Valve function and regurgitation are assessed, and additional balloon dilation performed if significant paravalvular MR is present (Figure 17.5). This TMVR approach has also been applied to patients with MAC and annuloplasty rings, with less success. The iatrogenic ASD may require closure.

Procedural steps for TS-TMVR in a *native* valve annulus are similar to a ViV implant and are shown in Figure 17.6. TSP is performed as described earlier, and TOE is used to guide the valve into the annular location and confirm fixation.

The Tendyne® valve (Abbott) is the most studied transcatheter MV replacement system (Figure 17.7). It is a TA-TMVR and secured by an apical tether and pad. TOE is used to confirm the site of the trans-apical puncture and to ensure the guidewire passes through the mitral orifice without chordal entanglement. Biplane imaging is ideal for guiding this step, and the technique is similar to positioning the inflow cannula of an LVAD (see Chapter 20). The delivery system is passed over the wire into the LA and then deployed. The position can be fine-tuned by adjusting the tension of the apical tether.

> ***Expert tip: Live multi-planar 3D is essential in ensuring proper position and rotation of the valve while being deployed.***

Post-procedure evaluation

While each device requires specific post-procedure TOE examination elements, all devices require a post-procedure assessment for:

- TMVR placement and seating
- Paravalvular or transvalvular MR

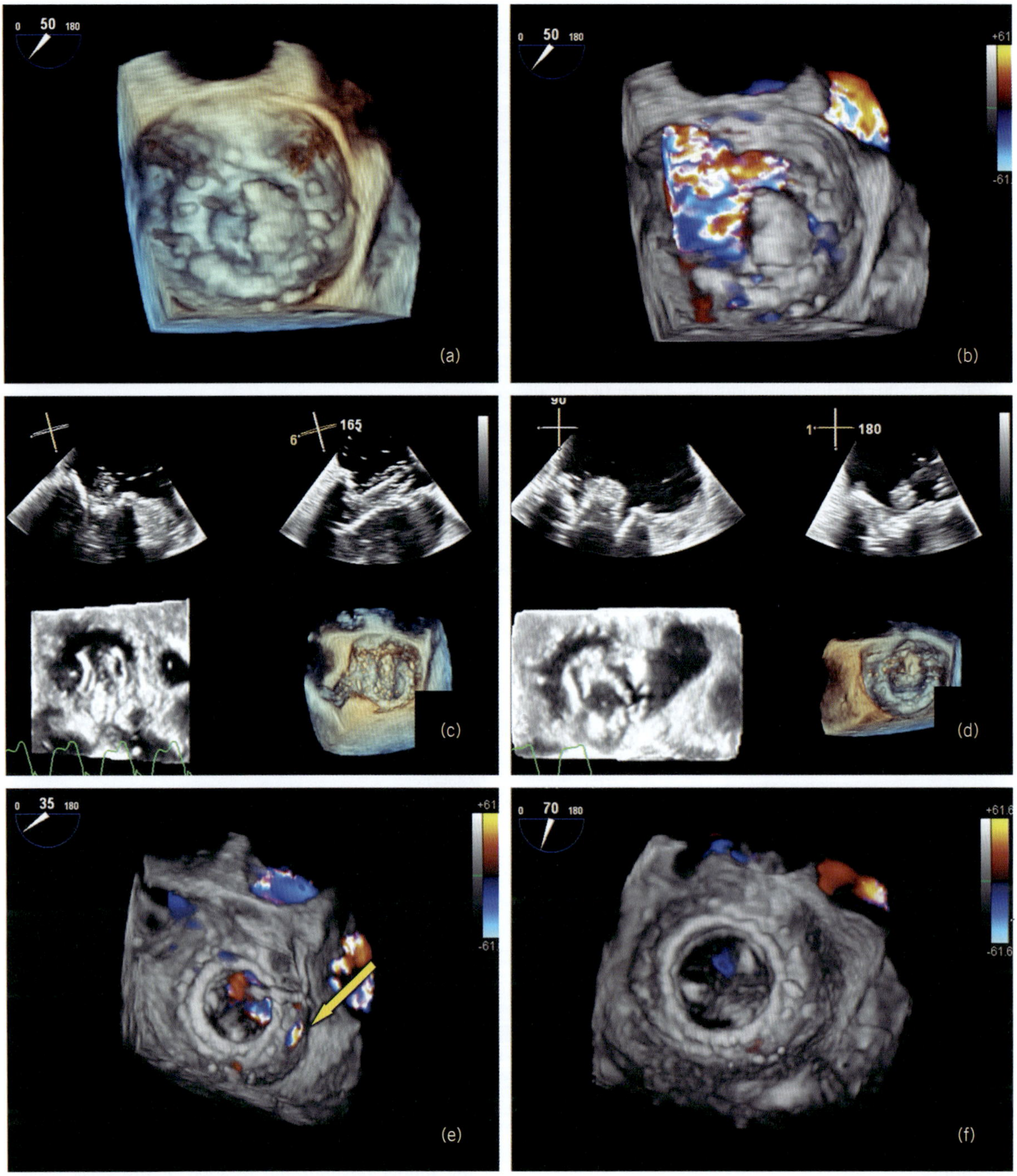

Figure 17.5 Valve-in-valve trans-catheter MV replacement. (a) 3D *en face* view of a degenerated bioprosthetic MV. (b) Same view with colour Doppler. (c) Balloon valvuloplasty under rapid pacing. (d) Valve deployment under rapid pacing. (e) Post-deployment 3D colour view showing medial paravalvular leak (arrow). (f) Same view, post-ballooning, showing no residual paravalvular leak. See Online appendix 9.5.2.

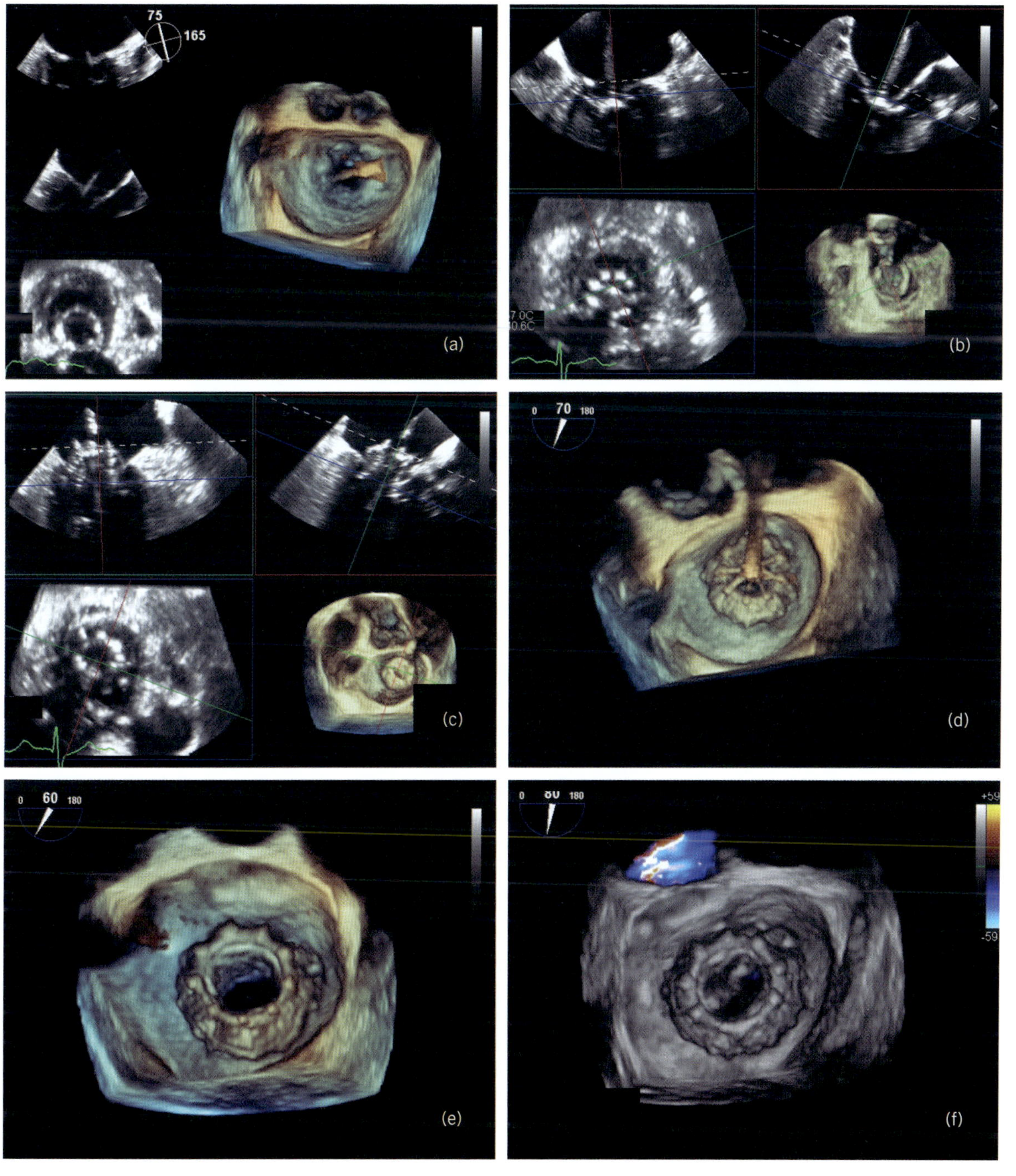

Figure 17.6 Trans-catheter replacement of a native MV. In this example, the Evoque Valve® (Edwards Lifesciences) is demonstrated. (a) 3D multi-planar view of the delivery system being in position within the valve. (b) Confirmation of the position of valve anchors. (c) Valve partial deployment. (d) Valve fully deployed, but still tethered to the delivery system. (e, f) 3D views of the deployed valve with and without colour Doppler. See Online appendix 9.5.3.

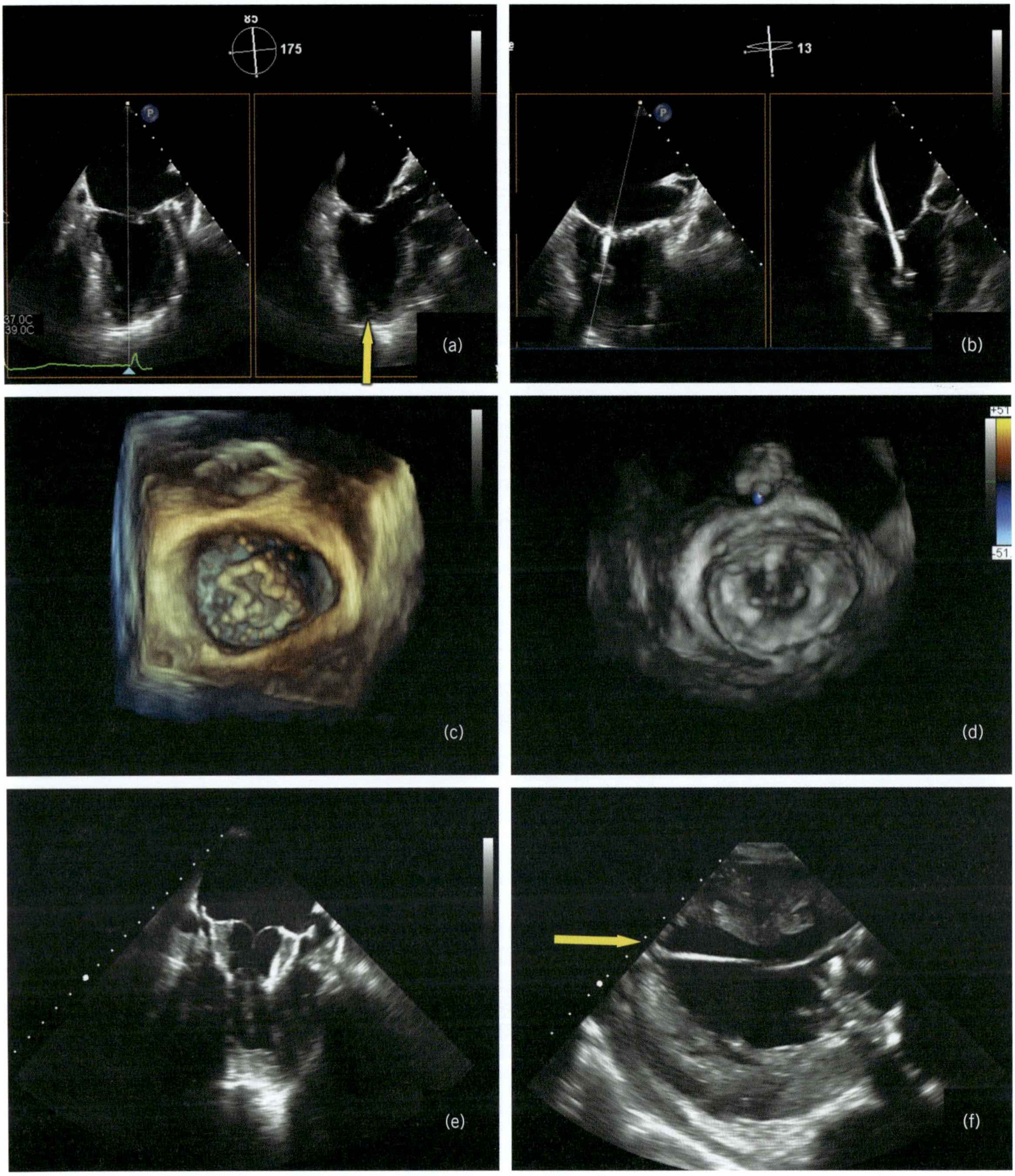

Figure 17.7 Trans-catheter MV replacement using the Tendyne® valve. (a) Orthogonal views of the LV showing the site of trans-apical puncture (arrow). (b) Catheter and balloon passed across the MV without chordal entanglement. (c) 3D LA view of the valve being deployed. (d). 3D colour LA view of deployed valve. (e) Deployed valve in the mid-oesophageal two-chamber view. (f) Transgastric LV long-axis view showing the apical tether (arrow).

- MV gradients
- Significant LVOTO
- LV systolic function
- Afterload mismatch (i.e. LV systolic failure due to complete elimination of MR)
- Mechanical complications (e.g. annular rupture, leaflet tear, papillary muscle avulsion).

Mitral valve balloon valvotomy

The first percutaneous balloon mitral valvotomies (BMVs) were performed in the 1980s as one of the earliest structural heart procedures. It is now the first-line treatment for patients with rheumatic MS and suitable valve morphology.

Screening

TOE should confirm the presence of severe MS (MVA ≤1.5 cm^2), assess the suitability of the valve for BMV, confirm the absence of significant MR (mild or less), rule out LA thrombus, and image the IAS to plan for a safe TSP. Valves that are heavily calcified and thickened with severe subvalvular involvement, severe commissural disease, and more than mild MR are generally not suitable for BMV. The Wilkins score is the most widely used BMV suitability scoring system,[10] but it does not include commissural assessment, which is critical to BMV success. Other scoring systems have been developed, which better predict MR and procedural success in patients with intermediate risk Wilkins' scores.[11,12] LAA thrombus is a contraindication, although some operators may choose to proceed in the presence of an *organized* LAA thrombus.

> ***Expert tip: MVA should be measured by 3D planimetry. Post-BMV pressure half-time is not reliable, and mitral gradients are flow-dependent. Particular attention should be paid to the commissures and subvalvular apparatus.***

Procedure

TSP is as described earlier. A single balloon mitral valvuloplasty catheter is most often used. Balloon sizing is based on the patient's height and/or mid-diastolic maximal intercommissural diameter. TOE imaging is used to position the balloon across the MV and exclude chordal entanglement. The balloon is quickly inflated and deflated. The valve is then assessed for commissural opening, MVA, and/or any increase in MR (Figure 17.8; see Online appendix 6.3.2). An optimal result is an increase in MVA of ≥50% or to >1.5 cm^2 with no more than moderate MR. If there has been no opening and no damage to the valve, then reballooning with incremental increases in balloon size can be performed. BMV should be stopped if:

- Indexed MVA is >1 cm^2/m^2
- Presence of complete opening of at least one commissure
- The valve is damaged
- Moderate or more-than-moderate MR.

Paravalvular leak closure

Clinically significant paravalvular leaks (PVLs) can occur after surgical valve replacement. Percutaneous PVL closure is indicated for high surgical risk patients with intractable haemolysis or advanced heart failure.[13] Newer purpose-specific devices, like the Amplatzer® Vascular Plug 3 (Abbott) and the Paravalvular Leak Device (Occlutech®, Schaffhausen, Switzerland), are designed to conform to the anatomy of PVLs.

Device closure of PVLs is performed with TOE and fluoroscopic guidance. Pre-procedural imaging should focus on the number and location of the defects, the shape and size of each defect, and the severity of the regurgitation. Location of mitral defects is described using a clock face, with the AV anteriorly at 12 o'clock, the middle of the posterior leaflet at 6 o'clock, the IAS at 3 o'clock, and the LAA at 9–10 o'clock (see Figures 13.12 and 13.13). For PVLs of the AV, defect location is usually described anatomically, referring to the position of the native right, left, or non-coronary cusps, or less commonly with a clock face (see Figure 13.14). For both valves, the severity of the PVL, measured in the short-axis view of the valve with colour Doppler at the level of the sewing ring, can be quantified based on the percentage of the circumference of the sewing ring (mild PVL <10% of total annular circumference, moderate 10–29%, and severe >30%).

> ***Expert tip: As with other instances where communication with the surgical/interventional team is required about the specific location of a lesion, it is extremely important that all members of the team thoroughly understand and use the same nomenclature and terminology to avoid confusion.***

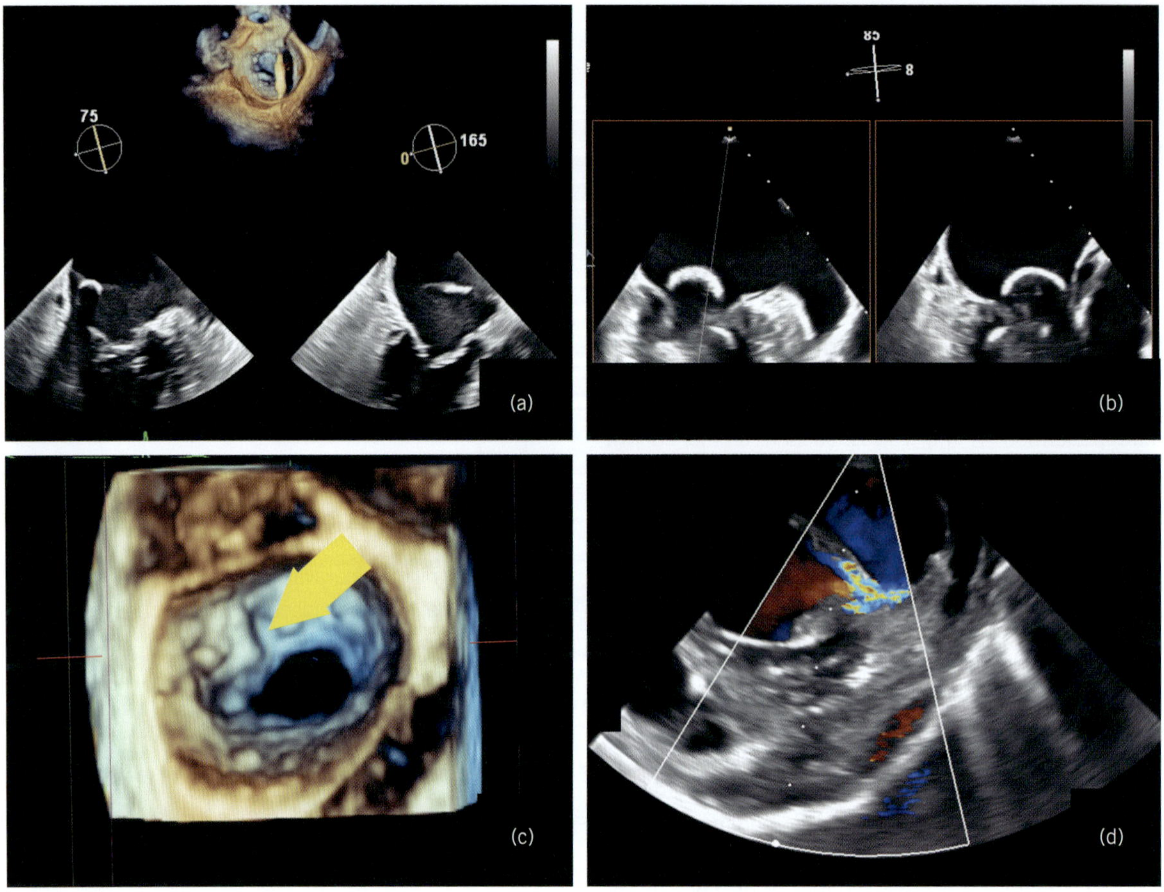

Figure 17.8 Balloon mitral valvuloplasty. (a) 3D multi-plane view showing balloon in the LA. (b) Biplane view during balloon inflation. (c) 3D *en face* view from the LA perspective, showing a tear in the anterior MV leaflet (arrow). (d) Transgastric short-axis view with colour Doppler showing MR at the site of the tear. See Online appendices 6.3.2.6–6.3.2.14 and 9.5.5.

A 3D view from the surgeon's perspective with and without colour is obtained (Figure 17.9a, b), and MPR of a colour 3D data set is used to display the vena contracta area and measure the size and shape of the defect(s) (Figure 17.9c, d). Real-time TOE guidance is essential for positioning of wires and devices. Mitral PVLs can be closed using an antegrade or retrograde approach. The defect is crossed with a guidewire; the delivery sheath is positioned, and the device is deployed (Figure 17.9e) An arteriovenous wire loop can be used to provide two-sided control of the wire and a stable 'rail' for the delivery sheath and device. Aortic PVLs are generally closed with a retrograde approach. Once the defect is crossed with a wire, the delivery sheath is advanced into the LV, and the closure device is deployed (Figure 17.9f). Multiple devices may be needed to close large or crescent-shaped leaks. Device interference with valve function needs to be ruled out prior to device release.

Left atrial appendage occlusion

Screening

Patients with atrial fibrillation who are intolerant of anti-coagulation are candidates for LAA occlusion (LAAO).[14] A TOE or CT scan is required ahead of the procedure to assess LAA morphology and for the absence of thrombus.[15] There are four prototypic LAA morphologies described in the literature (windsock, cactus, chicken wing, and cauliflower), which may be associated with altered stroke risk and can affect implantation difficulty (Figure 17.10).[16] The shape of the dominant lobe should be assessed, and the presence of accessory lobes should be noted, as this has implications on the choice of device and techniques of deployment.

Sizing the LAA is crucial and challenging, there are nuances in sizing across manufacturers, and the IFU of the device being placed should be consulted. The

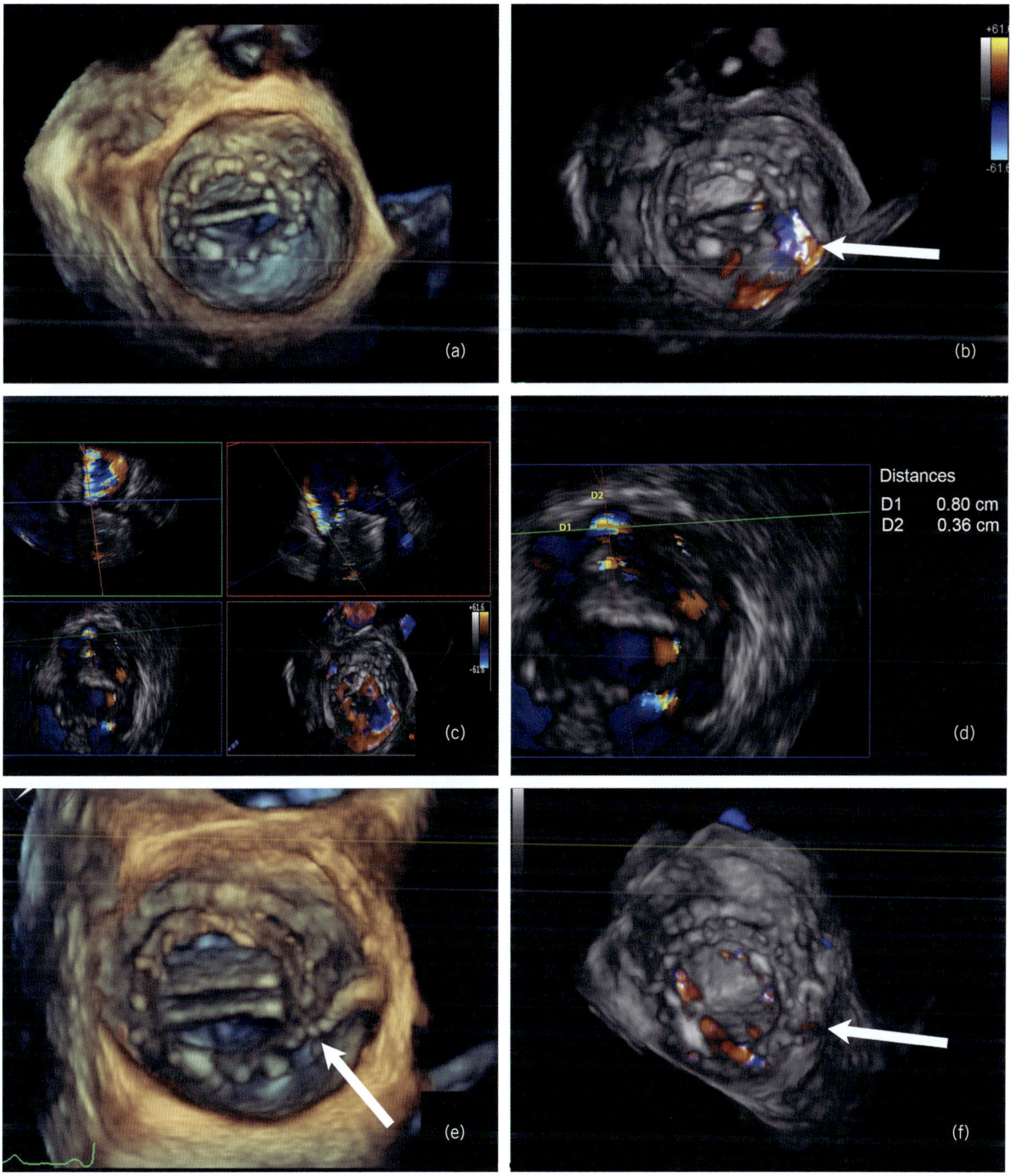

Figure 17.9 Trans-catheter closure of paravalvular leaks. (a, b) 3D surgical view of mechanical MV prosthesis with and without colour. The colour image shows a paravalvular leak at 5 o'clock (arrow). (c) Multi-plane image of colour 3D data set showing the paravalvular defect. Here the two long-axis planes are aligned with the PVL, and the short-axis plane (blue in this case) is moved to the level of the valve annulus. (d) The dimensions of the defect are measured. (e) 3D *en face* view from the LA side, showing the wire crossing the paravalvular leak at 5 o'clock (arrow). (f) Trivial MR (arrow) after deployment of the occluder.

relevant dimensions are the size of the os, the 'landing zone' (10–12 mm inside the os), and the depth of the LAA (from the os to the back wall of the LAA perpendicular to the axis of the os).

Sizing can be done with a stepwise 2D examination or with 3D. Using 2D, the required measurements are made by sweeping from 0° to 135° in 45° increments (Figure 17.11a). Ideally, the os of the appendage should

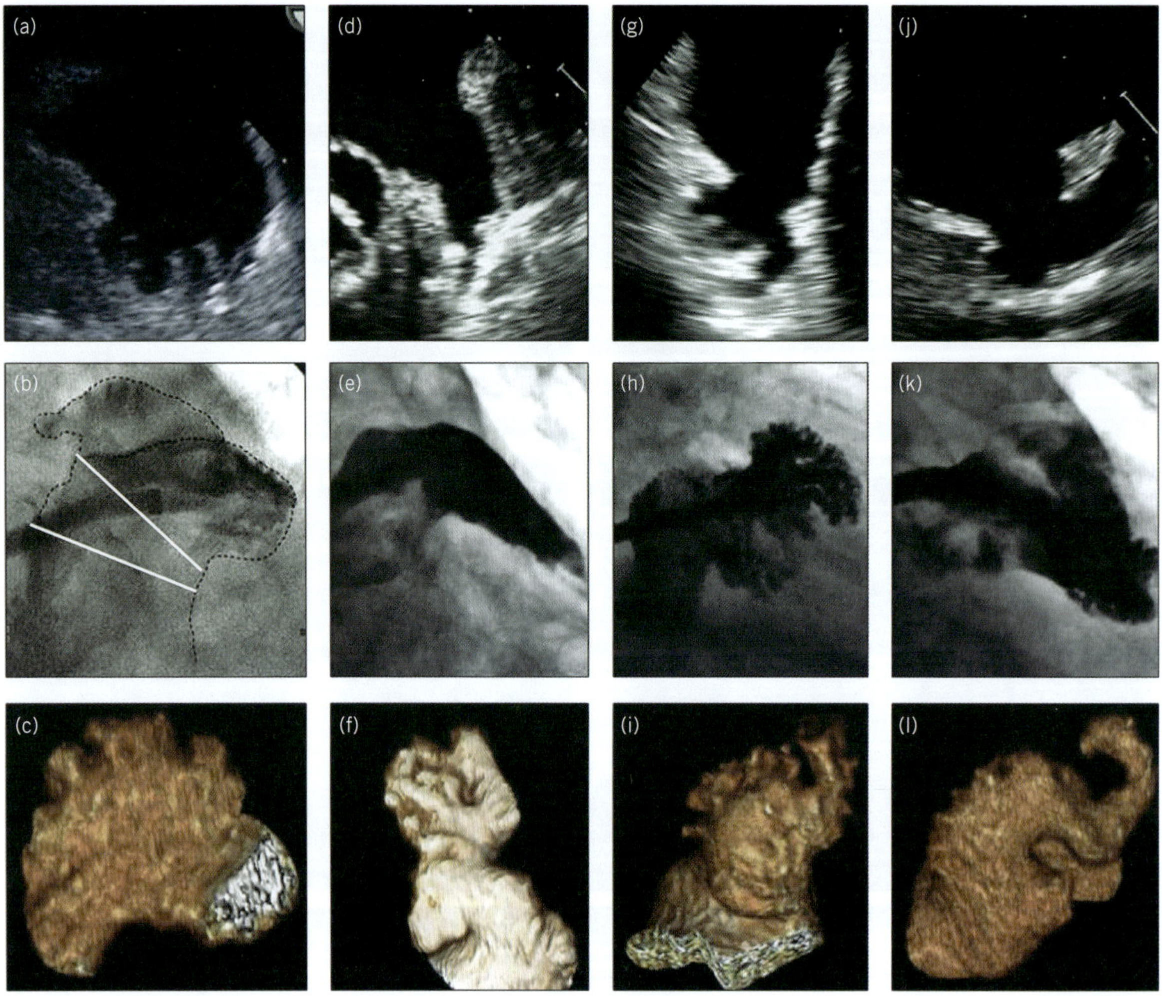

Figure 17.10 The four anatomic variants of the left atrial appendage: demonstrated with TOE (a, d, g, j), angiography (b, e, h, k), and 3D computed tomography (c, f, i, l). Cauliflower (a, b, c), windsock (d, e, f), cactus (g, h, i), and chicken wing (j, k, l).
Reprinted from *JACC: Cardiovascular Imaging*, **7**, 12, Beigel R *et al.*, The Left Atrial Appendage: Anatomy, Function, and Noninvasive Evaluation, pp. 1251–65, Copyright 2014, with permission from the American College of Cardiology Foundation. Published by Elsevier.

be aligned parallel to the ultrasound probe and centred in the imaging sector. This will reduce dropout of LAA walls and improve measurement accuracy. The smallest and largest diameters are measured, and the size of the device chosen according to the IFU.

Alternatively, a 3D data set of the LAA can be acquired, and the dimensions measured using multi-planar imaging (Figure 17.11b). The major and minor axes of the os and landing zone are measured, and a mean value calculated. An 'average' diameter can be calculated from the LAA perimeter in short-axis view, using the same technique used to calculate the mean aortic annular diameter (see Chapter 10).

Expert tips: Discrepancy between the mean diameter and the diameter calculated from the perimeter of the landing zone should prompt repeat imaging and measurements.

Procedure

A complete TOE should be performed to rule out intra-cardiac thrombus. LAA thrombus is not an absolute contraindication, but advanced techniques are required, which are beyond the scope of this discussion. Once TSP is performed as described earlier, LA pressure (LAP) is measured. LAA measurements are obtained only when

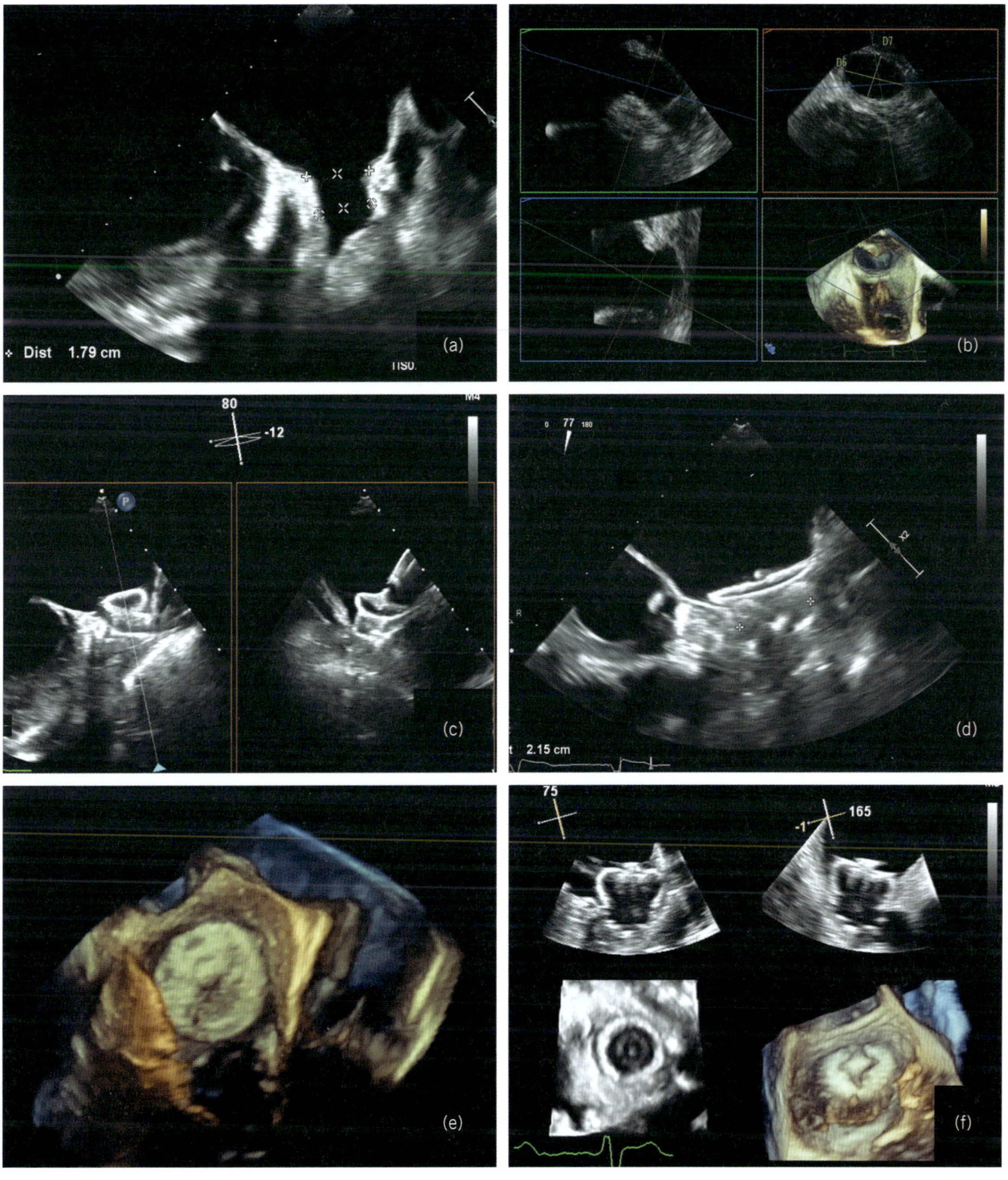

Figure 17.11 LAAO deployment. (a) 2D mid-oesophageal view, with the LAA parallel to the scanning plane, demonstrating sizing of the os and the landing zone, 10–12 mm inside the os. (b) Measurement using 3D MPR. The long-axis planes were aligned with the LAA, and the short-axis plane (red in this case) was positioned at the level of the landing zone. The minor and major axes were measured. Note that an average diameter can also be calculated from measuring the area of the os. (c) The occluder (in this case an Amulet®, Abbott) was deployed in the LAA, and the 'tug test' performed to verify stability. (d) Final positioning of the occluder. (e) 3D *en face* view of a deployed Amulet® *in situ*. (f) Multi-planar and 3D view of a deployed device (in this case, a Watchman® FLX, Boston Scientific).

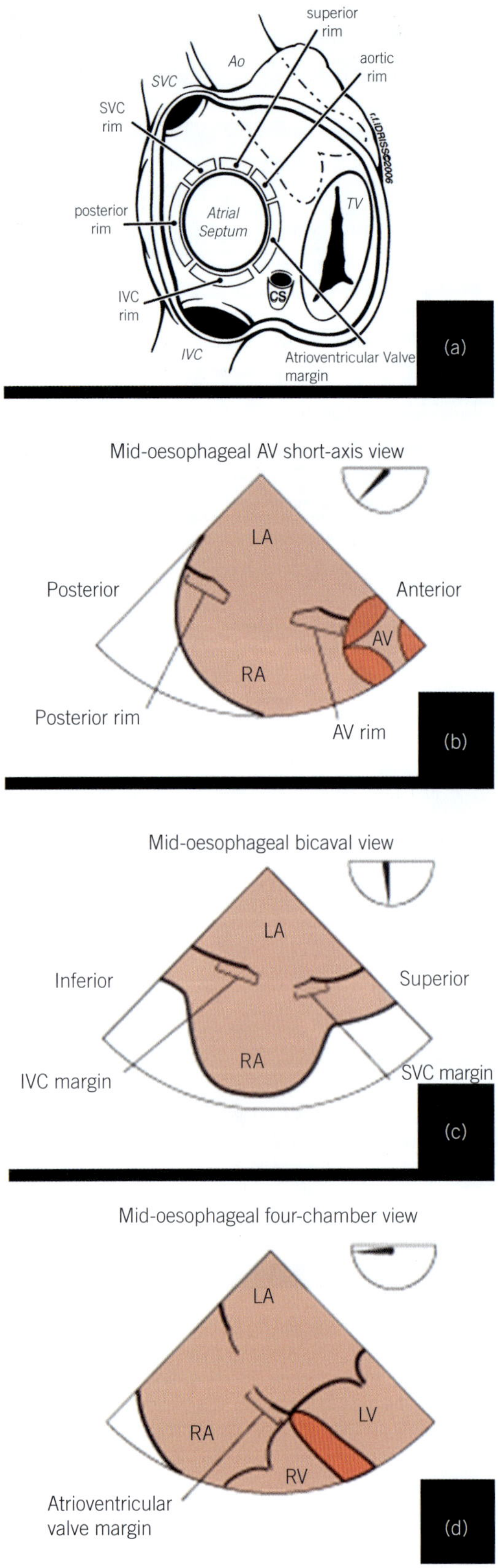

the LAP is ≥12 mmHg, so fluid loading may be required. Using a catheter-over-wire technique, a non-steerable curved catheter is inserted into the LAA. Fluoroscopy and LAA contrast injection at two imaging angles can be used to verify sizing. The device is advanced to the tip of the catheter, and the catheter retracted to deploy the device. Biplane imaging monitors the angle and depth of device deployment and allows the operator to correct the deployment in real time. The device is pulled (a 'tug test') to verify stability (Figure 17.12c).

Post-procedure evaluation

A stepwise (0–135° in 45° increments) examination of the device should be performed, assessing for:

- Device compression—maximal width at the centre of the device (Figure 17.12d)
- Residual leaks into the LAA—colour flow Doppler assessment *at a Nyquist limit of 25–35 cm/s*
- Deployment depth—measurement of the 'shoulder' of the device extending proximal to the circumflex artery
- Warfarin ridge capture (i.e. LA disc resting on the ridge, as opposed to inside the LAA)
- Interference with surrounding structures (e.g. MV, pulmonary vein).

Once IFU deployment criteria are met, the device is released and assessed for stability. If any movement occurs, the catheter can be advanced to tether the LAAO against the LAA wall until it can be retrieved using either transcatheter techniques or, rarely, surgery. The iatrogenic ASD rarely requires closure. Examination for pericardial effusion is also essential.

Figure 17.12 Evaluating the ASD and rim around the defect. (a) Schematic representation of a secundum ASD with surrounding rims and adjacent structures. (b) Mid-oesophageal short-axis view, (c) mid-oesophageal bicaval view, and (d) mid-oesophageal four-chamber view, used to measure the atrial septal rims and assess suitability for device closure. See text for details.

(a) Reprinted from *Journal of the American College of Cardiology*, 79, 22, Turner ME *et al.*, Transcatheter Closure of Atrial and Ventricular Septal Defects JACC Focus Seminar, pp. 2247–58, Copyright 2022, with permission from the American College of Cardiology Foundation. Published by Elsevier.

Patent foramen ovale and atrial septal defect closure

Secundum atrial septal defects represent the majority of ASDs and are the only ASDs amenable to percutaneous closure. ASDs cause intracardiac shunts, which may result in right heart enlargement, RV dysfunction, and pulmonary hypertension. In the absence of severe pulmonary hypertension, ASD closure is recommended for patients with haemodynamic (RA and/or RV enlargement) and/or clinical sequelae (arrhythmias, reduced functional capacity, or paradoxical embolism).[17]

Transcatheter closure of secundum ASDs is primarily performed under general anaesthesia with fluoroscopic and TOE guidance. Pre-procedure TOE evaluates the dimensions of the defect(s), and the tissue between the defect and adjacent anatomic structures ('rims') (Figure 17.12a).[18] A rim of 5 mm or greater is adequate for device closure. Corresponding 2D views for imaging the posterior, SVC, IVC, and AV rims are shown in Figure 17.12b–d. Using 3D MPR, the maximal and minimal dimensions of the defect can be measured (Figure 17.13a, b). An aortic rim of <5 mm can be closed as the discs can straddle the aortic root, whereas inferior rim deficiency is associated with device failure. Multiple defects or fenestrations can be closed, provided they are all within the FOv. Atrial septal aneurysms and Chiari network may complicate the procedure, while atrial thrombus may preclude the procedure altogether.

Closure devices consist of two discs with a central connecting waist. Depending on the device, defects with a maximal dimension of 40 mm are suitable for closure. Multiple defects or fenestrations may require multiple devices or one larger device.

A 'stop-flow' technique is used for sizing. A guidewire is placed through the ASD into the LA. A sizing balloon is then positioned to straddle the IAS. As the sizing balloon is inflated, the defect causes indentation of the balloon, which appears as a 'waist' on TOE and fluoroscopy (Figure 17.13c, d). When the inter-atrial shunting stops on colour Doppler, the waist is measured. For the Amplatzer Septal Occluder® (Abbott), the recommended size is equal to, or one size larger than, the stop flow diameter (Figure 17.13e).

The LA disc is deployed first, and if correctly positioned, the RA disc is then deployed. 2D and 3D imaging are performed to ensure all rims are captured and the discs are not impinging on surrounding structures. Residual flow is assessed with colour Doppler (Figure 17.13f), and the device is detached from the delivery system.

A patent foramen ovale (PFO) is present in 25–30% of adults, with a significantly higher incidence in patients who present with cryptogenic stroke. PFO closure for prevention of PFO-associated stroke is recommended.[19] Other potential indications include decompression sickness, migraines, and arterial deoxygenation syndromes. Tunnel length, presence of an atrial septal aneurysm, thickness of the septum secundum, and presence of additional septal defects should be assessed for. As with ASDs, guidance with TOE or intracardiac echocardiography (ICE) and fluoroscopy is used. Similar principles for device deployment and post-deployment evaluation are followed. Device-specific minimum distances (as per the manufacturer's IFU) between the PFO and the aortic root or SVC orifice are required for safe implantation.

Cardiovascular implantable electronic device lead removal

As the number of cardiovascular implantable electronic devices (CIEDs) increases, more patients will require lead extraction (LE). Infection and lead dysfunction are the two most common reasons for extraction. LE for abandoned functional leads, lead-related complications, and removal of non-MRI safe leads are less frequent indications.[20] The major risks associated with LE arise from fibrosis around lead material, which develops over time. This can cause dense, calcific adhesions along the course of the lead, most severe at the site of venous entry, in the SVC, and at the lead insertion into the myocardium. Increasingly, it is recognized that CIEDs are associated with tricuspid regurgitation (TR) due to lead adhesion, interference, or damage to the leaflets or subvalvular structures.[21]

A variety of techniques can be used to facilitate LE. Generally, a hierarchical approach is used, starting with simple transvenous lead traction and escalating to more complicated techniques with stylets, special wires, and sheaths, and ultimately laser or radiofrequency ablation. Major complications are rare, but catastrophic injury to large vessels and cardiac valves, perforation causing tamponade, and malignant arrhythmias can occur and be lethal. Intraprocedural TOE helps to monitor for these complications.

Expert tip: Thrombus or vegetations are often attached to the leads at the caval/atrial junction or at, or just above, the tricuspid valve. Particular attention should be paid to those areas. Also, the presence of any pericardial effusion pre-extraction should be noted, as the appearance of even small new effusions could be clinically significant.

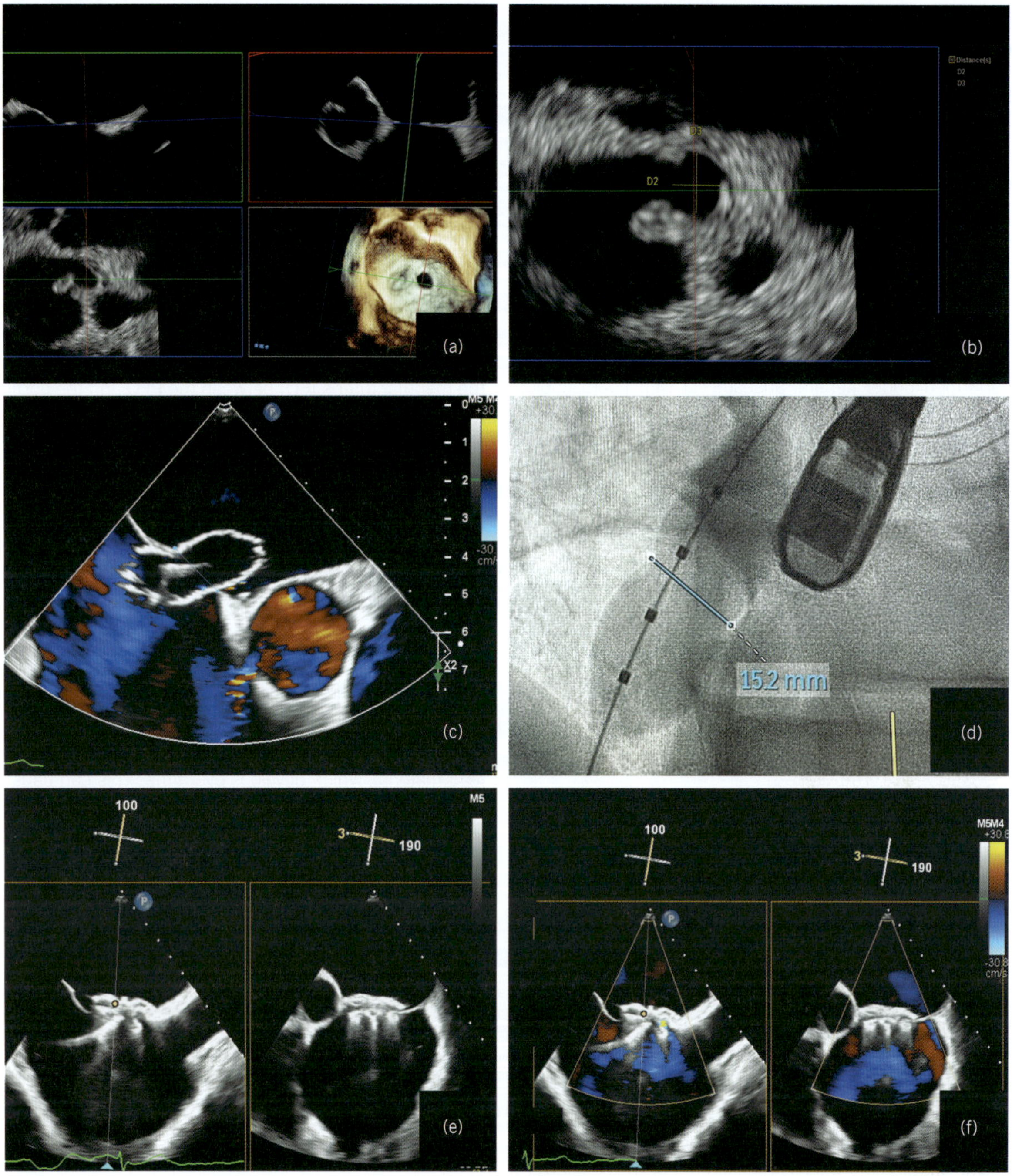

Figure 17.13 Device closure of secundum ASD. (a, b) Using 3D MPR, the maximum and minimum dimensions of the ASD are measured (note that the apparently 'open circle' in frame (b) is due to echo dropout). 'Stop flow' technique for balloon sizing with TOE (c) and fluoroscopy (d) (blue lines in each case). (e) Amplatzer® (Abbott) septal occluder positioned. (f) Trivial residual flow across the ASD occluder device, which is expected until endothelial cells cover the device. See Online appendices 10.1 and 10.2.

TOE examination should focus on areas where the leads contact other cardiac structures and on any masses attached to leads. 3D or short-axis TV views are particularly helpful in demonstrating lead adherence to TV or subvalvular structures. Continuous assessment is required throughout the procedure for perforation, tamponade, and leaflet avulsion (Figure 17.14). After extraction of infected leads, new lesions called 'ghosts' can be seen along the path of the lead. They are fibrous sheaths peeled from the lead, which can remain attached to other cardiac structures and are thought to be benign.[22]

Thrombus and endocarditis removal

Surgical thrombectomy to remove intracardiac thrombus remains the mainstay of therapy, but new devices permit the aspiration and removal of intracardiac and/or intravascular thrombus and vegetation in high surgical risk patients. Most experience has been with the AngioVac® system (AngioDynamics Incorporated, Latham, NY, USA). An aspiration cannula with a Nitinol expandable funnel tip is placed through a 26-French cannula inserted via the internal jugular or femoral vein. This is attached to an extracorporeal circuit with a filter to remove the aspirated material and a centrifugal pump to provide suction, and the aspirated blood is returned to the patient via a femoral 15- to 18-French cannula. Flows of 3–4 L/min can be attained. The AngioVac® is mainly used for the aspiration of IVC or right-sided cardiac thrombus, right heart vegetations or masses, or pulmonary emboli (Figure 17.15).[23] Rarely, it has been used for left heart lesions.

Procedure

TOE is used to confirm the presence of the material to be removed and assess cardiac pathology created by the material. Biplane imaging facilitates steering of the device towards the material to be aspirated. The cardiac response to aspiration and rapid retransfusion of the aspirated blood should be assessed throughout the procedure. TOE should also be used to monitor for suction events where cardiac chambers collapse and cause obstruction, and for damage to cardiac structures. Post-procedure TOE should focus on adequacy of material removal, damage to cardiac structures,

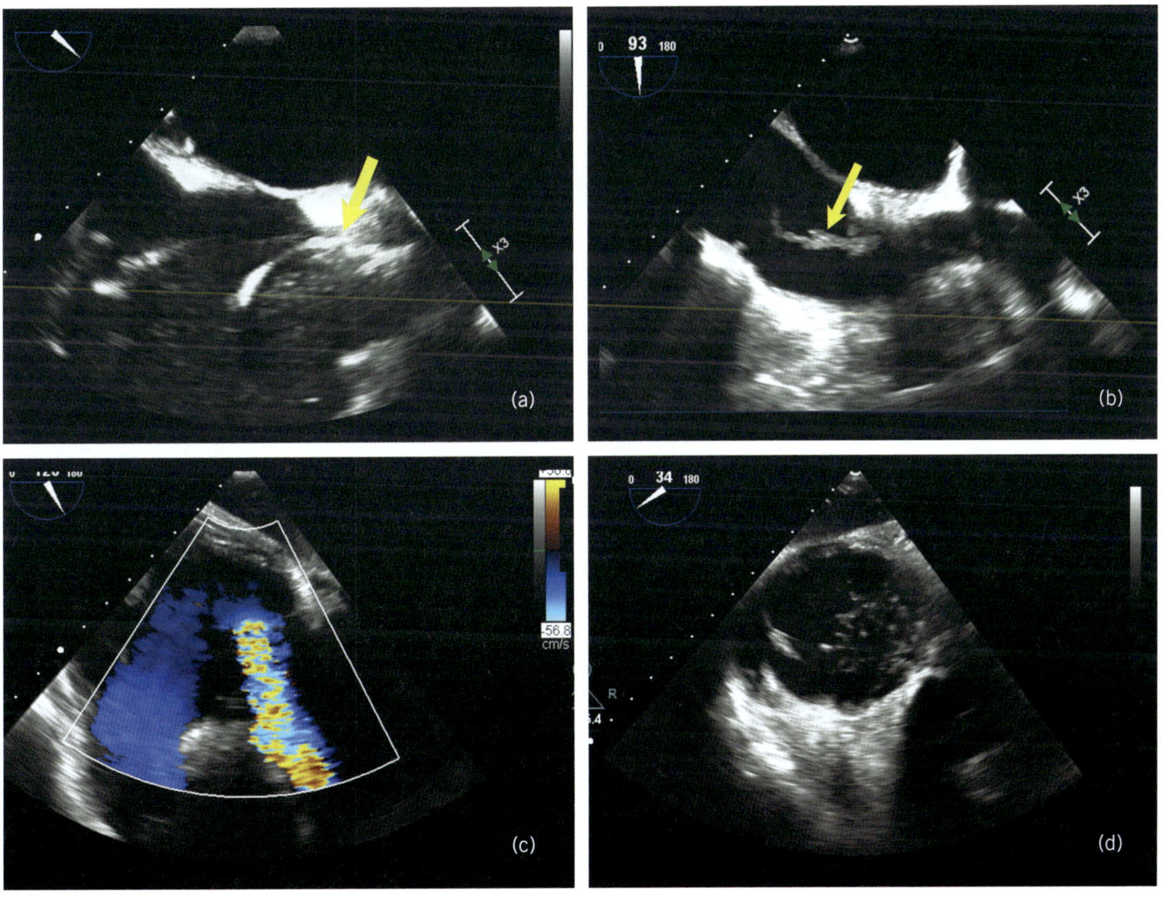

Figure 17.14 TOE for laser lead extraction. (a) Mid-oesophageal bicaval view showing multiple leads adherent to the IAS (arrow). (b) Same view showing 'ghost lesions' (arrow) in the LA after lead removal. (c) Mid-oesophageal inflow view zoomed on the TV, showing new TR after lead extraction in a patient with lead adherence to the TV. (d) Transgastric short axis-view showing multiple 'ghost lesions' on the TV in the same patient.

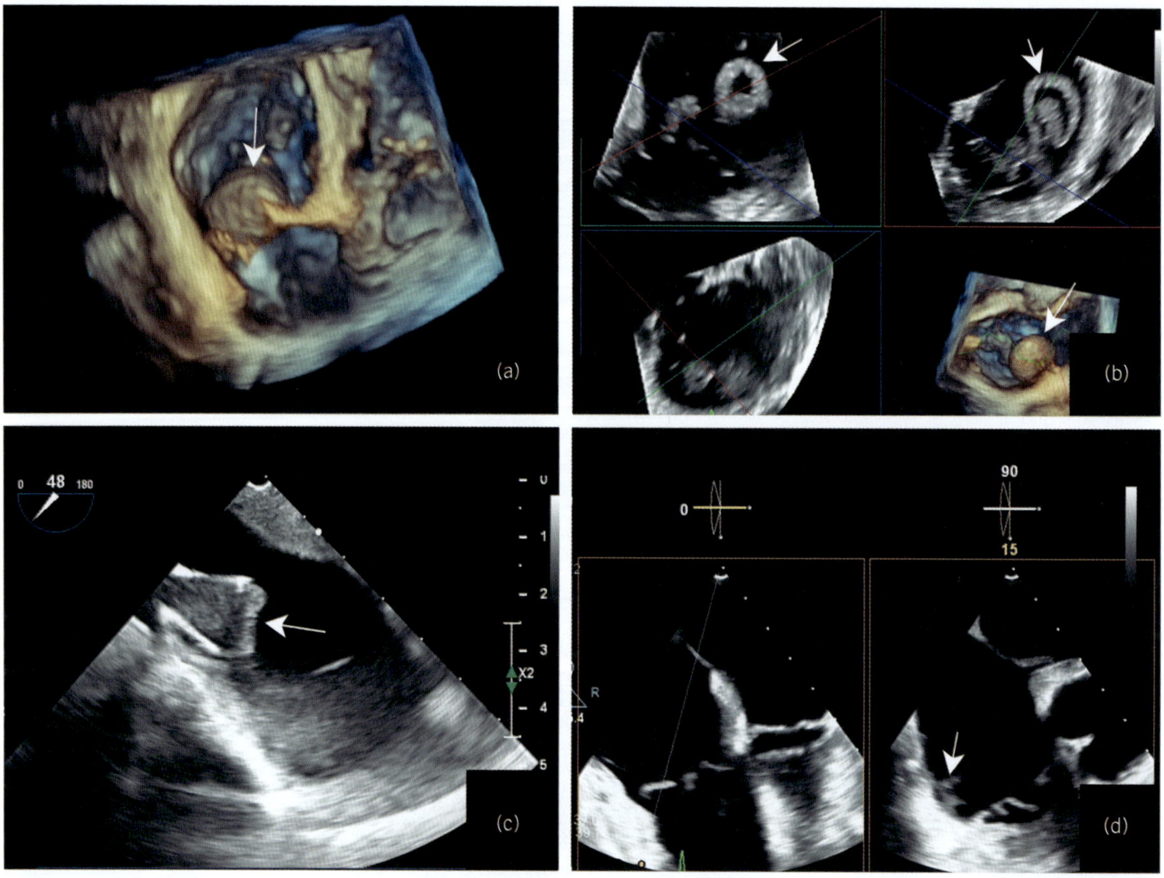

Figure 17.15 **Removal of tricuspid valve vegetations with the AngioVac®.** (a, b) 3D view of extensive TV vegetations (arrows). (c) AngioVac in the RA removing vegetation (arrow). (d) Biplane view of the RA showing small remaining vegetation (arrow). See Online appendix 9.5.6.

embolization of aspirated material, and pericardial effusion. For endocarditis cases, it is common to see a one-grade increase in valvular regurgitation after aspiration. Anything greater should prompt an examination for valve damage.

Edge-to-edge tricuspid valve repair

Screening

Since perioperative mortality associated with isolated surgical TV repair is high, a less invasive solution is appealing. Although there are other experimental approaches, trans-catheter edge-to-edge repair of the TV (TEER-TV) is currently the most widely used technique. While it does not improve mortality or hospitalizations, it has been shown to be safe and to improve quality of life at 1 year.[24] Relative contraindications are listed in Table 17.3.

Table 17.3 Relative contraindications for TEER-TV

Patient characteristics	Asymptomatic TR Severe pulmonary hypertension >60 mmHg Not on optimal medical therapy Other significant valvular disease Active endocarditis
Valve features	Previous tricuspid repair precluding clip placement Severe TR caused by CIED Coaptation gap >1 cm at site of target grasp Tricuspid stenosis
Atrial access	Presence of thrombus on CIED leads Thrombus in SVC, IVC, or RA
Imaging	Inadequate grasping views

TEER-TV presents unique challenges. Leaflet anatomy is highly variable, and a categorization scheme has been proposed to standardize the nomenclature (Figure 17.16).[25] In functional TR, the septal leaflet is often severely tethered, which increases the difficulty in imaging and grasping. Patients often present for TEER-TV at a late stage in their disease with severe annular dilation, large coaptation gaps, and multiple failures of coaptation. An expanded grading system has been proposed, which includes criteria for massive and torrential TR (Table 17.4).[26]

Good-quality images of the TV are critical. Leaflets must be visible for the entire length of coaptation throughout the cardiac cycle. A screening TOE must include an optimized transgastric short-axis view showing the TV leaflet edges, with and without colour flow Doppler, for leaflet morphology, coaptation gaps, and TR location.

Pre-procedure imaging involves a stepwise examination of the TV. Starting from a mid-oesophageal RV inflow–outflow view, with the TV in the centre of the screen, a biplane cursor is placed at the anterior-most position on the valve, showing simultaneous orthogonal planes, with and without colour. The cursor is moved to scan the entire valve from anterior to posterior in an incremental fashion, 3–5 mm at a time, looking at leaflet morphology, length, mobility, regurgitation, and coaptation gap at each point. (Figure 17.17).

Procedure

Under TOE guidance, the SGC is positioned and the clip is advanced into the RA. The tip of the clip is observed as it is steered towards the TV. Biplane imaging assists with this steering. Like in TEER-MV, biplane imaging and a 3D *en face* view are used to position the clip at its target location and to verify the orthogonal trajectory (Figure 17.18a). Independent grasper position is checked. A 3D *en face*

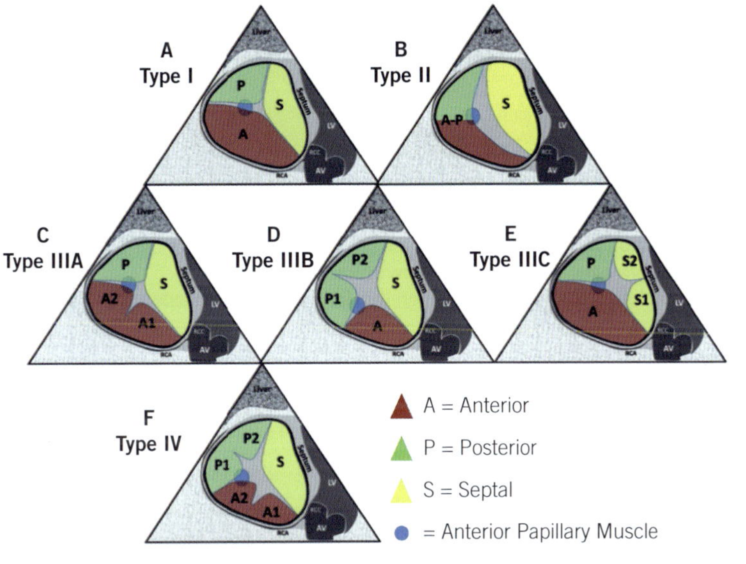

Figure 17.16 Proposed anatomic classification of highly variable tricuspid valve anatomy.

Reprinted from *JACC: Cardiovascular Imaging*, **14**, 7, Hahn RT *et al.*, Proposal for a Standard Echocardiographic Tricuspid Valve Nomenclature, pp. 1299–305, Copyright 2021, with permission from the American College of Cardiology Foundation. Published by Elsevier.

Table 17.4 Expanded TR grading system

	Mild	Moderate	Severe	Massive	Torrential
VC (biplane)	<3 mm	3–6.9 mm	7–13.9 mm	14–20.9 mm	≥21 mm
EROA (PISA)	<20 mm²	20–39 mm²	40–59 mm²	60–79 mm²	≥80 mm²
3D VCA or quantitative EROA			75–94 mm²	95–114 mm²	≥115 mm²

Reproduced from Hahn RT and Zamorano JL, 'The need for a new tricuspid regurgitation grading scheme', *European Heart Journal of Cardiovascular Imaging*, 2017, **18**, 12, pp. 1342–3, by permission of the European Society of Cardiology.[26]

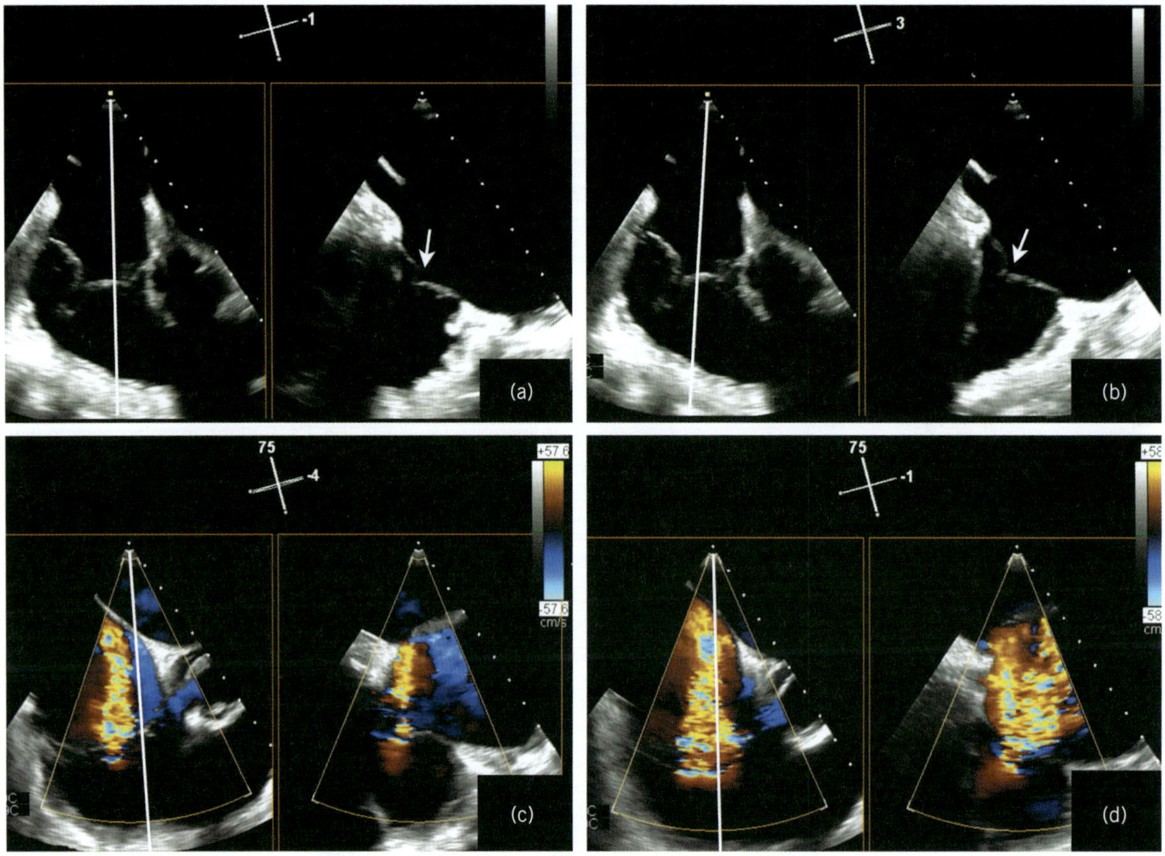

Figure 17.17 Screening examination for TEER-TV. Each frame shows a biplane view of the TV in the mid-oesophageal RV inflow–outflow view on the left, with the corresponding orthogonal view on the right. Between frames (a) and (b), the biplane cursor was moved slightly posteriorly, demonstrating a different coaptation gap (arrow) in the corresponding orthogonal view. Between frames (c) and (d), the biplane cursor was similarly moved slightly posteriorly, revealing more severe TR by colour Doppler at that site. The process is repeated for the entire valve. See also Figure 15.3.

view is used to rotate the open clip arms perpendicular to the line of coaptation at the target grasping site. Trajectory changes and rotation are monitored as the closed clip crosses the TV and opens in the RV. Positioning and rotation should be re-examined prior to a grasping attempt.

Using a TV view that best demonstrates the target leaflets in long axis, the leaflets are inserted along the entire length of the clip arms (Figure 17.18b). The grippers are dropped and can be seen 'bouncing' on the leaflet before clip closure (Figure 17.18c). As the clip is closed, it is important to monitor for leaflet slippage.

Using a combination of transgastric TV short-axis, biplane, and 3D imaging, the grasp is examined for appropriate location, rotation, and proper leaflet insertion. The clip is closed with colour Doppler to assess TR reduction (Figure 17.18d). The valve is assessed for residual TR and stenosis prior to release, and carefully observed for detachment during release. The clip delivery system is then safely retracted into the SGC.

Expert tip: 'Live' multi-planar 3D imaging gives real-time orientation and positional information, and can be used instead of repeatedly moving from transgastric to mid-oesophageal imaging.

Post-procedure evaluation

A complete study of the TV after each clip deployment should include the location and severity of residual TR and TV gradients. The procedure is complete with satisfactory TR reduction or when there are no remaining suitable targets to clip. A complete post-procedure TOE should be performed to rule out damage to cardiac structures, pericardial effusions, or clip detachment.

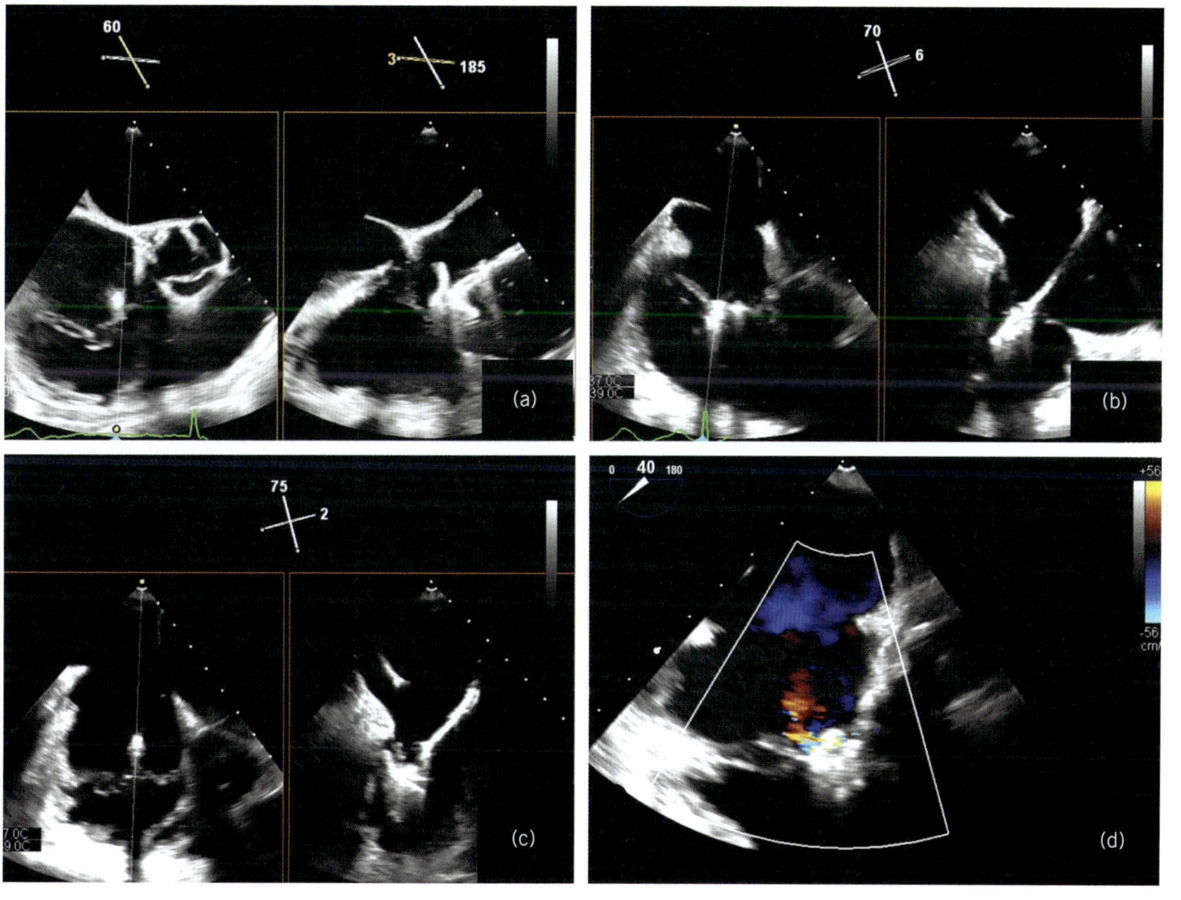

Figure 17.18 TOE imaging for TEER-TV, demonstrating a TriClip® (Abbott) placement. All frames are biplane images of mid-oesophageal RV inflow–outflow views, with corresponding orthogonal views. (a) The clip is opened above the valve, and the trajectories and orientation checked. (b) The clip is seen with its arms immediately below the tips of the tricuspid leaflets. (c) The septal and anterior leaflets are grasped with 'bouncing grippers'. (d) Colour Doppler zoomed view of the TV, showing minimal residual TR after placement of two clips.

Transcatheter aortic valve implantation

Indications for transcatheter aortic valve implantation (TAVI—also called TAVR for 'replacement' in certain parts of the world) have broadened as it provides comparable or better rates of stroke and mortality compared to surgical AV replacement. Age, technical or anatomical factors, comorbidities, and life expectancy are all evaluated by a multidisciplinary heart team prior to recommending TAVI.[27]

TAVI is indicated for patients with severe AS and elevated transvalvular gradients regardless of the severity of their symptoms. Patients with symptomatic low-flow low-gradient severe AS can also be considered.[27] All patients, regardless of the estimated surgical risk (low to prohibitive), can now be considered for TAVI over surgical valve replacement. Valve-in-valve TAVI is an option for patients who had prior bioprosthetic valves.

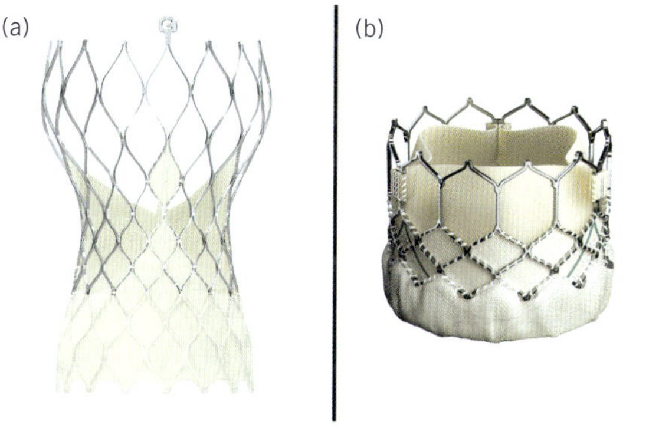

Figure 17.19 Transcatheter aortic valves. (a) Medtronic Evolut Pro+. (b) Edwards Sapien 3 Ultra.
(a) with kind permission from Medtronic and (b) courtesy of Edwards Lifesciences.

The primary TAVI valves in clinical use are the balloon-expandable Sapien® (Edwards Lifesciences) and the

Table 17.5 Procedural imaging steps for TAVI using TOE

Positioning of wires	Facilitate crossing of the AV Identify entrapment in the MV apparatus Exclude pericardial effusion Identify thrombus on wires or catheters
Balloon aortic valvuloplasty	Evaluate mobility of AV cusps and severity of aortic regurgitation Assess for new regional wall motion abnormalities Exclude pericardial effusion
Positioning and deployment of transcatheter valve	Balloon-expandable valve; confirm ventricular end 1–2 mm below annulus, and aortic end below sinotubular junction and covering cusps Self-expanding valve; confirm ventricular end 2–4 mm below annulus
Transapical cannulation	Confirm puncture site away from interventricular septum and RV Evaluate retrograde position of guidewire through AV Exclude entrapment of wire in MV apparatus
Post-deployment	Assess valve position, shape, transvalvular gradients, and aortic valve area Assess for central or paravalvular aortic regurgitation Exclude pericardial effusion

Adapted from *Journal of the American Society of Echocardiography*, **31**, 4, Hahn RT *et al.*, 'Echocardiographic Imaging for Transcatheter Aortic Valve Replacement', pp. 405–433, Copyright 2018, with permission from the American Society of Echocardiography.[28]

self-expandable Evolut® (Medtronic, Minneapolis, MN, USA) valves. The most recent generations are the Sapien 3 Ultra® and the Evolut Pro®+ (Figure 17.19). The Sapien® valves require balloon dilatation, are positioned intra-annularly, are not retrievable, and require rapid pacing for deployment. The Evolut® valves are self-expanding, are positioned supra-annularly, are recapturable, and do not require rapid pacing (although rapid pacing may be used to stabilize the implant position).

With advances in technology and experience, fluoroscopy-only procedures under conscious sedation now account for the vast majority of TAVI procedures, when the transfemoral approach is used. In such cases, the entire procedure is performed under fluoroscopy alone, and a focused TTE examination is used, instead of TOE, to evaluate the valve function after deployment. TOE is still of value for infrequent cases where patient factors preclude sedation, or in cases where a transfemoral approach is not possible due to severe peripheral vascular disease. Alternative approaches include trans-apical, direct trans-aortic, trans-subclavian, trans-carotid, and trans-caval. Such alternate approaches require general anaesthesia ± TOE.

Procedural imaging

When TOE is used, a comprehensive examination should be performed, with a focus on the LVOT and aortic root complex, using techniques described in Chapter 10. 3D multi-planar imaging is best to measure the LVOT, aortic annulus, and aortic root dimensions (see Figures 10.6 and 10.7). The distance from the annulus to the coronary ostia should be noted. For balloon-expandable prostheses, a distance of <10 mm carries a risk of coronary occlusion. TOE measurements should be compared to the preoperative CT findings. Depending on the TAVI valve, sizing by CT is based on the aortic annular perimeter, aortic annular area, and/or perimeter-derived diameter of the annulus.

Procedural imaging steps are outlined in Table 17.5.[28] Positioning and deployment of TAVI valves are primarily performed with fluoroscopic guidance. For balloon-expandable valves, the ventricular end should be positioned on the intervalvular fibrosa above the hinge point of the MV to avoid interference with the anterior leaflet of the MV. The aortic end should be below the sinotubular junction, as deployment that is too high in the aortic root can cause coronary occlusion. For self-expanding valves, the ventricular end should protrude minimally (2–4 mm) into the LVOT.

The implanted valve should be assessed for position, shape, peak and mean pressure gradients, and AV area. Quantifying the degree of AR is critical, as moderate or severe AR is associated with poor outcomes after TAVI. Key parameters for grading the severity of AR after deployment are outlined in Table 17.6.[29] Post-TAVI paravalvular

Table 17.6 Key parameters for grading the severity of paravalvular AR after TAVR

PAR severity	Mild	Moderate	Severe
Position of prosthesis	Usually normal	Variable	Frequently abnormal
Stent and leaflet morphology	Usually normal	Variable	Frequently abnormal
Proximal flow convergence (CD)	Absent	May be present	Often present
AR velocity waveform density (CWD)	Soft	Dense	Dense
Vena contracta width (cm) (CD)	<0.3	0.3–0.6	>0.6
Vena contracta area (cm^2) (2D/3D CD)	<0.1	0.1–0.29	≥0.3
Circumferential extent of PAR (%) (CD)	<10	10–29	≥30

PAR, paravalvular aortic regurgitation; CD, colour Doppler; CWD, continuous-wave Doppler.

Adapted from *Journal of the American Society of Echocardiography*, **32**, 4, Zoghbi WA *et al.*, 'Guidelines for the Evaluation of Valvular Regurgitation After Percutaneous Valve Repair or Replacement: A Report from the American Society of Echocardiography Developed in Collaboration with the Society for Cardiovascular Angiography and Interventions, Japanese Society of Echocardiography, and Society for Cardiovascular Magnetic Resonance', pp. 431–475, Copyright 2019, with permission from the American Society of Echocardiography.[29]

AR can be treated with balloon dilation or valve-in-valve replacement. It is important to distinguish paravalvular regurgitation from a 'twinkling' artefact—the latter is present in both systole and diastole, and does not extend into the LVOT.[28] Although transient haemodynamic instability occurs during valve deployment due to rapid pacing, TOE can rapidly identify causes of persistent hypotension such as cardiac tamponade or coronary ischaemia.

Multiple choice questions

Discover interactive multiple choice questions to test your knowledge on this chapter by searching for this book's title or ISBN (9780198873686) at **https://academic.oup.com/** and going to the online appendix at the end of the book. Use your scratch-off code on the inside cover to access the material.

References

1. Little SH, Rigolin VH, Garcia-Sayan E, *et al.* Recommendations for special competency in echocardiographic guidance of structural heart disease interventions: from the American Society of Echocardiography. *J Am Soc Echocardiogr.* 2023;**36**(4):350–65.
2. McNamara DA, Chopra R, Decker JM, *et al.* Comparison of radiation exposure among interventional echocardiographers, interventional cardiologists, and sonographers during percutaneous structural heart interventions. *JAMA Netw Open.* 2022;**5**(7):e2220597.
3. Patel KM, Desai RG, Trivedi K, Neuburger PJ, Krishnan S, Potestio CP. Complications of transesophageal echocardiography: a review of injuries, risk factors, and management. *J Cardiothorac Vasc Anesth.* 2022;**36**(8 Pt B):3292–302.
4. Faletra FF, Leo LA, Paiocchi VL, *et al.* Revisiting anatomy of the interatrial septum and its adjoining atrioventricular junction using noninvasive imaging techniques. *J Am Soc Echocardiogr.* 2019;**32**(5):580–92.
5. Katsiampoura A, Mufarrih SH, Sharkey A, *et al.* A sequential approach for echocardiographic guidance of transseptal puncture: the PITLOC Protocol. *J Cardiothorac Vasc Anesth.* 2022;**36**(8 Pt B):3257–64.
6. McInerney A, Marroquin-Donday L, Tirado-Conte G, *et al.* Transcatheter treatment of mitral regurgitation. *J Clin Med.* 2022;**11**(10):2921.
7. Feldman T, Foster E, Glower DD, *et al.* Percutaneous repair or surgery for mitral regurgitation. *N Engl J Med.* 2011;**364**(15):1395–406.
8. Arnold SV, Chinnakondepalli KM, Spertus JA, *et al.* Health status after transcatheter mitral-valve repair in heart failure and secondary mitral regurgitation: COAPT Trial. *J Am Coll Cardiol.* 2019;**73**(17):2123–32.
9. Hensey M, Brown RA, Lal S, *et al.* Transcatheter mitral valve replacement: an update on current techniques, technologies, and future directions. *JACC Cardiovasc Interv.* 2021;**14**(5):489–500.
10. Wilkins GT, Weyman AE, Abascal VM, Block PC, Palacios IF. Percutaneous balloon dilatation of the mitral valve: an analysis of echocardiographic variables related to outcome and the mechanism of dilatation. *Br Heart J.* 1988;**60**(4):299–308.
11. Nunes MC, Tan TC, Elmariah S, *et al.* The echo score revisited: Impact of incorporating commissural morphology and leaflet displacement to the prediction of outcome for patients undergoing percutaneous mitral valvuloplasty. *Circulation.* 2014;**129**(8):886–95.

12. Anwar AM, Attia WM, Nosir YF, *et al.* Validation of a new score for the assessment of mitral stenosis using real-time three-dimensional echocardiography. *J Am Soc Echocardiogr.* 2010;**23**(1):13–22.
13. Cruz-Gonzalez I, Antunez-Muinos P, Lopez-Tejero S, Sanchez PL. Mitral paravalvular leak: clinical implications, diagnosis and management. *J Clin Med.* 2022;**11**(5):1245.
14. January CT, Wann LS, Calkins H, *et al.* 2019 AHA/ACC/HRS focused update of the 2014 AHA/ACC/HRS Guideline for the management of patients with atrial fibrillation: a report of the American College of Cardiology/American Heart Association Task Force on clinical practice guidelines and the Heart Rhythm Society in collaboration with the Society of Thoracic Surgeons. *Circulation.* 2019;**140**(2):e125–51.
15. Beigel R, Wunderlich NC, Ho SY, Arsanjani R, Siegel RJ. The left atrial appendage: anatomy, function, and noninvasive evaluation. *JACC Cardiovasc Imaging.* 2014;**7**(12):1251–65.
16. Di Biase L, Santangeli P, Anselmino M, *et al.* Does the left atrial appendage morphology correlate with the risk of stroke in patients with atrial fibrillation? Results from a multicenter study. *J Am Coll Cardiol.* 2012;**60**(6):531–8.
17. Stout KK, Daniels CJ, Aboulhosn JA, *et al.* 2018 AHA/ACC Guideline for the management of adults with congenital heart disease: a report of the American College of Cardiology/American Heart Association Task Force on Clinical Practice Guidelines. *J Am Coll Cardiol.* 2019;**73**(12):e81–192.
18. Turner ME, Bouhout I, Petit CJ, Kalfa D. Transcatheter closure of atrial and ventricular septal defects: JACC focus seminar. *J Am Coll Cardiol.* 2022;**79**(22):2247–58.
19. Kavinsky CJ, Szerlip M, Goldsweig AM, *et al.* SCAI guidelines for the management of patent foramen ovale. *J Soc Cardiovasc Angiogr Interv.* 2022;**1**(4):100039.
20. Bongiorni MG, Burri H, Deharo JC, *et al.* 2018 EHRA expert consensus statement on lead extraction: recommendations on definitions, endpoints, research trial design, and data collection requirements for clinical scientific studies and registries: endorsed by APHRS/HRS/LAHRS. *Europace.* 2018;**20**(7):1217.
21. Addetia K, Harb SC, Hahn RT, Kapadia S, Lang RM. Cardiac implantable electronic device lead-induced tricuspid regurgitation. *JACC Cardiovasc Imaging.* 2019;**12**(4):622–36.
22. Caiati C, Luzzi G, Pollice P, Favale S, Lepera ME. A novel clinical perspective on new masses after lead extraction (ghosts) by means of intracardiac echocardiography. *J Clin Med.* 2020;**9**(8):2571.
23. Mhanna M, Beran A, Al-Abdouh A, *et al.* AngioVac for vegetation debulking in right-sided infective endocarditis: a systematic review and meta-analysis. *Curr Probl Cardiol.* 2022;**47**(11):101353.
24. Sorajja P, Whisenant B, Hamid N, *et al.* Transcatheter repair for patients with tricuspid regurgitation. *N Engl J Med.* 2023;**389**(9):865–6.
25. Hahn RT, Weckbach LT, Noack T, *et al.* Proposal for a standard echocardiographic tricuspid valve nomenclature. *JACC Cardiovasc Imaging.* 2021;**14**(7):1299–305.
26. Hahn RT, Zamorano JL. The need for a new tricuspid regurgitation grading scheme. *Eur Heart J Cardiovasc Imaging.* 2017;**18**(12):1342–3.
27. Asgar AW, Ouzounian M, Adams C, *et al.* 2019 Canadian Cardiovascular Society position statement for transcatheter aortic valve implantation. *Can J Cardiol.* 2019;**35**(11):1437–48.
28. Hahn RT, Nicoara A, Kapadia S, Svensson L, Martin R. Echocardiographic imaging for transcatheter aortic valve replacement. *J Am Soc Echocardiogr.* 2018;**31**(4):405–33.
29. Zoghbi WA, Asch FM, Bruce C, *et al.* Guidelines for the evaluation of valvular regurgitation after percutaneous valve repair or replacement: a report from the American Society of Echocardiography developed in collaboration with the Society for Cardiovascular Angiography and Interventions, Japanese Society of Echocardiography, and Society for Cardiovascular Magnetic Resonance. *J Am Soc Echocardiogr.* 2019;**32**(4):431–75.

18 Adult congenital heart disease

Congenital heart disease (CHD) is common, accounting for approximately 1% of live births.[1] Advances in paediatric cardiology and surgical care mean that the majority of those with moderate to severely complex CHD now survive to adulthood.[2] These individuals require lifelong surveillance and are unfortunately prone to developing long-term sequelae. Imaging is integral to guiding appropriate surveillance, care, and intervention. TOE plays an essential role in both the cardiac catheterization laboratory and the operating room, and this chapter aims to provide an overview of the most routine congenital heart defects that the echocardiographer may encounter in those settings. The chapter addresses lesions that are most commonly seen, before describing those of more moderate to severe complexity. ***It is important to note that this chapter is only a brief overview of some of the major congenital diseases that adult echocardiographers may encounter in their practice. Patients with moderate to severely complex conditions should always be evaluated and treated by individuals with appropriate training and clinical experience.***

Atrial septal defect

Atrial septal defects (ASDs) comprise about 10% of all congenital cardiac defects (excluding the bicuspid aortic valve). They are often diagnosed incidentally in older individuals when exercise intolerance, atrial arrhythmias, right-sided heart failure, or a paradoxical cerebrovascular accident CVA) is noted.

An ASD is defined as a communication between the left and right atria at the level of the inter-atrial septum. ASDs are classified by their location relative to the *fossa ovalis* (Figures 18.1 and 18.2). Regardless of the defect, all result in a left-to-right shunt. The degree of shunting is determined by: (1) the size of the defect; (2) the relative compliance of the left and right ventricles; and (3) the relative pressures between the left and right atria. This causes right heart overload with both RA and RV dilatation, as well as increased pulmonary blood flow. Any increase in LA pressure or decrease in LV compliance can increase the left-to-right shunt. Hypertension, ischaemic heart disease, cardiomyopathy, and aortic and MV disease can also influence this. A left-to-right shunt can decrease or reverse, driven by increasing RA pressure or decreasing RV compliance due to tricuspid disease, pulmonary stenosis, and/or pulmonary hypertension.

Classification of ASDs

Secundum ASD

Secundum ASDs account for 80% of all cases of inter-atrial communications and are located centrally within the inter-atrial septum at the level of the fossa ovalis (Figure 18.3). Embryologically, a secundum ASD is a defect in the septum primum that makes up the floor of the fossa ovalis. The size and nature of the defect can vary from complete absence of the atrial septal tissue to a minor defect and may include more than one defect, as in a fenestrated ASD (Figure 18.4).

Primum ASD

Primum ASDs account for 15% of ASDs and represent a form of partial atrioventricular septal defect. They are located anterior and inferior to the fossa ovalis, and no atrial septal tissue is present between the lower edge of the defect and the atrioventricular valves (see also atrioventricular septal defects later).

Sinus venosus defects

Though functionally identical to ASDs, sinus venosus defects result from abnormal development of the sinus venosus in relation to the systemic and pulmonary veins. In the embryonic heart, the sinus venosus is a cavity located between the venae cavae, and it later becomes incorporated into the wall of the RA. The superior sinus venosus defect is the most common and is located postero-superior to the fossa ovalis and connects the SVC to the LA. It accounts for 5% of all inter-atrial communications

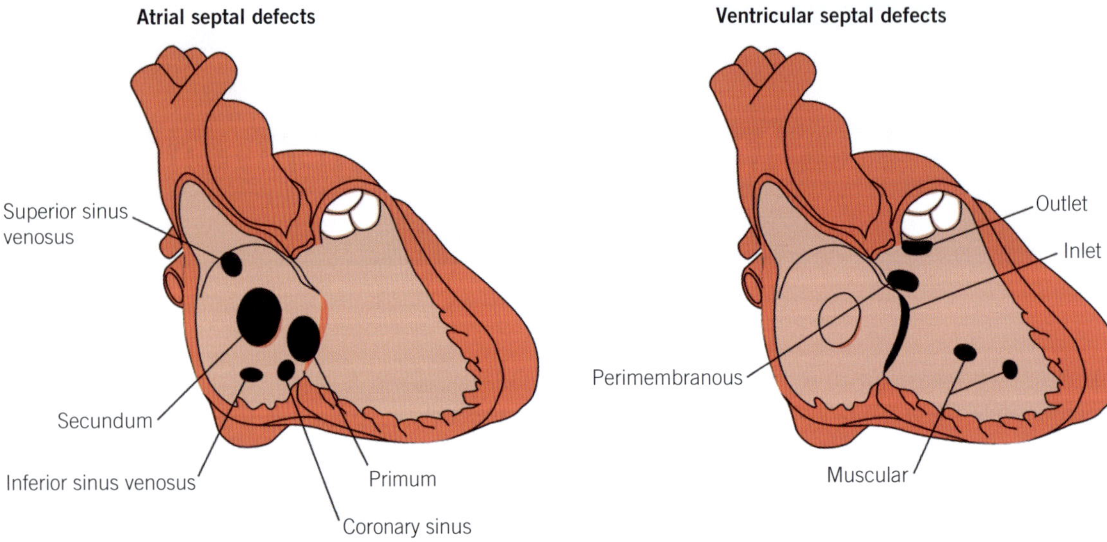

Figure 18.1 Schematic representation of ASDs and VSDs.

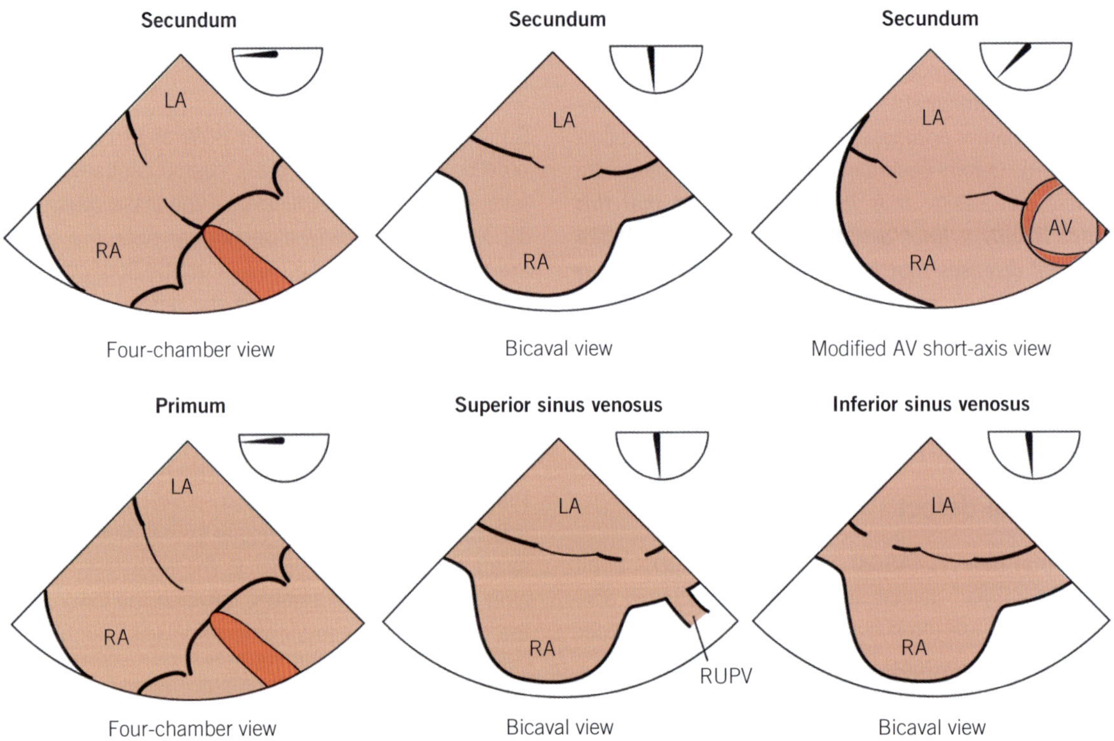

Figure 18.2 TOE views in which various types of ASDs are typically visualized. See text for details.

(Figure 18.5). It is often associated with anomalous pulmonary venous drainage of the right upper pulmonary vein (Figure 18.6). The much rarer inferior sinus venosus defect is postero-inferior to the fossa ovalis and connects the IVC to the LA; it accounts for <1% of cases.

Coronary sinus defect/unroofed coronary sinus

The rarest form of ASD is the unroofed coronary sinus. This defect is located inferior and anterior to the fossa ovalis at the usual position of the coronary sinus orifice. Either partial or complete deficiency of the wall separating

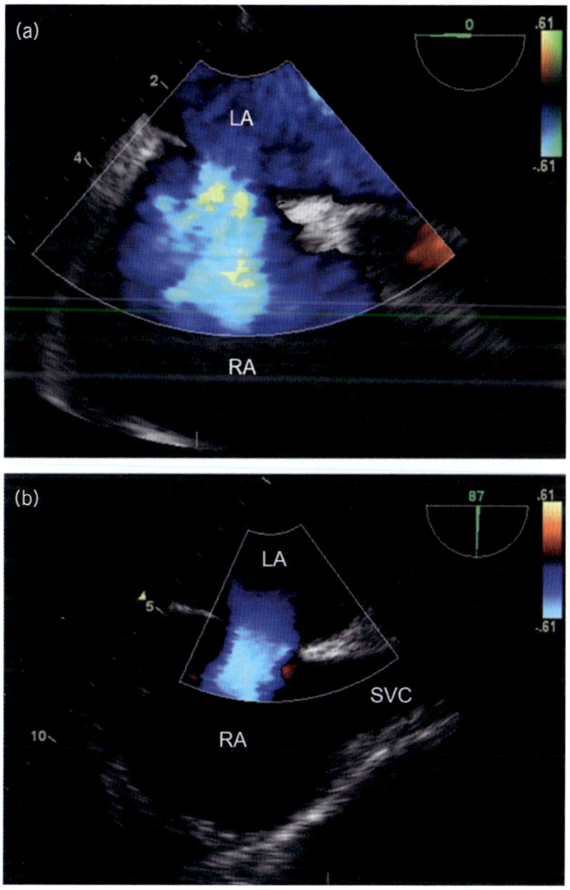

Figure 18.3 Secundum ASD. A large secundum ASD is demonstrated in a modified (rotated to the right) mid-oesophageal four-chamber view (a) and a mid-oesophageal bicaval view (b), with colour Doppler. Note that the flow is from the LA to the RA (away from the transducer) and it is of low velocity (i.e. there is no aliasing). See also Online appendix 10.1.

the coronary sinus from the LA is noted. It can be part of a more complex anomaly, including absence of the coronary sinus and a persistent left SVC.

> ***Expert tip: Sinus venosus ASD and coronary sinus defects are not always readily visible on standard views and can be easily missed if not sought after.***

Aims of imaging and treatment options

Excellent spatial and temporal imaging makes TOE the definitive imaging modality to assess the atrial septum. TOE views in which different types of ASDs are typically visualized are shown in Figure 18.2. TOE allows precise imaging of the fossa ovalis, sinus venosus septum, and pulmonary veins. An accurate assessment

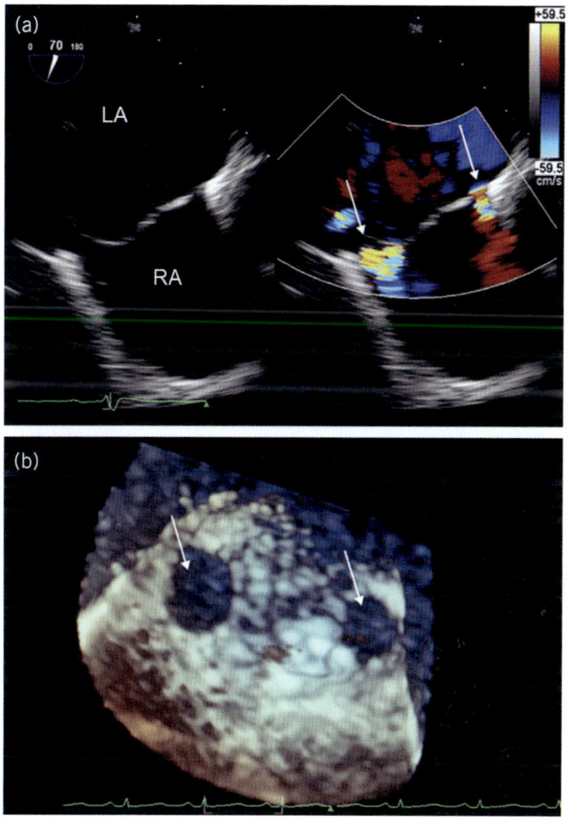

Figure 18.4 Fenestrated ASD. (a) is a modified bicaval view in a dual-screen layout. Two colour jets can be seen (arrows), indicating a fenestrated ASD. Flow is from the LA to the RA. (b) is a 3D view of the same atrial septum. Two defects (arrows) can be seen.

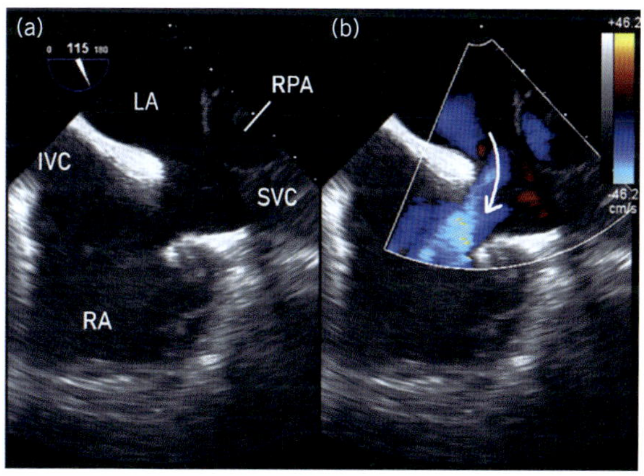

Figure 18.5 Superior sinus venosus ASD. The image is a modified mid-oesophageal bicaval view. From the standard position, the probe was slightly withdrawn and turned to the right to demonstrate the defect, located in the superior part of the inter-atrial septum close to the junction of the SVC (a). Flow is from the LA to the RA, as indicated by the arrow (b). RPA, right pulmonary artery. See also Online appendix 10.4.

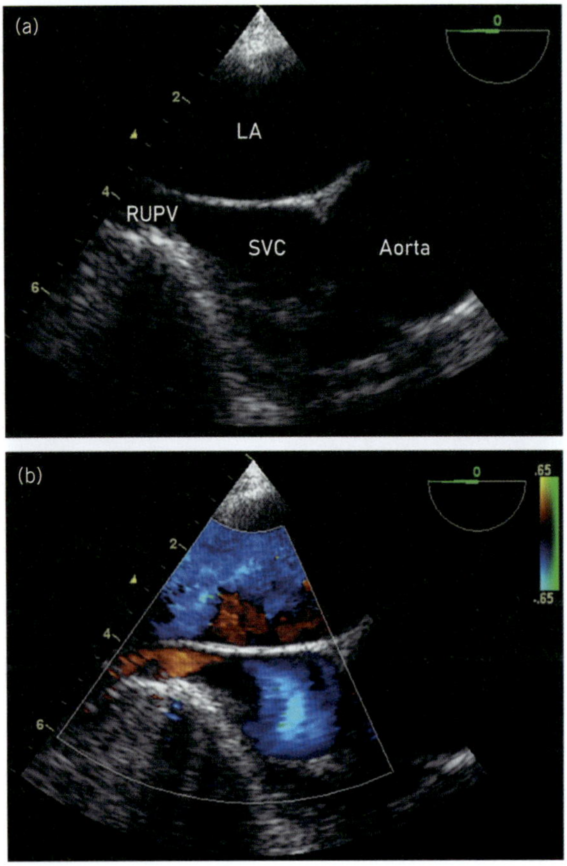

Figure 18.6 Anomalous drainage of the right upper pulmonary vein (RUPV). The images are mid-oesophageal ascending aorta short-axis views, without (a) and with (b) colour Doppler, demonstrating an anomalous connection between the RUPV and the SVC. The patient also had a superior sinus venosus ASD. See Online appendices 10.4.4 and 10.4.5.

of the defect size can be performed, and the residual septal morphology and rim sizes can be assessed. It is essential to demonstrate the relationship of the defect to the surrounding structures (atrioventricular valves, pulmonary and systemic veins). LV size and systolic function are also important to assess. 3D imaging is now a routine part of the assessment as it allows for better evaluation of defects than 2D imaging alone, including a better appreciation of the shape of the defect, which should not be assumed to be circular. 3D imaging also allows for better evaluation of RV volume and function. Atrial shunting occurs predominantly in diastole and is typically left-to-right. As the shunt velocity is typically low when interrogating the defect with colour flow Doppler, the Nyquist limit is best set to <30 cm/s.

Expert tip: For a shunt to be visible with colour Doppler, two things are needed: a defect and a pressure gradient across that defect. Absence of colour does not rule out a septal defect. If the LA and RA pressures are approximately equal, there may not be a colour jet visible, even if there is a defect.

In patients with evidence of RV volume overload and no pulmonary hypertension, ASD closure is recommended regardless of symptoms. Treatment of a secundum ASD is usually via percutaneous device closure, if the stretched diameter is no greater than 38 mm with adequate rims of approximately 5 mm, even without an adequate retro-aortic rim. TOE is used to guide device placement and demonstrates how the device relates to other cardiac structures (see Chapter 17 for details). Secundum defects that are too large to close percutaneously require surgery with the placement of a pericardial patch. All other types of defects require surgical correction and are not suitable for a percutaneous approach, with the exception of selected cases of sinus venosus defects, which may be suitable for a covered stent approach in experienced hands.

Patent foramen ovale

A patent foramen ovale (PFO) is not an ASD and is a normal variant, occurring in 20–34% of adults. Here, there is *no deficiency* of atrial tissue (i.e. no defect), but there is failure of anatomic fusion of the valve of the foramen ovale with the limbus (or border) of the fossa ovalis. Under normal physiological conditions, the PFO remains closed as the RA pressure is less than that of the LA, but during sneezing, coughing, or Valsalva manoeuvre when the pressure gradient is reversed, the PFO opens and blood is shunted right-to-left. Of note, left-to-right shunting can also occur at rest if dilatation or changes in atrial geometry render the valve incompetent.

Colour Doppler imaging of the atrial septum may reveal flow across a PFO (Figure 18.7), and the mid-oesophageal bicaval view is best to demonstrate it. Sometimes an agitated saline study may be required with physiological manoeuvres to demonstrate a PFO. To perform a saline contrast study, two syringes are connected via a three-way tap/stopcock to an intravenous (IV) line (either an antecubital IV or a central line). Ten millilitres of agitated saline with 2 mL of blood (optional) are mixed vigorously between two syringes and then rapidly injected via the IV line. Note that air is *not* required to produce high-quality contrast and should not be used. The mid-oesophageal four-chamber and bicaval views are best used to detect a shunt. Injection of agitated saline is timed with the release of a Valsalva manoeuvre—or a maximal inspiratory hold in a ventilated patient—which causes a sudden rise in venous return to the RA and increases the RA pressure. The test is positive when bubbles are clearly seen crossing through the PFO or with the appearance of bubbles in the LA within 3–5 cardiac cycles. Percutaneous closure is indicated in those who have had a cryptogenic stroke or who are suffering from platypnoea–orthodeoxia syndrome.

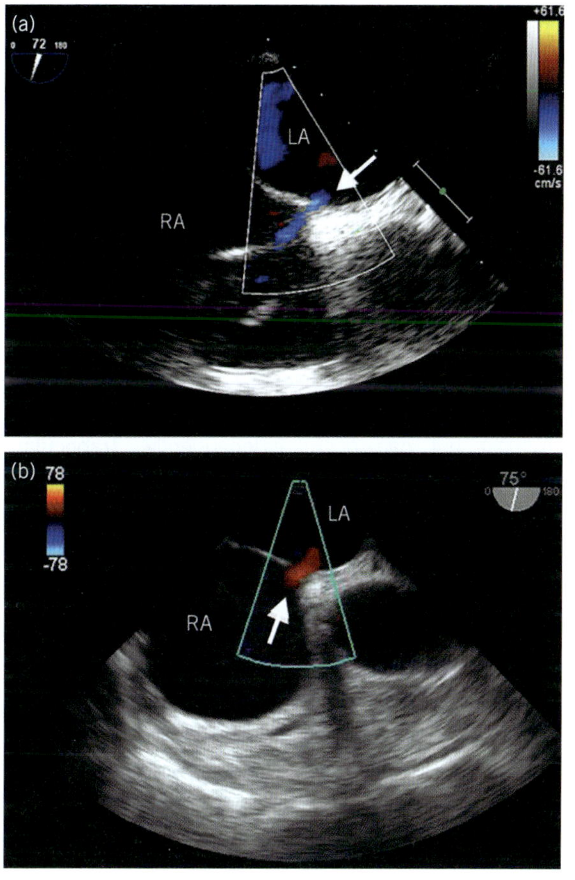

Figure 18.7 Patent foramen ovale. Both frames (a) and (b) are modified mid-oesophageal bicaval views demonstrating a PFO. The images are from two different patients. In (a), blood flow is from left to right (blue, away from the transducer), indicating LA pressure is greater than RA pressure. In (b), blood flow is from right to left (red, towards the transducer), indicating RA pressure is greater than LA pressure. See also Online appendix 10.1.1.

Ventricular septal defect

A **ventricular septal defect (VSD)** is a communication at the level of the interventricular septum (IVS). VSDs represent the most common cardiac congenital anomaly, accounting for 30% of all congenital cardiac cases (excluding the bicuspid aortic valve). They can occur as isolated lesions or as part of more complex lesions such as tetralogy of Fallot (ToF), transposition of the great arteries, common arterial trunk, or functionally univentricular heart.

The direction and magnitude of the shunt is determined by the size of the defect, the pulmonary vascular resistance, the systemic valvular resistance, and the presence of any associated abnormalities. Usually, a left-to-right shunt exists because of the higher LV pressure. A small restrictive VSD does not cause left heart dilatation, but this can be seen with moderate to large defects. If left untreated, a significant defect can increase pulmonary vascular resistance, causing a bidirectional shunt, which may eventually shunt right-to-left, leading to Eisenmenger syndrome with systemic oxygen desaturation.

Adults with a VSD typically have undergone a prior surgical repair or have a small restrictive defect. Repair of a large defect with associated severe pulmonary hypertension is contraindicated due to the high likelihood of RV failure, and these patients may require consideration of en bloc heart–lung transplant. Small restrictive defects can still result in long-term complications such as progressive AR and an increased risk of infective endocarditis.

Anatomy and classifications

The IVS consists of three portions: (1) the **inlet portion**, which lies posterior to the membranous septum and inferior to the atrioventricular valves; (2) the **trabecular portion**, which extends from the membranous septum to the cardiac apex; and (3) the **outlet portion**, which extends anteriorly from the membranous septum and lies above the trabecular septum and below the great arteries. The classification of VSDs has been contentious and numerous terms exist, which can cause confusion. The International Society for Nomenclature of Paediatric and Congenital Heart Disease categorizes VSDs by their location and the structures along their borders to unify the terminology.[3] This incorporates the two most popular classification approaches and provides a common language for describing each phenotype.

The four types of VSD are: (1) perimembranous; (2) outlet; (3) inlet; and (4) muscular or muscular–trabecular defects.

Perimembranous VSDs are the most common defect, accounting for approximately 80% of VSDs. They have fibrous continuity between the aortic and tricuspid valves. Due to their position adjacent to the septal leaflet of the tricuspid valve, the valve tissue can become adherent to the defect, limiting the amount of shunting. Perimembranous defects are associated with AV prolapse and subsequent regurgitation. They can extend into the inlet or outlet portion of the IVS. The incidence of **outlet VSDs** in European populations is low at 5% but account for 30% of cases in Asian populations. They have fibrous continuity with the aortic and pulmonic valves immediately below them. Right AV cusp prolapse is common, resulting in progressive AR. **Inlet VSDs** lie posteriorly and inferiorly to the AV plane. They are present in atrioventricular septal defects (AVSDs) but can occur independently. **Trabecular–muscular VSDs** are entirely located within the muscular IVS and account for 5–20% of cases. They can be single or multiple, and can be located mid muscular or apically. They can close spontaneously with time, but in those where surgery is indicated, determining the location relative to the conduction system is essential to prevent iatrogenic heart block. Acquired (ischaemic) VSDs are discussed in Chapter 6.

Aims of imaging and treatment options

The aim of echocardiography should be to determine the following features: (1) location and size of the VSD; (2) presence and severity of any valvular lesions (particularly AV prolapse and regurgitation, as well as TR); (3) ventricular function; (4) signs of pulmonary hypertension; and (5) presence of any other congenital heart lesions. A high-velocity jet across the VSD suggests a restrictive defect, whereas a large defect will be non-restrictive and may exhibit laminar flow with low velocities.

The TOE views in which the different types of VSD are typically visualized are shown in Figure 18.8. Perimembranous (Figure 18.9) and outlet (Figure 18.10) VSDs communicate with the LVOT and can be viewed in the mid-oesophageal RV inflow–outflow view and the mid-oesophageal AV long-axis view. In that view, *perimembranous* defects are adjacent to the *tricuspid* valve, whereas *outlet* defects are adjacent to the *pulmonic* valve (PV). The RV inflow–outflow view is also useful to differentiate between the perimembranous and outlet defects, with the latter being noted below the PV. Both of these defects can cause AV prolapse and regurgitation. 3D imaging is valuable for assessing the lesions in detail.

Atrioventricular septal defects

AVSDs are characterized by atrioventricular valve (A-V) abnormalities and a lack of A-V septation. In AVSDs, there is a common A-V junction with a common fibrous

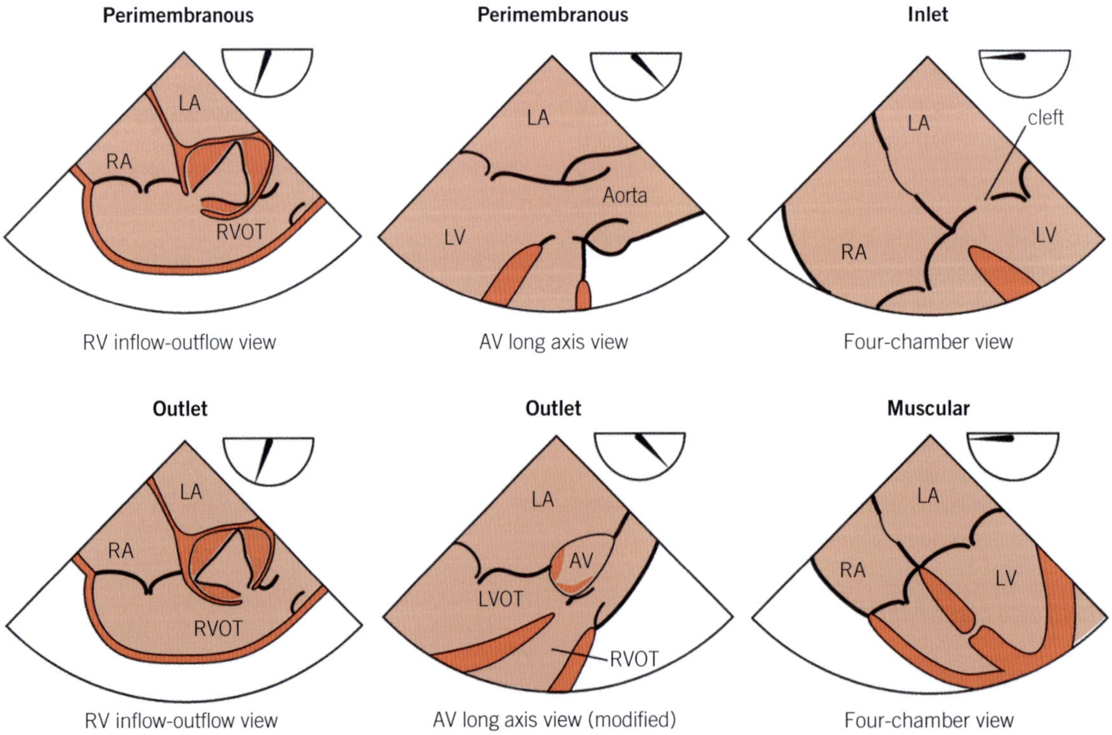

Figure 18.8 TOE views in which the different types of VSD are typically visualized. See text for details.

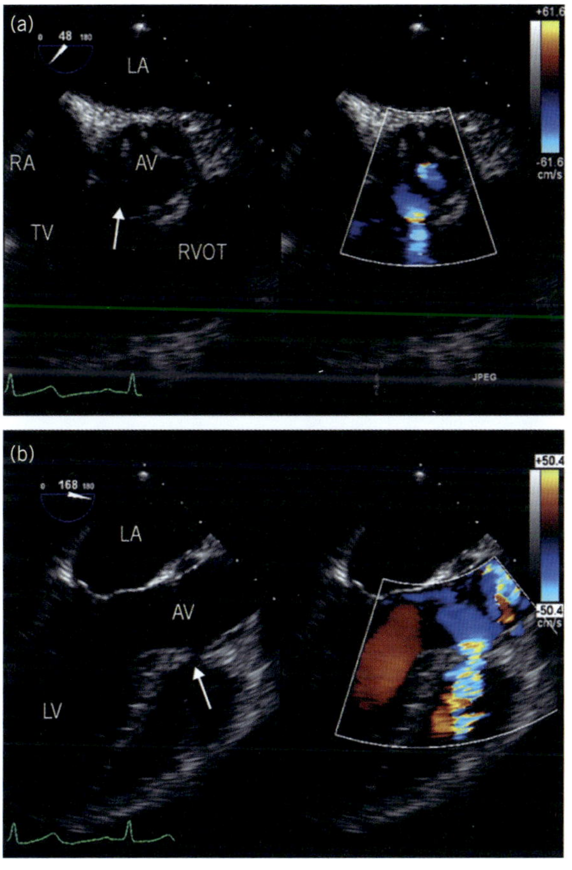

Figure 18.9 Perimembranous VSD. (a) is a mid-oesophageal RV inflow–outflow view in systole. Dual-screen layout has been used to visualize the defect, with and without colour Doppler. A VSD (arrow) can be seen adjacent to the TV. Its location adjacent to the TV indicates a perimembranous origin. (b) is a mid-oesophageal AV long-axis view from the same patient, also in systole using dual-screen layout. The defect can be seen below the AV. It is difficult to be sure in the AV long-axis view whether the defect is in the perimembranous or outlet portions of the ventricular septum. Flow is from left to right.

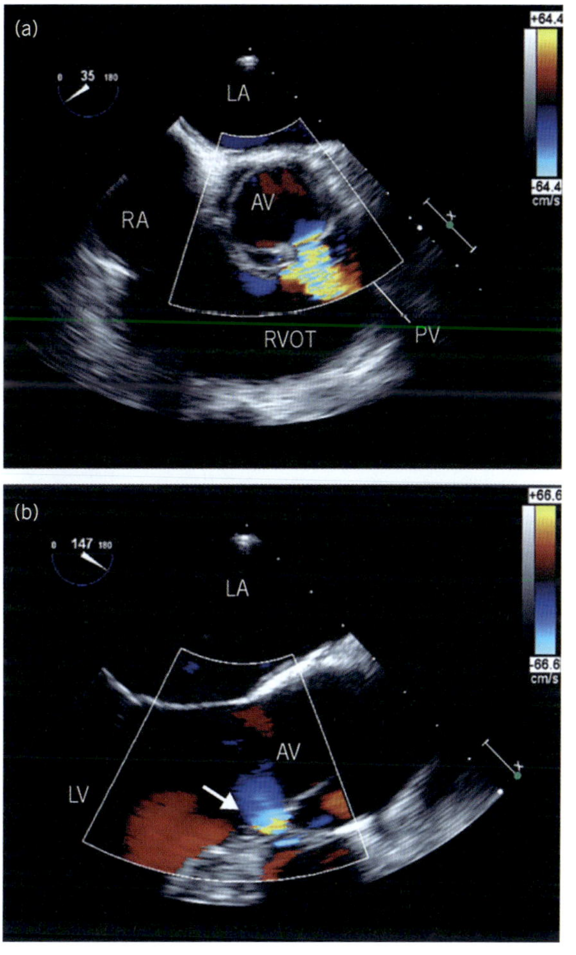

Figure 18.10 Outlet VSD. (a) is a mid-oesophageal RV inflow–outflow view in systole, with colour Doppler imaging. A VSD can be seen adjacent to the PV. Its location adjacent to the PV indicates its location is in the outlet portion of the septum. (b) is a mid-oesophageal AV long-axis view in systole, with colour Doppler imaging. A region of flow acceleration (arrow) can be seen below the AV. As stated in Figure 18.9, it may be difficult to ascertain in the AV long-axis view whether the VSD is in the outlet or membranous portions of the septum. Flow is from left to right.

ring. The prevalence of AVSDs is about 5% but increases to 15–30% in patients with Down syndrome. On echocardiography, this is demonstrated by the left and right A-V valves in the same anatomic plane (Figure 18.11a). The arrangement of the aorta is also changed, displaced anterosuperiorly, resulting in the LVOT being elongated and narrow (the 'gooseneck' deformity—Figure 18.11b). There are several classification systems for AVSDs, but they can be categorized as follows for simplicity:

- **Complete AVSD:** a complete AVSD has a primum ASD and an inlet VSD. A common A-V valve is present, which has *five* leaflets (superior and inferior bridging leaflets, left and right mural leaflets, and a right antero-septal leaflet).
- **Partial AVSD:** in a partial AVSD, there is a primum ASD, but no VSD. The five-leaflet common A-V valve is variably attached to the crest of the ventricular septum, resulting in the A-V valve being divided into separate right and left A-V valves. This results in a 'cleft' between the left A-V valve's superior and inferior bridging leaflets (Figure 18.12). It is important to note that there is *no true mitral or tricuspid valve, and*

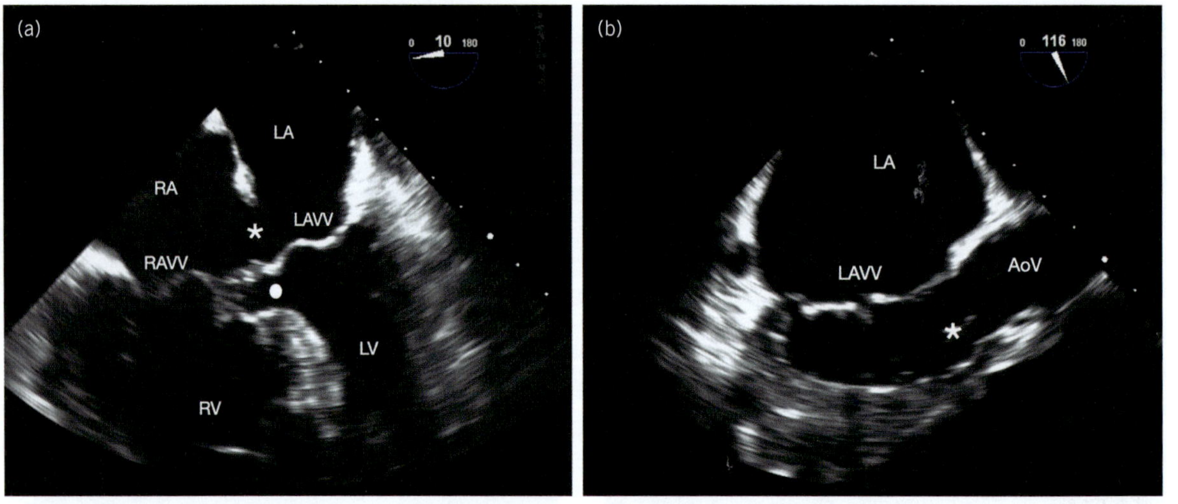

Figure 18.11 Atrioventricular canal defect. (a) Mid-oesophageal four-chamber view showing a large primum ASD (*) and a small inlet VSD (•), which is restricted by the subvalvular apparatus of the right atrioventricular valve (RAVV). (b) Mid-oesophageal AV long-axis view showing a long and slender LVOT (*), typical of the 'goose neck' appearance.

the valves should be correctly termed left and right A-V valves.

- **Transitional AVSD:** a transitional AVSD has a primum ASD and a restrictive VSD (the restriction is caused by partial occlusion from significant chordal attachments of the superior bridging leaflet). The left and right A-V valves are separate, as seen in the partial AVSD.

The effects of an AVSD are dependent upon the type and degree of shunting and valvular regurgitation if present. If an atrial shunt is predominant, it will cause right heart volume overload. A ventricular shunt will increase pulmonary blood flow and left heart volume overload.

The aims of imaging are to assess the anatomy and detect any residual lesions. Surgery is required to repair an AVSD, and given the complexity, only an experienced congenital cardiac surgeon should perform such procedures.[4] Surgical closure of a primum ASD is recommended in those with significant RV volume overload. The most frequent long-term problem noted in a repaired AVSD is left A-V valve regurgitation. As mentioned earlier, these valves are different from a mitral valve and are more difficult to repair. When surgical replacement is required, special consideration should be given to the resulting effect upon the LVOT. When a tissue valve is implanted, the echocardiographer should ensure that the struts do not impinge on the outflow tract and cause significant obstruction. Techniques to overcome such issues include placing the valve in a supra-annular position or undersizing the valve.

Right ventricular outflow tract obstruction

Right ventricular outflow tract obstruction (RVOTO) can be *sub-infundibular*, *infundibular*, *valvular*, or *supra-valvular* in nature. **Sub-infundibular stenosis**, or double-chambered right ventricle, results from hypertrophy of the septo-marginal trabeculation, resulting in a high-pressure inflow chamber and a lower-pressure infundibular chamber. The high-pressure RV inflow chamber commonly communicates with a VSD. **Infundibular stenosis** is commonly associated with other lesions (VSD, ToF, and pulmonary stenosis). Narrowing of the orifice during systole results in dynamic outflow obstruction.

Pulmonary stenosis (PS) accounts for approximately 9% of CHD. The PV is typically dome-like in shape, with a narrow central opening. Less frequently, the valve may be dysplastic and myxomatous, with poorly moving cusps. This pattern is often associated with Noonan syndrome. **Supra-valvular stenosis** is commonly associated with ToF, and Williams and Noonan syndromes. The narrowing can be at the level of the main pulmonary artery trunk or the pulmonary branches. Occasionally, it can be iatrogenic from scar tissue from prior pulmonary artery banding.

TOE provides detailed information about the RVOT, PV, and pulmonary artery. Turbulent accelerated flow demonstrated by colour Doppler can identify the level of the stenosis.

Accurate Doppler assessment of **RVOT obstruction** may be challenging. Poor Doppler alignment and/or RV dysfunction leads to underestimation of the severity,

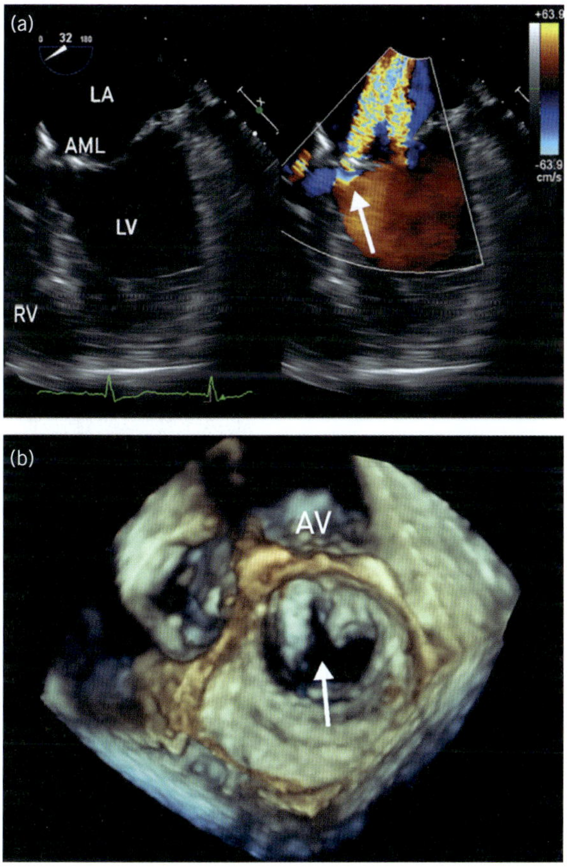

Figure 18.12 Left atrioventricular valve. (a) demonstrates two mid-oesophageal four-chamber views, with and without colour Doppler imaging in a dual-screen layout. Two jets of regurgitation can be seen. One jet arises from the coaptation line; a second jet (arrow) arises between the left atrioventricular valve's superior and inferior bridging leaflets. (b) shows a 3D view of the left atrioventricular valve from the atrial aspect in the surgical orientation (i.e. the aortic valve is at the 12 o'clock position). The large 'cleft' (arrow) can be seen between the left atrioventricular valve's superior and inferior bridging leaflets. This patient also had a primum ASD, which is not shown in these images.

whereas a long tubular narrowing can lead to overestimation. The severity of **pulmonary stenosis** is assessed with CW Doppler measurements (see Chapter 15). A peak velocity of <3 m/s suggests mild stenosis, and a velocity of >4 m/s represents severe PS; lesions with peak velocities of between 3 and 4 m/s are deemed moderate. Any chronic obstruction to RV outflow will lead to RV hypertrophy. The assessment of RV hypertrophy and RV function is discussed in Chapter 14.

Other imaging modalities are often required to assess RVOT anatomy, and CT and MRI are particularly useful in preoperative/interventional planning.[5] Balloon valvuloplasty is the intervention of choice in valvular PS. Regardless of symptoms, it is recommended for severe PS if the PV is anatomically suitable. Surgery is required for severe PS when patients are symptomatic or if they have evidence of one or more of the following: (1) decreasing exercise capacity; (2) decreasing RV function and/or progression to at least moderate TR; (3) a right ventricular systolic pressure (RVSP) of >80 mmHg; or (4) right-to-left shunting via an ASD or a VSD.

Peripheral pulmonary artery narrowing can be addressed with percutaneous balloon dilation. Stenting for dysplastic and hypoplastic pulmonary arteries surgery may be required.[4]

Tetralogy of Fallot

Tetralogy of Fallot (ToF) is the most common cyanotic CHD lesion. It is characterized by a large unrestricted VSD, RVOTO, an overriding aorta, and RV hypertrophy (Figure 18.13). All result from the antero-cephalic deviation of the outlet septum. ToF spans a spectrum of conditions, ranging from patients without any significant RVOTO to those with pulmonary atresia and a VSD. Associated anomalies include a right-sided aortic arch, anomalous coronary ostia, and ASD, as well as additional VSDs. Up to 25% of cases are associated with 22q11 deletion syndrome.

It is very unusual in industrialized nations to encounter an adult with ToF who has not undergone repair in childhood. Surgical repair in infancy involves patch closure of the VSD and relief of the RVOTO. Early repairs favouring an aggressive approach to RVOTO and trans-annular patches often resulted in severe pulmonary regurgitation. At present, the aim is to preserve the function of the PV. Techniques include pulmonary valvuloplasty, with patching limited to the infundibulum. However, in cases with a small PV annulus, a trans-annular patch may still be necessary to alleviate RVOTO. Other surgical techniques involve the implantation of a mono-cusp valve, a valved RV-to- pulmonary artery conduit, or a homograft valve.

Imaging adult patients with repaired ToF should focus on identifying the potential long-term complications. These include severe pulmonary regurgitation (PR—Figure 18.14), residual RVOTO (Figure 18.15), RV dilatation and dysfunction, residual VSD, an additional VSD not noted at the time of the initial repair, aortic root dilatation, AR, and LV dysfunction.

As the pulmonary valve itself is not always visible by TOE, severe PR can be diagnosed by a broad diastolic jet from the pulmonary artery to the RVOT (Figure 18.14), along with a dense signal with a rapid return to baseline on CW Doppler. Although echocardiography can assess

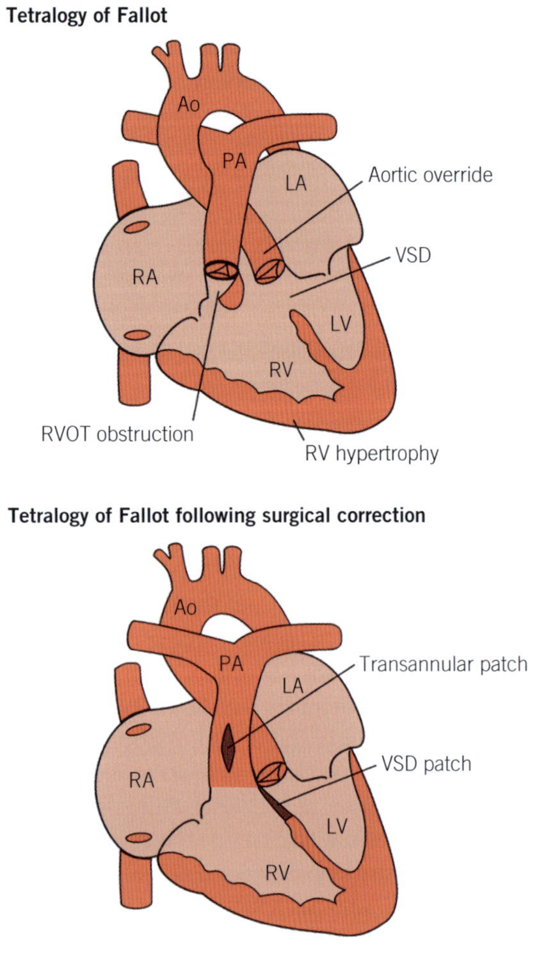

Figure 18.13 Schematic demonstrating tetralogy of Fallot before and after surgical correction. See text for details.

Reprinted from *Cardiothoracic Critical Care*, D Sidebotham, A McKee, M Gillham, JH Levy, Figures 15.1 and 15.3, pages 228 and 229, Copyright 2007, Elsevier.

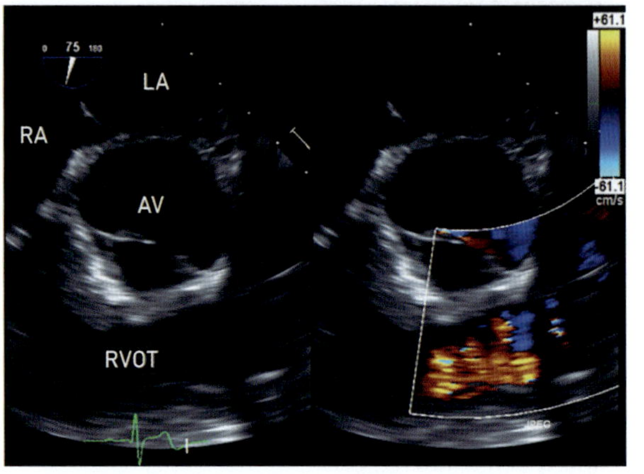

Figure 18.14 Pulmonary regurgitation following tetralogy of Fallot repair. Mid-oesophageal RV inflow–outflow view in diastole, showing the RVOT without and with colour Doppler in dual-screen layout. A large jet of pulmonary regurgitation is seen filling the RVOT in diastole.

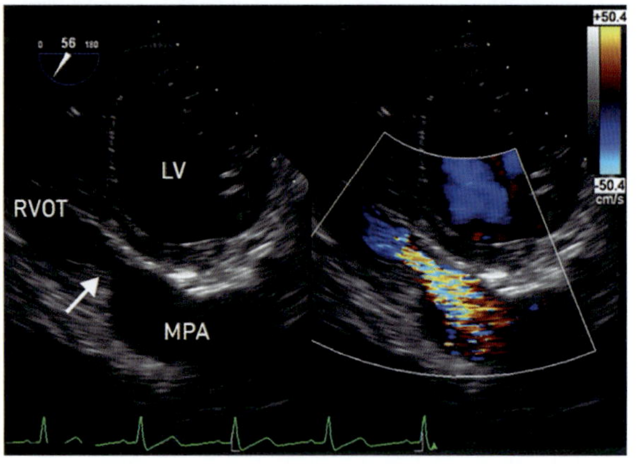

Figure 18.15 Stenosis of the RVOT following tetralogy of Fallot repair. Transgastric RV outflow view in systole, showing the RVOT without and with colour Doppler in dual-screen layout. The RVOT is narrowed (arrow) due to the presence of subvalvular muscle bundles. With colour Doppler imaging, marked turbulence is seen in the RVOT, consistent with RVOT stenosis.

RV size and function well, cardiac MRI is superior in the assessment of ventricular volumes and function, so it is the preferred modality to determine whether surgical replacement is required for severe PR.[5] PV replacement is recommended in symptomatic patients with severe PR. In patients with an RV-to-pulmonary artery conduit, a catheter-based intervention is preferred if it is anatomically feasible. In asymptomatic individuals with severe PR and/or RVOTO, a PV replacement may be considered if there is: (1) a decrease in exercise capacity; (2) progressive RV dilatation (RVESVi >80 mL/m^2 or RVEDVi >160 mL/m^2, where RVESVi is RV end-systolic volume index and RVEDVi is RV end-diastolic volume index); (3) progression to at least moderate TR; (4) progressive RV systolic dysfunction; or (5) an RVOTO with RVSP of >80 mmHg.[4]

Ebstein anomaly

Though **Ebstein anomaly** accounts for only 0.5% of congenital heart lesions, it is the most common congenital heart lesion of the tricuspid valve. Resulting from a failure of delamination of the valve tissue from the underlying myocardium, its severity depends on the degree to which this occurs. Severe forms have a poor prognosis, whereas mild forms may only be found incidentally in adulthood. The condition is characterized by apical displacement of the septal and posterior leaflets from the atrioventricular junction into the RV (Figure 18.16).

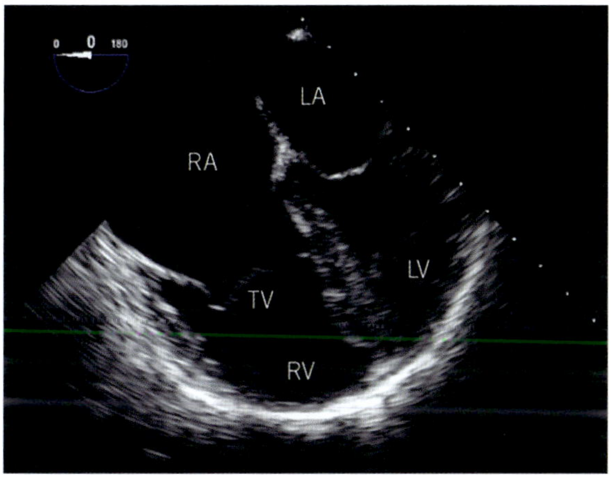

Figure 18.16 Ebstein anomaly, shown in a mid-oesophageal four-chamber view. Note the apical displacement of the TV (compare it with the much more basal attachment of the MV) and the 'atrialization' of part of the RV.

Apical displacement of the septal tricuspid leaflet of >8 mm/m^2 is diagnostic, and all of the TV leaflets are abnormal. The septal and posterior leaflets are dysplastic and adherent to the RV walls, often tethered by short anomalous cords. The 'sail-like' anterior leaflet is not usually displaced but is elongated and redundant. The anterior leaflet is often tethered to the ventricular free wall by chordal attachments, and the papillary muscles may be displaced. Fenestrations can be noted within the Ebstein valve, particularly within the anterior leaflet. The apical displacement of the valve results in reduction of the functional RV size, with 'atrialization' of the RV between the anatomical and functional tricuspid annulus. Ebstein anomaly is often associated with other lesions—an ASD or a PFO occurs in >50% of cases, and an accessory conduction pathway is present in approximately 25%. RVOTO, LV non-compaction, VSD, and coarctation of the aorta may also be associated.

Echocardiography helps to assess the severity of the disease and guide clinical decision-making. Surgery is indicated in patients with symptomatic severe TR and/or objective deterioration of exercise capacity. Patients with progressive right heart dilatation or reduction of RV systolic function should be considered for surgical intervention regardless of symptoms. Numerous views may be required to assess the TV in detail and appreciate the functional size of the RV (see Chapter 15). Imaging should aim to determine whether the valve tissue is sufficient for successful repair or whether a replacement is required. Surgery should be undertaken by an adult congenital surgeon with specific experience in Ebstein valve repair. Typically, surgery involves closure of the ASD or PFO if present, plication of the atrialized portion of the RV, and right atrioplasty. In some cases where the RV is particularly small, a bidirectional Glenn procedure is required to offload the RV.

Transposition of the great arteries

Transposition of the great arteries (TGA), also known as *D-transposition*, is characterized by discordant connection of the great arteries, such that the pulmonary trunk arises from the LV and the aorta arises from the RV. TGA is described as *simple* in the absence of other abnormalities, or *complex* when other abnormalities are present such as VSD, LVOT obstruction, pulmonary stenosis, and occasionally coarctation of the aorta. With TGA, the pulmonary and systemic circulations run *parallel to each other*, resulting in severe hypoxaemia, which is incompatible with life without adequate mixing of blood from a VSD, an ASD, or a patent ductus arteriosus (PDA) (Figure 18.17a). In the absence of a significant shunt, an atrial balloon septostomy is required in the first few days of life before definitive surgery is performed.

Historically, a **Mustard** or **Senning procedure** was performed to correct this lesion—also termed 'atrial switch procedures', these surgical repairs redirect venous return to the contralateral ventricle via the creation of atrial baffles. This results in physiologic correction of the circulation, but at the expense of the RV becoming the systemic ventricle, which results in RV hypertrophy and dilatation, and eventually systolic dysfunction. Atrial arrhythmias can occur, with the most common being cavo-tricuspid isthmus-dependent flutter, though atrial fibrillation also occurs. The atrial baffles are prone to becoming stenosed or to leaking, and TOE is particularly helpful in identifying these problems (Figure 18.17b).

In recent years, the 'arterial switch' or Jatene repair has become the preferred technique to correct TGA. Designed to restore the LV as the systemic ventricle, the aorta is removed from the RV and attached to the LV. The pulmonary artery is removed from the LV and attached to the RV. Reimplantation of the coronary arteries into the neo-aorta is then performed (Figure 18.17c). Long-term sequelae include neo-aortic root dilatation and resultant AR. Supra-valvular PS and pulmonary branch stenosis may also result from the position of the pulmonary bifurcation anterior to the ascending aorta. Rarely, proximal coronary artery disease can develop from prior reimplantation into the neo-aorta, resulting in LV dysfunction and ventricular arrhythmias.

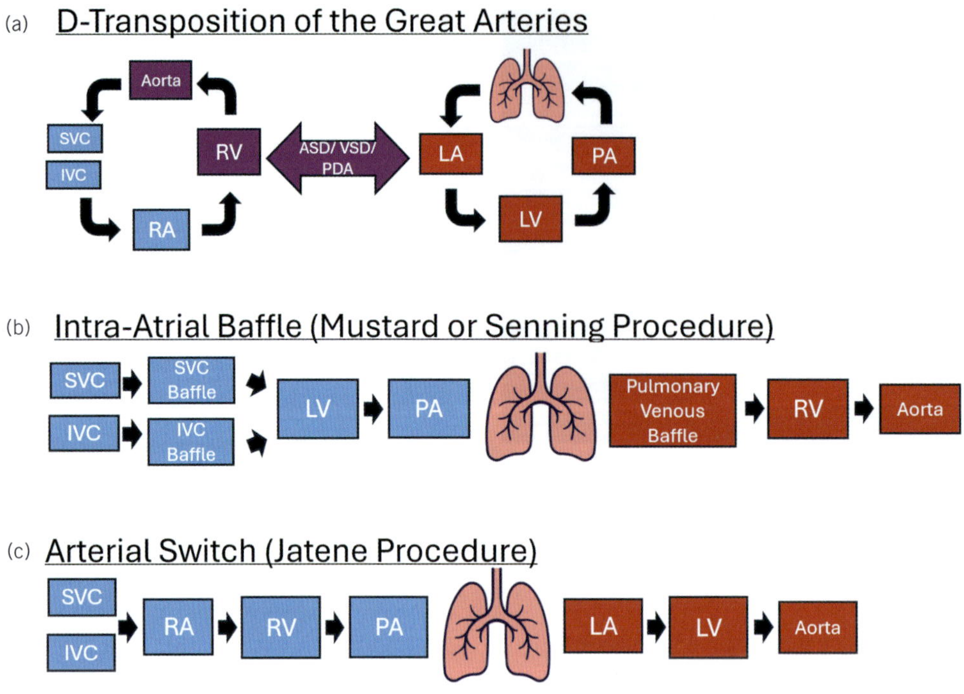

Figure 18.17 Transposition of the great arteries. Panel (a) illustrates the blood flow in a patient with uncorrected D-transposition of the great arteries, where the PA arises from the LV and the aorta arises from the RV. The systemic and pulmonary circulations operate in parallel, such that some shunting of blood between the two circuits (ASD, VSD, or PDA) must be present for the patient to survive. Panel (b) shows the blood flow following a Mustard or Senning procedure, where intra-atrial baffles are created to direct deoxygenated blood from the SVC/IVC to the LV, the PA, and the lungs (Mustard and Senning are the same correction, except Mustard uses prosthetic material to create the baffles, whereas Senning uses the patient's own tissues). This procedure corrects the hypoxaemia, but at the cost of making the RV the new systemic ventricle (see text for details). Panel (c) illustrates the blood flow following an arterial switch (or Jatene) procedure, where the aorta and pulmonary arteries are reconnected to their proper ventricles, thereby restoring the normal circulation. This has become the preferred technique to correct TGA.

Congenitally corrected transposition of the great arteries

Congenitally corrected transposition of the great arteries (ccTGA), also known as L-transposition, is rare, accounting for only 1% of congenital cardiac malformations. It is characterized by atrioventricular and ventriculoarterial discordance. The RA connects to the LV through the MV, and the LV then connects to the pulmonary artery. The LA connects to the RV through the TV, and the RV then ejects into the aorta. The RV is therefore the systemic ventricle. The most common associated lesion is an abnormal TV noted in 90% of autopsy findings, a perimembranous VSD present in 50%, and PS in 30–50%. Other reported lesions are coarctation of the aorta and conduction system abnormalities (the risk of complete heart block is 2–3% per year). The TV is the systemic A-V valve and is often dysplastic. The septal and posterior leaflets can be apically displaced. This malformation is often less amenable to repair than the Ebstein TV. The long-term prognosis of individuals with ccTGA is determined by the severity of the associated lesions and the degree of TR. Without other defects, an individual may remain undetected until adulthood, when the presentation is often secondary to conduction disease or heart failure.

The usual atrial arrangement is noted in the 0° mid-oesophageal four-chamber view, but with a reversed arrangement to the A-V valves and the ventricles (Figure 18.18). The TV and RV are where the MV and LV would be expected to be. The TV can be recognized by its apical displacement relative to the MV, and the morphologic RV by the presence of a *moderator band*. Note that mitral–aortic continuity will not be seen in the usual 120° mid-oesophageal view, and the great arteries will appear to run parallel. Careful assessment of the TV is required to determine the degree of regurgitation. The systemic–RV systolic function assessment by echocardiography can be challenging and is often estimated visually.

TV replacement is indicated in symptomatic individuals with severe TR and preserved or mildly impaired systemic–RV systolic function, and should be considered in asymptomatic patients with severe TR and progressive systemic–RV dilatation and/or mildly reduced systemic–RV systolic function.

Univentricular heart

The **single ventricle** or **univentricular heart** is a broad term that encompasses a variety of cardiac structural abnormalities, in which one ventricle is severely underdeveloped (Figure 18.19). Either the sub-pulmonic or the systemic ventricle fails to grow properly; there may be a deficient or an absent inlet, or an obstructive or absent outlet. In all these cases, the goal of surgical repair is to connect the functional ventricle with an outlet to the systemic circulation and to create cavo-pulmonary connections, so that blood can flow passively from the SVC and IVC directly into the pulmonary arteries.

Most adults with a single ventricle will have undergone a prior Fontan procedure, where the SVC connects to the pulmonary arteries via a superior cavo-pulmonary anastomosis or a Glenn procedure; it can connect to the right, left, or both pulmonary arteries. Visualizing the Glenn connection is challenging via TOE but can sometimes be achieved in the mid-oesophageal ascending aorta long-axis and the upper oesophageal aortic arch short-axis views. Clockwise or anticlockwise rotation is used to visualize the right- or left-sided connection. Flow at the connection is passive; therefore, turbulence suggests narrowing at the connection. The presence of a thrombus at the site should also be excluded.

In the current era of Fontan repair, flow from the IVC is directed to the pulmonary arteries via an intracardiac lateral tunnel or an extra-cardiac conduit. An older type of repair, the atrio-pulmonary connection, is still seen; the RA is significantly dilated in such cases. The IVC flow and connection to the Fontan conduit can be assessed in the usual IVC transgastric view. The mid-oesophageal bicaval view allows visualization of the baffle longitudinally.

The assessment of single-ventricle systolic function is challenging. Qualitative assessment from multiple mid-oesophageal and transgastric views is recommended to gain an overall impression of the systolic function. The biplane Simpson's method is inaccurate with a single ventricle and should not be used. 3D imaging can aid in interventional procedures, demonstrate thrombus within the Fontan circuit, and assess the A-V valve in detail.

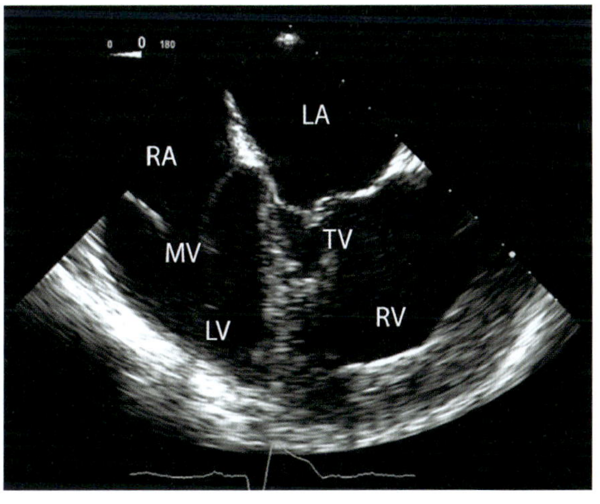

Figure 18.18 Congenitally corrected transposition of the great arteries. Mid-oesophageal four-chamber view demonstrating the anatomy of L-transposition of the great arteries. The RA connects to the right-sided LV via the MV, and the LA connects to the left-sided RV via the TV.

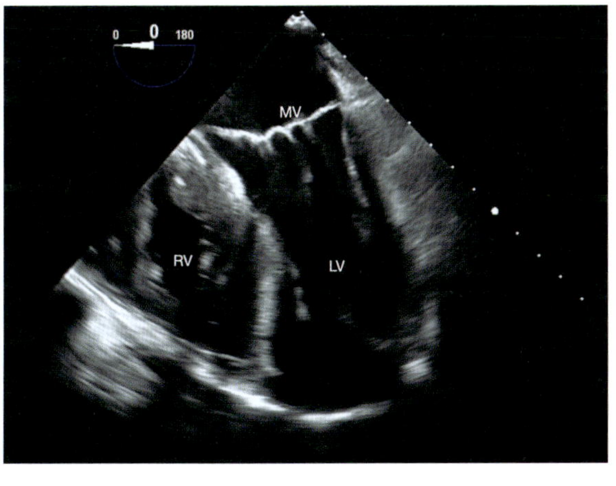

Figure 18.19 Double-inlet LV. This mid-oesophageal 'four-chamber' view shows a prominent LV and a small hypoplastic RV, which connects to the LV via a VSD (not shown in this image).

Multiple choice questions

Discover interactive multiple choice questions to test your knowledge on this chapter by searching for this book's title or ISBN (9780198873686) at **https://academic.oup.com/** and going to the online appendix at the end of the book. Use your scratch-off code on the inside cover to access the material.

References

1. Van Der Linde D, Konings EE, Slager MA, *et al.* Birth prevalence of congenital heart disease worldwide: a systematic review and meta-analysis. *J Am Coll Cardiol.* 2011;**58**(21):2241–7.

2. Moons P, Bovijn L, Budts W, Belmans A, Gewillig M. Temporal trends in survival to adulthood among patients born with congenital heart disease from 1970 to 1992 in Belgium. *Circulation.* 2010;**122**(22):2264–72.
3. Lopez L, Houyel L, Colan SD, *et al.* Classification of ventricular septal defects for the eleventh iteration of the International Classification of Diseases—striving for consensus: a report from the International Society for Nomenclature of Paediatric and Congenital Heart Disease. *Ann Thorac Surg.* 2018;**106**(5):1578–89.
4. Baumgartner H, De Backer J, Babu-Narayan SV, *et al.* 2020 ESC Guidelines for the management of adult congenital heart disease: the Task Force for the management of adult congenital heart disease of the European Society of Cardiology (ESC). Endorsed by: Association for European Paediatric and Congenital Cardiology (AEPC), International Society for Adult Congenital Heart Disease (ISACHD). *Eur Heart J.* 2021;**42**(6):563–645.
5. Di Salvo G, Miller O, Babu Narayan S, *et al.* Imaging the adult with congenital heart disease: a multimodality imaging approach—position paper from the EACVI. *Eur Heart J Cardiovasc Imaging.* 2018;**19**(10):1077–98.

19 Heart and lung transplantation

This chapter will review perioperative TOE imaging in the context of heart and lung transplantation. The first section will discuss heart transplantation, while the second section will review lung transplantation.

Heart transplantation

Assessment of potential donor heart

While cardiac transplantation is a definitive treatment for end-stage heart failure, echocardiographic assessment to establish donor heart suitability is critical. TTE or TOE may be used, although TOE may be preferred in mechanically ventilated donors. Comprehensive echocardiographic evaluation includes assessment of biventricular function, as well as identification of structural abnormalities precluding transplantation. The presence of intracranial pathology, inotropic support, and intravascular volume status should also be considered.

Ventricular function

Despite some regional differences across the world, acceptance criteria typically include a normal LVEF of >55% and an absence of regional wall motion abnormality (RWMA) or LV hypertrophy (LVH), defined as LV posterior wall or interventricular septal thickness of >11 mm.[1,2] The catecholamine surge secondary to brainstem death is followed by vasoplegia, which may result in transient myocardial stunning and ventricular dysfunction with RWMA. LV apical function is often preserved, but RWMA may include multiple coronary artery territories without angiographic evidence of coronary artery disease. Such changes are transient and gradually improve with donor optimization and transplantation. Dobutamine stress echocardiography may be necessary to distinguish between reversible ventricular dysfunction and RWMA due to neurologic death, versus irreversible LV dysfunction.

Historically, one of the most common reasons for declining a donor heart was poor LV systolic function and/or the presence of LVH. However, as the demand for donor hearts increases, acceptance criteria have expanded in some centres to include hearts with LVEF of <45% or LV wall thickness of 11–13 mm. Recipient mortality at 1 year appears unchanged with donor hearts with mild LV dysfunction or mild LVH.[3,4] However, LVH of >14 mm, donor age of >55 years, and ischaemic time of >4 hours are associated with worse outcomes.[1,4]

Structural abnormalities

Significant valvular abnormalities are generally uncommon in potential donor hearts. Mild central MR is the most prevalent lesion and is not a contraindication to transplantation in the absence of structural valvular abnormalities. Moderate to severe TR or mild stenosis of a bicuspid AV are less common but are typically contraindications to transplantation. As acceptance criteria expand, a case-by-case analysis of donor suitability with bench repair or replacement of valvular abnormalities at the time of transplantation may be considered. A patent foramen ovale (PFO) or small ASD is not a contraindication to transplantation but should be noted (and repaired), as the potential for shunting may occur post-operatively. Structural compromise of the right heart secondary to external resuscitative compressions should also be ruled out.

Intraoperative assessment of the recipient's native heart

Recipients with end-stage heart failure may have concurrent mechanical assist devices, transvenous pacemakers, and defibrillators *in situ*. LA or LV thrombus may be present and require minimizing handling of the native heart to prevent inadvertent embolization. Structural cardiac and great vessel abnormalities may be present due to previous cardiac surgery, catheter-based interventions, pre-existing congenital lesions, or cardiac compressions (Figure 19.1; see Online appendix 11.6.4). Placement of invasive monitoring, such as arterial lines, central venous, and pulmonary artery catheters, may be impacted. The

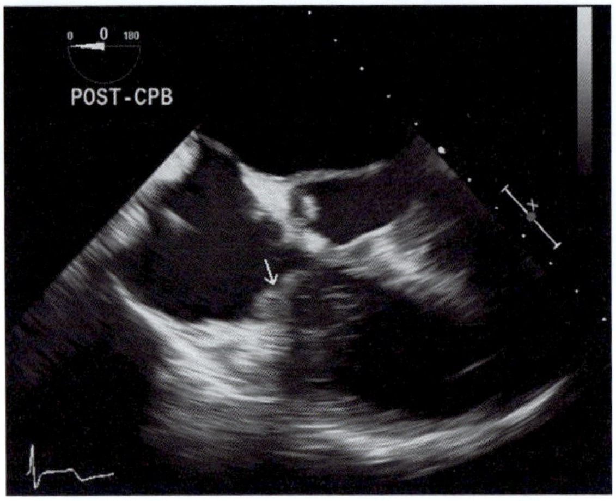

Figure 19.1 Right atrial clot in the newly transplanted heart. This mid-oesophageal four-chamber view focused on the right heart demonstrates a thrombus in the RA, just above the TV (arrow). Return to CPB and inspection of the RA revealed a cardiac contusion that led to the adjacent thrombosis, presumed to have been caused by external cardiac compressions in the donor. See Online appendix 11.6.4.

presence of aortic atheroma should be assessed in case an intra-aortic balloon pump is needed post-transplantation. The degree of pulmonary hypertension should be evaluated by CW Doppler interrogation of the TR jet, and the presence of pleural effusions should be noted and can be drained intraoperatively.[5]

Early assessment following heart transplantation

Prior to separation from CPB, adequacy of de-airing should be ensured, particularly at the LV apex or anastomotic sites (see Chapter 6 for discussion on intracardiac air). Positioning of the patient in Trendelenburg prior to cross-clamp removal may minimize air emboli to the head vessels. Once ejection of the transplanted heart has been established, a preliminary assessment of gross ventricular and valvular morphology and function should be performed. During weaning from CPB, attention should be directed to preload, systolic function, and valvular function. If significant ventricular or valvular dysfunction is noted, optimization of pharmacologic support and plans for potential mechanical circulatory support may be required prior to successful separation from CPB. A comprehensive assessment of the transplanted heart should be conducted once successfully separated from CPB.

LV function

LV systolic dysfunction may be due to the combined effects of brain death and suboptimal myocardial protection, and it generally resolves over the following hours to days. Pacing of the heart may result in septal wall motion abnormalities. Primary graft dysfunction (PGD) can occur within the first 24 hours of transplantation and clinically can result in cardiogenic shock. Other causes of shock, such as cardiac tamponade or inadequate filling status, may be differentiated by echocardiography. LV mass may initially appear to be increased due to underfilling or tissue oedema. Global longitudinal strain (GLS) (see Chapter 6) has been shown to be an independent predictor of all-cause mortality and major adverse cardiovascular events, with incremental prognostic value, even when compared with established post-orthotopic cardiac transplant clinical predictors such as history of rejection, LVEF/right ventricular ejection fraction (RVEF), and cardiac allograft vasculopathy. The predictive value of GLS remains significant in the face of preserved LVEF and in the absence of obvious myocardial damage by late gadolinium enhancement, and thus GLS may play a larger role in the evaluation of the transplanted heart in the future.[6]

Assessment of LV diastolic function may be complicated by an elevated heart rate in the denervated heart and resultant E–A-wave fusion. Biatrial anastomoses may result in dual RA activity with pulmonary venous flow reflecting the recipient's own atrial activity. Diastolic function may be altered due to ischaemia of the graft or precapillary pulmonary hypertension of the recipient. Therefore, restrictive physiology is common in the immediate post-transplant period and has no prognostic value.[7]

RV function

Immediately post-operatively, RV dysfunction is common due to the physiologic effects of neurologic death, suboptimal myocardial protection, elevated pulmonary vascular resistance (PVR) in the recipient, possible size mismatch, and potential air emboli to the right coronary artery. RV volumes tend to be elevated initially as well, again due to elevated PVR of the recipient. Over the next few months, RV size decreases concurrently as PVR decreases.[7]

Immediate post-transplant RV systolic function measured by classical echocardiographic methods such as tricuspid annular plane systolic excursion (TAPSE), FAC, and GLS of the free wall all trend lower than normal accepted values. Furthermore, echocardiographic values for RV function are no longer sensitive markers in the long-term assessment of a transplanted heart when compared to cardiac MRI. FAC remains the most correlative value in longer-term assessments of RV function.[8]

Assessment of surgical anastomoses

The surgical technique affects echocardiographic findings. Bicaval anastomoses should not affect atrial geometry.[7] Biatrial/modified biatrial suture lines may appear as echo-dense ridges in the right or left atria (Figure 19.2). Acquired cor triatriatum and mid-atrial stenosis due to tense suture lines may be identified with PW Doppler and/or 3D imaging. SVC, IVC, pulmonary venous, pulmonary arterial, and aortic anastomotic sites should all be assessed with colour Doppler and PW Doppler to rule out stenoses—aliasing flow by colour Doppler at an anastomotic site warrants careful examination. Once the chest is closed, localized pericardial effusions and/or tamponade may indicate bleeding from atrial suture lines.

Valvular abnormalities

Although significant structural valvular disease is usually a reason to decline a donor heart, new functional MR due to impaired LV function and papillary muscle oedema is common in the early post-CPB period and should improve over time. Significant functional TR secondary to RV dysfunction, pulmonary arterial hypertension, or fluid overload reduces 5-year survival, and donor bench TV annuloplasty may improve the prognosis.[9]

Late assessment following heart transplantation

Pericardial fluid

As the (normal-size) transplanted heart is often inserted into an enlarged pericardial sac caused by dilation of the recipient's failing native heart, post-operative pericardial collections are common. Small to moderate pericardial effusions are observed in two-thirds of patients at 3 months post-operatively and remain present in one-quarter of patients at 6 months.[7] Serial imaging to assess for changes in size and location of effusions should be performed. Causes of enlarging effusions or new-onset effusions include graft rejection, RV perforation post-endomyocardial biopsy, infection, or neoplasm.

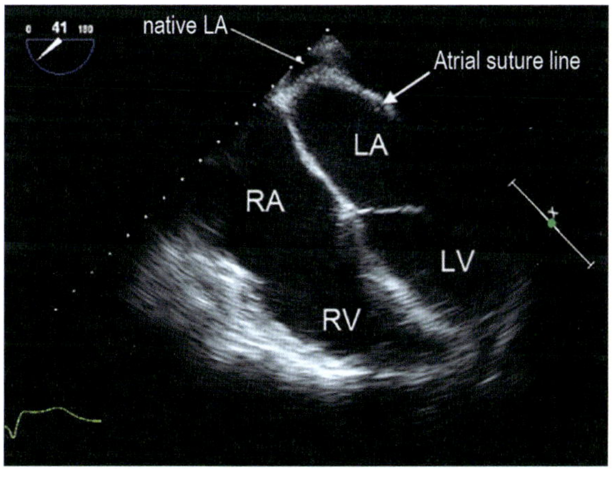

Figure 19.2 Atrial suture line. This is a mid-oesophageal four-chamber view (obtained at 40° of transducer rotation in this freshly transplanted heart) demonstrating the atrial suture line as a bright ridge in the LA, with the native LA above and new donor LA below the ridge. See also Online appendices 11.6.1 and 11.6.2.

Acute rejection

Acute graft rejection is the leading cause of mortality in the first year post-heart transplantation.[10] Endomyocardial biopsy is the gold standard for diagnosis, but echocardiography is often used to assess the need for biopsy as early acute rejection may be associated with changes in diastolic filling patterns. Restrictive patterns—with reduced e', a', and s' on TDI of the MV—correlate with rejection; however, such patterns are not necessarily specific and may be pre-existing due to the physiology of the denervated transplanted heart.[11] Graft rejection is usually a focal process and leads to segmental myocardial dysfunction. Reduction in LV segmental and global strain rates may occur due to diminished global systolic function.[7] Other abnormalities such as new or enlarging pericardial effusions, new valvular regurgitation, and ventricular dilatation may be present.

Cardiac allograft vasculopathy

Chronic rejection is due to cardiac allograft vasculopathy (CAV), a diffuse process that affects coronary epicardial and microvasculature. Stress echocardiography is often used as a screening tool for CAV. Given the challenge of reaching a target heart rate in a denervated heart, exercise stress echocardiography has a low sensitivity. However, dobutamine stress echocardiography has a sensitivity of between 70% and 80% for detecting RWMA due to angiographically significant CAV. Systolic function is generally preserved, even in advanced forms of CAV.[11]

Lung transplantation

Patients undergoing lung transplantation are vulnerable to haemodynamic instability perioperatively due to various patient and surgical factors. The most common indications for lung transplantation are interstitial lung disease (ILD), advanced chronic obstructive pulmonary disease (COPD), cystic fibrosis (CF), and pulmonary arterial hypertension (PAH).[12] Pre-existing pulmonary vascular hypertension, RV dysfunction, and limited cardiorespiratory

Table 19.1 Pre-transplant TOE assessment

IAS	• Identify PFO/ASD • Colour Doppler/contrast assessment of shunt
RV morphology	• Size: mid-oesophageal four-chamber minor axis <3.5 cm • Wall thickness: transgastric short-axis inferior wall <5 mm
RV function	• Fractional area change: mid-oesophageal four-chamber view (normal >35%) • TAPSE: using M-mode (normal >16 mm): deep transgastric view • RIMP*: using PW Doppler (normal <0.4) • Septal position and motion (flattening, bulging to the left in systole and/or diastole) • Transgastric mid-papillary short-axis view • Baseline RVSP: using CW Doppler of TR jet (normal <2.8 m/s)[5] in RV inflow–outflow view/bicaval view
LV function	• Systolic function transgastric short-axis view
Pulmonary veins	• Baseline diameter (normal >5 mm) • Baseline velocity (normal <100 cm/s)

* RIMP = IVCT + IVRT/ET.

RIMP, right ventricular index of myocardial performance; IVCT, isovolumic contraction time; IVRT, isovolumic relaxation time; ET, ejection time.

Adapted from Evans A *et al.*, 'Intraoperative echocardiography for patients undergoing lung transplantation', *Anesthesia and Analgesia*, **118**, 4, pp. 725–30, copyright 2014, International Anesthesia Research Society https://journals.lww.com/anesthesia-analgesia/pages/default.aspx

reserve are common in these patients, and the time span between initial listing for transplant and organ availability warrants careful assessment of the LV and RV function to detect interim deteriorations. In addition, the inter-atrial septum and pulmonary veins should be imaged to identify the presence of an intracardiac shunt or abnormal pulmonary venous morphology (Table 19.1).

Lung transplantation can be performed with or without CPB or extracorporeal membranous oxygenation (ECMO), and may require one-lung ventilation. The posterior anatomical location of the hilum requires frequent intraoperative manipulation of the heart, resulting in rapid fluctuations in preload and afterload. These fluctuations, coupled with the need to balance fluid administration to minimize acute lung injury in the setting of pre-existing RV systolic dysfunction, necessitate a comprehensive initial TOE examination and constant monitoring throughout the operative period.

Intraoperative assessment

RV function

Chronic and acute RV dysfunction is prevalent in patients undergoing lung transplantation. A comprehensive assessment of the right heart, as well as continuous monitoring throughout, is useful in guiding management and for early recognition of potential complications.

Evidence of RV systolic dysfunction may include RV dilation, reduced TAPSE and FAC, moderate to severe functional TR, and reduced TDI velocities or strain rates. Signs of RV pressure overload include RV hypertrophy, elevated right ventricular systolic pressure (RVSP), leftward bowing of the inter-atrial septum, and paradoxical motion of the interventricular septum during systole.[13]

Acute RV failure and haemodynamic collapse may be precipitated by ventilatory or oxygenation challenges. Induction of anaesthesia, positive pressure ventilation and/or one-lung ventilation, surgical manipulation of the heart (particularly during left lung implantation), unclamping of the pulmonary arteries, reperfusion of the lungs, and sternal closure can all lead to acute changes in RV preload, afterload, and function. Ongoing TOE monitoring of the RV at these time points is critical in guiding fluid management, titration of pharmacological RV support, optimization of gas exchange, and/or reinstitution of CPB/ECMO (Table 19.2).

Assessment of structural abnormalities

The presence of a PFO or an ASD, as well as the direction of shunt, should be evaluated by TOE. The presence of a PFO does not mandate closure but should be evaluated against the possibility of shunt-related hypoxaemia and haemodynamic instability.

Baseline evaluation with visualization and Doppler interrogation of the pulmonary arteries and all four pulmonary veins should be performed for comparison post-transplant.

LV function and preload

Assessment of LV function and preload may be challenging in patients undergoing lung transplantation, as RV dilation and pressure overload can cause leftward shifting of the interventricular septum and may result in a small or underfilled LV. Fluid management and titration of pharmacological support may be guided to a greater degree by assessment of the RV. Electrocardiographic changes and transient RWMA can occur due to compression, or even torsion, of coronary arteries during surgical manipulation of the heart.

Table 19.2 Intraprocedural assessment

Assess RV response to pulmonary artery cross-clamping	• Reassess size for chamber dilatation • Reassess TAPSE for contractility • Reassess TR jet for estimation of PA systolic pressure
If PFO present	• Colour Doppler assessment of reversibility of shunt

Adapted from Evans A *et al.*, 'Intraoperative echocardiography for patients undergoing lung transplantation', *Anesthesia and Analgesia*, **118**, 4, pp. 725–30, copyright 2014, International Anesthesia Research Society https://journals.lww.com/anesthesia-analgesia/pages/default.aspx

Assessment post-lung transplantation

(See Table 19.3.)

Assessment of surgical anastomoses

Pulmonary venous obstruction is an uncommon, but serious, complication of lung transplantation (Figure 19.3). Recipients with smaller thoracic cavities, such as those with small body habitus or restrictive lung disease, are at higher risk. Stenosis can arise from torsion, kinking, or external compression of the left- or right-sided tissue of atrial cuffs. Pulmonary venous obstruction or thrombosis may result in hypoxaemia, pulmonary oedema, and graft dysfunction.[14] Once both lungs are reperfused, visualization of all four pulmonary veins may be difficult, but at least one pulmonary vein from each operative lung should be assessed. A pulmonary venous diameter of <0.5 cm, peak systolic velocity of >1 m/s, loss of systolic flow dominance (S > D), and pulmonary vein-to-LA pressure gradient of >10–12 mmHg are all suggestive of clinically significant obstruction. A pulmonary vein diameter of <0.25 cm has been described as a threshold for graft failure. Surgical revision may be warranted if visible obstruction or thrombosis is noted.[15,16,17]

Persistent PAH due to narrowing of the pulmonary artery anastomoses is exceedingly rare. As the anastomoses may be too distal to be adequately visualized via TOE, epi-arterial echocardiography may be used.

Assessment of RVOT obstruction

Decreasing pulmonary artery pressures and reduction in RV cavity size may result in dynamic RV outflow tract obstruction, especially in the presence of RV hypertrophy. RVOT flow velocities of >2.0 m/s or the presence of an RV

Table 19.3 Post-transplant assessment

Pulmonary vein assessment (examine all four veins if possible)	• Diameter (normal >5 mm) • Laminar versus turbulence flow: colour Doppler • Velocity (normal <100 cm/s): PW Doppler
Pulmonary artery anastomosis	• Look for thrombus and air • Diameter (>75% of proximal pulmonary artery) • Laminar versus turbulence: colour Doppler in upper oesophageal ascending aorta short-axis view
Right ventricle assessment	• Right ventricular end-diastolic volume (look for dilatation) • TAPSE • Septal position • Reassess RVSP • RIMP*
Left ventricle assessment	• Preload • Systolic function • Presence of air
Flow across PFO (if exists)	• Determine direction of flow

* RIMP = (IVCT + IVRT)/ET.

RIMP, right ventricular index of myocardial performance; IVCT, isovolumic contraction time; IVRT, isovolumic relaxation time; ET, ejection time.

Adapted from Evans A *et al.*, 'Intraoperative echocardiography for patients undergoing lung transplantation', *Anesthesia and Analgesia*, **118**, 4, pp. 725–30, copyright 2014, International Anesthesia Research Society https://journals.lww.com/anesthesia-analgesia/pages/default.aspx

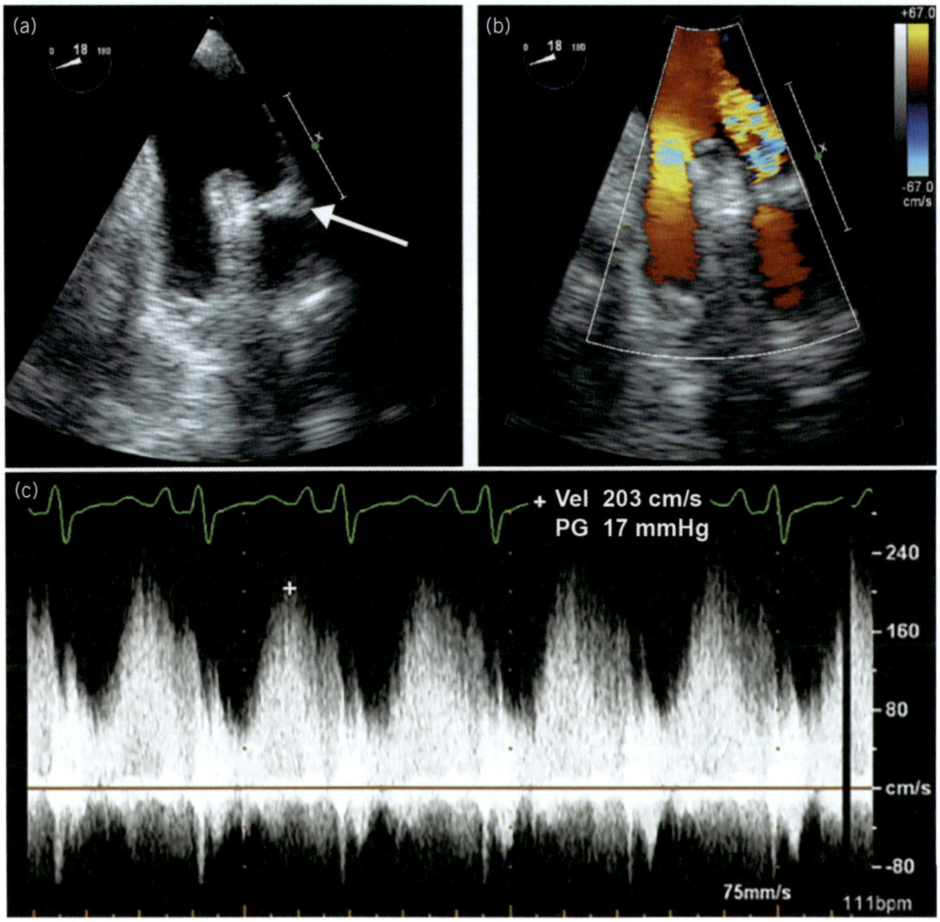

Figure 19.3 Obstructed pulmonary vein flow following lung transplantation. (a) and (b) are zoomed views of the left-sided pulmonary veins following lung transplantation. (a) 2D imaging shows an obstruction in one of the veins, which is probably the left upper vein. (b) With colour Doppler imaging, aliasing can be seen in the same pulmonary vein, suggesting an obstruction. (c) shows a PW Doppler waveform through the obstructed vein. The velocity (2.03 m/s) and calculated peak pressure gradient (17 mmHg) are significantly elevated. See also Online appendices 11.7.1 and 11.7.2.

systolic-to-PA systolic gradient of >25 mmHg is suggestive of RVOT obstruction.[18] Ongoing clinical management of RV function post-transplantation may be challenging in the presence of RVOT obstruction.

Assessment of hypoxaemia

The presence of pulmonary vein obstruction, persistent intra-cardiac right-to-left shunting from a new or residual PFO, and pleural effusions may be detected on TOE to aid in the diagnosis and optimization of the management of post-transplant hypoxaemia.

Multiple choice questions

Discover interactive multiple choice questions to test your knowledge on this chapter by searching for this book's title or ISBN (9780198873686) at **https://academic.oup.com/** and going to the online appendix at the end of the book. Use your scratch-off code on the inside cover to access the material.

References

1. Copeland H, Knezevic I, Baran DA, *et al.* Donor heart selection: evidence-based guidelines for providers. *J Heart Lung Transplant.* 2023;**42**(1):7–29.
2. Copeland H, Hayanga JWA, Neyrinck A, *et al.* Donor heart and lung procurement: a consensus statement. *J Heart Lung Transplant.* 2020;**39**(6):501–17.
3. Chen CW, Sprys MH, Gaffey AC, *et al.* Low ejection fraction in donor hearts is not directly associated with increased recipient mortality. *J Heart Lung Transplant.* 2017;**36**(6):611–15.
4. Bombardini T, Arpesella G, Maccherini M, *et al.* Medium-term outcome of recipients of marginal donor hearts

selected with new stress-echocardiographic techniques over standard criteria. *Cardiovasc Ultrasound*. 2014;**12**(1):12–20.
5. Neethling E, Moreno Garijo J, Mangalam TK, *et al.* Intraoperative and early postoperative management of heart transplantation: anesthetic implications. *J Cardiothorac Vasc Anesth*. 2020;**34**(8):2189–206.
6. Raman SV, Jarori U. Strain and long-term prognosis after heart transplantation: a necessary advance in the pursuit of sufficient understanding. *JACC Cardiovasc Imaging*. 2020;**13**(9):1943–4.
7. Masarone D, Kittleson M, Gravino R, Valente F, Petraio A, Pacileo G. The role of echocardiography in the management of heart transplant recipients. *Diagnostics*. 2021;**22**(12):2338.
8. Simsek E, Nalbantgil S, Ceylan N, *et al.* Assessment of right ventricular systolic function in heart transplant patients: correlation between echocardiography and cardiac magnetic resonance imaging. Investigation of the accuracy and reliability of echocardiography. *Echocardiography*. 2017;**34**(10):1432–8.
9. Bacusca AE, Tarus A, Burlacu A, Enache M, Tinica G. A meta-analysis on prophylactic donor heart tricuspid annuloplasty in orthotopic heart transplantation: high hopes from a small intervention. *Healthcare (Basel)*. 2021;**9**(3):306.
10. Lund LH, Edwards LB, Kucheryavaya AY, *et al.* The registry of the international society for heart and lung transplantation: thirty-first official adult heart transplant report—2014; focus theme: retransplantation. *J Heart Lung Transplant*. 2014;**33**(10):996–1008.
11. Olymbios M, Kwiecinski J, Berman DS, Kobashigawa JA. Imaging in heart transplant patients. *JACC Cardiovasc Imaging*. 2018;**11**(10):1514–30.
12. Chambers DC, Perch M, Zuckermann A, *et al.* The International Thoracic Organ Transplant Registry of the International Society for Heart and Lung Transplantation: thirty-eighth adult lung transplantation report—2021; focus on recipient characteristics. *J Heart Lung Transplant*. 2021;**40**(10):1060–72.
13. Rudski LG, Lai WW, Afilalo J, *et al.* Guidelines for the echocardiographic assessment of the right heart in adults: a report from the American Society of Echocardiography. Endorsed by the European Association of Echocardiography, a registered branch of the European Society of Cardiology, and the Canadian Society of Echocardiography. *J Am Soc Echocardiogr*. 2010;**23**(7):685–713.
14. McIlroy DR, Sesto AC, Buckland MR. Pulmonary vein thrombosis, lung transplantation, and intraoperative transesophageal echocardiography. *J Cardiothorac Vasc Anesth*. 2006;**20**(5):712–15.
15. Gentile F, Manterof A, Lippolis A, *et al.* Pulmonary venous flow velocity patterns in 143 normal subjects aged 20 to 80 years old. An echo 2D colour Doppler cooperative study. *Eur Heart J*. 1997;**18**(1):148–64.
16. González-Fernández C, González-Castro A, Rodríguez-Borregán JC, *et al.* Pulmonary venous obstruction after lung transplantation. Diagnostic advantages of transesophageal echocardiography. *Clin Transplant*. 2009;**23**(6):975–80.
17. Evans A, Dwarakanath S, Hogue C, *et al.* Intraoperative echocardiography for patients undergoing lung transplantation. *Anesth Analg*. 2014;**118**(4):725–30.
18. Zeng YH, Calderone A, Rousseau-Saine N, *et al.* Right ventricular outflow tract obstruction in adults: a systematic review and meta-analysis. *CJC Open*. 2021;**3**(9):1153–68.

20

Echocardiography for mechanical support

TOE is an essential tool in the management of patients receiving mechanical circulatory support: intra-aortic balloon pumps (IABPs), extracorporeal membrane oxygenation (ECMO), and ventricular assist devices (VADs).

Intra-aortic balloon pumps

TOE may be used to assess the indications and contraindications for IABP, monitor insertion, identify complications, and evaluate efficacy. Echocardiography has several advantages over chest radiography and fluoroscopy for IABP placement, including the ability to visualize structures in real time, superior portability, and lack of exposure to ionizing radiation.[1]

Considerations prior to IABP insertion

A comprehensive TOE examination should be performed to confirm the indications for, and exclude any contraindications to, IABP use (Table 20.1). Treatable causes of haemodynamic instability may be identified such as hypovolaemia, vasoplegia, or cardiac tamponade. The examination should then focus on the AV and the thoracic aorta.

The AV is examined in the mid-oesophageal AV short- and long-axis views. Aortic dimensions should be measured, and any AR quantified. IABPs should not be used in patients with moderate or severe AR, as they worsen regurgitation severity and do not improve diastolic coronary perfusion pressure in this circumstance. IABPs may be used in the presence of mild AR, albeit with reduced efficacy. IABPs reduce LV afterload and can therefore worsen dynamic LVOT obstruction and systolic anterior motion of the MV (see Chapter 6) in patients predisposed to this problem.

The aortic root, ascending aorta, aortic arch, and descending thoracic aorta should be examined to exclude severe atheroma, aneurysmal dilatation, dissection, or other abnormalities. The left subclavian artery aids in correctly positioning the IABP, with the IABP tip just distal to the vessel origin. This is identified in the upper oesophageal aortic arch short-axis view (see Figure 4.8). The presence of severe atheroma (especially mobile) in the aortic arch or descending thoracic aorta is associated with a risk of embolization of atheromatous material during insertion and use of IABPs, and it is a contraindication to their use. With large aneurysms of the descending aorta, there is an increased risk of aortic rupture or disruption of atheromatous plaque. With aortic dissection, it is possible to place

Table 20.1 Indications and contraindications to IABPs

Indications	Contraindications
• Cardiogenic shock • Acute myocardial ischaemia • Mechanical complications of myocardial infarction • Refractory ventricular arrhythmias • Preoperative support of high-risk cardiac surgical patients (acute ischaemia or LVEF<25%) • Support during high-risk cardiac catheterization • Weaning from CPB • LV systolic failure following cardiac surgery • RV failure	**Absolute** • Severe AR • Severe atheroma in descending thoracic aorta • Aortic dissection • Severe occlusive disease in distal arteries **Relative** • Dynamic LVOT obstruction • Low systemic vascular resistance • Systemic–pulmonary shunts (e.g. patent ductus arteriosus) • Large aneurysm of descending aorta • Aortic coarctation

an IAPB in the false lumen, to extend the dissection, or to exacerbate malperfusion of abdominal organs; therefore, aortic dissection is an *absolute* contraindication to the use of an IABP.

Considerations during IABP insertion

IABPs are most commonly inserted via a Seldinger technique into the femoral artery. TOE imaging is useful for confirming the presence of the guidewire in the aorta and subsequent advancement and optimal positioning of the IABP catheter. Effective function of an IABP depends on optimal positioning of the balloon, with the tip situated approximately 2 cm distal to the origin of the left subclavian artery and the proximal portion of the balloon above the diaphragm (Figure 20.1). A higher position in the aorta may occlude the left subclavian artery, while a lower position provides less cardiac augmentation and may intermittently occlude the mesenteric or renal arteries.

As the catheter is advanced, the echo-dense and thick distal tip of the catheter and the lucent body of the balloon (Figure 20.2) can be distinguished from the echo-dense thin wire. The origin of the left subclavian artery is visualized, and the tip of the IABP advanced until 2 cm below this point. If the origin of the left subclavian artery is not visualized, the inferior margin of the aortic arch may be used as a landmark and the IABP tip positioned just distal to this point.

Expert tip: A simple technique to confirm positioning may be used. In the descending aorta short-axis view, the tip of the balloon is identified. The echocardiographer places their fingertips on the TOE probe at the level of the patient's teeth, and the probe is gradually withdrawn until the origin of the subclavian artery comes into view. The distance from the echocardiographer's fingers to the patient's teeth is the distance from the balloon tip to the origin of the subclavian artery.

Considerations following IABP insertion

Complications of IABPs that can be identified with TOE include venous insertion, aortic injury, atheroma

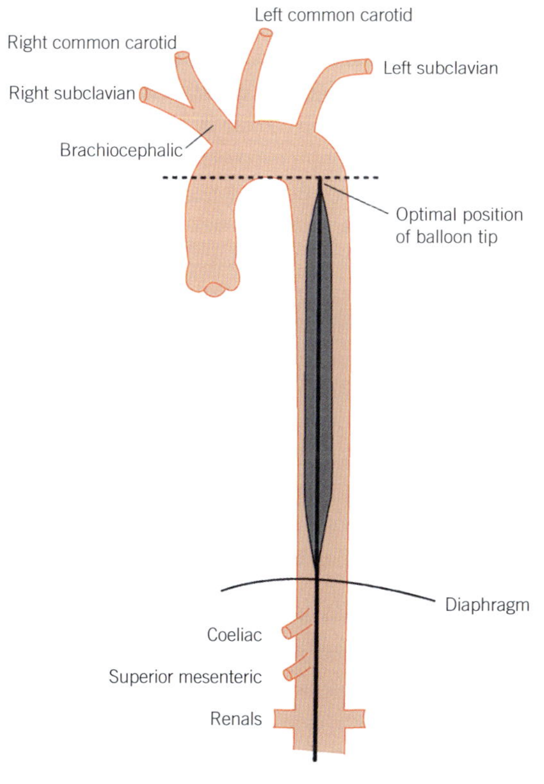

Figure 20.1 Schematic showing the correct position of an IABP in the descending thoracic aorta.

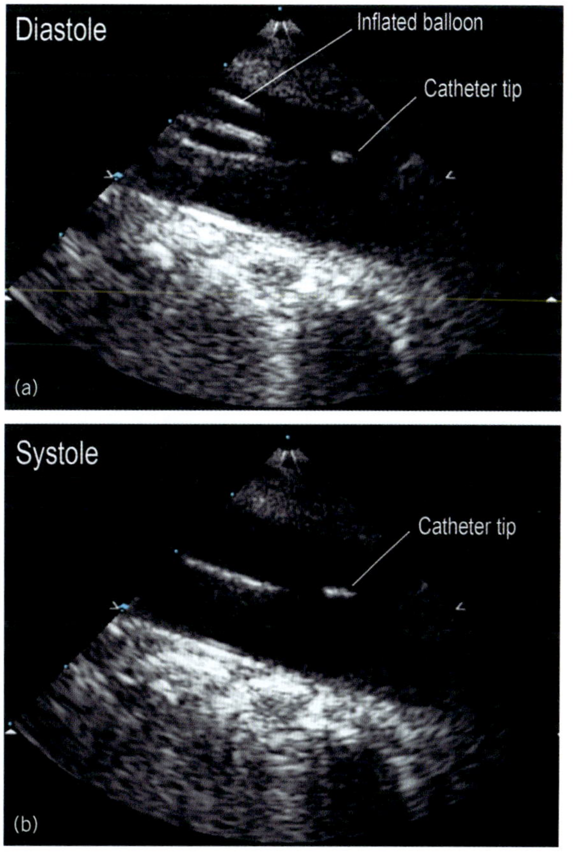

Figure 20.2 Descending aorta long-axis view showing an IABP. (a) In diastole, the balloon is inflated, and the catheter tip and the balloon can be seen. (b) In systole, the balloon is deflated, and only the central catheter and catheter tip can be seen.

disruption and embolism, thrombosis/thromboembolism, and balloon rupture. Using TOE to guide insertion may minimize the development of complications and allow early recognition when they occur.

Following insertion, TOE may be used to assess IABP efficacy. Cardiac output, ventricular dimensions, LVEF, and the effect on coronary blood flow and regional wall motion abnormalities (RWMAs) should be assessed (see Chapters 6 and 21).

Extracorporeal membrane oxygenation

ECMO is used to treat acute respiratory, cardiac, or combined cardiorespiratory failure that is unresponsive to conventional therapies.[2,3,4] The two most common types of ECMO are veno-venous (VV) and veno-arterial (VA). VV ECMO is used to support isolated respiratory failure, while VA ECMO is used to support isolated cardiac failure or combined cardiorespiratory failure.[5]

With VV ECMO, deoxygenated blood is drained from the patient's venous system (typically the IVC), passed through an external membrane gas exchanger, and returned to the patient's RA as oxygenated blood. This oxygenated blood mixes with the patient's systemic venous return and then passes to the pulmonary circulation and then to the left heart. VV ECMO is typically established peripherally, with cannulae advanced from the femoral veins or right internal jugular vein. Separate cannulae may be used for drainage and return or, alternatively, a double-lumen single cannula system may be used. If a two-cannula technique is used, the drainage cannula is typically advanced into the IVC from a femoral vein and the return cannula is advanced from the right internal jugular vein to the RA. Alternatively, a long cannula for venous return can be placed in the femoral vein and advanced into the IVC or RA. The tips of the drainage and return cannula may lie close together, with the return cannula design mitigating against recirculation. For the double-lumen single cannula technique, the cannula is advanced from the right internal jugular vein to the RA and IVC.

With VA ECMO, deoxygenated blood is drained from the patient's venous system (typically the IVC and RA), passed through an external membrane gas exchanger, and returned as oxygenated blood at systemic pressure to the patient's arterial system. VA ECMO can provide support for the left and right ventricles and the lungs, similar to conventional CPB. VA ECMO can be established centrally or peripherally. With peripheral cannulation, the venous drainage cannula is typically advanced from a femoral vein into the RA, and the arterial return cannula placed in a femoral artery. Central cannulation is usually performed via a sternotomy incision. The venous cannula is placed directly into the RA, and the arterial cannula is placed in the ascending aorta. Thus, central cannulation for VA ECMO is anatomically and physiologically similar to CPB.

Considerations prior to, and during, institution of ECMO

A comprehensive TOE examination should be performed to confirm the indications for ECMO, exclude contraindications, and aid in selecting the appropriate mode of support. During cannulation, TOE is useful to guide cannula placement and determine optimal positioning.

Assessing ventricular function to help determine the mode of ECMO support

Pivotal in selecting the appropriate mode of ECMO support (VA vs VV) is an assessment of ventricular function. Isolated severe respiratory failure, with normal haemodynamics, is managed with VV ECMO. However, many patients with severe respiratory failure also develop progressive haemodynamic instability. In this circumstance, haemodynamic instability is typically related to one or more of the following: (1) RV dysfunction secondary to aggressive mechanical ventilation and acutely raised pulmonary vascular resistance (PVR); (2) LV or RV dysfunction secondary to sepsis or underlying cardiac disease; (3) vasodilation secondary to sepsis; or (4) hypovolaemia.[6] RV dysfunction is common in patients with severe respiratory failure due to the combined effects of raised intrathoracic pressure and acutely raised PVR (acute cor pulmonale), which occurs as a consequence of pulmonary inflammation, hypoxaemia, and acidosis. RV dysfunction due to raised intrathoracic pressure and acute cor pulmonale usually resolves with institution of ECMO and reduction of mechanical ventilation to rest settings, and can therefore be managed with VV ECMO support. Similarly, when the cause of the haemodynamic instability is excessive vasodilation, VV support combined with vasopressor therapy is usually sufficient. VA ECMO is indicated when LV or RV dysfunction is severe.

Identifying cardiac lesions that complicate ECMO

Significant aortic or mitral regurgitation can lead to acute LV distension in patients receiving VA ECMO who have minimal LV ejection (see Online appendices 11.5.6–11.5.8). Therefore, careful evaluation of aortic and mitral valve function prior to institution of VA ECMO is important.

Severe aortic disease, such as dissection or aneurysm, is a contraindication to VA ECMO due to the risk of aortic rupture and, with dissection, inadvertent placement of the arterial return cannula in the false lumen. Severe aortic atheroma is also a relative contraindication to VA ECMO due to the increased risk of systemic embolization of atheroma by the sand-blasting effect of blood flow from the return cannula. Intracardiac shunts (e.g. PFO or ASD) may complicate VV ECMO because of the possibility of systemic embolization of thrombus or gas. However, a PFO is not a contraindication to ECMO.

Cannula positioning

Cannulation for peripheral ECMO is commonly performed percutaneously via a Seldinger technique. After cannulation of the femoral vein or artery, passage of a guidewire into the IVC or aorta can be confirmed with TOE. The IVC is visualized by advancing the probe from a modified mid-oesophageal bicaval view (see Figure 4.7); the thoracic aorta can be seen in the descending aortic long- and short-axis views. From the right internal jugular vein, passage of the guidewire through the SVC and into the RA can be confirmed from the mid-oesophageal bicaval view (Figure 20.3; see Online appendix 11.2.2). Once the guidewire is confirmed as being in the appropriate vessel, percutaneous dilatation and passage of the ECMO cannula are more safely and confidently performed. In extracorporeal cardiopulmonary resuscitation (ECPR) for refractory cardiac arrest, peripheral venous and arterial cannulation is used.[7]

With VV ECMO using separate drainage and return cannulae, the optimum position of the return cannula tip is within the RA, ideally with the jet of oxygenated blood directed towards the TV (see Online appendices 11.2.4 and 11.2.5S). The correct position for the drainage cannula varies according to cannula choice and configuration. For jugular–femoral configuration, the drainage cannula tip position should be within the IVC, as to avoid recirculation, it is important the tips of drainage and return cannulae are separate from each other. Thus, the tip of the drainage cannula should remain outside the RA, ideally at the level of the hepatic veins (see Online appendix 11.2.6). For femoral–femoral configuration, the drainage cannula tip may be positioned within the IVC, or advanced into the RA when a cannula with a flow profile designed to mitigate recirculation is used. The correct position of a double-lumen single cannula is with the drainage lumen within the IVC, just beyond the hepatic veins (Figure 20.4), and the return lumen within the RA, directing flow towards the TV.

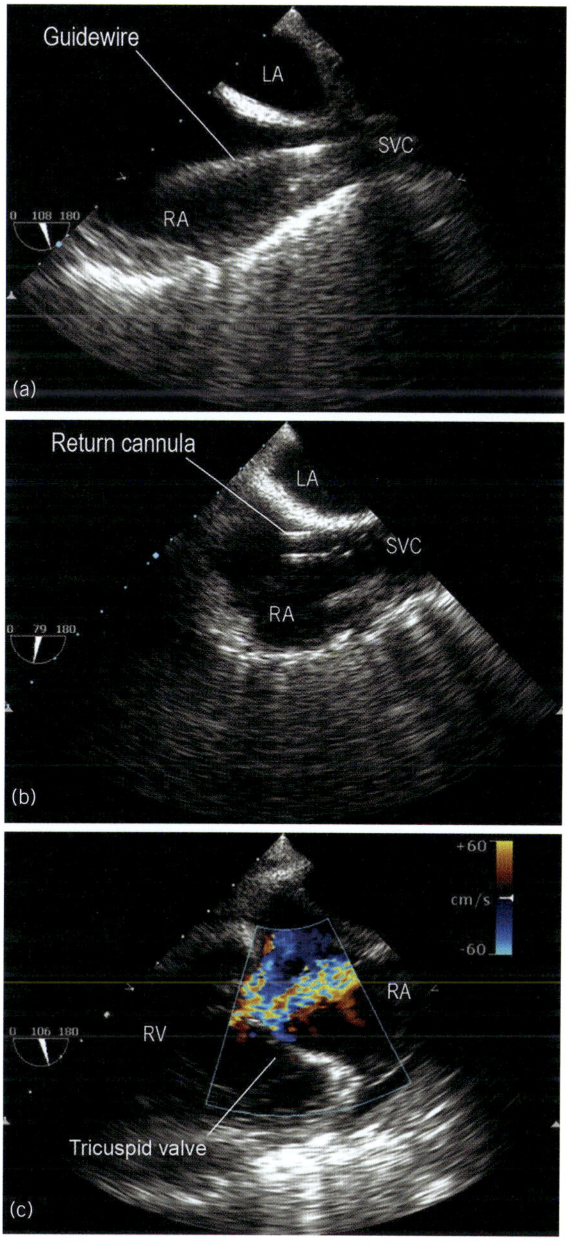

Figure 20.3 Return cannula for VV ECMO. (a) and (b) are mid-oesophageal bicaval views. (c) is a modified bicaval TV view (see Figure 4.4). In (a), a guidewire was advanced from the right internal jugular vein into the RA. In (b), the return cannula was inserted over the guidewire and the wire was withdrawn. The tip of the return cannula is positioned in the centre of the RA. (c) was obtained during VV ECMO support using a two-cannula technique. The high-velocity jet from the return cannula can be seen traversing the TV. The return cannula has been withdrawn slightly from the position shown in (b) and can no longer be seen.

For VA ECMO, there is no risk of recirculation; therefore, the drainage cannula can be advanced up the IVC into the RA (see Online appendix 11.2.9). The femoral arterial cannula is not seen on TOE.

Considerations following institution of ECMO

Careful ongoing assessment is required in order to avoid the following complications:

- Immediate obstruction of cannulae due to malposition (VV or VA ECMO)
- Recirculation (VV ECMO)
- LV distension and pulmonary oedema (VA ECMO)
- Upper body hypoxaemia (peripheral VA ECMO)
- Thrombus formation in the heart or great vessels (VV or VA ECMO)
- Cardiac tamponade (central VA ECMO post-cardiac surgery).

Cannula malposition

Malposition or migration of cannulae can result in partial obstruction by vascular walls or cardiac structures, resulting in low circuit flows. A malpositioned cannula may be seen impinging on a vascular or cardiac structure with 2D imaging or be identified by the presence of a high-velocity, turbulent jet on colour Doppler imaging. Immediate repositioning of the cannula under echocardiographic guidance is indicated.

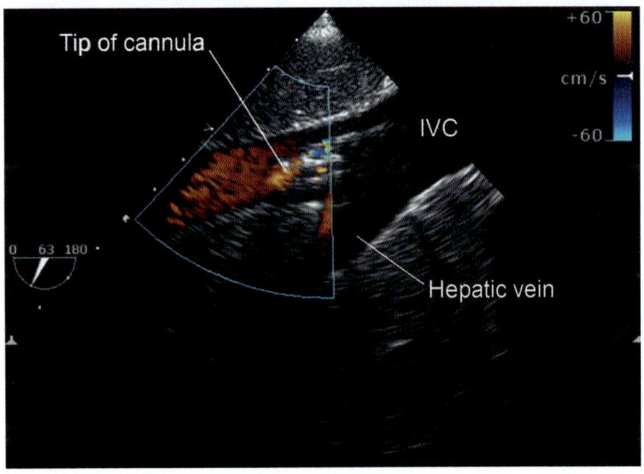

Figure 20.4 Drainage cannula for VV ECMO. In this example, VV ECMO was performed using a double-lumen single-cannula technique. The cannula was advanced from the right internal jugular vein. The return lumen is in the RA, with the flow ideally directed towards the TV. The distal end of the drainage lumen is in the IVC. This image is the transgastric IVC view (see Figure 4.7), showing the tip of the drainage lumen is just distal to a large hepatic vein. Velocity into the drainage lumen is of much lower velocity than flow out of the return lumen. Compare to Figure 20.3.

Recirculation during VV ECMO

Recirculation occurs when oxygenated blood from the return cannula is entrained into the drainage cannula, bypassing the lungs, resulting in arterial hypoxaemia. TOE is very useful to confirm the diagnosis. The tips of the drainage cannulae should be identified with 2D imaging. The high-velocity jet from the return cannula should be interrogated with colour Doppler imaging. Ideally, the jet is directed towards the TV. Recirculation is likely if the high-velocity colour jet is directed down the IVC (Figure 20.5;

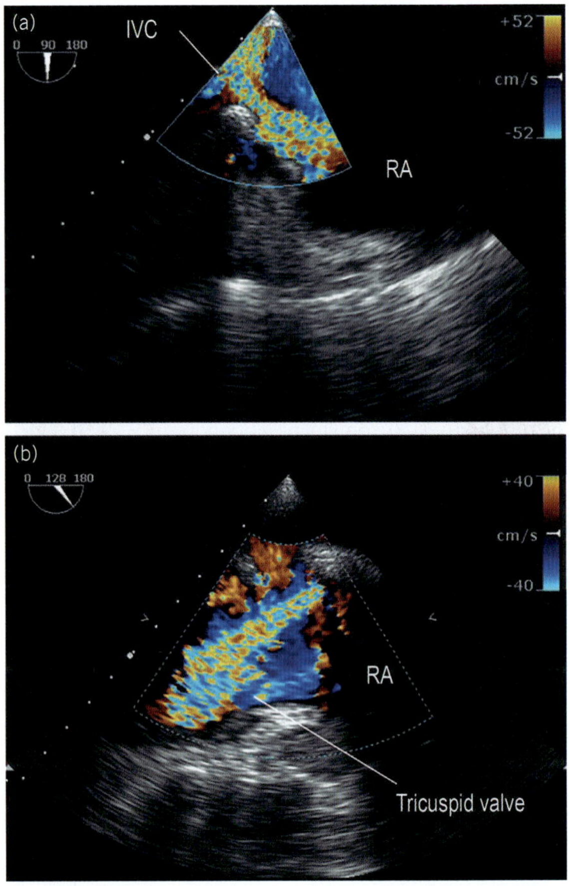

Figure 20.5 Adjustment of the return cannula to treat recirculation. In this case, VV ECMO was performed using a two-cannula technique. The return cannula was advanced from the right internal jugular vein into the RA. The drainage cannula was advanced from the femoral vein into the IVC (not shown). (a) is a mid-oesophageal bicaval view showing the inferior part of the RA and the origin of the IVC. The high-velocity jet from the return cannula can be seen entering the IVC. There was clinical evidence of recirculation. (b) is a modified mid-oesophageal bicaval TV view (see Figure 4.4). The return cannula was withdrawn and rotated. Now the jet of oxygenated blood from the return cannula can be seen traversing the TV.

see Online appendices 11.3.1–11.3.3) or includes the tip of the drainage cannula (Figure 20.6). Recirculation can also occur with a double-lumen cannula if blood from the return cannula is directed towards the IVC.

If recirculation is identified, adjustment of the positions of the drainage and return cannulae under echocardiographic guidance is indicated. This may involve withdrawing either the drainage or return cannulae and/or repositioning the return cannula, so blood flow is directed towards the IV (see Online appendices 11.3.4 and 11.3.5).

LV distension during VA ECMO

Acute LV distension is a potential problem in patients with minimal or no LV ejection who are receiving VA ECMO.[8] The problem is exacerbated by pre-existing mitral and (particularly) aortic regurgitation.[9] Clinically, acute LV distension maybe indicated by a non-pulsatile arterial waveform and the development of acute pulmonary oedema. On TOE, there is marked LV distension, minimal systolic contractility, minimal or absent opening of the AV, marked LA distension, and usually significant MR (see Online appendices 11.5.1–11.5.3). Severe LV distension causes pulmonary oedema, delays myocardial recovery, and results in intracardiac stasis, predisposing to intracavity thrombus formation. Possible solutions to decompress the left heart include indirect drainage methods (such as promoting LV ejection with inotropes or IABP, or performing an atrial septostomy; Figure 20.7) or direct 'active' drainage methods (such as use of an Impella® device, surgical drainage vent via a small thoracotomy, or percutaneous drainage catheters). There are regional differences around the world in how to address this serious problem. TOE is extremely useful in guiding an atrial septostomy puncture, positioning various external devices, and evaluating the subsequent reduction in LV and LA dimensions.

Thrombotic and bleeding complications

Thrombus formation within the ECMO circuit may manifest as a reduction in ECMO flow. TOE may detect thrombus on cannulae (Figure 20.8). Intracardiac thrombus may also develop, particularly during VA ECMO when

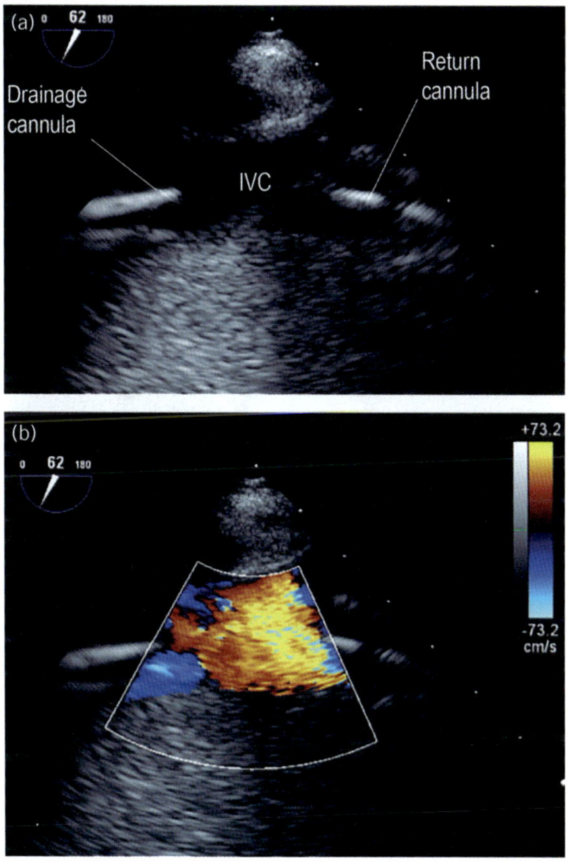

Figure 20.6 Severe recirculation. In this case, VV ECMO was performed using the two-cannula technique described in Figure 20.5. Frames (a) and (b) show the IVC just below the IVC–RA junction. The return cannula was inadvertently advanced into the IVC and lies very close to the tip of the drainage cannula. With colour Doppler imaging (b), the high-velocity jet from the return cannula is directed at the drainage cannula, causing severe recirculation. Withdrawing the return cannula into the RA resolved the problem.

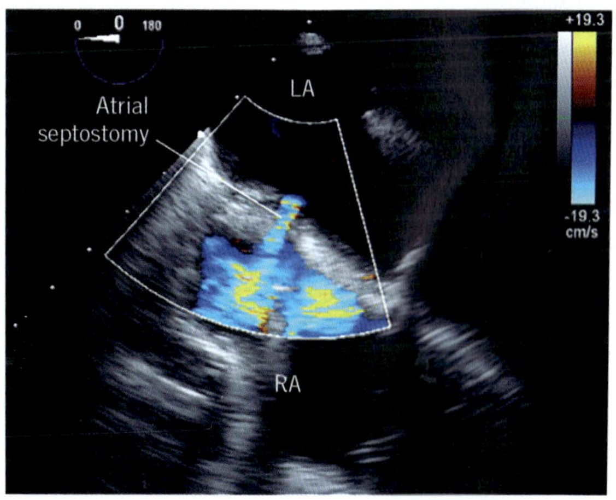

Figure 20.7 Atrial septostomy in a patient receiving VA ECMO. The image is a modified mid-oesophageal four-chamber view. The patient had been placed on peripheral VA ECMO for fulminant myocarditis. Following initiation of ECMO, severe pulmonary oedema developed due to LV akinesis. Percutaneous atrial septostomy was performed in the catheter laboratory. Colour Doppler imaging shows left-to-right flow across the atrial septum. The LA now appears decompressed. The LV was also decompressed but is not seen in this frame.

blood flow through the heart is reduced, leading to stasis (Figure 20.9; see Online appendices 11.5.9–11.5.10). Dense spontaneous echo contrast or thrombus may be visible within the cardiac chambers.

Cardiac tamponade may occur in patients receiving VA ECMO following cardiac surgery but may be difficult to diagnose in a timely manner. Because the ECMO circuit largely bypasses blood flow through the heart, tamponade may be initially reasonably well tolerated. However, increasing pericardial pressure eventually causes collapse of the RA, impairing flow into the drainage cannula and reducing ECMO circuit flow. Raised central venous pressures and low circuit flows during central VA ECMO strongly suggest cardiac tamponade. The diagnosis is confirmed with echocardiography.

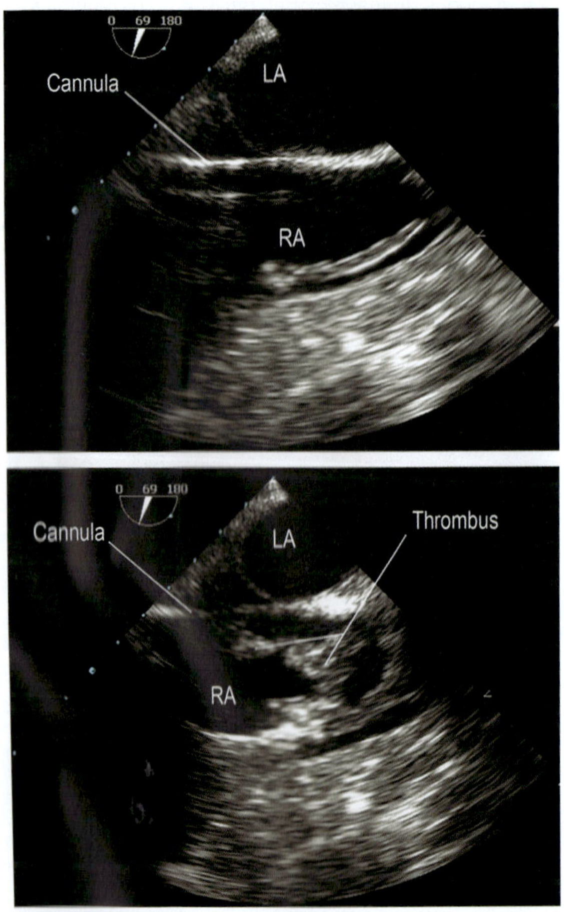

Figure 20.8 Thrombus attached to a double-lumen ECMO cannula. The image is a mid-oesophageal bicaval view. The patient was receiving VV ECMO via a double-lumen single cannula advanced from the right internal jugular vein. The cannula and the thrombus were not simultaneously visible, so the two frames were obtained at different points in the cardiac cycle. Thrombus was intermittently seen in the RA but was attached to the cannula distally in the IVC.

Expert tip: One should have a low threshold for re-evaluation with TOE following institution of ECMO, as complications are common and may be difficult to detect early.

Weaning from ECMO

TOE is very useful during weaning from VA ECMO. Serial evaluation of ventricular function during staged reductions in ECMO flow (ideally to <1.5 L/min) can be used to evaluate the likelihood of successful weaning from VA ECMO (see Online appendix 11.4). Echocardiographic predictors of successful weaning from VA ECMO are not firmly established; however, an LVEF >25%, a velocity–time integral measured across the AV with CW Doppler >10 cm, and a lateral mitral annular peak systolic velocity >6 cm/s measured with TDI have all been associated with an increased likelihood of successful weaning.[10,11]

Echocardiography is not usually required for weaning from VV ECMO. However, TOE assessment of right heart function—in particularly for the presence of acute cor pulmonale—is prudent prior to weaning, particularly if lung compliance remains poor and high ventilatory pressures are likely to be required.

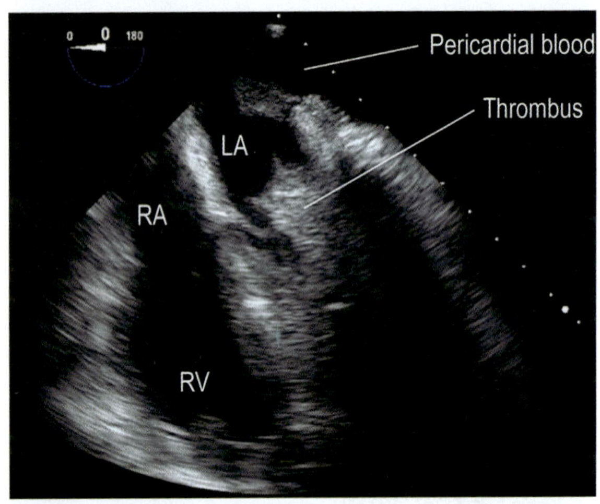

Figure 20.9 Intracardiac thrombus in a patient receiving VV ECMO. The image is a mid-oesophageal four-chamber view. Thrombus can be seen in the region of the MV. In addition, there is an echolucent space around the LA, which was unclotted blood. The patient had been placed on ECMO following cardiac surgery. Several hours later, he developed cardiac tamponade, which was associated with reduced blood flow through the heart. Blood stasis combined with no anticoagulation—due to high chest tube drainage—resulted in the formation of intracardiac thrombus. The patient was urgently taken to the operating room, where the pericardial blood was evacuated. CPB was initiated and the intracardiac thrombus was removed.

Ventricular assist devices

VADs are mechanical systems used to provide full or partial circulatory support for patients with severe cardiac failure.[12] There are several VADs currently in clinical use, each with different mechanisms and configurations. Several components are common to all VADs:

- A pump providing continuous flow
- An inflow cannula, which drains blood from the patient to the VAD
- An outflow cannula, which delivers blood from the VAD to the patient
- A controller, which is located externally and connected to the patient via a driveline.

VADs are implanted in parallel with the native circulation, in either a left-sided (LVAD) or right-sided (RVAD) configuration. VADs may be temporary (designed for days to weeks of use) or durable (designed for weeks to years of use). With LVADs, the inflow cannula typically drains blood from the LV apex, and the outflow cannula typically returns blood to the ascending aorta in an end-to-side anastomosis (Figures 20.10 and 20.11). VADs are used for temporary support as a bridge to recovery or, more commonly, for longer-term support as a bridge to transplantation or as destination therapy (i.e. permanent support). The Heartmate 3™ LVAD (Abbott, Abbott Park, IL, USA) is currently the predominant device used for durable VAD support worldwide, having superseded other devices due to improved outcomes.[13] With RVADs, the inflow cannula drains blood from the RA and the outflow cannula returns blood to the pulmonary artery.

Most patients undergoing VAD implantation for long-term support receive an LVAD. Occasionally, two devices are implanted (LVAD and RVAD) for long-term biventricular support (BiVAD). Not infrequently, a temporary RVAD is required at the time of LVAD implantation. The

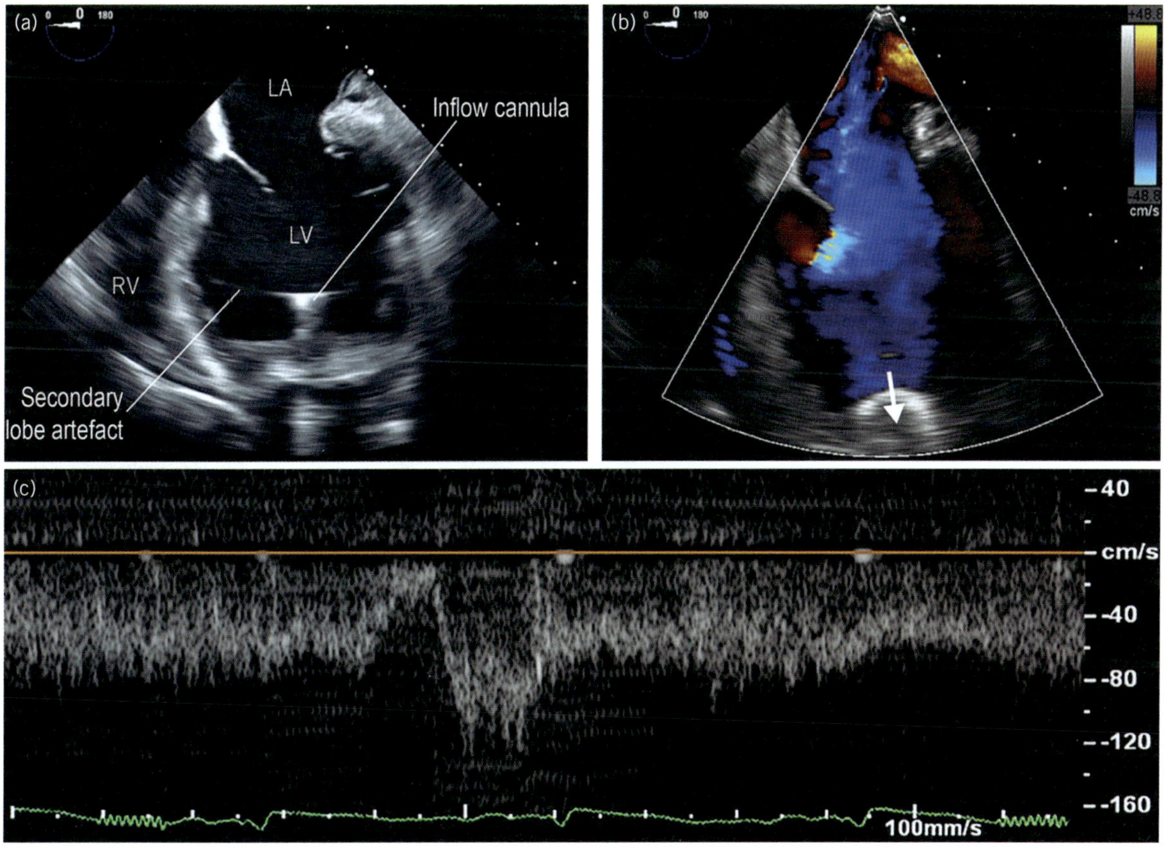

Figure 20.10 Normal appearances of LVAD inflow cannula. The image is a mid-oesophageal four-chamber view in diastole, without (a) and with (b) colour Doppler. The inflow cannula is positioned in the LV apex and is directed towards the MV. Flow towards the cannula is laminar and of low velocity (dark blue). The ventricular septum is displaced to the right, suggesting LVAD pump speed may need to be increased. (c) shows the CW Doppler of a HeartMate 3 device when the beam is directed through the inflow cannula. Flow is continuous throughout the cardiac cycle, with an occasional cardiac contraction. The peak velocity of the continuous component is approximately 1 m/s, which is normal.

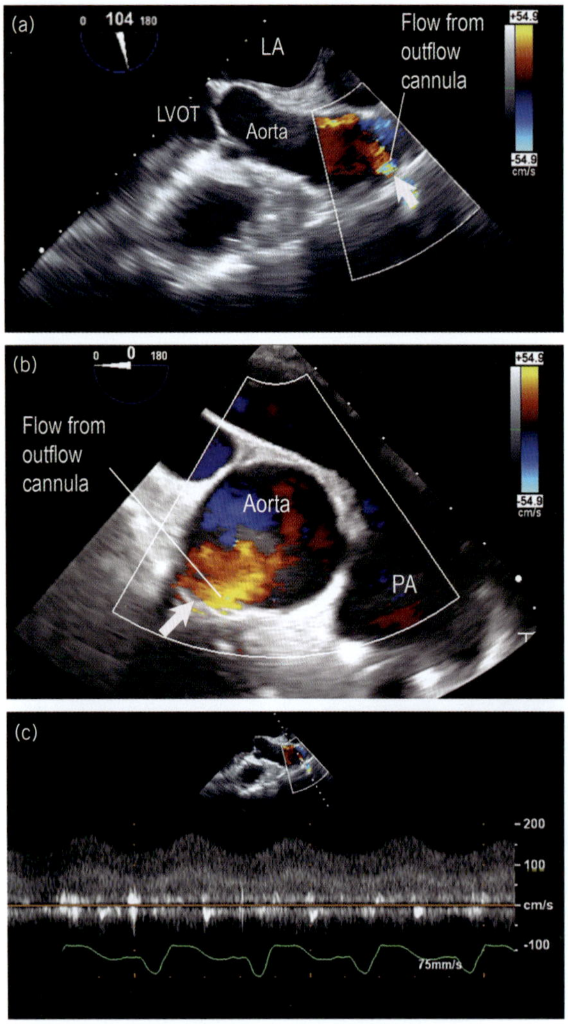

Figure 20.11 Normal appearance of LVAD outflow cannula. (a) is a mid-oesophageal ascending aorta long-axis view, showing an LVAD outflow cannula. The colour jet from the outflow cannula is seen (arrow). (b) is a mid-oesophageal ascending aorta short-axis view, showing another outflow cannula (from a different patient), with the flow entering the ascending aorta (arrow). (c) is a CW Doppler through an outflow cannula. Peak velocity is <1.5 m/s, which is normal. Note the peak velocity is approximately three times the colour alias velocity (0.54 m/s), which is why (a) shows aliased flow in the cannula. See also Online appendices 11.1.8 and 11.1.9.

American Society of Echocardiography has published guidelines on the use of echocardiography in the management of patients with LVADs.[14]

Considerations prior to VAD insertion

Prior to VAD implantation, TOE examination is focused on assessment of LV size, left and right ventricular function, and identification or exclusion of important cardiac abnormalities and pathologies (Box 20.1).

Box 20.1 Echocardiographic examination prior to VAD insertion

- Ventricular assessment:
  - LV function and dimensions
  - RV function and dimensions
  - LV or RV scarring or aneurysm at the cannulation sites
- Intracardiac thrombus
- Valvular abnormalities:
  - AR (LVAD)
  - MS
  - TR
  - Pulmonary regurgitation (RVAD)
- Aorta:
  - Ascending aortic atherosclerosis or aneurysm
- Intracardiac shunts (patent foramen ovale, ASD, VSD)

Intracardiac shunts

Once LVAD support is initiated, LA pressure falls below RA pressure, and right-to-left shunting can occur across a patent foramen ovale (PFO) or ASD, with the potential for arterial hypoxaemia or systemic embolization of right-sided gas or thrombus. Similarly, flow from right to left across a VSD may occur. Thus, it is essential to identify the presence of a PFO, ASD, or VSD prior to implantation, and, if present, to close it as part of the surgical procedure. The technique for identifying a PFO is outlined in Chapter 18 (and see Online appendices 8.1.11,10.1.1, and 11.1.2). Because a PFO may be difficult to detect prior to initiation of LVAD support, despite provocative manoeuvres, re-examination of the atrial septum should be performed after LVAD support is commenced. However, not all right-to-left shunting in the post-CPB period is due to a missed PFO, and traumatic injuries to the atrial septum can also occur. Detection of an intracardiac shunt following initiation of LVAD support usually necessitates return to CPB and closure of the defect.

AV pathology

AR may result in LVAD recirculation, whereby blood enters the aorta from the outflow cannula, flows back into the LV across the incompetent AV, and back into the LVAD inflow cannula. While mild AR is well tolerated, moderate or severe AR limits the efficacy of LVAD support. Surgical correction of moderate or severe AR should be performed prior to initiating LVAD support. If the LVAD is being used as a bridge to recovery, the AV should ideally be repaired; if the LVAD is used as a bridge to transplantation or as destination therapy, the AV may be sutured closed. If repair or closure is not possible, the valve must be replaced. However, there is an increased risk of prosthetic valve thrombosis and systemic thromboembolism with prosthetic AVs due to blood stasis within the region of the valve. This risk is greatest for mechanical valves. Therefore, if AV replacement is required prior to LVAD placement, a bioprosthesis is recommended.[14]

In patients with end-stage LV failure, the severity of AR may be underestimated with colour Doppler imaging due to diastolic pressure equalization between the aorta and the LV. Assessment of AR while on CPB most accurately reflects the trans-aortic gradient that will occur following LVAD placement, and patients with previously competent AVs may develop new AR following LVAD insertion. Therefore, an assessment of AR severity while on CPB should be performed, along with further assessment at different pump speeds following LVAD activation. The width of the vena contracta and the ratio of the jet width-to-LVOT width are appropriate techniques for quantifying AR in this context. The pressure half-time method and the presence of holodiastolic flow reversal in the thoracic aorta are not reliable methods during CPB or following LVAD placement due to their dependence on loading conditions and aortic pulse pressure, and due to the altered timing of AR, which may be continuous or variable throughout the cardiac cycle.

> ***Expert tip: LV vent flows on CPB during LVAD insertion can provide information on the significance of any AR. The requirement for high LV vent flows may point to clinically significant AR that will reduce the efficacy of LVAD support.***

AS is usually of little clinical importance in LVAD insertion and support. However, in patients receiving an LVAD for partial circulatory support (in whom ongoing LV ejection through the AV is required), AS may preclude the implantation of such a device or require surgical correction.

MV pathology

MS can restrict LVAD flow if the inflow cannula is positioned in the LV apex. If present, stenosis that is moderate or severe should be surgically corrected during LVAD insertion.

Tricuspid regurgitation

TR may contribute to RV dysfunction following LVAD insertion and is a marker of post-operative RV failure. Moderate or severe regurgitation should be surgically corrected at the time of LVAD implantation.[14]

Intracardiac thrombi

The left heart should be inspected for the presence of thrombus, particularly at the LV apex (see Online appendices 3.1.10 and 3.1.11) and within the LA appendage (see Online appendices 3.1.5–3.1.7). Thrombus at the LV apex necessitates clot removal during device implantation but is not an absolute contraindication to implantation. If thrombus is seen in the LA appendage, the appendage may be ligated or removed to reduce the risk of post-operative thromboembolism.

RV function

RV dysfunction is common in patients with end-stage LV failure, and effective functioning of an LVAD is dependent on adequate RV contractility. Severe RV dysfunction following LVAD implantation may necessitate RVAD support, and implantation of this concurrently with LVAD implantation, rather than in a delayed manner, is associated with improved outcomes.[14] As noted above, in most circumstances, RVAD support is temporary.

Careful aggregate assessment of RV function, including quantitative measures where possible, is therefore important prior to LVAD implantation (see Chapter 14). Preoperative risk factors for the development of severe RV dysfunction following LVAD implantation include moderate or severe TR, tricuspid annular plane systolic excursion (TAPSE)<7.5 mm, and a short-to-long-axis ratio of the RV ≥0.6.[15,16] There is, however, no single reliable parameter predictive of post-operative RV failure. Severe post-operative RV dysfunction may be difficult to predict, and can develop even if RV function was relatively normal in the preoperative assessment.

Aorta

The presence of calcified plaque, severe atheroma, aneurysmal dilatation, or dissection of the ascending aorta should be identified. If atheroma or calcified plaque is seen, the anastomotic site of the outflow cannula should be adjusted. The presence of an aneurysmal ascending aorta may necessitate graft replacement before the end-to-side anastomosis of the outflow cannula.

Box 20.2 Echocardiographic assessment during and following VAD insertion

- De-airing:
  - VAD
  - Great vessels
  - Cardiac chambers
- LV decompression and function
- AV:
  - Opening
  - Regurgitation
- RV function
- Tricuspid regurgitation
- Intracardiac shunts
- Cannulae and VAD:
  - Positioning and alignment of inflow and outflow cannulae
  - Flow patterns and velocities of inflow and outflow cannulae
- Aortic dissection
- Pericardial tamponade

Considerations during and following VAD insertion

Examination after LVAD activation should be used to optimize VAD performance, and detect and manage any complications. The examination should focus on assessing left and right ventricular function, the position and function of the VAD cannulae, the adequacy of de-airing, and AV function (Box 20.2).[14] Low cardiac output following LVAD placement has several causes (Box 20.3), all of which can be identified with TOE.

De-airing

Following VAD implantation, air may be present in the heart, great vessels, pump, or cannulae. Air typically collects in the LV, the LA, the pulmonary veins, and the ascending aorta. Meticulous de-airing manoeuvres are important, both to avoid coronary artery air embolism (see Chapter 6) and to avoid pump failure due to air lock. TOE can guide the surgeon to the location of air pockets and assess the efficacy of de-airing manoeuvres. TOE may also identify air entrainment along suture lines when negative pressure is generated by an LVAD, such as can occur during periods of hypovolaemia, RV failure, inflow cannula obstruction, or excessive pump speed.

Box 20.3 Causes of low cardiac output following LVAD implantation

Early causes of low cardiac output

- RV dysfunction
- Hypovolaemia
- Arrhythmias
- Excessive VAD speed causing LV suckdown
- Inadequate VAD speed
- Malposition of inflow cannula
- Occlusion of inflow cannula (thrombus, cardiac tissues)
- Malposition or compression of outflow cannula
- Air lock
- Cardiac tamponade

Late causes of low cardiac output

- RV dysfunction
- Obstruction of inflow or outflow cannula (thrombus, pannus, infective vegetations)
- Device failure

LV function

Compared with pre implantation, the LV should no longer be distended, and the ventricular septum should be flat and in a neutral position (Figure 20.12a). The LV should be adequately filled, however, and it is important to adjust the LVAD speed and patient volume status to maintain ventricular filling and avoid collapse of the LV, known as a 'suction event' or 'ventricular suckdown' (Figure 20.12c). A completely collapsed LV causes inflow cannula obstruction, decreased LVAD output, RV dysfunction, and arrhythmias, and may cause air entrainment.[17]

Ramp studies may be performed to determine the optimal LVAD pump speed.[14] The LVAD is set to a minimum speed, then gradually increased while TOE monitors ventricular size and function, the position of the ventricular septum, and AV opening. Ideal LVAD speed is identified by a flat septum, an adequately filled, but not overdistended, LV, and intermittent opening of the AV. Leftward bowing of the ventricular septum or LV suckdown identifies excessive ('maximum') LVAD speed, while rightward bowing of the septum indicates LVAD speed is too low ('minimum') (Figure 20.12b). Ramp studies may also be used following LVAD implantation to assess for potential problems such as pump thrombosis, new or worsening valvular regurgitation, or RV failure.[14]

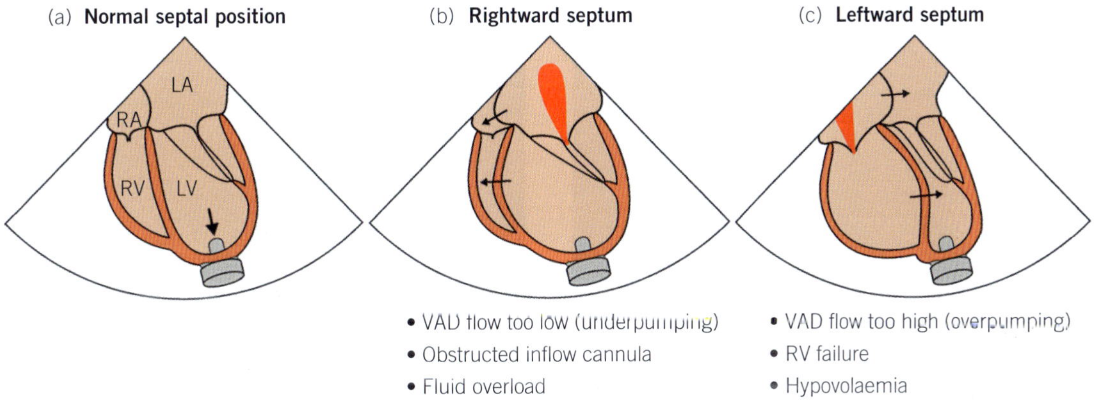

Figure 20.12 Schematic representation of normal and abnormal positions of the ventricular and atrial septa during LVAD support. (a) With normal LVAD function, the ventricular septum should be flat, in a neutral position. The atrial septum may demonstrate mild leftward bowing, as RA pressure is often slightly higher than LA pressure with LVAD support. (b) Marked rightward displacement of the ventricular septum indicates that the LV is inadequately decompressed. The atrial septum is also displaced rightward. MR is common. (c) Marked leftward displacement of the ventricular septum is associated with collapse of the LV and LA, termed 'suction event' or 'ventricular suckdown'. The atrial septum is also displaced leftward. The RV is typically severely dilated and TR is common. The common causes of these abnormalities are listed in the text.

RV function

RV dysfunction is common following LVAD placement, and may be transient or persistent. RVAD support may be required for severe refractory RV failure.

Although LVAD support reduces RV afterload, RV function does not always improve post-operatively. There are several reasons for this. CPB depresses RV function, as do the administration of large volumes of fluid and transfusion of blood products. PVR may be chronically elevated in severe LV failure and therefore may not normalize when the LV is decompressed. The LVAD may also provide a much greater (i.e. normalized) RV preload than previously, overwhelming the capacity of the RV. Finally, altering the loading conditions and geometry of the LV may adversely affect the RV, which depends on a loaded LV to generate contractile force.

Echocardiographic signs of acute RV failure include severe RV and RA dilatation, reduced TAPSE, marked leftward bowing of the atrial and ventricular septa, and severe TR (see Chapter 14). Persistent LV collapse and suckdown despite low LVAD speeds are also a sign of acute severe RV failure and may indicate the need for RVAD support.[14] Less severe RV failure may be managed by reducing LVAD speed, reducing RV afterload, and increasing inotropic support.

Temporary RVAD

Temporary support for the RV may be provided by a surgically grafted RVAD (e.g. CentriMag™, Abbott, Abbott Park, IL, USA) or by the Protek Duo® (LivaNova, London, UK), a percutaneously placed dual-lumen cannula inserted via the right internal jugular vein. The Protek Duo® has a proximal inflow lumen with the tip in the RA, and a distal outflow lumen with the tip in the proximal main pulmonary artery. Flows of up to 4.5 L/min may be generated. TOE is integral to the placement of the device in real time. Colour flow Doppler should be used to confirm the inflow and outflow positions, using a modified mid-oesophageal RV inflow–outflow view (Figure 20.13). The upper oesophageal aortic arch views may also be used to assess device placement.

RVAD dysfunction or inadequate positioning can be identified with TOE in a timely fashion. As with all forms of mechanical support, any deterioration in haemodynamic state should be assessed with TOE, with specific attention to cannula malposition or occlusion.

AV function

Intermittent opening of the AV is expected with continuous-flow devices, ideally at least once every 3–5 beats, demonstrating some native LV function and reducing the risk of blood stagnation and thrombosis in the aortic root. The presence of new AR should be sought following LVAD implantation. Moderate or severe AR necessitates surgical correction. The HeartMate 3™ LVAD uses programmed rhythmic flow changes to mimic normal physiology, and reduced stasis and thrombosis.[13]

Assessment of VAD cannulae

A combination of 2D, colour Doppler, and CW Doppler imaging should be used to assess the inflow and outflow

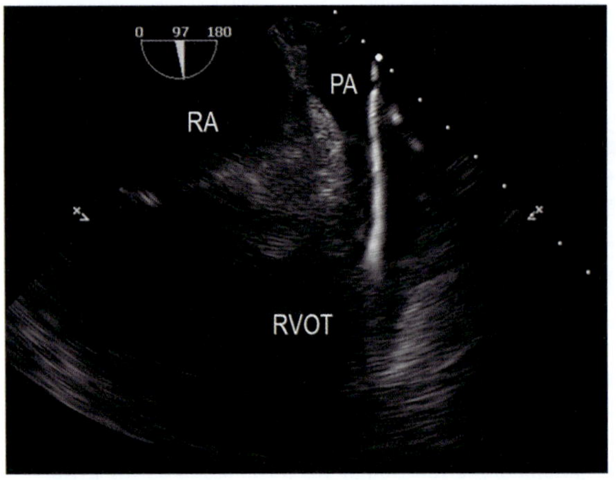

Figure 20.13 Protek Duo® RVAD. Modified mid-oesophageal right ventricular inflow–outflow view showing the cannula advanced from the internal jugular vein, with the tip positioned in the main pulmonary artery.

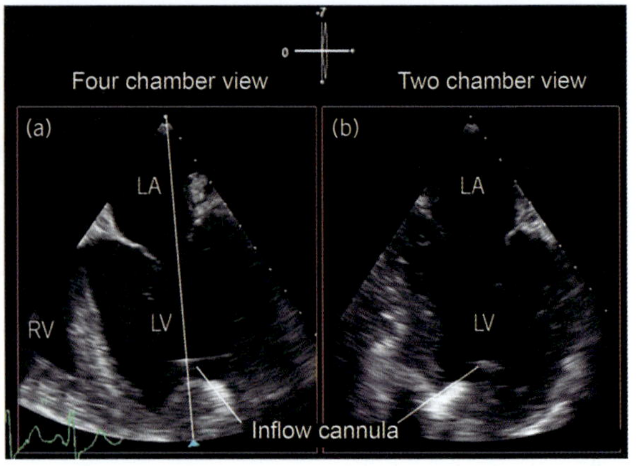

Figure 20.14 Orthogonal views of an LVAD inflow cannula with biplane imaging. The starting image (a) is a mid-oesophageal four-chamber view. (b) is an orthogonal (i.e. two-chamber) view. The plane of (b) is shown as a white line on (a). The inflow cannula is directed towards the centre of the MV in both views, indicating correct orientation.

cannulae. The LVAD inflow cannula is usually placed in the LV apex but is sometimes positioned in the LA (via the pulmonary veins). An apical inflow cannula can usually be visualized in the mid-oesophageal LV views (Figure 20.10). Imaging the position and flow pattern of the inflow cannula is essential to rule out obstruction or malposition. The inflow cannula should be orientated along the long axis of the LV, such that flow is aligned with the MV, and not directed towards the LV wall or ventricular septum, as this may lead to obstruction.

Expert tip: To confirm correct orientation, the inflow cannula should be imaged in two orthogonal long-axis views, using biplane (x-plane) imaging from the mid-oesophageal four-chamber view (Figure 20.14).

The LVAD outflow cannula is usually attached to the ascending aorta with an end-to-side anastomosis. The outflow cannula can usually be visualized in modified mid-oesophageal AV long-axis view or in the ascending aorta short-and long-axis views (Figure 20.11).

Colour Doppler imaging of the cannulae should demonstrate laminar, non-turbulent flow (Figures 20.10 and 20.11). Blood flow in the ascending aorta often shows some aliasing. PW and CW Doppler imaging should be used to interrogate the velocity profiles in both cannulae. The velocity waveform within the inflow cannula typically demonstrates a continuous component and a superimposed pulsatile component primarily due to cardiac contraction, if present (Figure 20.10c). For the inflow cannula, the peak velocity of the continuous component of flow is typically <1.5 m/s.[14,18] For the outflow cannula, the peak velocity is usually <1–2 m/s (Figure 20.11). Although the outflow velocity varies considerably with pump speeds and device, outflow velocities >2 m/s may indicate flow obstruction and warrant further evaluation.[14]

Obstruction of the inflow cannula of an LVAD at the time of device implantation is most commonly due to the cannula impinging on the LV wall, but may be due to entrapment of the trabeculated myocardium or mitral subvalvular apparatus. Ventricular suckdown is another important early cause of inflow cannula obstruction. Late obstruction may result from thrombus, pannus, or infective vegetations. Inflow cannula obstruction results in an aliased pattern on colour Doppler and increased velocity with interrupted diastolic flow on CW Doppler imaging. If the cause of the obstruction is malposition, the cannula may appear to be directed towards the ventricular septum or lateral LV wall, rather than aligned with the MV.

Early obstruction of the outflow cannula of an LVAD is most commonly due to cannula malposition or kinking (sometimes as a result of chest closure or patient positioning). Late obstruction may be due to thrombus formation or infective vegetations. Turbulent high-velocity flow is typically seen on spectral Doppler imaging. Because of the risk of obstruction to, or movement of, the cannulae at the time of chest closure, it is important to reinterrogate both the inflow and outflow cannulae flow patterns at this time. Note that flow in both cannulae should be *unidirectional*.

To optimize the LVAD following implantation, it is necessary to interpret echocardiographic data in the context of the LVAD display console. The flow (L/min) is dependent upon pump speed (revolutions per minute, rpm) and the gradient across the pump. Devices are preload-dependent and afterload-sensitive, and flow is derived from speed and power use. Higher speed and power use result in greater estimated flow. Speed (rpm) can be adjusted in conjunction with TOE monitoring to allow for adequate LV filling. Power (W) is proportional to flow and takes a higher value in the presence of AR for a given flow. Sudden increases in flow may indicate pump thrombosis. Reduced power consumption is seen with decreased preload and cannula obstruction. Pulsatility index is dimensionless and estimates LV pulsatility. A low value indicates low intravascular volume or minimal native cardiac function.

Other complications

The aorta should be re-examined after LVAD insertion to exclude iatrogenic dissection. Bleeding and tamponade are common following VAD implantation. Tamponade typically presents with clinical signs of low cardiac output, low VAD flows, and a high central venous pressure. Echocardiography is essential to distinguish tamponade from other causes of low cardiac output, particularly RV dysfunction. Late complications that may be detected with echocardiography include infective vegetations, thrombus formation, AR, thromboembolism, and device failure.

Surveillance

A surveillance echocardiography study is recommended once LVAD settings and the patient are stable, to establish baseline parameters and potentially allow early detection of complications, or to monitor recovery of LV function. The ASE recommends further surveillance echocardiography at 2 weeks post-implantation, then at 1, 3, 6, and 12 months post-operatively and every 6–12 months thereafter.[14]

Temporary ventricular assist devices

The use of temporary mechanical circulatory support devices as a bridge to recovery, bridge to decision, or bridge to more durable therapy is increasing. Common indications include support during high-risk percutaneous revascularization or electrophysiological ablation procedures, cardiogenic shock (including post-cardiotomy shock), acute decompensation of heart failure, and venting of the LV during peripheral VA ECMO support.[19]

The Impella® (Abiomed, Danvers, MA, USA) is a commonly used temporary VAD, with several models able to provide partial or full support for the left or right heart, approved for ≤4 days (Impella® 2.5, Impella® CP, and Impella® RP) or ≤14 days (Impella® 5.0 and Impella® LD). Consisting of an axial pump (with an Archimedes screw design), mounted on a flexible catheter and connected to a drive line, all Impella® models function in the same manner—with the inlet of the pump in the LV and the outlet portion of the pump in the ascending aorta (or inlet in the RV and outlet in the pulmonary artery for Impella® RP). Since effective cardiac support depends on the location of the pump components, TOE is essential to ensure correct positioning of the pump and assessment of device malfunction.

First, contraindications to Impella® use must be ruled out: mechanical AV, LV thrombus, moderate to severe AI, AV area <0.6 cm² (the size of the device), post-infarct VSD or LV rupture, or significant RV failure. During insertion, TOE is used to confirm wire advancement (from the femoral or axillary arterial vessels) up the ascending aorta and across the AV into the LV. Standard long- and short-axis views of the aorta and AV are used. It is important to identify entrapment of the guidewires in the MV apparatus or AV leaflets, as this will require withdrawal and repositioning of the guidewire. The Impella® pump is then advanced over the guidewire, with TOE monitoring in the mid-oesophageal long-axis view. The motor inlet of the Impella® (a teardrop shape) should be identified in the LV using 2D and 3D Doppler imaging. The optimal position of the motor inlet should be about 3.5 cm from the AV (Figure 20.15; see Online appendix 11.1.12). Note that the device has a pigtail tip that extends beyond the

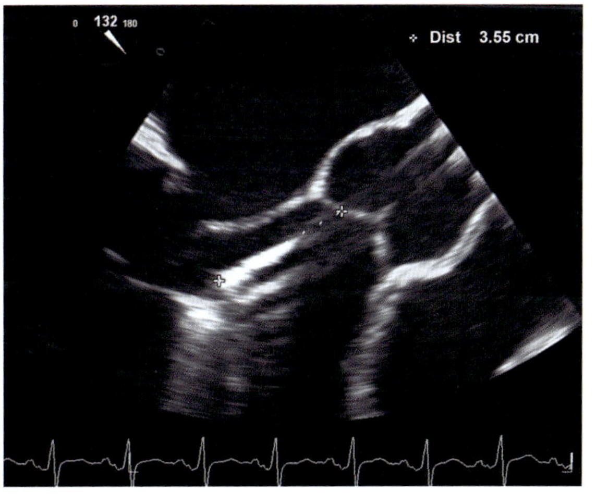

Figure 20.15 Impella® device. This mid-oesophageal long-axis view demonstrates an Impella® device advanced from the femoral artery across the AV and into the LV. The distance between the tip of the device and the AV should be 3–4 cm but may be less in small ventricles.

inlet and it should not be included in the measurement. The pump outlet is also identified in the ascending aorta using colour Doppler. MV and AV function should then be reinterrogated, the aorta reassessed to exclude injury, and the pericardium assessed for any new pericardial collections.

Similar to long-term VADs, ongoing assessment includes monitoring to ensure optimal Impella® support and assessment for causes of any ongoing shock. The interventricular septum should be neutral (near the mid-line)—bowing to the right indicates inadequate Impella® support (managed by increased speed or inotrope therapy), whereas bowing to the left (or, in the extreme, suction events) indicates RV failure, hypovolaemia, or excessive Impella® speed.

New valvular lesions can occur during Impella® support—mechanical complications due to the Impella® catheter, but also mechanical complications due to the underlying disease (e.g. MR due to ischaemic rupture of a papillary muscle). Ventricular arrythmias may occur if the Impella® contacts the LV endocardium, either due to migration of the device into the LV or as improving LV function results in increased LV contraction. Contact with the LV may cause entrainment of the papillary muscle or chordae into the pump inlet, resulting in occlusion. Finally, Impella® support will be inadequate if the device is withdrawn into the ascending aorta. TOE can identify all these elements, assess the response to management, and monitor cardiac recovery.

Multiple choice questions

Discover interactive multiple choice questions to test your knowledge on this chapter by searching for this book's title or ISBN (9780198873686) at **https://academic.oup.com/** and going to the online appendix at the end of the book. Use your scratch-off code on the inside cover to access the material.

References

1. Klopman MA, Chen EP, Sniecinski RM. Positioning an intraaortic balloon pump using intraoperative transesophageal echocardiogram guidance. *Anesth Analg.* 2011;**113**(1):40–3.
2. Sidebotham D, McGeorge A, McGuinnessS, Edwards M, WillcoxT, BecaJ. Extracorporeal membrane oxygenation for treating severe cardiac and respiratory failure in adults: part 2—technical considerations. *J Cardiothorac Vasc Anesth.* 2010;**24**(1):164–72.
3. Sidebotham D, Allen SJ, McGeorge A, Ibbott N, Willcox T. Venovenous extracorporeal membrane oxygenation in adults: practical aspects of circuits, cannulae, and procedures. *J Cardiothorac Vasc Anesth.* 2012;**26**(5):893–909.
4. Combes A, Peek GJ, Hajage D, *et al.* ECMO for severe ARDS: systematic review and individual patient data meta-analysis. *Intensive Care Med.* 2020;**46**(11):2048–57.
5. Charlesworth M, Garcia M, Head L, *et al.* Venoarterial extracorporeal membrane oxygenation for postcardiotomy cardiogenic shock—a six-year service evaluation. *Artif Organs.* 2020;**44**(7):709–16.
6. Zochios V, Charlesworth M. Protecting the right ventricle in COVID-19 pneumonitis: a missing piece of the puzzle?*Anaesthesia.* 2022;**77**(7):739–42.
7. Suverein MM, Delnoij TSR, Lorusso R, *et al.* Early extracorporeal CPR for refractory out-of-hospital cardiac arrest. *N Engl J Med.*2023;**388**(4):299–309.
8. Cevasco M, Takayama H, Ando M, Garan AR, Naka Y, Takeda K. Left ventricular distension and venting strategies for patients on venoarterial extracorporeal membrane oxygenation. *J Thorac Dis.* 2019;**11**(4):1676–83.
9. Sidebotham D, Allen S, McGeorge A, Beca J. Catastrophic left heart distension following initiation of venoarterial extracorporeal membrane oxygenation in a patient with mild aortic regurgitation. *Anaesth Intensive Care.* 2012;**40**(3):568–9.
10. Aissaoui N, Luyt CE, Leprince P, *et al.* Predictors of successful extracorporeal membrane oxygenation (ECMO) weaning after assistance for refractory cardiogenic shock. *Intensive Care Med.* 2011;**37**(11):1738–45.
11. Ortuno S, Delmas C, Diehl JL, *et al.* Weaning from veno-arterial extra-corporeal membrane oxygenation: which strategy to use?*Ann Cardiothorac Surg.* 2019;**8**(1):E1–8.
12. Allen SJ, Sidebotham D. Postoperative care and complications after ventricular assist device implantation. *Best Pract Res Clin Anaesthesiol.* 2012;**26**(2):231–46.
13. MehraMR, Uriel N, Naka Y, *et al.* A fully magnetically levitated left ventricular assist device—final report. *N Engl J Med.*2019;**380**(17):1618–27.
14. Stainback RF, Estep JD, Agler DA, *et al.* Echocardiography in the management of patients with left ventricular assist devices: recommendations from the American Society of Echocardiography. *J Am Soc Echocardiogr.* 2015;**28**(8):853–909.
15. Potapov EV, Stepanenko A, Dandel M, *et al.* Tricuspid incompetence and geometry of the right ventricle as predictors of right ventricular function after implantation of a left ventricular assist device. *J Heart Lung Transplant.* 2008;**27**(12):1275–81.
16. Puwanant S, Hamilton KK, Klodell CT, *et al.* Tricuspid annular motion as a predictor of severe right ventricular failure after left ventricular assist device implantation. *J Heart Lung Transplant.*2008;**27**(10):1102–7.
17. Mauermann WJ, Rehfeldt KH, Park SJ. Transesophageal echocardiography in a patient in hemodynamic compromise after Jarvik 2000 implantation: the suckdown effect. *Anesth Analg.* 2008;**107**(3):791–2.
18. Chumnanvej S, Wood MJ, MacGillivray TE, Melo MF. Perioperative echocardiographic examination for ventricular assist device implantation. *Anesth Analg.* 2007;**105**(3):583–601.
19. Crowley J, Cronin B, Essandoh M, D'Alessandro D, Shelton K, Dalia AA. Transesophageal echocardiography for Impella placement and management. *J Cardiothorac Vasc Anesth.* 2019;**33**(10):2663–8.

21 Haemodynamic instability

Haemodynamic instability is common after cardiac surgery. In the perioperative environment, echocardiography is an essential tool for assessing the haemodynamic state and for investigating the cause of haemodynamic instability. Assessing the haemodynamic state refers to measuring the cardiac output (CO), intravascular pressures, and volume status. Investigating haemodynamic instability refers to determining the cause(s) of hypotension and low (or pathologically high) CO. TOE has advantages over TTE, including ease of imaging in mechanically ventilated patients with surgical drains and dressings, and the quality of images for left heart structures, prosthetic valves and devices, the pericardium, and the pleural spaces.

When making haemodynamic assessments, it is important to integrate TOE-derived data with information obtained from other sources (e.g. clinical assessment, invasive pressure monitors, central oximetry) and to appreciate the strengths and limitations of TOE, compared to other techniques. Review of previous echocardiographic imaging is helpful to understand the baseline and post-surgical anatomy.

Assessing the haemodynamic state

Systemic arterial pressure and central venous pressure are routinely measured with invasive catheters in cardiac surgical patients. TOE can provide useful information on CO, LA pressure, and PA pressure. Additionally, TOE can help assess intravascular volume status.

Stroke volume

In the absence of regurgitation or intracardiac shunting, flow through a cardiac chamber or valve during a single heartbeat represents the stroke volume (SV) and is quantified as the product of the velocity–time integral (VTI) and cross-sectional area (CSA) (Equation 21.1):

$$\text{Stroke volume} = VTI \times CSA \qquad \text{Equation 21.1}$$

The most widely used site to estimate the CO with TOE is the LVOT. The uniform shape allows the CSA of the LVOT to be measured reasonably accurately (see later), while the low velocity profile of blood flow in the LVOT allows PW Doppler sampling of velocities to accurately represent average instantaneous velocities. VTI is recorded using the transgastric long-axis view or the deep transgastric five-chamber view. The PW sample volume is usually positioned 0.5–1.0 cm proximal from the AV (see Online appendix 1.6.12). Practically, the sample volume may be initially placed at the level of the AV and then slowly moved into the LVOT until a smooth Doppler envelope is obtained with minimal spectral broadening. The LVOT CSA should be measured at the same distance from the AV as the VTI measurement, in mid systole in the mid-oesophageal AV long-axis view (see Online appendices 1.6.12 and 7.3.13).

In mechanically ventilated patients, all VTI measurements should be measured at end-expiration or during a period of brief apnoea, to minimize the cardiorespiratory impact of mechanical ventilation. Assuming normal values for LVOT CSA (3–5 cm^2) and SV (60–75 mL), typical normal values for LVOT VTI are in the range of 15–20 cm. VTI values <15 cm are indicative of low SV, and values >20 cm of high SV.

> ***Expert tip: In practice, because the LVOT diameter does not change, changes in the VTI reflect changes in the stroke volume.***

While useful clinically, there are several potential problems with the technique. In a small number of patients, it is not possible to achieve adequate Doppler alignment with the blood flow in the LVOT. Off-axis imaging underestimates VTI, and hence SV. Conversely, placing the sample volume too close to the AV in a region of flow acceleration (e.g. due to AS) overestimates VTI and SV. In patients with AS, colour Doppler imaging can be used to ensure the PW Doppler sample volume is positioned proximally in the LVOT, away from the zone of flow acceleration. As the technique measures the volume of blood passing through the LVOT in systole, but does not measure regurgitant volume in diastole (which will reduce net forward flow), the technique will overestimate CO in patients with more than mild AR, and should not be used in this circumstance. The LVOT is oval-shaped, not circular, with the shorter axis typically visualized in the 2D mid-oesophageal AV long-axis view. Measuring the shorter axis of the LVOT underestimates SV. When 3D imaging is used to estimate the CSA of the LVOT (see Chapter 10), values for CO are approximately 10% higher than with standard 2D imaging.[1] Finally, when SV varies significantly between heartbeats (e.g. due to atrial fibrillation, hypovolaemia, or cardiac tamponade), multiple VTI measurements over several heartbeats should be obtained and the results averaged. When SV varies from beat to beat (e.g. atrial fibrillation), choosing only the largest waveform for analysis overestimates CO.

LA pressure

LA pressure cannot be measured directly with TOE, but evidence of abnormal LA pressure may be inferred from 2D assessment of atrial septal motion and Doppler evaluation of the trans-mitral velocity waveform and mitral annular motion.

Increasing LA pressure results in an increased trans-mitral E-wave velocity measured by PW Doppler. Mitral annular e' velocity also increases with increased preload, but the effect is modest, as e'-wave velocity is less influenced by preload, particularly when myocardial relaxation is impaired (see Chapter 7).[2] Because the effect of preload on the mitral annular e'-wave velocity is less than on the trans-mitral E-wave, the E/e' ratio provides a useful measure of LA pressure in patients with abnormal relaxation. In spontaneously breathing subjects assessed with TTE, an E/e' ratio >15 is usually associated with elevated LA pressure and an E/e' ratio <8 is usually associated with normal filling pressure.[2,3] E/e' ratios between 8 and 15 are indeterminate and not predictive. These cut-off values are not valid in patients with normal myocardial relaxation[2] (see Chapter 7) and are unreliable in patients with advanced decompensated heart failure.[4] Mitral annular e'-wave velocity is influenced by mitral annular calcification, mitral prostheses, and MS; therefore, the E/e' ratio is not valid in patients with these conditions.

E/e' can also be assessed by TOE in ventilated patients, but the technique is not well validated. TDI measurements should be made from the lateral mitral annulus (mid-oesophageal four-chamber view), as adequate alignment between the Doppler signal and the medial annulus is frequently not possible. In general, a lower TOE-derived E/e' ratio is predictive of raised LA pressure in ventilated patients; however, the data are inconsistent. Combes and colleagues demonstrated that an E/e' ratio >7.5 predicted a pulmonary artery wedge pressure (PAWP) of >15 mmHg, with a sensitivity of 86% and a specificity of 81%.[5] Vignon and colleagues demonstrated an E/e' ratio ≤8 predicted a PAWP of ≤18 mmHg, with a sensitivity of 83% and a specificity of 88%.[6] By contrast, Haji and colleagues found the E/e' ratio could not reliably predict PAWP in a group of ventilated cardiac surgical patients, but that fixed rightward bowing of the atrial septum was strongly predictive of raised LA pressure, with a sensitivity of 81% and a specificity of 98% for PAWP ≥17 mmHg.[7]

In ventilated patients with normal atrial pressures, the atrial septum bows predominantly rightward throughout the cardiac cycle, with a brief reversal in mid systole during both inspiration and expiration (Figure 21.1). Loss of the normal mid-systolic reversal and exaggerated rightward bowing of the septum indicate raised LA pressure. Kusumoto *et al.* demonstrated that loss of mid-systolic reversal predicts an LA pressure of ≥15 mmHg, with a sensitivity of 89% and a specificity of 95%.[8] Excessive motion and systolic buckling of the atrial septum indicate low LA pressure. However, care must be taken to not misdiagnose excessive septal motion as low LA pressure when the actual cause is an aneurysmal atrial septum. Motion of the atrial septum is also influenced by severe mitral and tricuspid regurgitation, the presence of which may render these signs unreliable.

Other echocardiographic features of raised LA pressure are a tense, enlarged LA on 2D imaging, a pseudonormal or restrictive pattern on the trans-mitral PW Doppler waveform, and an S-wave < D-wave (i.e. S/D <1) on the pulmonary venous PW Doppler waveform.

Pulmonary artery pressure

Application of the simplified Bernoulli equation allows RV systolic pressure (RVSP) to be obtained from the peak velocity of the TR jet (V_{TR}) and RA pressure (RAP) (Equation 21.2):

$$RVSP - RAP = 4(V_{TR})^2 \qquad \text{Equation 21.2}$$

In the absence of PV stenosis, PA systolic pressure (PAP_S) is equivalent to RVSP (Equation 21.3):

$$PAP_s = 4(V_{TR})^2 + RAP \qquad \text{Equation 21.3}$$

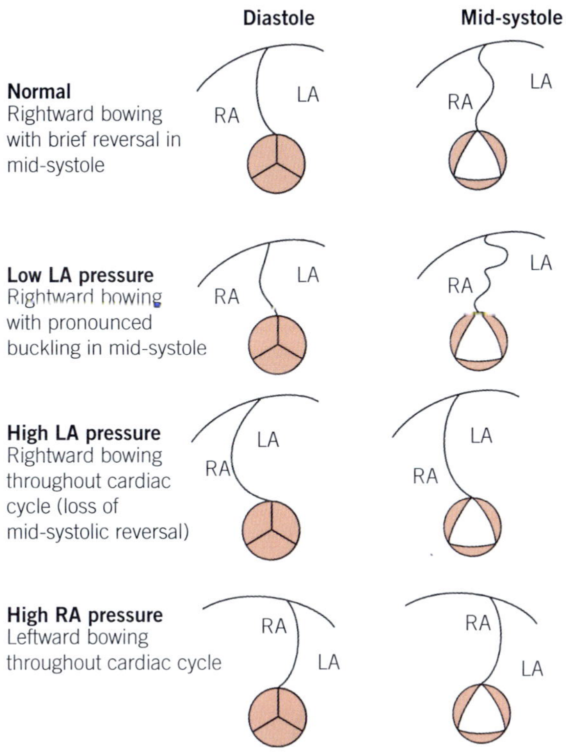

Figure 21.1 Patterns of atrial septal motion. Examples of abnormal motion of the atrial septum are demonstrated in Online appendix 8.1.

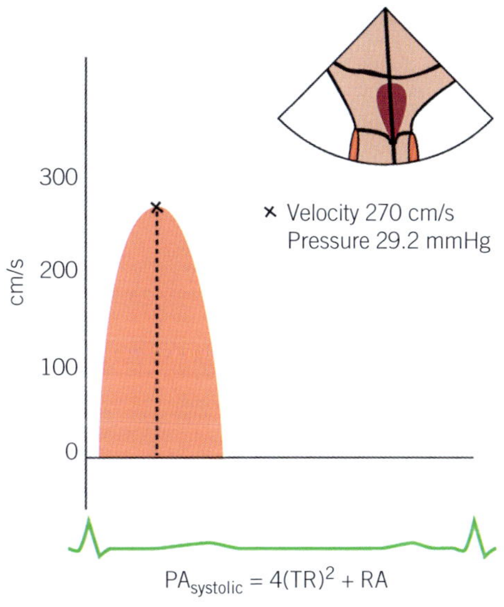

Figure 21.2 Technique for measuring pulmonary artery systolic pressure with CW Doppler, using the modified Bernoulli equation. The TR velocity is measured from the mid-oesophageal modified bicaval TV view or similar. See example in Online appendix 10.1.7.

The peak TR jet velocity can usually—but not always—be obtained using CW Doppler from the mid-oesophageal four-chamber, bicaval, or modified bicaval TV view (Figure 21.2). A peak TR jet velocity of 2.5 m/s yields a systolic PA pressure of 25 mmHg (+ RAP), and therefore, this value provides a useful upper normal limit for TR jet velocity. Poor alignment (>20°) between the TR jet and the Doppler beam leads to significant underestimation of RVSP. Note also that TR jet velocity is not necessarily related to regurgitation severity (see Chapter 15).

Volume responsiveness

Assessment of volume responsiveness is an important component of evaluation of haemodynamic instability. The parameters used to evaluate volume responsiveness are generally categorized into static and dynamic parameters.[9] Static parameters are single measurements at a specific point in time (e.g. central venous pressure, LV end-diastolic area (LVEDA)). Dynamic parameters are measurements of changes in haemodynamic parameters over time (e.g. SV variation, VTI).

The general principle of assessment of volume responsiveness using static parameters is to measure at baseline, administer a fluid bolus, and then repeat the measurement to assess any increment. Changes in LVEDA (a static parameter) using the transgastric mid-papillary short-axis view can be used to monitor changes in preload and to guide LV filling. Advantages of this method include the simplicity (standard 2D views are used) and the ease of image acquisition in the intraoperative setting. End-diastole is identified as the point at which the LV area is maximal. The 'blood pool' is included in the calculated area, meaning the trace should go around the papillary muscles (see Figure 6.5). LVEDA can be classified as normal (8–14 cm^2), large (>14 cm^2), or small (<8 cm^2).

Up to a certain point, intravenous fluid administration increases LVEDA and, by the Frank–Starling mechanism, SV. However, beyond that point, further fluid administration results in little change in LVEDA, no increase in SV, and a disproportionate increase in LV end-diastolic pressure (Figure 21.3). Optimal preload is the LVEDA at which SV is maximal. However, several factors influence LVEDA, in addition to preload. In particular, LV compliance (i.e. diastolic function), LV systolic function, pericardial pressure, intrathoracic pressure, and RV size and function (ventricular interdependence) all influence LVEDA, independent of preload. For this reason, there are no absolute values for LVEDA that relate to intravascular volume

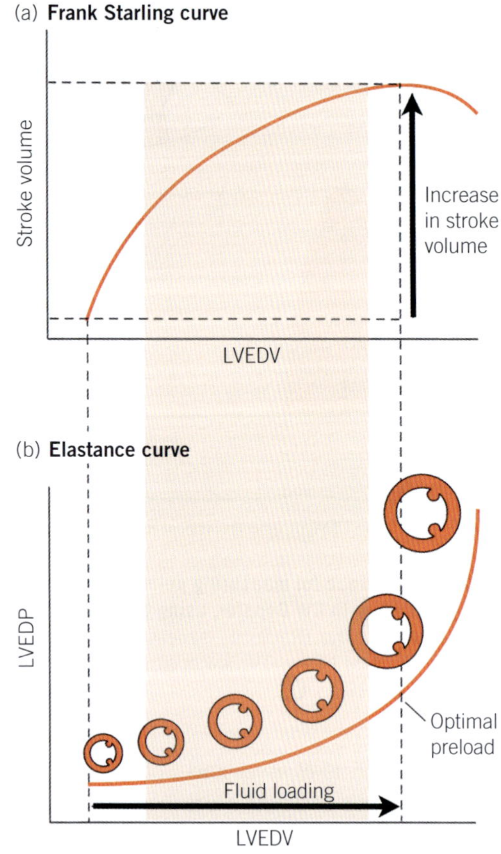

Figure 21.3 Changes in LV end-diastolic pressure (LVEDP), LV end-diastolic volume (LVEDV), and stroke volume in response to fluid loading. (a) shows a diastolic elastance (ΔP/ΔV) curve for the LV. (Compliance (ΔV/ΔP) is the reciprocal of elastance.) LVEDV (and LV end-diastolic area) is a surrogate for preload. Up to a certain point, increasing preload increases stroke volume by the Frank–Starling mechanism. (b) Optimal preload is the LVEDV at which the stroke volume is maximal. Further fluid loading beyond this point results in a disproportionate increase in LVEDP. The shaded area represents the normal working range for the ventricle. The slope of the Frank–Starling curve is fairly constant over the working range of the LV. The slope of the curve (SV/LVEDV) is the ejection fraction (see Chapter 6). Thus, over the normal working range of the LV, ejection fraction is fairly independent of preload.

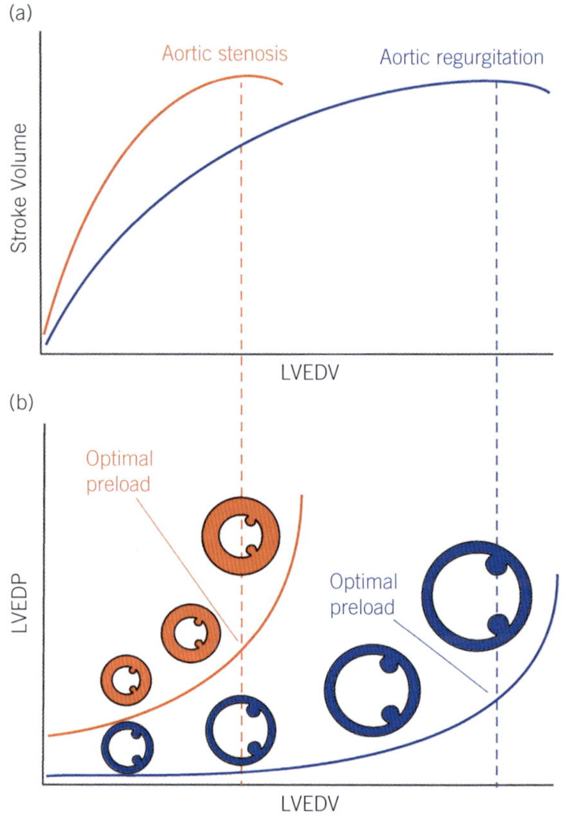

Figure 21.4 Comparison of Frank–Starling curves (a) with diastolic elastance (b) in AS and AR. With chronic AS, the diastolic elastance curve is shifted upwards and leftwards (reduced compliance), compared to normal. With chronic AR, the curve is shifted downwards and rightwards (increased compliance), compared to normal. Optimal preload occurs at a higher LV end-diastolic volume (LVEDV) and lower LV end-diastolic pressure (LVEDP) with AR, compared to AS.

status. For instance, in a patient with chronic AS, who has normal LV systolic function, but reduced LV compliance, optimal preload may occur at LVEDA <10 cm^2, whereas a patient with chronic AR, who has severely impaired LV systolic function and increased LV compliance, optimal preload may occur at LVEDA >30 cm^2 (Figure 21.4). Notwithstanding these caveats, for an individual patient, monitoring changes in LVEDA in response to fluid loading may help to optimize preload. However, a note of caution is warranted. When LV compliance is reduced, optimal preload may be associated with an unacceptably high LA pressure. Thus, the fact that a patient is fluid-responsive (i.e. not optimally preloaded) does not mean that fluid is indicated. In general, due to the above-mentioned reasons, change in LVEDA is unreliable to estimate volume responsiveness in patients on mechanical ventilation.[10,11]

In contrast to static parameters, dynamic parameters help to determine whether the ventricle is in the preload-dependent or preload-independent part of the Frank–Starling curve using the cardiorespiratory interaction during mechanical ventilation. Cardiorespiratory changes during positive pressure ventilation give rise to respiratory variations in dynamic parameters.[12] The inspiratory phase of mechanical ventilation is accompanied by increased intrathoracic pressure, leading to a reduced RV preload

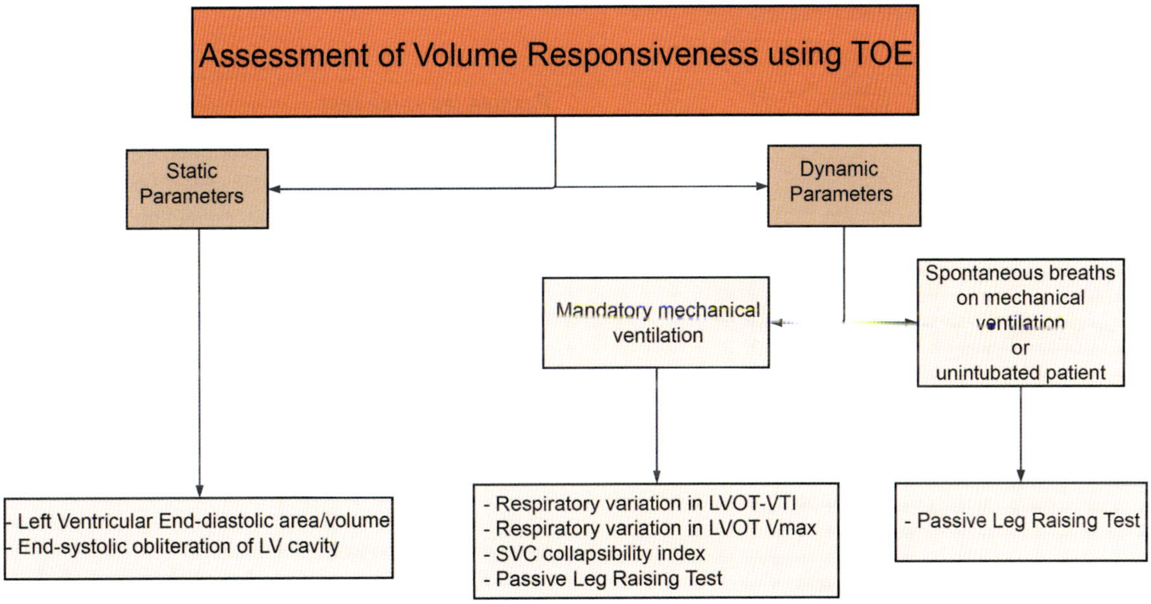

Figure 21.5 Assessing fluid responsiveness with static and dynamic parameters using TOE. See text for details. SVC, superior vena cava.

and an increased RV afterload. The cumulative effect is reduced RV cardiac output. Concomitantly, increased intrathoracic pressure causes increased LA preload and reduced LV afterload, with increased LV cardiac output. During expiration, these changes reverse. In patients with hypovolaemia, these respiratory variations are exaggerated; thus, an increase in respiratory variation is suggestive of volume responsiveness. A non-echocardiographic example of a dynamic parameter is the presence of pulse pressure variations on the arterial waveform. Several echocardiographic parameters that vary with ventilation have been investigated as absolute markers of fluid responsiveness. These include the 'SVC collapsibility index', variation in LVOT VTI or LVOT V_{max} with respiration, and passive leg raise test (Figure 21.5). Caveats for use of the SVC collapsibility index and the LVOT VTI variation measurements exist, and include validation only for mechanically ventilated patients with no spontaneous respiration, tidal volume >8 mL/kg ideal body weight, and normal respiratory rate, with sinus rhythm and without significant RV dysfunction.

SVC collapsibility index

The SVC can be visualized, as outlined in Figure 21.6. The SVC diameter reduces during inspiration with positive pressure ventilation, and returns to baseline with expiration. Changes in the diameter of the SVC are best appreciated using M-mode imaging (Figure 21.7). The extent of respiratory variation in the SVC diameter can be quantified by calculating the collapsibility index (Equation 21.4):

$$\text{Collapsibility Index} = \frac{SVC_{MAX} - SVC_{MIN}}{SVC_{MAX}} \times 100 \quad \text{Equation 21.4}$$

In one study of ventilated septic patients, a collapsibility index >36% identified fluid responders from non-responders, with a sensitivity of 90% and a specificity of 100%.[13]

Variation in LVOT V_{max} or LVOT VTI

The cyclical variation in blood flow across the LVOT with respiration is measured, using the transgastric long-axis view or the deep transgastric five-chamber view. A 12% increase in LVOT V_{max} and a 9% increase in SV with inspiration are suggestive of fluid responsiveness.[14,15] Accurate Doppler beam alignment is important to ensure the maximum variation is measured (Equations 21.5 and 21.6):

$$\Delta LVOT\ V_{max} = \frac{LVOT\ V_{max} - LVOT\ V_{min}}{LVOT\ V_{mean}} \times 100$$

Equation 21.5

$$\Delta LVOT\ V_{max} = \frac{\text{maximum}\,SV - \text{minimum}\ SV}{\text{mean}\ SV} \times 100$$

Equation 21.6

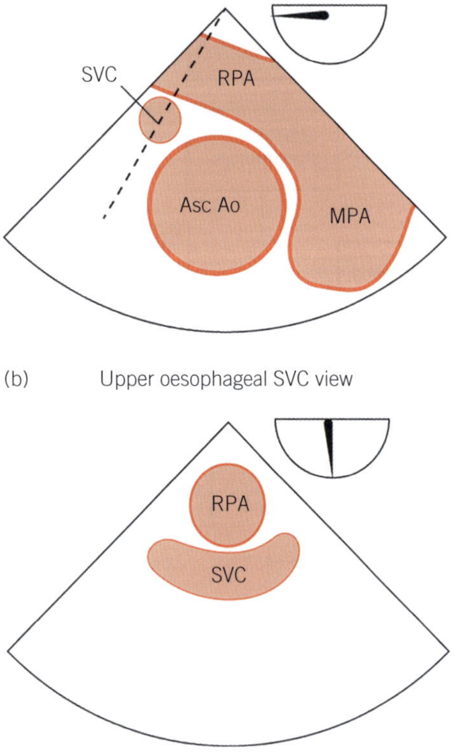

Figure 21.6 Upper oesophageal long-axis view of the SVC. From the mid-oesophageal ascending aorta short-axis view (a), the probe is turned to the right to centre the image on the SVC. The probe is then slightly withdrawn, and the sector scan forward-rotated to about 90°, until a long-axis image of the SVC is seen (b). The dashed line in (a) indicates the image plane in (b). M-mode imaging is used to visualize changes in the diameter of the SVC with ventilation.

Passive leg raise test

Using the transgastric long-axis or deep transgastric five-chamber view, SV or CO is calculated using LVOT VTI. The patient's leg is raised by 45°, directing approximately 300–500 mL of blood to the central venous return. After 1 minute, SV or CO is remeasured. It is important to place the range gate in the same position in the LVOT throughout the sequence of measurements.

A 10% increase in SV on passive leg raise will result in an approximate 15% increase in SV with a 500-mL fluid challenge. Advantages of the passive leg raise test are that it can be used in spontaneously breathing patients, as well as patients with mechanical ventilation, and the measurement is reliable in patients with atrial fibrillation.[9] Additionally, there is no fluid challenge given to patients who are non-responders. The passive leg raise test should not be used in patients with intra-abdominal hypertension, or those with restrictions on positioning. Note also patients with severe hypovolaemia may be misclassified as non-responders, as there is less blood for auto-transfusion.

Investigating haemodynamic instability

The potential causes of haemodynamic instability in cardiac surgical patients are listed in Box 21.1. Note that evaluation of the pleural spaces is an essential part of

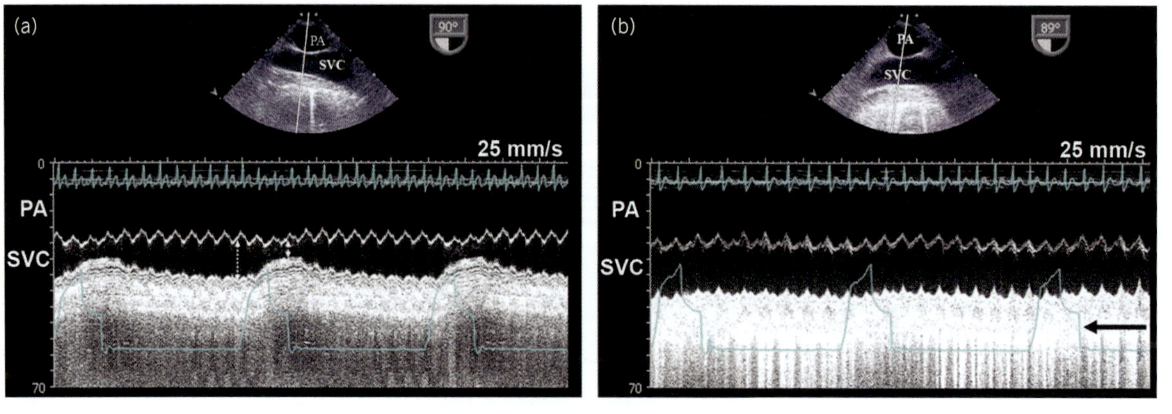

Figure 21.7 Upper oesophageal view of the SVC using M-mode imaging in a ventilated patient. Airway pressure is superimposed in blue on the screen (identified by the solid arrow). The SVC is subject to intrathoracic pressure, and therefore during positive pressure ventilation, its diameter is maximal during expiration and minimal during inspiration. At baseline (a), partial collapse of the SVC can be seen during inspiration, suggestive of fluid responsiveness. Following fluid resuscitation (b), respiratory variability is greatly reduced, suggesting a lack of further fluid responsiveness.

Box 21.1 Causes of acute haemodynamic instability in cardiac surgical patients

- Arrhythmias and heart block
- Hypovolaemia
- Low LV afterload
- LV systolic dysfunction
- LV diastolic dysfunction*
- RV dysfunction
- Cardiac tamponade
- Acute valvular regurgitation
- Dynamic LVOT obstruction
- Raised intrathoracic pressure:
  - Patient–ventilator dyssynchrony
  - Tension pneumothorax
  - Dynamic pulmonary hyperinflation
  - Massive haemothorax

* Unlikely to be an isolated cause, but an important contributory factor.

the examination, as pleural collections may also give rise to haemodynamic instability in post-cardiac surgery patients.

Hypovolaemia and low LV afterload

Hypovolaemia and low LV afterload are common following cardiac surgery, have similar echocardiographic appearances, and often coexist. Consequently, the two conditions can be difficult to tell apart. Hypovolaemia occurs due to fluid loss (e.g. blood loss), inadequate fluid intake, or redistribution from the vascular space (e.g. capillary endothelial leak). Causes of low LV afterload include excessive arteriolar vasodilation, MR, and systemic-to-pulmonary shunts. Excessive arteriolar vasodilation and capillary endothelial leak both occur in association with systemic inflammatory response syndrome (SIRS), which can occur as a consequence of CPB, sepsis, anaphylaxis, and other causes (see Online appendix 5.2).

Echocardiographic appearances

Hypovolaemia and low LV afterload are best assessed in the transgastric mid-papillary short-axis view (Figure 21.8). Both conditions are characterized by reduced LV end-systolic area (LVESA). Severely reduced LVESA results in end-systolic cavity obliteration and 'kissing' papillary muscles. Hypovolaemia and low afterload may be distinguished by evaluating LVEDA—LVEDA is normal with low LV afterload, and reduced with hypovolaemia. Thus, with low afterload, the LV fills normally and empties more completely, whereas with hypovolaemia, the LV only partially fills and also empties more completely than normal. FAC is increased in both conditions—but more so with low LV afterload—imparting a hyperdynamic appearance to LV function.

Hypovolaemia is associated with a reduced PW Doppler trans-mitral E-wave velocity, an increased A-wave, and a reduced E/A ratio compared with 'normal' for that patient (see Chapter 7). The effect with low LV afterload is dependent on volume status.

Measuring CO helps to distinguish hypovolaemia from low LV afterload. With low LV afterload, CO is usually high, whereas with hypovolaemia, CO is usually low.

Considerations

There are several reasons why hypovolaemia and low afterload are difficult to distinguish echocardiographically. First, as noted previously, the two conditions frequently coexist. Second, reduced end-systolic area is more readily appreciated than reduced end-diastolic area, particularly when there is end-systolic cavity obliteration—which is visually striking—or tachycardia. Third, when assessing LVEDA and LVESA, the echocardiographer must take into account the expected 'normal' values for these parameters in a particular individual. Thus, hypovolaemia in a patient with severe AS will appear very different from that in a patient with severe AR. Also, the presence of LV hypertrophy by virtue of increased wall thickness relative to cavity size—can mimic the appearances of hypovolaemia (Figure 21.9). Both hypovolaemia and low afterload make the LV look hyperdynamic and make the systolic function appear better than it actually is.

LV systolic dysfunction

LV systolic dysfunction may be pre-existing or due to intraoperative factors (e.g. prolonged CPB duration, coronary air embolus, inadequate myocardial protection, injury to coronary arteries). The primary indices of LV systolic function that are measurable with TOE are LVEF and FAC. The impact of LV systolic dysfunction on the haemodynamic state is strongly influenced by ventricular dimensions, LV afterload, and LA pressure (see Online appendix 5.3).

Echocardiographic appearances

The most useful view for assessing global LV systolic function is the transgastric mid-papillary short-axis view; however, complete imaging of the LV using the mid-oesophageal and additional transgastric views is

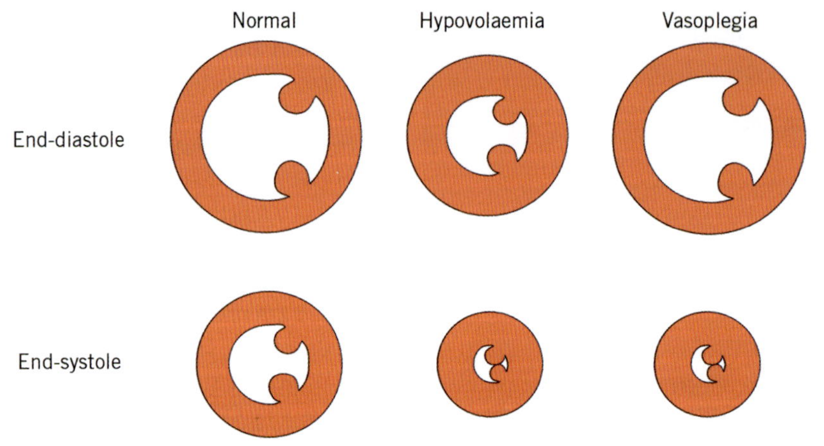

Figure 21.8 Hypovolaemia, compared with low LV afterload. Changes in end-diastolic and end-systolic areas in the transgastric mid-papillary short-axis view are shown. End-systolic area is reduced in both conditions, compared to normal. With hypovolaemia, end-diastolic area is reduced, whereas with low LV afterload, end-diastolic area is normal. With hypovolaemia, increased wall thickness relative to cavity size at end-diastole can create the false impression of LV hypertrophy. See also Online appendix 5.2.

important to avoid missing regional wall motion abnormalities (RWMAs).

Chronic LV dysfunction is associated with increased ventricular dimensions, often significantly so. LVESA is increased out of proportion to LVEDA, resulting in decreased LVEF and FAC. Because of the effects of ventricular remodelling, wall motion and thickening tend to be globally affected, even when the original problem was regional. Thus, for chronic ischaemic cardiomyopathy, RWMAs may be absent or difficult to discern.

With acute LV dysfunction, LVEDA is typically normal or only mildly increased. Reduced LVEF and FAC result from increased LVESA. RWMAs are common, particularly if the underlying cause is ischaemia; however, RWMAs are also present in viral myocarditis. Following MV surgery, a new RWMA may indicate a circumflex artery injury as the course of the circumflex artery runs very close to the MV annulus. A new RWMA following AV surgery should prompt interrogation of coronary artery blood flow for any occlusion to the coronary ostium by the prosthetic valve struts.[16]

Diastolic parameters are frequently abnormal. Severe end-stage cardiomyopathy is typically associated with a restrictive filling pattern on trans-mitral PW Doppler analysis. Impaired relaxation or a pseudo-normal pattern may be seen with acute or chronic LV dysfunction. The E/e' ratio will depend on whether LA pressure is elevated.

In patients with haemodynamic compromise secondary to LV systolic dysfunction, echocardiographic signs of MR, raised LA pressure, and pulmonary hypertension should also be sought.

Considerations

The increased ventricular volumes associated with chronic LV systolic dysfunction help to preserve CO, despite reduced LVEF. For instance, if LVEF is 30%, but left ventricular end-diastolic volume (LVEDV) is increased to 240 mL, SV is 70 mL, which is relatively normal (at rest). LA pressure is typically normal in this circumstance also. However, chronically dilated LVs are very sensitive to changes in afterload. If LV afterload significantly increases (e.g. due to administration of a vasopressor or repair of a regurgitant MV), CO may fall and LA pressure may rise. Conversely, reduced LV afterload (e.g. due to administration of a vasodilator or the presence of severe MR) improves LV systolic function, as noted previously.

With acute LV systolic dysfunction (e.g. following anterior myocardial infarction), ventricular dilation has not occurred. In this circumstance, low LVEF is frequently associated with low CO.

A further consideration is the effect of inotropic drugs on LV performance. A normal LV under the influence of an inotropic agent will appear hyperdynamic, and an impaired LV may appear 'normal'.

LV diastolic dysfunction

LV diastolic dysfunction can be defined as a reduced ability of the LV to fill at normal LA pressures. The primary clinical consequence of LV diastolic dysfunction is high LA pressure, which can precipitate pulmonary oedema. Conversely, 'normal' LA pressure in a patient with severe diastolic dysfunction may represent hypovolaemia and

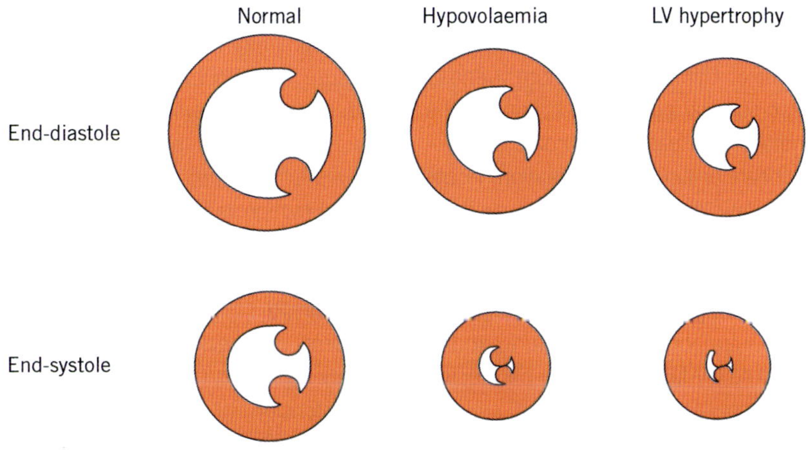

Figure 21.9 Hypovolaemia, compared with LV hypertrophy. Changes in end-diastolic and end-systolic areas in the transgastric mid-papillary short-axis view are shown. End-diastolic and end-systolic areas are reduced with both hypovolaemia and LV hypertrophy, compared to normal. End-diastolic wall thickness is increased with LV hypertrophy, but not with hypovolaemia.

lead to low CO/hypotension. Hence, evaluation of LV diastolic dysfunction is important when assessing haemodynamic instability.

Diastolic dysfunction may occur in isolation or in conjunction with systolic dysfunction. Diastolic dysfunction with preserved systolic function is associated with LV hypertrophy (e.g. due to poorly controlled hypertension or AS) and hypertrophic cardiomyopathy. Diastolic dysfunction with impaired systolic function occurs with end-stage dilated cardiomyopathy and with restrictive cardiomyopathy. Impaired diastolic filling of the LV can also result from RV dysfunction, RV volume overload (due to leftward displacement of the interventricular septum during diastole), and raised pericardial (i.e. pericardial tamponade or constriction) and/or intrathoracic pressures.

As explained in Chapter 7, patients with mild diastolic dysfunction (i.e. impaired relaxation) are typically preload-tolerant. LA pressure is usually relatively normal, and LVEDV is below the optimal preload (Figure 21.3). Preload augmentation results in increased CO. By contrast, patients with severe diastolic dysfunction (i.e. pseudo-normal or restrictive filling) are usually preload-intolerant. LA pressure is increased, and LVEDV may be above the optimal preload. In this circumstance, preload augmentation does not result in increased CO and may precipitate pulmonary oedema.

Echocardiographic appearances

Assessment of diastolic dysfunction in the perioperative setting is challenging. Current guidelines for assessment of diastolic dysfunction are TTE-based, with measurements validated in spontaneously breathing, non-ventilated patients. Some measurements acquired routinely with TTE (e.g. LA volume) cannot be determined accurately with TOE.

The common features of isolated diastolic dysfunction are small ventricular volumes, normal or increased LVEF (and FAC), and LV hypertrophy. These appearances are similar to those seen with hypovolaemia (Figure 21.9). However, in contrast to hypovolaemia, LA pressure is normal or high. The LA may appear 'tense', with abnormal rightward bowing of the atrial septum. The trans-mitral E- and A-wave waveforms are abnormal, typically demonstrating pseudo-normalization or restrictive filling. The mitral E/e' may be increased. Depending on the intravascular volume status and the severity of diastolic dysfunction, CO may be normal or low.

RV dysfunction

RV dysfunction is a frequent, and often unexpected, finding when echocardiography is performed for haemodynamic instability. Transient RV dysfunction occurs in most patients undergoing CPB and, in a small subset of patients, is associated with marked haemodynamic compromise (see Online appendix 8.1).

Perioperative RV dysfunction mainly occurs as a consequence of primary RV systolic failure or decompensated RV pressure overload. Common causes of RV systolic failure in cardiac surgical patients include poor myocardial protection during CPB, air embolus to the right coronary artery, and RV myocardial infarction. RV pressure overload may be acute or chronic and virtually always reflects increased pulmonary vascular resistance (PVR). The exception is pulmonary valve (PV) stenosis, in which

RV pressure overload occurs in the absence of elevated PVR. When RV pressure overload results in RV failure, it is termed 'cor pulmonale'. Chronic RV pressure overload is common in cardiac surgical patients, occurring in the context of long-standing MV disease and chronic lung disease, and following heart or lung transplantation. Acute decompensation of chronic stable RV pressure overload can occur during the perioperative period. Common causes of acute decompensation include adverse effects of hypoxia, hypercarbia, and SIRS on PVR, high ventilatory pressures, raised intra-abdominal pressure, and/or large haemothorax. Acute RV failure can also be precipitated by massive pulmonary embolism.

Occasionally, RV dysfunction is due to primary RV volume overload (e.g. due to an ASD or primary TR). Primary TR (e.g. due to endocarditis or carcinoid disease) is a *cause* of RV dysfunction, whereas secondary (or functional) TR is a *consequence* of RV dysfunction. Both primary RV systolic failure and pressure overload are associated with secondary RV volume overload, as this is the primary compensatory mechanism for the failing RV.

Echocardiographic appearances

The fact that the RV lies in the far field and has a non-geometric shape makes it hard to assess with TOE. The right heart should be imaged in a range of views to visualize the RV inflow and TV, the RV free wall and apex, and the RVOT and PV (see Chapter 14).

Impaired RV contractility is a feature of both primary RV systolic failure and decompensated RV pressure overload (i.e. cor pulmonale), and is evidenced by reduced tricuspid annular plane systolic excursion (TAPSE) (<17 mm), reduced tricuspid annular tissue Doppler velocity (<10 cm/s, although this parameter is difficult to measure with TOE due to poor Doppler alignment), and reduced thickening of the RV free wall. TAPSE is often reduced after cardiac surgery (with an unclear mechanism); however, studies using 3D echocardiography have shown that RV ejection fraction (RVEF) in these patients are unaltered.[17] Hence, TAPSE should be used with caution to quantify RV function in the post-operative period. Other non-specific signs of RV dysfunction include raised RA pressure, RV dilatation, and functional (i.e. secondary) TR. Increased RA pressure causes leftward bowing of the inter-atrial septum, present throughout the cardiac cycle (Figure 21.1). The RA may appear enlarged and 'tense'.

The echocardiographic distinction between RV systolic failure and decompensated pressure overload is the presence or absence of specific signs of pressure overload. Chronic RV pressure overload is associated with RV hypertrophy (end-diastolic RV wall thickness >6 mm) and prominent muscular trabeculations. The ventricular septum is flattened and typically moves paradoxically (i.e. rightward) in systole, reflecting the centre of mass of the heart having shifted to the RV. (Normally, the septum moves leftwards in systole, towards the LV.) Paradoxical septal motion is best visualized in the mid-oesophageal four-chamber view or transgastric mid-papillary view. Potential causes of paradoxical septal motion are listed in Table 21.1. The LV is often small and underfilled. If present, the velocity of the TR jet is usually significantly increased (>3.5 m/s), reflecting severe pulmonary hypertension.

With acute RV pressure overload (e.g. due to pulmonary embolism), elevated RV pressure causes prolongation of RV systole beyond LV systole, which, in turn, results in flattening and paradoxical (i.e. leftward) motion of the ventricular septum, commencing at end-systole.[18] The abnormal position of the ventricular septum is maintained into diastole. Significant RV hypertrophy is not present with acute pressure overload, and the peak TR jet velocity is only moderately increased (2.5–3.5 m/s).

Cardiac tamponade

Pericardial tamponade is a common cause of haemodynamic instability following cardiac surgery. However, the clinical and echocardiographic features in this group of patients frequently differ from those with medical causes of tamponade discussed in Chapter 16. This is because tamponade following cardiac surgery usually develops acutely, and even small collections can cause marked haemodynamic compromise. Additionally, the accumulating blood may clot and cause localized

Table 21.1 Causes of paradoxical motion of the interventricular septum

Aetiology	Timing and direction of abnormal motion
Chronic RV pressure overload	Systole, rightward
Acute RV pressure overload	End-systole, leftward
Chronic RV volume overload	Diastole, leftward
Pericardial tamponade	Early diastole, leftward
Constrictive pericarditis	Early diastole, leftward
RV epicardial pacing	Early systole, rightward
Left bundle branch block	Early systole, rightward

compression of a specific area, leading to regional tamponade. Tamponade can be a difficult diagnosis to make in the perioperative environment—first, the classical clinical features of tamponade may not be readily apparent following cardiac surgery; second, the presence of vasoactive medications, mechanical ventilation, and occasionally mechanical cardiac support devices like ECMO or LVAD can compensate and temporarily mask the diagnosis (see Online appendix 4.1).

Echocardiographic appearances

Unclotted blood appears as an echolucent (i.e. black) space around the heart. Circumferential blood collections are associated with the classical echocardiographic and haemodynamic features of tamponade and may be graded as small (<0.5 cm), moderate (0.5–2 cm), or large (>2 cm) at its maximum extent. As little as 1 cm of circumferential blood can cause marked haemodynamic compromise in post-operative cardiac surgical patients. Small fibrinous strands may be seen within the fluid. Pericardial fat is also echolucent and has similar echocardiographic appearances as haemopericardium, but it is not circumferential. The ventricular cavity typically appears underfilled and wall thickness is increased, so-called pseudo-hypertrophy.[19] The vena cavae appear distended.

In contrast, clotted blood appears echo-dense (i.e. grey/white) and has similar appearances to ventricular myocardium and atelectatic lung. Clotted blood is usually confined to a specific region such as behind the LA (in the oblique pericardial sinus), posterolateral to the RV, or compressing the RA free wall (Figure 21.10). RA compression may be sufficiently severe to produce virtual cavity obliteration; in this situation, the injection of agitated saline into a central venous line can help to define the atrial border. Clotted blood adjacent to the LV or RV can easily be mistaken for thickened akinetic ventricular wall—particularly collections that lie in the far field of the echocardiographic image. This is distinct from pseudo-hypertrophy, in which compression from fluid surrounding the heart causes the ventricular walls to be thicker.

The distinction between pericardial and pleural collections is usually straightforward. However, in the context of bleeding from the internal mammary bed with an open pleural space, it can be difficult to differentiate among pleural, pericardial, and combined collections. A useful landmark is the space between the LA and the descending aorta, which lies within the pericardium (Figure 21.11). Pericardial fluid will splay the gap between these two structures, whereas pleural fluid will not.

Tamponade physiology

Tamponade physiology occurs when pericardial pressure exceeds the pressure in one or more cardiac chambers and typically produces a number of echocardiographic findings. These findings are well validated in spontaneously breathing subjects in whom large liquid collections have accumulated slowly. In ventilated cardiac surgical patients, in whom blood collections accumulate rapidly or are localized, the standard echocardiographic indices

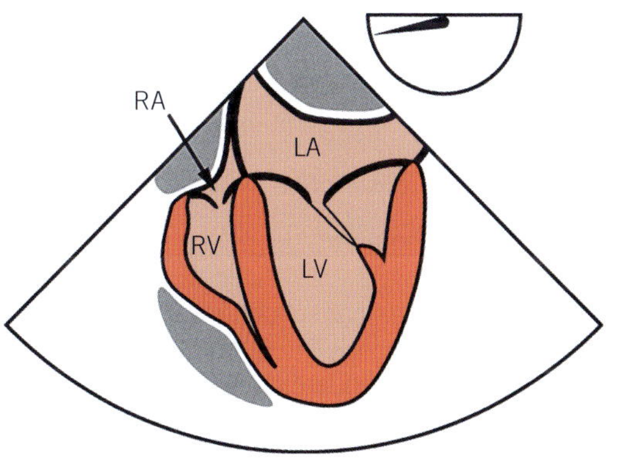

Figure 21.10 Regional tamponade. Schematic representation of a mid-oesophageal four-chamber view, demonstrating the three common sites where pericardial clot tends to accumulate and cause compression: overlying the RA; behind the LA in the oblique pericardial sinus; and overlying the RV free wall. Clotted blood appears echo-dense (i.e. grey/white). See examples in Online appendix 4.1.

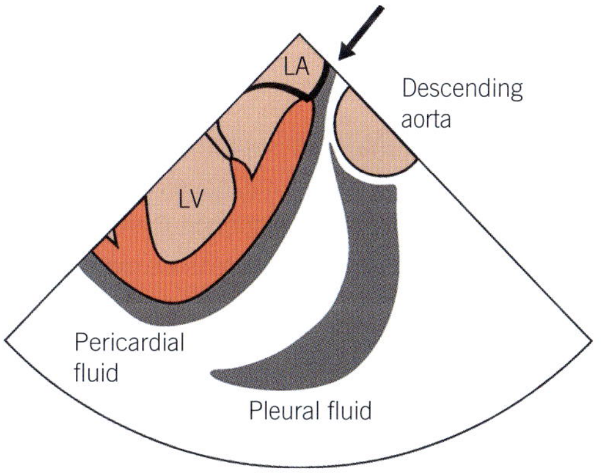

Figure 21.11 Pericardial versus pleural fluid. In this schematic illustration, the probe has been turned to the left from a standard mid-oesophageal four-chamber view, to display the descending thoracic aorta. Unclotted fluid in the left pleural space is seen as an echolucent (black) space in the shape of a 'tiger claw', pointing to the left of the screen. Fluid lying in the recess between the LA and the descending aorta lies within the pericardium.

of tamponade physiology are different (due to the effects of mechanical ventilation), frequently absent, and incompletely understood.

Unclotted circumferential blood may cause cyclical collapse of the atria or RV timed to the cardiac cycle. RV collapse occurs during ventricular diastole, when RV chamber pressure is lowest. LV diastolic pressure is typically higher than pericardial pressure, and therefore, LV collapse is rare. Atrial pressure is lowest during ventricular systole. However, pericardial pressure is also lowest in systole (when the ventricles are empty). Atrial collapse is typically maximal at end-diastole. Exceptions to this are patients with severe pulmonary hypertension with RV hypertrophy and RA dilatation, in whom LA and LV chamber compression occurs prior to RA/RV compression.

In spontaneously breathing patients, cardiac tamponade and constrictive pericarditis are both associated with exaggerated normal respiratory variations in peak E-wave velocity across the mitral (>5%) and tricuspid (>20%) valves. During spontaneous inspiration, maximal trans-tricuspid velocity increases due to enhanced systemic venous return, while during spontaneous expiration, maximal trans-mitral velocity increases due to enhanced pulmonary venous return. It is intuitive to expect that the opposite patterns would be seen with positive pressure ventilation. While there is evidence that the opposite pattern is seen in mechanically ventilated patients with constrictive pericarditis (see Chapter 16), the principle does not appear to hold for cardiac tamponade. Data are limited; however, in an animal model of acute tamponade, mechanical ventilation was associated with reduced maximal transmitral E-wave velocity during both inspiration and expiration, with reduced cyclical variation compared to normal.[20]

Cardiac tamponade is associated with paradoxical motion of the ventricular septum during early diastole (septal bounce). In circumstances where there is increased ventricular interdependence (cardiac tamponade, constrictive pericarditis), RV pressure may transiently exceed LV pressure in early diastole, resulting in a brief period of paradoxical (i.e. leftward) motion of the ventricular septum that rapidly normalizes, giving the appearance of 'septal bounce'. With mechanical ventilation, septal bounce is most marked during expiration, when RV filling is augmented.

Expert tip: Perioperative tamponade can be defined as 'haemodynamic instability in the presence of increased intra-pericardial pressure'. TOE can identify causes and signs of increased pericardial pressure; however, tamponade remains a clinical diagnosis. In the face of haemodynamic instability and pericardial blood/clot, definitive treatment should not be delayed because of absent or equivocal echocardiographic signs of tamponade.

Valve dysfunction

Rarely, acute valve dysfunction may be diagnosed while assessing the cause of haemodynamic dysfunction. In patients following valve replacement, it is particularly important to evaluate the prosthetic valve for any acute prosthetic valve dysfunction. Any new valvular dysfunction will need to be evaluated in detail, as surgical correction may be the only option to address their haemodynamic instability.

The difficult diagnosis

Sometimes the cause of haemodynamic instability is not readily apparent with TOE—'the heart looks fine, but the patient looks terrible'. It is important to remember that haemodynamic instability frequently occurs in the presence of vigorous systolic function (Box 21.2) and that some causes may be difficult to diagnose with echocardiography alone (Box 21.3). In many circumstances, the cause of haemodynamic instability is multifactorial. The

Box 21.2 Causes of haemodynamic instability in which LV systolic function may appear hyperdynamic

- Hypovolaemia
- Low LV afterload
- LV diastolic dysfunction
- Pericardial tamponade
- Dynamic LVOT obstruction
- Acute mitral regurgitation

Box 21.3 Causes of haemodynamic instability with a reassuring echocardiographic examination

- Low LV afterload
- Arrhythmias
- Patient–ventilator dyssynchrony
- Tension pneumothorax
- Dynamic pulmonary hyperinflation
- Massive haemothorax

following should be considered when the diagnosis is not obvious on echocardiographic examination.

Multifactorial causes

Hypovolaemia frequently coexists with other pathology, including diastolic dysfunction, systolic dysfunction, low LV afterload, and pericardial tamponade. In the presence of a secondary condition (e.g. systolic LV dysfunction), small pericardial collections that would normally be benign can lead to marked haemodynamic compromise. RV dysfunction can result in impaired filling of the LV due to leftward displacement of the interventricular septum during diastole (ventricular interdependence). Subclinical valvular lesions may exacerbate the haemodynamic consequences of other pathology such as low LV afterload or myocardial ischaemia.

The effect of inotropic agents

It is usual for hypotensive patients to be receiving inotropic support during the echocardiographic examination. These agents give the ventricular motion a 'snappy' appearance, which can mask poor systolic function and low CO. It is useful to formally measure the LVEF or FAC in this setting. A 'normal' heart appears hyperdynamic under the influence of inotropic agents and in the presence of sepsis.

The effect of sepsis and systemic inflammatory response syndrome

Sepsis and SIRS typically produce a hyperdynamic, dilated circulation with a high CO. Conditions that reduce cardiovascular reserve (e.g. chronic LV dysfunction, pericardial fluid, or RV dysfunction) may limit CO to less than this. Thus, the heart may look vigorous, but the patient may be in a relatively low CO state.

The effect of rhythm disturbances

Rhythm disturbances are an important cause of haemodynamic compromise, and the diagnosis is not always immediately obvious from the electrocardiogram, particularly loss of atrioventricular synchrony or nodal rhythm. With echocardiography, the LV may appear hyperdynamic, despite the presence of low CO or hypotension. Atrial pressures are typically high. A clue to the presence of a rhythm disturbance is provided by the loss of the normal E- and A-wave pattern on the trans-mitral PW Doppler waveform and signs of raised LA pressure. Treating with antiarrhythmic agents and adjusting epicardial pacing settings may improve haemodynamics. In patients with LVAD, a malpositioned inflow cannula can be the cause of triggering arrhythmias. If this is identified, surgical options for readjusting the position of the inflow cannula of LVAD will merit discussion.

Multiple choice questions

Discover interactive multiple choice questions to test your knowledge on this chapter by searching for this book's title or ISBN (9780198873686) at **https://academic.oup.com/** and going to the online appendix at the end of the book. Use your scratch-off code on the inside cover to access the material.

References

1. Montealegre-Gallegos M, Mahmood F, Owais K, Hess P, Jainandunsing JS, Matyal R. Cardiac output calculation and three-dimensional echocardiography. *J Cardiothorac Vasc Anesth*. 2014;**28**(3):547–50.
2. Nagueh SF, Smiseth OA, Appleton CP, *et al*. Recommendations for the evaluation of left ventricular diastolic function by echocardiography: an update from the American Society of Echocardiography and the European Association of Cardiovascular Imaging. *J Am Soc Echocardiogr*. 2016;**29**(4):277–314.
3. Ommen SR, Nishimura RA, Appleton CP, *et al*. Clinical utility of Doppler echocardiography and tissue Doppler imaging in the estimation of left ventricular filling pressures: a comparative simultaneous Doppler-catheterization study. *Circulation*. 2000;**102**(15):1788–94.
4. Mullens W, Borowski AG, Curtin RJ, Thomas JD, Tang WH. Tissue Doppler imaging in the estimation of intracardiac filling pressure in decompensated patients with advanced systolic heart failure. *Circulation*. 2009;**119**(1):62–70.
5. Combes A, Arnoult F, Trouillet JL. Tissue Doppler imaging estimation of pulmonary artery occlusion pressure in ICU patients. *Intensive Care Med*. 2004;**30**(1):75–81.
6. Vignon P, AitHssain A, François B, *et al*. Echocardiographic assessment of pulmonary artery occlusion pressure in ventilated patients: a transoesophageal study. *Crit Care*. 2008;**12**(1):R18.
7. Haji DL, Ali MM, Royse A, Canty DJ, Clarke S, Royse CF. Interatrial septum motion but not Doppler assessment predicts elevated pulmonary capillary wedge pressure in patients undergoing cardiac surgery. *Anesthesiology*. 2014;**121**(4):719–29.
8. Kusumoto FM, Muhiudeen IA, Kuecherer HF, Cahalan MK, Schiller NB. Response of the interatrial septum to transatrial pressure gradients and its potential for predicting pulmonary capillary wedge pressure: an intraoperative study using transesophageal echocardiography in patients during mechanical ventilation. *J Am Coll Cardiol*. 1993;**21**(3):721–8.

9. Vignon P. Preload and fluid responsiveness. In: McLean A, Huang S, Hilton A, editors. *Oxford Textbook of Advanced Critical Care Echocardiography.* Oxford: Oxford University Press; 2020, pp. 141–52.
10. Rex S, Brose S, Metzelder S, *et al.* Prediction of fluid responsiveness in patients during cardiac surgery. *Br J Anaesth.* 2004;**93**(6):782–8.
11. Hofer CK, Müller SM, Furrer L, Klaghofer R, Genoni M, Zollinger A. Stroke volume and pulse pressure variation for prediction of fluid responsiveness in patients undergoing off-pump coronary artery bypass grafting. *Chest.* 2005;**128**(2):848–54.
12. Pinsky MR. Cardiopulmonary interactions: physiologic basis and clinical applications. *Ann Am Thorac Soc.* 2018;**15**(Suppl 1):S45–8.
13. Vieillard-Baron A, Chergui K, Rabiller A, *et al.* Superior vena caval collapsibility as a gauge of volume status in ventilated septic patients. *Intensive Care Med.* 2004;**30**(9):1734–9.
14. Feissel M, Mangin I, Ruyer O, Faller J-P, Michard F, Teboul J-L. Respiratory changes in aortic blood velocity as an indicator of fluid responsiveness in ventilated patients with septic shock. *Chest.* 2001;**119**(3):867–73.
15. Slama M, Masson H, Teboul JL, *et al.* Respiratory variations of aortic VTI: a new index of hypovolemia and fluid responsiveness. *Am J Physiol Heart Circ Physiol.* 2002;**283**(4):H1729–33.
16. Kondo N, Hirose N, Kihara K, Tashiro M, Miyashita K, Orihashi K. Intraoperative transesophageal echocardiography for coronary artery assessment. *Circ Rep.* 2020;**2**(9):517–25.
17. Grønlykke L, Korshin A, Holmgaard F, *et al.* Severe loss of right ventricular longitudinal contraction occurs after cardiopulmonary bypass in patients with preserved right ventricular output. *Int J Cardiovasc Imaging.* 2019;**35**(9):1661–70.
18. Jardin F, Dubourg O, Bourdarias JP. Echocardiographic pattern of acute cor pulmonale. *Chest.* 1997;**111**(1):209–17.
19. Feinberg MS, Popescu BA, Popescu AC, *et al.* Assessment of pseudohypertrophy as a measure of left-ventricular compression in patients with cardiac tamponade. *Cardiology.* 2000;**94**(4):213–19.
20. Faehnrich JA, Noone RB Jr, White WD, *et al.* Effects of positive-pressure ventilation, pericardial effusion, and cardiac tamponade on respiratory variation in transmitral flow velocities. *J Cardiothorac Vasc Anesth.* 2003;**17**(1):45–50.

Index

For the benefit of digital users, indexed terms that span two pages (e.g., 52–53) may, on occasion, appear on only one of those pages.

Tables, figures, and boxes are indicated by an italic *t*, *f*, and *b* following the page number.